The Integrative Action of the Autonomic Nervous System

Almost all bodily functions are dependent on activity of the autonomic nervous system – from the cardiovascular system, the gastrointestinal tract, the evacuative and sexual organs, to the regulation of temperature, metabolism and tissue defense. Balanced functioning of each aspect of this system is an important basis of our life and well-being. In this long-awaited second edition, the author, a leading figure in this field, provides an up-to-date and detailed description of the cellular and integrative organization of the autonomic nervous system, covering both peripheral and central aspects. The book exposes modern neurobiological concepts that allow us to understand why this system normally runs so smoothly and why its deterioration has such disastrous consequences. This broad overview will appeal to researchers and advanced undergraduate students of the various biological and medical sciences studying how the autonomic nervous system works and to clinicians and physical therapists whose practice involves systems dependent on autonomic functions.

Wilfrid Jänig is Professor Emeritus of Physiology at the Christian-Albrechts University in Kiel, Germany. He has conducted neurobiological research on the autonomic nervous system since 1973. He combined research in Kiel with research at universities in Australia (Brisbane, Melbourne, Sydney), at the Hebrew University in Jerusalem, and at the University of California, San Francisco. His experiments, in which electrical signals in single sympathetic nerve fibers were recorded during natural and reflex activity, have established the principle of selective control of peripheral organs by the brain and the involvement of the sympathetic nervous system in various types of pain and in inflammation.

"This is the ultimate resource for anyone interested in autonomic neurosciences. Professor Jänig has tastefully updated a classic book which manages to distill a vast body of knowledge that will continue to be cherished by students as well as established scientists."

Kalyanam Shivkumar MD PhD, Professor of Medicine, The University of California, Los Angeles (UCLA), and President, International Society for Autonomic Neuroscience (ISAN 2022)

"Wilfrid Jänig has produced an outstanding synthesis of the state of knowledge of the autonomic nervous system (ANS). The book is far more than a summary of knowledge; Jänig has drawn out important principles from experimental work and his deep understanding of physiology. He shows how the ANS, in partnership with endocrine hormones, purposefully maintains cells, tissues, and organs in their optimal functional states.
He points out that the definitions of the sympathetic and the parasympathetic nervous systems are based on the specialized anatomical arrangement of the autonomic outflow from the central nervous system to peripheral target tissues. Jänig points out forcefully that to speak of sympathetic or parasympathetic 'functions' generates misunderstandings and gives the wrong impression of how the ANS works. He writes instead of the many function-specific autonomic pathways (channels) that supply controls to tissues and organs. Jänig discusses in detail the old, but persistent, idea of a type of unitary discharge of the 'sympathetic' (or 'parasympathetic') system, which he concludes to be counter to what actually occurs. A nuanced ANS control dependent on sensory information from all organs, and the environment, as well as on emotional influences, is explained, that is, *The Integrative Action of the Autonomic Nervous System* to maintain bodily homeostasis.

The book is beautifully illustrated, especially with diagrams of autonomic circuits. Also very helpful are the conclusions paragraphs at the ends of chapters.
The book is essential reading for the seriously engaged physiologist and physician."

John B. Furness, Professor of Anatomy and Physiology, The University of Melbourne and The Florey Institute of Neuroscience and Mental Health

"For me, this is the 'Workshop Manual' of how the autonomic nervous system works. The *integrative* aspect of this book is quite superb. Jänig has avoided the traditional, and unhelpful, silo approach where bodily systems are separated in distinct chapters. This is inconsistent with how the body works. This new edition leaves no 'autonomic' stone unturned, covering endplates to emotion, credits the historical facts that have stood the test of time but kicks those into touch that have not. So pleasing was to see that the book challenges old/outdated dogma and sets the facts straight by reviewing the most current evidence. For instance, Jänig refutes respectfully Cannon's ideas on antagonism prevalence within the autonomic nervous system that corrupts so many of our students minds when reading their textbooks. I know that my copy of this book will spend its life being read and not on a shelf; it will be poured over by professors and students alike. The illustrations require a mention: they are exceptional – clear, concise, and comprehensive. I believe this book will put the autonomic nervous system front and center in the field of neuroscience."

Julian F.R. Paton PhD FRSNZ, Professor of Translational Physiology, University of Auckland, New Zealand

The Integrative Action of the Autonomic Nervous System

Neurobiology of Homeostasis

Wilfrid Jänig

Christian-Albrechts Universität zu Kiel, Germany

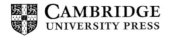

CAMBRIDGE
UNIVERSITY PRESS

CAMBRIDGE
UNIVERSITY PRESS

University Printing House, Cambridge CB2 8BS, United Kingdom

One Liberty Plaza, 20th Floor, New York, NY 10006, USA

477 Williamstown Road, Port Melbourne, VIC 3207, Australia

314–321, 3rd Floor, Plot 3, Splendor Forum, Jasola District Centre,
New Delhi – 110025, India

103 Penang Road, #05–06/07, Visioncrest Commercial, Singapore 238467

Cambridge University Press is part of the University of Cambridge.

It furthers the University's mission by disseminating knowledge in the pursuit of
education, learning, and research at the highest international levels of excellence.

www.cambridge.org
Information on this title: www.cambridge.org/9781108478632
DOI: 10.1017/9781108778411

First published 2006
First printed digitally 2008
Second edition 2022

Printed in the United Kingdom by TJ Books Limited, Padstow Cornwall

A catalogue record for this publication is available from the British Library.

Library of Congress Cataloging-in-Publication Data
Names: Jänig, Wilfrid, author.
Title: The integrative action of the autonomic nervous system : neurobiology of
homeostasis / Wilfrid Jänig, Christian-Albrechts Universität zu Kiel, Germany.
Description: 2 edition. | Cambridge, United Kingdom ; New York, NY : Cambridge
University Press, 2022. | Includes bibliographical references and index.
Identifiers: LCCN 2021049182 (print) | LCCN 2021049183 (ebook) | ISBN 9781108478632
(hardback) | ISBN 9781108778411 (ebook)
Subjects: LCSH: Autonomic nervous system.
Classification: LCC QP368 .J36 2022 (print) | LCC QP368 (ebook) | DDC 612.8/9 – dc23/eng/
20211008
LC record available at https://lccn.loc.gov/2021049182
LC ebook record available at https://lccn.loc.gov/2021049183

ISBN 978-1-108-47863-2 Hardback
ISBN 978-1-108-74598-7 Paperback

Additional resources for this publication at https://www.cambridge.org/janig.

For UTE, my beloved wife.
Without her this book would never have appeared in the World of Science

Contents

All references cited in the text are available online at
www.cambridge.org/janig.

Foreword to the Second Edition

Elspeth M. McLachlan, Prince of Wales Medical Research Institute and the University of New South Wales, Sydney, NSW, Australia.

Cardiac and smooth muscles, exocrine glands, fat stores, primary and secondary immune organs, etc. throughout the bodies of vertebrates are innervated by autonomic pathways. The first edition of Wilfrid Jänig's book *The Integrative Action of the Autonomic Nervous System* (2006) brought together what was known about the anatomy, physiology and pharmacology of this system, at the level of organs, tissues and cells. The book has become the mainstay of current information on the neural control of autonomic function. In the first edition, Wilfrid compiled and extended knowledge of how central nervous integration is transformed within sympathetic and parasympathetic pathways to regulate the peripheral organs and tissues, including the cellular mechanisms by which the central signals are transmitted to the effector tissues. Information about research in autonomic function, using classical and modern techniques in neurophysiology, neuroanatomy, pharmacology and biochemistry, was integrated with the fundamental understanding of this system accumulated over more than 100 years and summarized in a complete and accessible way.

Over many years, Wilfrid's own laboratory has concentrated on the ongoing and reflex electrophysiological activity of sympathetic outflows, mainly postganglionic, in limb and visceral nerves supplying a variety of organs. Recently they have examined the effects of nerve injury on this activity, and the mechanisms underlying neuropathic pain. In addition, Wilfrid has recruited an international autonomic community to analyze at a cellular level, using cellular anatomy and topography, neurochemistry, ganglionic and neuroeffector transmission, and sympathetic involvement in nociception and inflammation. The results of this research by him and his collaborators underpin the philosophy of his book. However, his wider interests encompass the central pathways involved in the control of autonomic outflows and he has sought to synthesize what is known about these pathways as well. Gaps in knowledge have been defined and the most significant questions to be answered clearly identified.

In the 16 years since the first edition, many of the important questions have been addressed using newer techniques in molecular biology, genetic manipulation and ontogenetics, and it is time to re-evaluate the material. This new edition of the book incorporates many of the more recent data into the stories told in the previous edition and outlines the new ideas that have been developed over this period. The questions still to be answered have been reconsidered and are posed for the current cohort of researchers to investigate.

Wilfrid has spent half a century lecturing to medical students, postgraduate researchers and clinical practitioners about the functioning of the autonomic nervous system and the results of modern research. His expertise in concisely summarizing the concepts in each area of study with simple clear diagrams reflects this long experience and the popularity of his approach. He has not only trained dozens of medical and science graduates in the methodology of research, but has also written, revised and updated many chapters in textbooks addressed to the next generation of basic and clinical physiologists. This combination of teaching and research was much influenced by his interactions with Robert Schmidt, his mentor at the onset of his career in the 1960s, and follows the German tradition of the "unity of research and teaching" (*Einheit von Forschung und Lehre*) formulated and propagated by Wilhelm von Humboldt. This second edition has benefitted from this extensive experience in rethinking and improving the contents of this very valuable and comprehensive book. This revised and updated version will bring Wilfrid's special interpretation of current knowledge of the regulation of autonomic function to the next generation of readers.

Foreword to the First Edition

Elspeth M. McLachlan, Prince of Wales Medical Research Institute and the University of New South Wales, Sydney, NSW, Australia.

The autonomic nervous system carries the signals from the central nervous system to all organs and tissues of the body except skeletal muscle fibers. It is made up of preganglionic and postganglionic neurons linked together in functionally distinct pathways. The postganglionic terminals have specific relationships with their target tissue. As well as distributing centrally derived command signals, this system can also integrate reflex interactions between different parts of the peripheral nervous system, even without involving the spinal cord. All of these activities are specific for each organ system and attempts to generalize have often proved incorrect. The breadth and scope of involvement of this system in body function are obvious. The autonomic nervous system controls not only the quantity and quality of tissue perfusion in response to varying needs, and the maintenance of secretions for protection of the body's orifices and the lining of the gastrointestinal tract, but it also regulates the usually intermittent but complex functions of the abdominal viscera and pelvic organs, the mechanical aspects of the eye and the communication between the nervous system and the immune system. Many autonomic pathways are continuously active but they can also be recruited when the environmental and/or emotional situation demands it. This system is essential for homeostasis – hence the subtitle of this book.

Despite its enormous importance for the maintenance of normal physiology in all vertebrate species, and for the understanding of many clinical symptoms of disease, the autonomic nervous system has not, even transiently, been the center of attention in neuroscience research internationally over the past 40 years. Many seem to think that this system has been worked out and there is nothing new to investigate. The discovery of neuropeptides as putative transmitters was probably the only interlude that triggered widespread excitement. Others simply forget that the system exists except for emergencies.

Two views about the autonomic nervous system are often encountered:

1. that this system is similar to the endocrine system and its functions can all be explained by the pharmacological actions of the major neurotransmitters, noradrenaline and acetylcholine, possibly involving modulation by cotransmitters and neuropeptides, or
2. that the functions of this system are not important as life continues without them.

For anyone who thinks about it, at least the latter of these concepts is obviously not true. Life can be maintained in a cocoon in individuals with autonomic failure but the ability to cope with external stressors severely compromises their quality of life. The extent to which the practical difficulties of daily life for people with spinal cord injury, which disrupts the links between the brain and the autonomic control of the body's organs, absorb personal energy and resources should not be underestimated by those who take their bodies for granted. Elderly people face similar problems as some of their autonomic pathways degenerate.

On the other hand, the former of the above two concepts dominates almost all current textbooks of physiology and neuroscience. It is true that some of the effects of autonomic nerve activity can be mimicked by the application of neurotransmitter substances locally or systemically. However, the mechanisms by which the same substances released from nerve terminals produce responses in the target tissue have proved to be quite different in most cases so far analyzed. This helps to explain the failure of many pharmaceutical interventions based on this simplistic idea as outlined above. What is important here is that the present volume collates the evidence against both these ideas and develops the factual and conceptual framework that describes how an organized system of functional nerve connections that operate with distinct behaviors is coordinated to regulate the workings of the organ systems of each individual.

Nevertheless, over the past 40 years, there have been remarkable strides in our understanding. Technical problems limit how the complexities of this system can be unraveled. There are enormous challenges involved in investigating a complex interconnected system made up of small neurons that are not always packaged together in precisely the same way between individuals. Even in the spinal cord, the neuroanatomical distribution and apparent imprecision have been daunting. To study this system requires patience and persistence in the development of manipulative and analytical skills. These attributes are relatively rare.

Fortunately, over this period, a small but steady stream of researchers has persisted in their endeavors to clarify how this functionally diverse system works. One of the most significant players has been Wilfrid Jänig. Wilfrid and his many students and collaborators at the Christian-Albrechts-Universität in Kiel have pursued a major and uniquely productive approach to understanding how sympathetic pathways work. This has been to apply the technique of extracellular recording from single identified axons dissected from peripheral nerves projecting to particular target tissues and therefore acting in known functional pathways. Over the 40 years, this work, originally in cats and latterly in rats, has revealed the principles underlying reflex behavior of sympathetic axons in the anesthetized animal. The characteristic behavior of pre- and postganglionic neurons in over a dozen functional pathways has been defined. As the reader progresses through the book, it will become clear that many of these reflexes are also present in humans. The parallel technique of microneurography, pioneered by Hagbarth, has been implemented over a similar period in the sympathetic pathways of conscious humans by Gunnar Wallin and his colleagues in Göteborg. While pathways to the viscera are currently too hard to study in humans because they are less accessible, the principles of their organization can be deduced from Wilfrid's data on pre- and postganglionic discharge patterns and from the analyses of ganglionic and neuroeffector transmission conducted by him and others.

Over the 40 years, Wilfrid's various interests have been broad but always focused. They have taken him to many places to answer questions about the structure and function of sympathetic pathways. His earliest training in single unit recording was in sensory neurophysiology and this background has been the basis of his parallel studies of visceral afferent behavior and nociception. Early in his career, he was interested in integrative autonomic control at the higher levels of the nervous system and developed a passion to follow on the work of Philip Bard. After returning to Germany from New York in the 1970s, he conducted experiments on decorticate and decerebrate cats in which he created behaviors such as sham rage during which he planned to record and analyze the sympathetic outflow. These experiments did not progress because of limited resources, but instead he undertook a most detailed analysis of the distinctive behavior of skin and muscle sympathetic vasoconstrictor axons. These results provided evidence that strongly rejected popular ideas that a general level of "sympathetic tone" was the determinant of peripheral vascular resistance. It was clear that the reflex connectivity of the pathways involved in cutaneous and skeletal muscle blood flow are largely independent. This concept was more dramatically confirmed in recordings from humans where it is possible to demonstrate the strong emotional drive that modulates cutaneous vasoconstrictor activity (see Subchapter 4.1.2 in this book). Subsequently Wilfrid's laboratory has extended this type of analysis to over a dozen different pathways that they have studied in anesthetized animals.

I first met Wilfrid in 1979 when he came to give a seminar in Edinburgh where I was on sabbatical leave at the time. As my original background was in cardiovascular physiology, I had naturally read his work on vasoconstrictor discharge patterns and had lots of questions to ask him. Wilfrid invited me to visit Kiel on my way home (it was very cold and wet in November) and then he came to Melbourne to work with me to trace the peripheral sympathetic pathways quantitatively. In my laboratory at Monash University, I had established the retrograde tracing technique using horseradish peroxidase to identify the location of preganglionic neurons in the spinal cord as a prelude to recording intracellularly from them. He worked hard with me cutting and mounting thousands of sections and soon after I spent a similar period in Kiel helping his group establish the technique there. This quantitative work dovetailed well to explain how the axons that his group sampled in their recordings related to the entire population.

It has been my great privilege to continue to work with Wilfrid and his colleagues, particularly up to the early 1990s, undertaking studies for which he and I received the Max-Planck Forschungspreis for international collaboration in 1993. Since that time, and in various parts of Australia as I have moved between universities, we have worked together and in parallel on aspects of the interactions between the sympathetic and sensory systems that may be involved in neuropathic pain after nerve injury. We have continued to communicate frequently and his younger colleagues, notably Ralf Baron, Ursula Wesselmann and Joachim Häbler, have spent time in Australia working in my laboratory. I hope and expect that these interactions will continue.

Wilfrid's early studies of sympathetic activity were made when Robert Schmidt was in Kiel and were conducted in parallel with studies of somatosensory, particularly nociceptive, afferents. This anteceded his interest in visceral afferent function to which he applied the same technical expertise to unravel the behavior of these neurons, particularly in pelvic organ reflexes. His interests in nerve injury were pursued in part with Marshall Devor in Jerusalem. This involved extended studies of the ectopic activity of sensory neurons after peripheral nerve lesions and the role of sympathetic activity in triggering this. His laboratory has also conducted a wide range of studies on the effects of various nerve lesions on the properties of sympathetic and afferent axons. As Wilfrid appreciated that the problem of neuropathic pain was probably related to inflammation, he sought out Jon Levine in San Francisco where he was exposed to a very strong research community involved in pain and inflammation research. He has a prodigious output from Jon's laboratory deciphering the components of the neuroimmune interactions using rigorous and systematic approaches to identify the pathways and sites at which the hypothalamo–pituitary–adrenal axis (HPA) intervenes in inflammation and in nociception, in some cases with sympathetic involvement. More recently, Wilfrid and Ralf Baron have worked with the clinical community worldwide on clarifying the misnamed concept of "reflex sympathetic dystrophy" and developing the newer definitions of various "complex regional pain syndromes" to help to clarify the diagnosis of the mechanisms underlying chronic neuropathic pain.

When visiting my laboratories at Monash and the Baker Institute in Melbourne, and subsequently at the Universities of New South Wales and Queensland, and more recently at the Prince of Wales Medical Research Institute in Sydney, Wilfrid has been able to visit many neuroscientists around Australia where research on the neurobiology of the autonomic nervous system and on central cardiovascular control is prolific by world standards. He has seized upon these opportunities to learn what the community of Australian autonomic researchers is doing and has established strong relationships with the leaders of many active laboratories including those of David Hirst, Ian Gibbins and Judy Morris, John Furness, Marcello Costa, Christopher Bell, Janet Keast, Sue Luff, James Brock, Roger Dampney, Robin McAllen, Bill Blessing, Paul Korner, Dick Bandler, Paul Pilowsky and Dirk van Helden. This extensive Australian involvement in autonomic neuroscience arose in part from the students who trained with Geoff Burnstock and Mollie Holman in Melbourne in the 1960s and 1970s and who have taken their skills across the country and have been training the next generations since that time. Despite the divergence of their specific interests, this community continues to be one of the largest internationally working in the autonomic nervous system. Wilfrid's exposure to the cellular, pharmacological and neuroanatomical aspects of ganglionic and junctional transmission in the peripheral pathways gave him a very wide view of autonomic effector systems, which he has so cleverly incorporated into this book.

Throughout these years, Wilfrid has been a prodigious author of textbook chapters and review articles. Although many of the former have been written in German, he has also developed and expounded his ideas about neural control of vasoconstriction, pain and the sympathetic nervous system, the consequences of nerve injury, the involvement of the HPA axis in inflammation and nociception, and on clinical aspects of these topics. This book arises from this lifetime of synthetic writing and from his reflection on the wider issues of this area of science. It also is the product of his frustration, which I share, with the limited availability of publications that summarize the scientific background and present the current status of our understanding of how the autonomic nervous system works. As in his experiments, he has dissected the system into the major functional pathways in which reflex behavior and cellular mechanisms have been well investigated. He reviews and synthesizes the available information on the spinal cord and brain stem components of autonomic reflexes and then re-synthesizes these output systems into a complex package that includes the control of autonomic discharge patterns from the midbrain and higher centers. He has extracted the key information yielded by both classical and modern technical approaches used to study these components of the nervous system. He has incorporated the conceptual background behind each area of research. Finally, he discusses how the old "unifying" concepts of Cannon and Hess misrepresented the diversity of autonomic outflow patterns that the brain recruits during the various behaviors that function to conserve the body in a range of environmental circumstances. This philosophical base needs to replace the widely held views mentioned earlier if we are to progress our understanding of this important set of control systems. The present *tour de force* has involved discussion and input from many of Wilfrid's collaborators and colleagues around the world whose contributions have ensured that the final product really contains the most up-to-date summary of our current knowledge of autonomic function.

Despite, or because of, this diversity of inputs, this book provides Wilfrid Jänig's unique overview of the autonomic nervous system. Without his driving fascination with how the whole autonomic system works in the body, this book would never have been written. No-one else currently has the conceptual breadth and capacity to integrate so many aspects to compose this amalgam. He has collected all the available data from the past and the present and fitted them together with what is known of the central control and spinal integration that determine the activity patterns in each outflow pathway. He has taken the knowledge from Langley's time, through Cannon, Hess and Bard, Burnstock and Holman, to the recent application of cellular biology and molecular genetics to collate a truly comprehensive compendium. I am delighted that he has committed himself to drawing together so many diverse aspects of autonomic function in one place and to give us a truly integrated overview of what is known at the beginning of the twenty-first century. He has made very clear what he feels are the major questions that remain to be answered. I know that Wilfrid will contribute to many of those answers.

Preface

In the late 1960s, while I was working in Robert F. Schmidt's laboratory in the Department of Physiology of the University of Heidelberg, conducting experiments on cutaneous primary afferent neurons and presynaptic inhibition in the spinal cord, Robert introduced me to the sympathetic nervous system. We worked on somatosympathetic reflexes and other spinal reflexes, some of the work being conducted with Akio Sato. At this time, I tried to understand *The Wisdom of the Body* by Walter Bradford Cannon (Cannon 1939) and *Vegetatives Nervensystem* by Walter Rudolf Hess (Hess 1948). However, from 1971 to 1974, I continued with my experimental work on the somatosensory system and concentrated with Alden Spencer on the cuneate nucleus and thalamus in the Department of Neurobiology and Behavior of the Public Health Institute of the City of New York (directed by Eric Kandel).

While working in New York I came into contact with Chandler McCuskey Brooks (Downstate Medical Center, State University of New York). He invited me to attend the Centennial Symposium "The Life and Influence of Walter Bradford Cannon, 1871–1945: The Development of Physiology in this Century" (Brooks et al. 1975). Chandler encouraged me to concentrate scientifically on the autonomic nervous system; he remained very supportive until his death 17 years later. This influence and particularly the books of Cannon and Hess led to my decision to leave the somatosensory field and redirect my research, after my return to Germany, to investigations of the sympathetic nervous system. The books by Cannon and Hess, and the published papers on which they are based, aroused from the beginning my opposition on the one hand and my secret admiration for these authors on the other. This ambiguity in my scientific attitude towards Cannon and Hess has always been in the background of the scientific activities in my laboratory, of my teaching and of my writing on the autonomic nervous system.

I am particularly grateful to two persons who have kept me going on the scientific path amidst trials and tribulations to unravel some of the mysteries of the autonomic nervous system. Robert Schmidt has made me invest time in writing textbook chapters on the autonomic nervous system since 1971. Elspeth McLachlan has always been extremely supportive and virtually carried me through some periods of doubt and despondency throughout the 40 years we have worked experimentally and scientifically together. She introduced me to Australian Autonomic Neuroscience and is responsible for this book being in some ways an Australian book (see below). Finally, the many young students in my laboratory, some now professors, influenced me by their enthusiasm despite my being entirely uncompromising, which was sometimes hard for them to digest.

The German Research Foundation has fully supported my research over more than 45 years. Without this continuous funding, for research that was often methodologically, and as regards content, not in the mainstream, I never would have been able to continue my research on the autonomic nervous system for so many years. So I am deeply grateful to the many anonymous referees of the German Research Foundation for their fair judgment.

Finally, and most important, on a very personal level, the research over these decades, and still continuing, could never have happened without the never-ending tolerance and support of my wife Ute and our sons Nils and Volker. My family life has sustained my research more than anything else.

I want this book to be a forum for ongoing discussion. I strongly encourage young scientists to invest their time in research on the autonomic nervous system. While writing the book I was in continuous discourse with many scientists in Australia, Europe and the United States addressing various scientific aspects of the book. These scientists have made a major contribution.

- I would particularly like to thank those who undertook to read and comment on chapters or subchapters of the book. AUSTRALIA: Richard Bandler (Sydney), Bill Blessing (Adelaide), James Brock (Melbourne), Roger Dampney (Sydney), John Furness (Melbourne), Ian Gibbins (Adelaide),

Robin McAllen (Melbourne), Elspeth McLachlan (Sydney), Judy Morris (Adelaide), Julian Paton (Aukland, New Zealand), Paul Pilowsky (Sydney), Dirk van Helden (Newcastle). *EUROPE*: Niels Birbaumer (Tübingen, Germany), John Coote (Birmingham, UK), Sue Deuchars (Leeds, UK), Henry Evrard (Tübingen, Germany), Peter Holzer (Graz, Austria), Michael Illert (Kiel, Germany), Winfried Neuhuber (Erlangen, Germany), Hans-Georg Schaible (Jena, Germany), Gunnar Wallin (Göteborg, Sweden). *NORTH AMERICA*: Arthur (Bud) Craig (Phoenix, Arizona), Chet de Groat (Pittsburgh, Pennsylvania), Patrice Guyenet (Charlottesville, Virginia), Gerlinda Hermann (Baton Rouge, Louisiana), John Horn (Pittsburgh, Pennsylvania), Jon Levine (San Francisco, California), Arthur Loewy (St. Louis, Missouri), Larry Schramm (Baltimore, Maryland), Orville Smith (Seattle, Washington), Terry Smith (Reno, Nevada), Alberto Travagli (Baton Rouge, Louisiana).

- I am thankful to those who never hesitated to think about and answer my questions. *AUSTRALIA*: David Hirst (Melbourne), Phil Jobling (Newcastle), Ida Llewellyn-Smith (Adelaide), Susan Luff (Melbourne), Vaughn Macefield (Sydney). *EUROPE*: Jean-François Bernard (Paris, France), Uwe Ernsberger (Frankfurt, Germany), Björn Folkow (Göteborg, Sweden), Andrew Todd (Glasgow, Scotland). *NORTH AMERICA*: Susan Barman (East Lansing, Michigan), Lori Birder (Pittsburgh, Pennsylvania), Kevan McKenna (Chicago, Illinois), Shaun Morrison (Portland, Oregon), Michael Panneton (St. Louis, Missouri), Terry Powley (West Lafayette, Indiana), Clifford Saper (Boston, Massachusetts), Ann Schreihofer (Fort Worth, Texas), Ruth Stornetta (Charlottesville, Virginia).

Eike Tallone (Kiel) has my very special thanks. She is responsible for the graphical work in almost all figures of this book. Without her, the figures would not be of such high quality.

Finally, I thank Professor Markus Bleich, Professor Thomas Baukrowitz and Professor Peer Wulff (Directorate of the Physiologisches Institut of the Christian-Albrechts-Universität zu Kiel) for their continuous support. This support allowed me to use the infrastructure of the institute and to have an office with my own library after my retirement.

Abbreviations

The main abbreviations used are listed below. Special abbreviations related to anatomical structures in the lower brain stem or hypothalamus are listed in the legends of the figures and tables, particularly Figures 10.2, 11.13, 11.14 and Tables 8.2 and 8.3.

AC	anterior commissure
ACC	anterior cingulate cortex
ACh	acetylcholine
Ag/AgCl	silver-silver chloride
AG	antigen
AHN	anterior hypothalamic nucleus
AM	adrenal medulla
AN	arcuate nucleus
ANS	autonomic nervous system
ANU	autonomic neural unit
AP	area postrema
ATP	adenosine triphosphate
BAT	brown adipose tissue
BC	bulbocavernous (muscle)
BDNF	brain-derived neurotrophic factor
BK	bradykinin
BMP	bone morphogenetic protein
BN	Barrington's nucleus
BNST	bed nucleus of the stria terminalis
BötC	Bötzinger complex
BP	blood pressure
BV	blood vessel
c, C	cervical (segment)
CA	central autonomic nucleus
Ca^{2+}	calcium ion
cAMP	cyclic adenosine monophosphate
CBF	cerebral blood flow
cc	central canal
CC	corpus callosum
CCK	cholecystokinin
CE	external carotid artery
CeAM	central nucleus of the amygdala
CG	celiac ganglion
cGMP	cyclic guanosine monophosphate
CGRP	calcitonin gene-related peptide
ChAT	choline acetyltransferase
CI	internal carotid artery
CL/cl	centrolateral nucleus (thalamus)
CM	circular musculature (gastrointestinal tract)
CNS	central nervous system
CoCa	common carotid artery
CPA	caudal pressor area
CRG	central respiratory generator
CRH	corticotropin-releasing hormone
CRPS	complex regional pain syndrome
CSN	carotid sinus nerve
CSP	carotid sinus pressure
CST	cervical sympathetic trunk
CT	chromaffin tissue
CTb	cholera toxin subunit B
CVC	cutaneous vasoconstrictor (neuron)
CVD	cutaneous vasodilator (neuron)
CVLM	caudal ventrolateral medulla
cVRG	caudal ventral respiratory group
CVS	cardiovascular system
DA	dopamine
DBH	dopamine-β-hydroxylase
DC	dorsal column (spinal cord)
DCN	dorsal commissural nucleus (spinal cord)

DH	dorsal horn (spinal cord, trigeminal)	GiV	gigantocellular reticular nucleus ventral
DLF	dorsolateral funiculus (spinal cord)	GLP-1	glucagon-like peptide 1
DMH or DM	dorsomedial hypothalamus	GnRH	gonadotropin-releasing hormone
DMN	dorsomedial nucleus (of the hypothalamus)	GR	gray ramus
		GRP	gastrin-releasing peptide
DMNX	dorsal motor nucleus of the vagus	GSR	galvanic skin response
		HGN	hypogastric nerve
DOPA	dihydroxyphenylalanine	HPA axis	hypothalamo–pituitary–adrenal axis
dpINS	dorsal posterior insula		
DR	dorsal root	HPC	heat pinch (noxious) cold
DRG	dorsal root ganglion	HR	heart rate
DVC	dorsal vagal complex	HRP	horseradish peroxidase
DYN	dynorphin	5-HT	5-hydroxytryptamine (serotonin)
ECG	electrocardiogram		
EJC	excitatory junction current	HVPG	hypothalamic visceral pattern generator
EJP	excitatory junction potential	IAS	intrinsic anal sphincter
		IC	intercalated spinal nucleus
el	external lateral nucleus (parabrachial complex)	ICC	interstitial cell of Cajal
		ICNS	intrinsic cardiac nervous system
EMG	electromyogram		
ENDC	endocrine cell	IEG	immediate early gene
ENK	enkephalin	IGL	intraganglionic laminar ending (enteric nervous system)
ENS	enteric nervous system		
EPSC	excitatory postsynaptic current	IJP	inhibitory junction potential
EPSP	excitatory postsynaptic potential	IL	interleukin
		ILf	funicular part of the intermediolateral nucleus
EUS	external urethral sphincter		
EW	nucleus Edinger–Westphal		
FB	Fast Blue	ILp	principal part of the intermediolateral nucleus
FG	Fluoro-Gold		
FN	facial nucleus		
GABA	γ-aminobutyric acid	IMA	intramuscular array (enteric nervous system)
GAL	galanin		
GALT	gut-associated lymphoid tissue	IMG	inferior mesenteric ganglion
GH	growth hormone	IML	intermediolateral nucleus (spinal cord)
GHRH	growth hormone-releasing hormone	IN	interneuron
		INA	integrated nerve activity
GiA	gigantocellular reticular nucleus alpha	INCS	intrinsic cardiac nervous system
GIT	gastrointestinal tract		

INS	inspiratory/inspiration-type sympathetic neuron	LT	low threshold
		LTB	leukotriene B
		LTC	leukotriene C
INSP	inspiratory/inspiration	LTF	lateral tegmental field
IO	inferior olive nucleus	MAP	mean arterial blood pressure
IPAN	intrinsic primary afferent neuron (enteric nervous system)	MaSN	major splanchnic nerve
IP_3	inositol 1,4,5-triphosphate	MBO	mammillary body
		MC	mast cell
IPS	inferior periinsular sulcus	MCC	middle cingulate cortex
IPSP	inhibitory postsynaptic potential	MCG	middle cervical ganglion
		MDvc	ventral portion of the medial dorsal nucleus (thalamus)
IRH	inhibitory releasing hormone		
i.v.	intravenous	ME	median eminence
IVLM	intermediate ventrolateral medulla	MePO	median preoptic nucleus
		MiSN	minor splanchnic nerve
IZ	intermediate zone (spinal cord)	MMC	migrating myoelectric complex (enteric nervous system)
JGA	juxtaglomerular apparatus (kidney)		
KF	Kölliker–Fuse (nucleus)	MP	myenteric plexus (enteric nervous system)
I, L	lumbar (segment)		
LAH	long afterhyperpolarization	MPN	medial preoptic nucleus
LC	locus ceruleus	MR	motility-regulating (neuron)
LCN	local circuit neuron		
LF	lateral funiculus (spinal cord)	mRNA	messenger ribonucleic acid
LFN	lateral funicular nucleus	MVC	muscle vasoconstrictor (neuron)
LH	lateral hypothalamus		
LHA	lateral hypothalamic area	MVD	muscle vasodilator (neuron)
LHRH	luteinizing-hormone-releasing hormone		
		N	neurotensin
LM	longitudinal musculature (enteric nervous system)	NA	nucleus ambiguus
		NA_C	compact formation of the NA
LPGi	nucleus paragigantocellularis lateralis	NA_e	external formation of the NA
LPN	lateral preoptic nucleus	NA_L	loose formation of the NA
LPS	lipopolysaccharide		
LRN	lateral reticular nucleus	NA_{SC}	subcompact formation of the NA
LSN	lumbar splanchnic nerve		
LST/LSC	lumbar sympathetic trunk/lumbar sympathetic chain	nAChR	nicotinic acetylcholine receptor
		NAd	noradrenaline

NANC	non-adrenergic non-cholinergic	PMC	pontine micturition center
NAR	nucleus arcuatus	PMNL	polymorphonuclear leukocyte
NFP	neurofilament protein	PNMT	phenylethanolamine-N-methyl transferase
NK1/NKA	neurokinin 1/A		
NMDA	N-methyl-D-aspartate (acid)	PP	pancreatic polypeptide
NO	nitric oxide	preBötC	preBötzinger complex
NOS	nitric oxide synthase	PRV	pseudorabies virus
NPY	neuropeptide Y	PSC	pontine storage center
NS	nociceptive specific (neuron)	PSCN	presuprachiasmatic preoptic nucleus
NSF	N-ethylmaleimide-sensitive factor	PSDC	postsynaptic dorsal column
NTAP	nerve terminal action potential	PSN	pelvic splanchnic nerve
		PT	primary transmitter
NTS	nucleus tractus solitarii	PVH	paraventricular nucleus of the hypothalamus
NTS$_{cen}$	pars centralis of the NTS		
OT	optic tract	PYY	peptide YY
OVLT	organum vasculosum laminae terminalis	REM	rapid eye movement
		RESP	respiration
PACAP	pituitary adenylate cyclase-activating peptide	RH	releasing hormone
		RN	raphe nuclei
		RNA	ribonucleic acid
PaCO$_2$	arterial CO$_2$ pressure	Rob/pal	raphe obscurus/pallidus
PAF	platelet-activating factor	RVC	renal vasoconstrictor (neuron)
PAG	periaqueductal gray	RVLM	rostral ventrolateral medulla
PAN	primary afferent neuron		
PaO$_2$	arterial O$_2$ pressure	rVRG	rostral ventral respirator group
para	parasympathetic	s,S	sacral (segment)
PBC/PB	parabrachial complex/parabrachial nucleus	SAH	synaptic afterhyperpolarization
PCM	parasympathetic cardio-motor (neuron)	SALT	skin-associated lymphoid tissue
PE	plasma extravasation	SCG	superior cervical ganglion
Pf	parafascicular nucleus (thalamus)	SCM	sympathetic cardiomotor (neuron)
PGE	prostaglandin E	SCN	suprachiasmatic nucleus
PHA	posterior hypothalamic area	SCO	subcommissural organ
PHA-L	phaseolus vulgaris leuko-agglutinin	sEPSP	slow excitatory postsynaptic potential
PHR	phrenic nerve	SEPT	septum
PM	pilomotor (neuron)	SI/SII	primary/secondary somatosensory cortex

S.E.M	standard error of mean	VH	ventral horn (spinal cord)
SFO	subfornical organ	VIP	vasoactive intestinal peptide
SG	stellate ganglion		
SI	primary somatosensory cortex	vl	ventrolateral nucleus (parabrachial)
SII	secondary somatosensory cortex	VLM	ventrolateral medulla
		VM/VMN	ventromedial nucleus (hypothalamus)
sIPSP	slow inhibitory postsynaptic potential	VMH	ventromedial hypothalamus
SIS	skin immune system		
SK channel	small-conductance Ca^{2+}-activated channel	VMM	ventromedial medulla
		VMb	basal part of the ventromedial nucleus (thalamus)
SKP	skin potential		
SKT	skin temperature		
SM	sudomotor (neuron)	VMpo	posterior part of the ventromedial nucleus (thalamus, primate)
SMC	smooth muscle cell		
SMP	submucosal plexus (enteric nervous system)	VPI	ventral posterior inferior nucleus (thalamus)
SOM	somatostatin		
SP	substance P	VPL	ventral posterior lateral nucleus (thalamus)
SPL	splanchnic nerve		
Sp5	spinal trigeminal nucleus	VPM	ventral posterior medial nucleus (thalamus)
sp5	spinal trigeminal tract		
SS	somatostatin		
STT	spinothalamic tract	VPpc	ventral posterior parvicellular nucleus of the thalamus (rat)
Sy	sympathetic		
t,T	thoracic (segment)	VR	ventral root
TH	tyrosine hydroxylase	VRC	ventral respiratory column
TK	tachykinin		
TNF	tumor necrosis factor	VRG	ventral respiratory group
		VTA	ventral tegmental area
TRH	thyrotropin-releasing hormone	VVC	visceral vasoconstrictor (neuron)
TRP	transient receptor potential	WDR	wide dynamic range (neuron)
TS	tractus solitarius	WHBP	working-heart-brain-stem preparation
TTX	tetrodotoxin		
UB	urinary bladder	WR	white ramus
VAChT	vesicular acetylcholine transporter	X	vagus nerve/nucleus
		ZI	zona incerta

The Autonomic Nervous System and the Regulation of Body Functions

Autonomic Adjustments of the Body and Behavior

All living organisms interact continuously with their environment. They receive multiple signals from the environment via their sensory systems and respond by way of their somatomotor system. Both sensory processing and motor actions are entirely under the control of the central nervous system. The brain represents the extracorporeal space, the somatic body domains, the executive motor programs and programs for the diverse patterns of behavior initiated from higher centers. It generates complex motor commands on the basis of these central representations leading to movements of the body in its environment against different internal and external forces. The tools for performing these actions are the effector machines, the skeletal muscles and their controlling somatomotoneurons.

The body's motor activity and behavior are only possible when its internal milieu is controlled to keep the component cells, tissues and organs (including the brain and skeletal muscles) maintained in an optimal state for their function. This enables the organism to adjust its performance to the varying internal and external demands placed on the organism. The mechanisms involved include the control of:

- fluid matrix of the body (fluid volume regulation, osmoregulation),
- gas exchange with the environment (regulation of airway resistance and the pulmonary circulation),
- ingestion and digestion of nutrients (regulation of the gastrointestinal tract and of energy balance),
- transport of gases, nutrients and other substances throughout the body to supply organs, including the brain, to maintain consciousness (regulation of blood flows and blood pressure by the cardiovascular regulation),
- excretion of substances (disposal of waste),
- body temperature (thermoregulation),
- reproductive behavior (mechanics of sexual organs),
- defensive behaviors,
- body recovery (control of circadian rhythms, of sleep and wakefulness),
- development and maintenance of body organs and tissues,

- body protection at the cellular and systems level (regulation of inflammatory processes, control of the immune system).

These body functions responsible for maintaining the internal milieu are controlled by the brain. The control is exerted by the autonomic nervous system and the endocrine system. Specifically, the brain acts on many peripheral target tissues (smooth muscle cells of various organs, cardiac muscle cells, exocrine glands, endocrine cells, metabolic tissues, immune cells, etc.). The *efferent signals* from the brain to the periphery of the body by which this control is achieved are *neural* (by the autonomic nervous system) and *hormonal* (by the neuroendocrine systems). The time scales of these controls may differ by orders of magnitude; changes in autonomic regulation are normally fast and occur within seconds, and neuroendocrine regulation is relatively slow (over tens of minutes, hours or even days). The *afferent signals* from the periphery of the body to the brain are neural, hormonal (e.g., hormones from both endocrine organs and the gastrointestinal tract, cytokines from the immune system, leptin from adipocytes) and physicochemical (e.g., blood glucose level, blood temperature, etc.).

The maintenance of physiological parameters such as concentrations of ions, blood glucose, arterial blood gases, body core temperature in a narrow range (but around predetermined "set points") is called *homeostasis*. Homeostatic regulation involves autonomic systems, endocrine systems and gas exchange (respiration). The concept of homeostasis was formulated by Walter Bradford Cannon (1929) based on the idea of the fixity of the internal milieu of the body (Claude Bernard 1957, 1974) (Note 1). However, this concept is too narrow and static to understand how the organism is able to maintain the parameters in the body stably and to temporarily adapt them during environmental changes. To understand how the internal milieu is maintained stably during changes in the body or in the environment, the concept of allostasis has been developed. This extends the concept of homeostasis and describes the temporary changes of set points of homeostatic regulation during large changes in the body or in the environment. It distinguishes between systems that are essential for life (e.g., the concentrations of ions and pH in the extracellular and intracellular fluid compartments; homeostasis in the narrow sense) and systems

that maintain these systems in balance ("allostasis") as the environment changes. This is achieved by the autonomic nervous systems and the endocrine systems and is fully dependent on a functioning central nervous system, notably the hypothalamus and the cerebral hemispheres (Sterling and Eyer 1988; McEwen 2001b, 2007; McEwen and Wingfield 2003; Schulkin 2003a, b; Schulkin and Sterling 2019).

Autonomic Nervous System and Brain

The somatomotor system and the somatosensory system form "sensorimotor programs" for the control of movement of the organism in its environment. These somatic sensorimotor programs are represented in the spinal cord, brain stem and hypothalamus and are under the control of the telencephalon (Figure 0.1 right). By analogy, autonomic motor systems and neuroendocrine motor systems, together with interoceptive afferent neural, hormonal and humoral input systems that monitor the conditions of the inner milieu of the body, form autonomic and neuroendocrine "sensorimotor programs" for the regulation of the inner milieu of the body. Similarly, these autonomic and neuroendocrine sensorimotor programs are represented in the spinal cord, brain stem and hypothalamus and are under control of the telencephalon (Figure 0.1 left). Integration within the brain, between the centers that are involved with the autonomic, neuroendocrine and somatomotor as well as interoceptive sensory input systems, is essential for the coordination of the behavior of the organism within its environment.

The explanatory model in Figure 0.2 outlines the role of the autonomic nervous system in the generation of behavior. It is based on the "Four System Network Model" of Larry Swanson (Swanson 2012, 2013, Card and Swanson 2013). The four systems are the motor system, the sensory system, the cortical system and the state system. Behavior is defined as the purposeful motor action of the body in the environment. It is generated by coordinated activation (1) of somatomotor neurons to move the body in the environment and (2) of autonomic and neuroendocrine motor neurons to prepare and adjust the internal milieu and body organs enabling the body to move. Thus, under the motor system we subsume

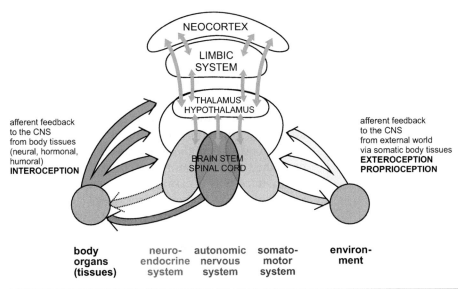

body organs (tissues) **neuro-endocrine system** **autonomic nervous system** **somato-motor system** **environ-ment**

Figure 0.1 Autonomic nervous system, brain and body. *Right*, somatic nervous system (somatomotor system and sensory systems to spinal cord and brain stem) and environment. *Left*, autonomic nervous system, neuroendocrine system and body organs. In the *middle*, spinal cord, brain stem, hypothalamus, limbic system and neocortex. The interoceptive afferent feedback from the body is neuronal, hormonal and humoral (physicochemical; e.g., glucose concentration, osmolality) and of other modalities (e.g., body temperature). *Solid-line arrows*, neuronal; *dotted-line arrow*, hormonal. Limbic system is anatomically descriptive and a collective term denoting brain structures common to all mammals that include hippocampus, dentate gyrus with archicortex, cingulate gyrus, septal nuclei and amygdala. These forebrain structures are functionally heterogeneous and not a unitary system (as the term "limbic system" may imply). They are involved in the generation of emotional and motivational aspects of behavior (see LeDoux [1996]). Note the reciprocal communication between hypothalamus, limbic system and neocortex (symbolized by the green double arrows) indicating that the centers of the cerebral hemispheres control the autonomic regulation. Modified from Jänig and Häbler (1999) with permission.

the three divisions, the somatic, the autonomic and the neuroendocrine motor systems (Swanson 2000; Watts and Swanson 2002; Card and Swanson 2013):

- The three divisions of the motor system are closely integrated in the spinal cord, brain stem and hypothalamus. Both somatomotor and autonomic motor systems are hierarchically organized; their integration occurs at each level of the hierarchy. The neuroendocrine motor system is represented at the top of this hierarchy (in the hypothalamus).
- The motoneuron pools (final motor pathways) extend from the midbrain to the caudal end of the spinal cord for the somatomotor system and the autonomic system (the latter with gaps in the cervical and lower lumbar spinal cord). The neuroendocrine motor neurons are located in the periventricular zone of the hypothalamus.
- The activity of the motor system generating behavior is dependent on three major classes of input: (1) exteroceptive and interoceptive sensory systems,

(2) cortical systems and (3) behavioral state systems (Figures 0.1 and 0.2).

- The sensory systems monitor events in the body (*interoceptive* in Figure 0.2) or in the environment (*exteroceptive* in Figure 0.2). They are closely welded to the motor hierarchy and generate on all levels of this hierarchy reflex behavior (*reflex* in Figure 0.2).
- The cerebral hemispheres initiate and maintain behavior based on cognition and affective-emotional processes (*cortical* in Figure 0.2).
- The behavioral state system consists of intrinsic neural systems that control circadian timing of all body functions, sleep and wakefulness, arousal, attention, vigilance (*state* in Figure 0.2). This system modulates the somatic, autonomic and neuroendocrine motor systems.
- The three global input systems to the motor system interact with each other too.

This way of looking at the autonomic nervous system shows that the activity in the autonomic

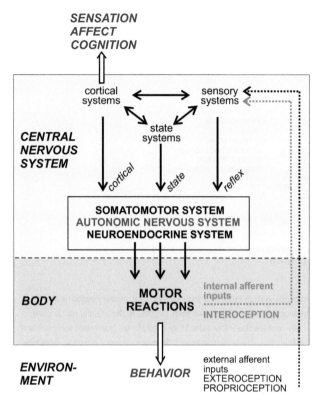

SENSATION
AFFECT
COGNITION

CENTRAL
NERVOUS
SYSTEM

cortical
systems

sensory
systems

state
systems

cortical

state

reflex

SOMATOMOTOR SYSTEM
AUTONOMIC NERVOUS SYSTEM
NEUROENDOCRINE SYSTEM

BODY

MOTOR
REACTIONS

internal afferent
inputs

INTEROCEPTION

ENVIRON-
MENT

BEHAVIOR

external afferent
inputs
EXTEROCEPTION
PROPRIOCEPTION

Figure 0.2 Functional organization of the nervous system to generate behavior. The motor system, consisting of the somatomotor, the autonomic (visceromotor) and the neuroendocrine systems, controls behavior. It is hierarchically organized in the spinal cord, brain stem and hypothalamus. The motor system receives three general types of synaptic input: (1) from the sensory systems monitoring processes in the body or the environment to all levels of the motor system generating reflex behavior (*reflex*); (2) from the cerebral hemispheres responsible for cortical control of the behavior based on neural processes related to cognitive and affective-emotional processes (*cortical*); (3) from the behavioral state system controlling attention, arousal, sleep/wakefulness, circadian timing (*state*). The three general input systems communicate bidirectionally with each other (upper part of the figure). Modified from Swanson (2012, 2013) and Card and Swanson (2013).

neurons is dependent on the intrinsic structure of the sensorimotor programs of the motor hierarchy and on its three global input systems. Any change in these input systems should be reflected in the activity of the neurons of the final autonomic pathways and therefore in autonomic regulation of different organ systems.

Precision of Autonomic Regulation and its Failure in Disease

The precision and biological importance of the control of peripheral target organs by the autonomic nervous system are silently accepted, but the mechanisms by which they come about are not generally understood. Both of these aspects become quite obvious when the regulatory functions fail. Failure of autonomic control may occur at a time when the somatomotor and the sensory systems are functioning normally (Low 1993; Appenzeller 2000; Robertson et al. 2012; Buijs and Swaab 2013; Mathias and Bannister 2013). It may develop:

- when the peripheral (efferent) autonomic neurons are damaged (e.g., as a consequence of metabolic disease, such as long-term diabetes in which peripheral autonomic neurons are destroyed), resulting in the failure of regulation of the cardiovascular system, the gastrointestinal tract, pelvic organs (sexual organs, urinary bladder, hindgut) or other organs;
- when certain types of peripheral autonomic neurons are inherently absent such as the rare cases of *pure autonomic failure* in which most neurons in the autonomic ganglia are absent or in which one enzyme for synthesis of the transmitter noradrenaline, dopamine-β-hydroxylase, is deficient or absent (Mathias and Bannister 2013); or in *Hirschsprung's disease* in which some of the inhibitory motor neurons of the enteric nervous system of the gut are missing (Christensen 1994);
- when the *spinal cord* is *lesioned* leading to interruption of the control of these spinal autonomic circuits by supraspinal autonomic centers to the spinal autonomic circuits;
- when the efferent sympathetic and afferent pathways in the peripheral somatic tissues are disrupted after trauma (with or without nerve lesions), leading to abnormal relationships between sympathetic and afferent systems and consequently to pain syndromes such as complex regional pain syndrome type I or type II (Stanton-Hicks et al. 1995; Jänig and Stanton-Hicks 1996; Harden et al. 2001; Jänig and Baron 2002, 2003; Jänig 2020);
- when hypothalamic functions are impaired (e.g., in anorexia nervosa or as a consequence of a tumor or trauma);

- during severe infectious diseases, when central regulation of the cardiovascular system or gastrointestinal tract fails;
- quite commonly in *old age* when peripheral autonomic neurons may die and autonomic regulation may be reduced in effectiveness.

Functional diseases, involving the autonomic nervous system and neuroendocrine systems, may also develop when allostatic responses, which are physiologically rapidly mobilized during external and internal perturbations ("stress") and then turned off when no longer needed, remain active over a longer time. These maintained allostatic responses are called *allostatic load* or *overload* and are believed to contribute to various types of functional diseases, such as hypertension, myocardial infarction, obesity, type II diabetes, atherosclerosis and metabolic syndrome (Folkow et al. 1997; McEwen 2001a; McEwen and Wingfield 2003; Robertson et al. 2012).

Although we can in principle live without the function of large parts of the autonomic nervous system, the lifestyle of an individual in such a state becomes severely constrained so that many of the activities for which our biology equips us, such as being sexually active, playing tennis, running a marathon, climbing mountains, diving in the sea, living in the tropics or in arctic climates, or being involved in intellectual activities, are not possible. All vertebrates are endowed with autonomic systems in order to meet extreme environmental challenges such as very cold or hot climates, high altitudes, extreme body motor activity, extreme states of starvation or extreme dry climates. These examples illustrate the dynamic plasticity of autonomic regulation. This plasticity may have been essential for the evolution of mammals, humans probably being one of the most adaptable mammals. Development, anatomical differentiation and functional differentiation of the autonomic nervous system evolved in association with the behavioral repertoire of the different vertebrate species. Thus, the complexity of autonomic regulation increased with the complexity of the behavioral repertoire (Nilsson 1983; Nilsson and Holmgren 1994; Holmgren and Olsson 2011; see Subchapter 1.5). This is fully in line with the concept of functioning of the hierarchically organized motor system that includes the somatomotor, the autonomic and neuroendocrine systems as outlined above (Figure 0.2).

Autonomic regulation of body functions requires the existence of specific neuronal pathways in the periphery and specific organization in the central nervous system; otherwise it would not be possible to have the precision and flexibility of control that higher vertebrates possess for rapid adjustments during diverse behaviors. This implies that the various autonomic systems must be centrally integrated and have multiple, but distinct, peripheral motor pathways. These pathways are defined according to the function they mediate in the target cells they innervate. The effector cells of the autonomic nervous system are anatomically and functionally very diverse while those of the somatic efferent system are not, i.e., it consists of skeletal muscle fibers. From this point of view, it is clear that the autonomic nervous system is the major efferent component of the peripheral nervous system and outweighs the somatic efferent pathways in the diversity of its functions and its size.

Organization and Aims of the Book

In this book, I will describe the principles of organization of the properties of autonomic circuits and of single autonomic neurons in the context of their biological functions in vivo. This description should help to explain why the brain is able to adapt and coordinate the different functions of the body so precisely during our daily activities, as well as during extreme exertion and physiological stress. The book is organized in five parts:

1. *The Autonomic Nervous System: Functional Anatomy and Interoceptive Visceral Afferents.* I describe the neuroanatomical basis for the precise regulation of the peripheral autonomic target organs in higher vertebrates. This provides definitions and lays the groundwork for this book. It also includes a general description of the anatomy and physiology of *interoceptive afferent neurons*, which are closely associated with the functioning of the autonomic nervous system, with interoceptive sensations and general feelings triggered from the body tissues and, finally, also with emotions.

2. *Functional Organization of the Peripheral Autonomic Nervous System.* This section describes the functional organization of sympathetic and parasympathetic pathways in the periphery and the

principles of the organization of the enteric nervous system.

3. *Transmission of Signals in the Peripheral Autonomic Nervous System.* I describe the "tools" by which the signals generated in the brain are transmitted by the autonomic pathways to the effector cells. This description includes the neurotransmitters and their receptors, ganglionic transmission and neuroeffector transmission.

4. *Representation of the Autonomic Nervous System in Spinal Cord and Lower Brain Stem.* I describe some principles of organization of the autonomic control systems in the spinal cord and lower brain stem. This description will have its reference in the functional organization of the peripheral autonomic pathways that has been extensively described in the two previous parts.

5. *The Centers of Homeostasis in the Mesencephalon and Hypothalamus and their Telencephalic Control.* I will discuss how the functions of autonomic systems that are represented in the spinal cord and lower brain stem are integrated in complex regulatory circuits involving somatomotor, autonomic and neuroendocrine systems (Figure 0.2) that are represented in the mesencephalon, the hypothalamus and the telencephalon. I will paraphrase Walter Bradford Cannon as expressed in his most influential book *The Wisdom of the Body* (Cannon 1939).

For the detailed physiology of the various autonomic control systems, as well as their specific organization in the spinal cord, brain stem and hypothalamus, the reader is referred, *first*, to the series of volumes on the Autonomic Nervous System edited by Burnstock and by several volume editors (see under volume editors) (Note 2), *second*, to textbooks covering the autonomic nervous system or parts of it (Note 3) and, *third*, to selected review articles (Note 4). The approach used here should also lead to a better understanding of primary disorders of the autonomic nervous system and of autonomic disorders that are secondary to, rather than causative of, various diseases (Note 5). This book is not intended to extensively describe special fields of the neurobiology of the autonomic nervous system, such as regulation of the cardiovascular system, body temperature, pelvic organs, gastrointestinal tract, etc. Furthermore, it is not intended to discuss the pathophysiology of the autonomic nervous system. However, it is of course the basis to understanding pathophysiological changes in autonomic functions.

Suggested Reading

Cannon, W. B. (1939) *The Wisdom of the Body, 2nd Revised and Enlarged Edition*, Norton, New York.

Swanson, L. W. (2012) *Brain Architecture: Understanding the Basic Plan, 2nd Edn*, Oxford University Press, Oxford.

Swanson, L. W. (2013) Basic plan of the nervous system. In *Fundamental Neuroscience, 4th Edn* (Squire, L. R., Berg, D., Bloom, F. E., et al., eds.) pp. 15–38, Elsevier Academic Press, Amsterdam.

All references cited in the text are available online at www.cambridge.org/janig.

Notes

1. Claude Bernard was the first to formulate the idea of the fixity of the internal milieu of the body. This formulation was not so much based on experimental observations; however, it related to the experiments he had conducted over tens of years (Bernard 1878). Physiologists became aware of the universal importance of this concept in the frame of experimental physiology and medicine when it was applied to regulation of acid-base balance in the first half of the last century.

2. Burnstock and Hoyle (1992); Hendry and Hill (1992); Maggi (1993); Nilsson and Holmgren (1994); McLachlan (1995); Bennett and Gardiner (1996); Shepherd and Vatner (1996); Unzicker (1996); Barnes (1997); Jordan (1997); Morris and Gibbins (1997); Burnstock and Sillito (2000); Brookes and Costa (2002).

3. Randall (1984); Loewy and Spyer (1990); Ritter et al. (1992); Low (1993); Rowell (1993); Shepherd and Vatner (1996); Appenzeller and Oribe (1997); Blessing (1997); Appenzeller (1999); Undem and Weinreich (2005); Llewellyne-Smith and Verberne (2011); Mathias and Bannister (2013).

4. Jänig (1985, 1986, 1988a, 1995a, 1996a); Jänig and McLachlan (1987); Guyenet (1990, 2006, 2014); Dampney (1994, 2016); Häbler et al. (1994a); Spyer (1994); Kirchheim et al. (1998); Jänig and Häbler (1999, 2003); Folkow (2000); Schreihofer and Sved (2011); Guyenet and Bayliss (2015); reviews in Romanovsky (2018).

5. Low (1993); Robertson and Biaggioni (1995); Appenzeller and Oribe (1997); Appenzeller (2000); Robertson et al. (2012); Buijs and Swaab (2013); Mathias and Bannister (2013).

Part I

The Autonomic Nervous System: Functional Anatomy and Interoceptive Afferents

Before developing the general neurobiological concepts of the function of the autonomic nervous system I will describe some aspects of the anatomy and function of this system on the macroscopic level and explain the limitations of our present understanding of the autonomic nervous system and its functioning. Furthermore, I will provide some definitions. This conventional approach is necessary to help to convey what is meant when we speak of how the peripheral autonomic nervous system behaves and to lay the groundwork for the description of the functions in which the autonomic nervous system is involved.

The brain continuously receives messages from internal organs and somatic tissues of the body. These afferent messages are neuronal, hormonal, chemical and physical in nature (see Figure 0.1). The continuous afferent feedback to the brain conveys information about the state of body organs and tissues (e.g., the mechanical, thermal, metabolic and inflammatory states; the degree and composition of filling of the gastrointestinal tract; the state of pelvic organs; the state of the cardiovascular system, etc.),

the state of parameters regulated homeostatically (e.g., the concentrations of glucose, oxygen and bicarbonate in the blood; the size of fat stores by the concentration of leptin in the blood), the activity of endocrine glands (by the concentration of circulating hormones secreted by these glands) and the state of peripheral protective mechanisms of the body (e.g., by activity in nociceptive afferent neurons, by signals from immune tissues [cytokines acting directly on the brain or indirectly via vagal afferents]). The multiple afferent feedback signals to the brain from the organs and tissues of the body are essential to achieve the precision of the homeostatic short- and long-term regulation in which the autonomic nervous systems are involved. This afferent feedback connects to all levels of the autonomic motor hierarchy, to the centers of the cerebral hemispheres, which are responsible for conscious sensations and cognitive inputs to the motor hierarchy, and to the behavioral state system (Swanson 2000, 2012, 2013; see Introduction and Figure 0.2; see Subchapters 11.4 and 11.6).

Chapter 1

Functional Anatomy of the Peripheral Sympathetic and Parasympathetic Systems

1.1 Definitions and Limitations

Langley (1900, 1903a, b, 1921) originally proposed the generic term *autonomic nervous system* to describe the system of nerves that regulates the function of all innervated tissues and organs throughout the vertebrate body except striated muscle fibers; that is, the innervation of the viscera, vasculature, exocrine and some endocrine glands, and some other tissues. This term is synonymous with the term *vegetative nervous system*, which has become obsolete in Anglo-American countries. However, the latter is still the preferred term in German ("vegetatives Nervensystem"; Jänig and Baron 2019), French ("système végétative"), Italian ("sistema neurovegetativo"), Spanish ("sistema nervioso vegetativo") and Russian ("vegetativnaia nervnaia sistema"). In Chinese and Japanese the terms "Zizhu shenjing xitong" and "Jiritsu shinkei-kei", respectively, are translations of the term "autonomic nervous system."

Langley (1921) divided the autonomic nervous system into three parts: the parasympathetic nervous system, the sympathetic nervous system and the enteric nervous system. This definition has stood the test of time and is now universally used in descriptions of the autonomic nervous system in vertebrates (Nilsson 1983; Gibbins 1994).

The definition of the *sympathetic* and the *parasympathetic nervous systems* is based on the specialized neuroanatomical arrangement of the autonomic outflow from the central nervous system to the peripheral target tissues (see Figure 1.1). This outflow is separated into a tectal (mesencephalon), bulbar (medulla oblongata) and sacral system (collectively called the craniosacral system = parasympathetic system; see Figures 1.1 and 1.4) and a thoracolumbar system (sympathetic system). The separation made by Langley was based on several criteria: the distribution of innervated target organs, the opposing effects of nerve stimulation, embryological development and the effects of exogenously applied substances (e.g., adrenaline, nicotine, pilocarpine, atropine) on effector organs (Langley 1903a). The main feature distinguishing sympathetic and parasympathetic spinal outflow is their separation by the cervical and lumbar enlargements of the spinal cord (which contain the somatomotor innervation and neural circuits related to the upper and lower limbs, respectively), and so the definition is primarily an *anatomical* one. Thus, there is sympathetic innervation of the limbs

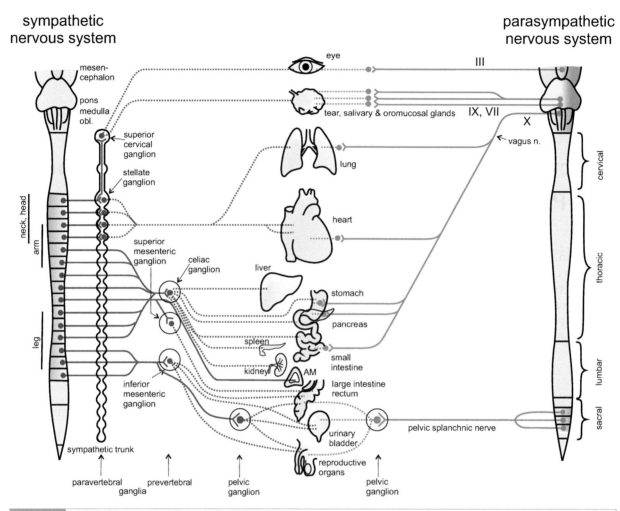

Figure 1.1 The sympathetic and parasympathetic nervous system in humans. Continuous lines, preganglionic axons; dotted lines, postganglionic axons. The sympathetic outflow to skin and deep somatic structures of the extremities (upper extremity, T2 to T5; lower extremity T12 to L3) and of the trunk are not shown. AM, adrenal medulla; III, oculomotor nerve; VII, facial nerve; IX, glossopharyngeal nerve; X, vagus nerve (with permission from Jänig and Baron 2019).

and trunk but not parasympathetic innervation. In rats, cats and some other mammalian species, the spinal parasympathetic outflow to the pelvic organs also originates from the last lumbar spinal segment.

In some lower vertebrates, the distinction between sympathetic outflow and sacral parasympathetic outflow to pelvic organs cannot be made (see Subchapter 1.5). Therefore it has been proposed to use the terms *cranial autonomic outflow* and *spinal autonomic outflow* rather than the terms *sympathetic* and *parasympathetic* (Nilsson, 1983). Although there is some merit in this nomenclature, I will not use it in this book.

Espinosa-Medina et al. (2016) have studied several transcription factors and molecular markers in either cranial or spinal preganglionic neurons and associated autonomic ganglia in mouse embryos at various embryological stages. This interesting study shows that the "transcriptional fingerprints" of sacral and thoracolumbar preganglionic neurons are similar but different from those of the cranial (bulbar) preganglionic neurons (here in the dorsal vagal motor nucleus). Furthermore, it shows that pelvic ganglia, just like sympathetic ganglia, develop independently of the outgrowing preganglionic axons. The authors conclude from their findings that the sacral auto-nomic (parasympathetic) system is the "caudal out-post of the sympathetic outflow," thus proposing a simple dichotomy of parasympathetic (cranial) and sympathetic (spinal) systems which would replace Langley's classical concept. This proposed re-classification of the peripheral autonomic nervous system, based on molecular-genetic criteria, was vig-orously opposed and considered not to be justified; it would compromise the sophisticated neurobiology of the regulation of pelvic organs (Horn 2018; Jänig et al. 2017, 2018; Neuhuber et al. 2017).

Throughout the book I will use the terms *sympa-thetic* and *parasympathetic* as defined *anatomically* by Langley (1903a, b, 1921). When peripheral autonomic neurons or neuron populations cannot unambigu-ously be assigned to one of these systems (as is the case for some neurons in pelvic ganglia), I will speak of autonomic neurons. I will not use the terms *sympa-thetic* and *parasympathetic* in a global functional sense, as may be inferred from the work of Cannon (1939), Hess (1948) and others, and is still commonly done in the literature, because it leads to generalizations that are not justified in view of the neurobiological and functional differentiation of the autonomic nervous system. Thus, to speak of sympathetic or parasympa-thetic "functions" generates misunderstandings and gives the wrong impression of how these systems work. This point will be discussed in more detail in Subchapter 11.1 and will be clarified in Part II. Finally, I will not apply these terms to visceral primary affer-ent neurons at equivalent spinal levels nor to vagal afferents as the autonomic nervous system is entirely efferent in function (see Subchapter 2.1).

1.2 Gross Anatomy of the Peripheral Sympathetic and Parasympathetic Nervous Systems

The basic feature of the peripheral sympathetic and parasympathetic systems is that each consists of two populations of neurons, which are arranged in series and which are connected at synapses in the periph-ery. The sympathetic and parasympathetic neurons that innervate the target tissue lie entirely outside the central nervous system. The cell bodies of these auto-nomic neurons are grouped in structures called *auto-nomic ganglia*. Their axons project from these ganglia

to the target organs and tissues. Therefore, these neurons are called *ganglion neurons* or *postganglionic neurons*. The efferent neurons that send axons from the spinal cord or brain stem into the ganglia and form synapses on the dendrites and cell bodies of the postganglionic neurons are called *preganglionic neurons*. The cell bodies of the preganglionic neurons lie in the spinal cord or in the brain stem. In Subchapters 1.2 and 1.3, some aspects of the macro-anatomical organization and function of the two autonomic systems are described. Further details of the anatomical organization can be found in the lit-erature (Pick 1970; Gray's Anatomy 2016; Brodal 1998) (Note 1).

Langley defined the spinal levels of the functional outflow to different organs by examining organ func-tions in response to stimulation of the ventral root at each segmental level. He then localized ganglionic synapses in each pathway by direct application of nicotine, a substance that excites postganglionic cell bodies. In this way, all the major efferent functional pathways to the peripheral tissues of several species of laboratory animal (cat, dog and rabbit) were defined. It was evident that every organ receives a supply from one or both of the sympathetic and parasympathetic outflows, and that the effects on each organ system are discrete and appear in some cases to be opposing each other. These experiments led to the concept of control of function of the auto-nomic target organs by independent peripheral auto-nomic pathways.

By the end of his life, Langley had also described the *enteric nervous system*, which is intrinsic to the wall of the gastrointestinal tract and is distinct from the sympathetic and parasympathetic nervous systems (see Chapter 5).

The transmission of signals from preganglionic neurons to postganglionic neurons and from post-ganglionic neurons to the effector cells is chemical. All preganglionic neurons are cholinergic and use *acetylcholine (ACh)* as transmitter. All postganglionic parasympathetic neurons are potentially cholinergic in that they contain the enzyme choline acetyltrans-ferase (ChAT), the enzyme used at the final step in the synthesis of ACh (Note 2). However, not all postgan-glionic parasympathetic neurons seem to use acetyl-choline as a transmitter. The major effects of some postganglionic parasympathetic pathways appear to be mediated by cotransmitters such as nitric oxide (NO) and vasoactive intestinal polypeptide (VIP), which are synthesized in the same neurons. Whether acetylcholine present in the same neurons has another effect as yet unidentified remains to be clarified (see Subchapters 1.4, 4.8 and 7.1 and Table 1.2). Most postganglionic sympathetic neurons are adrenergic and use *noradrenaline* (*NAd*) as a transmitter in mammals; some sympathetic postganglionic neurons, most prominently sudomotor neurons, are cholinergic. Synaptic transmission in the peripheral sympathetic and parasympathetic systems will be described in Chapters 6 and 7.

1.2.1 Sympathetic Nervous System

Sympathetic Postganglionic Neurons

Most sympathetic postganglionic neurons are aggregated in the paravertebral ganglia or in the prevertebral ganglia. The sympathetic ganglia are usually discrete in laboratory and smaller domestic animals but some may become more like plexuses in larger species like humans (particularly the prevertebral ganglia and the lumbosacral sympathetic chains). This plexus-like organization probably contributed to the erroneous belief that the sympathetic nervous system is diffusely organized (Note 3).

The *paravertebral ganglia* are interconnected by nerve trunks to form a chain on either side of the vertebral column, extending from the base of the skull to the sacrum. These chains are called *sympathetic trunks* (or *sympathetic chains*). The *prevertebral ganglia* (celiac, aorticorenal, superior mesenteric and inferior mesenteric) (Note 4) lie in front of the vertebral column. They consist of right and left lobes that are often fused to a variable extent and are mostly arranged around the origin of the major branches of the abdominal aorta.

All sympathetic ganglia lie remotely from the organs they supply, so that their postganglionic axons are long. The *axons of postganglionic neurons* are unmyelinated and conduct action potentials at less than 1 m/s. Sympathetic postganglionic axons do not branch in the projection course to their target tissue. They exhibit multiple branches close to their target cells. These terminal branches have up to thousands of varicosities (small swellings), which contain the biochemical machineries for synthesis, inactivation, storage, release and reuptake of the transmitter(s).

- Overall, there is generally one pair of paravertebral ganglia per thoracic, lumbar and sacral segment. Macroscopically sympathetic chains are sometimes fused at the lumbar level in rodents but rarely in humans.

- The paravertebral ganglia are connected to the spinal nerves by white and gray rami (Note 5). Preganglionic neurons project exclusively through the white rami, which connect the spinal nerves with the sympathetic trunk. Most postganglionic neurons in the paravertebral ganglia project through the gray rami to the spinal nerves, some project through the white rami to the spinal nerves and some through splanchnic nerves to viscera.

- The paravertebral ganglia are named according to the spinal nerve from which the white ramus comes. For the thoracic chain ganglia T1 to T10, the gray rami project to the same spinal nerve (e.g., gray ramus T5 to spinal nerve T5). Due to some rearrangement of white and gray rami in the thoracic segments T10 to T12, the gray rami of the lumbar and sacral chain ganglia project to the spinal nerve one segment further caudally (e.g., gray ramus from paravertebral ganglion L3 projects to spinal nerve L4). Very often there are two or more white and/or gray rami per segment. Other variations in the arrangement also exist (Pick 1970; Baron et al. 1985a, 1988, 1995).

- At the rostral end of the cervical sympathetic trunk (CST) lies the *superior cervical ganglion* (*SCG*), which contains the postganglionic neurons projecting to the head and to the upper half of the neck. This ganglion results from the fusion of several cervical ganglia. A small middle or intermediate cervical ganglion may exist between the SCG and the stellate ganglion, but this is inconsistent across species. In large animals, including human beings, a middle cervical ganglion is present along the CST.

- At the rostral end of the thoracic sympathetic trunk lies the *stellate ganglion* (*SG*), which is a combination of the lower cervical and the two or three most rostral thoracic paravertebral ganglia. This ganglion contains the postganglionic neurons projecting to the upper extremity in the brachial plexus and to the thoracic organs. These postganglionic neurons project through cardiac branches to the heart, through other branches to the lung, and through gray rami or the vertebral nerve to the cervical spinal nerves C4 to C8 (Note 6). There is no evidence that postganglionic neurons in the stellate ganglion project to intra- and extracranial target tissues (Pick 1970).

- At the caudal end, both sympathetic trunks join and sometimes form the ganglion "impar." In animals with tails, cells in the ganglion impar supply the vasculature of the distal tail.
- Most postganglionic neurons in the paravertebral ganglia project through the gray rami, the respective spinal nerves and the peripheral nerves to the effector cells in the somatic tissues. They may ascend or descend one or two segments in the chain before they leave. There is no experimental or clinical evidence that postganglionic sympathetic neurons in paravertebral ganglia project to the extremities along the major blood vessels, such as the subclavian and iliac arteries, as is erroneously shown in some anatomy texts (Brodal 1998). The projection of postganglionic neurons in paravertebral ganglia is shown for the innervation of the head, upper extremity and lower extremity in Figure 1.2. However, the postganglionic axons may project for a few centimeters (depending on the size of the animal species) along a blood vessel before branching into terminals on that vessel.

Some postganglionic neurons in the paravertebral ganglia project through the splanchnic nerves to the viscera (Baron et al. 1985c).
- Postganglionic neurons in the SCG that project to the target organs in the head travel in perivascular bundles (with the internal and external carotid and pharyngeal arteries and their branches) and join the cranial nerves that project to the target organs in the head. Some postganglionic neurons in the SCG project through special gray rami to the upper three or four cervical spinal nerves (Lichtman et al. 1979) or through several small branches to some other structures in the neck.
- Postganglionic neurons in the prevertebral ganglia project in nerve bundles that accompany the relevant blood vessels (e.g., the branches of the celiac, superior and inferior mesenteric arteries) or sometimes in special nerves (e.g., the hypogastric nerves) to the organs in the abdominal and pelvic cavity.
- Some aggregations of sympathetic postganglionic cell bodies are found more peripherally in ganglia in the vicinity of the pelvic organs (e.g., urinary

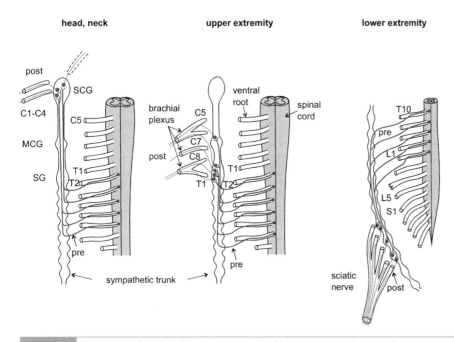

head, neck   **upper extremity**   **lower extremity**

Figure 1.2 Innervation of head, neck, upper extremity and lower extremity by sympathetic postganglionic neurons and preganglionic neurons in humans. Preganglionic neurons in the thoracolumbar spinal cord project through the ventral roots and white rami (see Figure 1.3) to postganglionic neurons in the sympathetic trunk. Postganglionic neurons project through the corresponding gray rami (see Figure 1.3) to the spinal nerves or along the internal carotid artery to the head, C1, C5, T1, etc., segmental ventral root or spinal nerve. For the lower extremity only the projections in the sciatic nerve are shown. MCG, middle cervical ganglion; pre, preganglionic; post, postganglionic; SCG, superior cervical ganglion; SG, stellate ganglion. Highly schematized. Modified from Brodal (1998) who took the figure from Haymaker and Woodhall (1945). With permission.

bladder, rectum, vas deferens, seminal vesicle, prostate). These ganglia belong to the pelvic plexus, which includes neurons that are innervated by *either* sympathetic *or* parasympathetic preganglionic axons or probably rarely by both (i.e., these latter neurons are simply autonomic since they receive convergent synaptic input from preganglionic sympathetic and parasympathetic neurons) (Keast 1995). The preganglionic sympathetic axons to these postganglionic neurons project through the hypogastric nerves (or plexuses).

The *effector cells and organs* of the sympathetic nervous system are the smooth musculature of all organs (blood vessels, erector pili muscles, iris, lung, evacuative organs, sphincters of the gastrointestinal tract), the heart and some glands (sweat, salivary and digestive glands). In addition, sympathetic postganglionic fibers innervate adipose tissue (white and brown), liver cells, the pineal gland and lymphatic tissues (e.g., thymus, spleen, lymph nodes and Peyer's patches in the gastrointestinal tract). Finally, activity of the enteric nervous system is modulated by postganglionic sympathetic neurons. Thus, the effects of sympathetic postganglionic neurons on gastrointestinal motility and secretion are usually mediated by at least three neurons in series (Figure 5.16).

Cells in the *adrenal medulla* are ontogenetically homologous to sympathetic postganglionic neurons. These cells are synaptically innervated by thoracic preganglionic neurons that project through the splanchnic nerves, bypassing the celiac ganglion. The adrenal medulla is an endocrine gland made up of cells that release either adrenaline or noradrenaline directly into the blood, which circulates to reach tissues throughout the body. The responses of these tissues depend on the characteristic adrenoceptors and postreceptor events that are present in each, and their interaction with the innervation. However, whether this is important under physiological conditions for tissues innervated by sympathetic postganglionic fibers is questionable (see Subchapter 4.5).

Sympathetic Preganglionic Neurons

The cell bodies of the preganglionic sympathetic neurons lie in the *intermediate zone* of the *thoracic* and *upper lumbar spinal cord* (the upper two to five lumbar segments, depending on the species). The axons of

these neurons are either myelinated or unmyelinated and conduct action potentials at 0.5 to 15 m/s. They leave the spinal cord in the ventral roots and white rami communicantes, and project (Figure 1.3):

1. either through the sympathetic chains, terminating in the bilateral *paravertebral ganglia*;
2. through the sympathetic chains and various splanchnic nerves (major, lesser, minor, lumbar) and terminate in the (largely unpaired) *prevertebral ganglia* in the abdomen (celiac, aorticorenal, superior mesenteric and inferior mesenteric ganglion or plexus); or

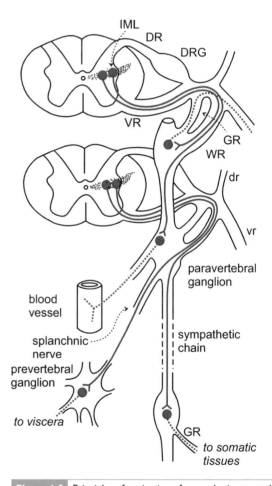

Figure 1.3 Principles of projection of sympathetic preganglionic neurons to postganglionic neurons in para- and prevertebral ganglia. Dotted area in spinal cord, intermediate zone; IML, intermediolateral nucleus; DR, dorsal root; DRG, dorsal root ganglion; VR, ventral root; GR, gray ramus; WR, white ramus; dr, dorsal ramus of spinal nerve; vr, ventral ramus of spinal nerve.

3. further through the hypogastric nerves, terminating in the *pelvic ganglia* (plexus hypogastricus inferior).

A sympathetic preganglionic axon may travel through several paravertebral ganglia before making its main synaptic contacts (e.g., with postganglionic neurons in the SCG to the head or in lumbar paravertebral ganglia to the hindlimb). However, each preganglionic axon usually forms synapses with postganglionic neurons in several paravertebral ganglia. There is no indication that individual preganglionic axons that innervate postganglionic neurons to the head or extremities project both up and down in the sympathetic chain, although they may do so in the midthoracic region. Furthermore, there is no evidence that individual preganglionic axons branch to form synapses on postganglionic neurons in paravertebral as well as prevertebral ganglia. Finally, almost all preganglionic neurons projecting to paravertebral ganglia terminate only in ipsilateral ganglia. About 80% of the preganglionic neurons projecting to prevertebral ganglia terminate on the ipsilateral side and about 20% on the contralateral side (Baron et al. 1985b, c; Jänig and McLachlan 1986a, b).

Location of Sympathetic Pre- and Postganglionic Neurons With Respect to Organs

Pre- and postganglionic neurons exhibit distinct topographical locations with respect to different organs. This has been detailed for various organs, skin and skeletal muscle of the head and neck, the upper extremity and the lower extremity in humans in Table 1.1. The locations of these neurons in humans have been worked out with classical anatomical techniques. These locations have been fully confirmed in anatomical studies on animals (mostly cat and rat) using modern tracer techniques (see Chapter 8 and Tables 8.1, 8.2 and 8.3).

Approximately 90% of the cell bodies of sympathetic postganglionic neurons projecting through the dorsal cutaneous nerves to the dorsal skin of the trunk or through the intercostal nerves are located in the paravertebral ganglion corresponding to the dorsal root ganglion and in the next caudal paravertebral ganglion (Baron et al. 1995).

1.2.2 Parasympathetic Nervous System

The cell bodies of preganglionic parasympathetic neurons are situated in the *brain stem* (dorsal motor nucleus of the vagus, nucleus ambiguus, superior and inferior salivary nuclei, visceral efferent oculomotor [Edinger–Westphal] nucleus [Note 7]) and in the *intermediate zone* of the *sacral spinal cord* (Table 1.1). They project through the third (oculomotor), seventh (facial and intermediate) or ninth (glossopharyngeal) cranial nerves to the parasympathetic ganglia associated with the intraocular smooth muscles and glands of the head, through the tenth cranial (vagal) nerve to the ganglia associated with the target organs in the thoracic and abdominal cavity and through the pelvic splanchnic nerves to the ganglia associated with the pelvic organs. The preganglionic axons can be very long and are either myelinated or unmyelinated.

Discrete *parasympathetic ganglia* containing the postganglionic parasympathetic neurons are found in the head region. Figure 1.4 schematically shows these ganglia, the location of the preganglionic neurons in the brain stem, the nerves through which these preganglionic neurons project and the target organs of the postganglionic neurons (ciliary ganglion: eye; pterygopalatine ganglion: lacrimal, nasal and palatal glands; otic and submandibular ganglion: salivary glands). Discrete ganglia are also found near or in the wall of the effector organs (heart: cardiac plexus [discrete small ganglia innervating different groups of effector cells, e.g., pacemaker cells in the sinus venosus, atrial muscle cells, atrioventricular pacemaker cells]; airways: ganglia on the membranous part; pancreas [exocrine, endocrine]; gallbladder; organs in the pelvic cavity: ganglia in the pelvic plexus, see McLachlan [1995]). Preganglionic neurons that project to the gastrointestinal tract synapse with neurons that are part of the enteric nervous system (Figure 1.4; see Chapter 5). The sacral parasympathetic outflow to the hindgut (in particular the rectum) largely consists of three populations of neurons connected synaptically in series (Fukai and Fukuda 1985; Olsson et al. 2006): preganglionic neurons in the sacral spinal cord, postganglionic neurons in the pelvic ganglia and neurons of the enteric nervous system (neurons in the myenteric plexus or serosal neurons) (Table 1.1). However, some neurons in the pelvic ganglion appear to innervate smooth muscles in the rectum directly (Luckensmeyer and Keast 1998).

The parasympathetic system innervates the exocrine glands of the head, the intraocular smooth muscles, the smooth muscles and glands of the airways, the smooth musculature, exocrine glands and

Table 1.1 | Location of sympathetic and parasympathetic preganglionic and postganglionic neurons in humans

Organ	The sympathetic system		The parasympathetic system	
	Preganglionic neurons	Postganglionic neurons	Preganglionic neurons	Postganglionic neurons
Eye	T1–2	Superior cervical ganglion	Edinger–Westphal nucleus	Ciliary ganglion
Lacrimal gland	T1–2	Superior cervical ganglion	Superior salivary nucleus	Pterygopalatine ganglion
Nasal, small lingual, oromucosal glands	T1–2	Superior cervical ganglion	Superior salivary nucleus	Pterygopalatine ganglion
Submandibular and sublingual glands	T1–2	Superior cervical ganglion	Superior salivary nucleus	Submandibular ganglion
Parotid gland	T1–2	Superior cervical ganglion	Inferior salivary nucleus	Otic ganglion
Heart	T1–4 (T1–T5)	Stellate ganglion, upper thoracic ganglia (superior and middle cerv. ganglion)	Nucleus ambiguus; dorsal motor nucleus of the vagus nerve (lateral part)	Cardiac plexus
Bronchi, lungs	T2–7 (T2–T4)	Stellate ganglion and upper thoracic ganglia	Nucleus ambiguus	Pulmonary plexus
Esophagus (smooth muscle portion)	(T5–T6)	Stellate ganglion and upper thoracic ganglia	Dorsal motor nucleus of the vagus nerve	Myenteric plexus
Stomach	T6–10	Celiac ganglion	Dorsal motor nucleus of the vagus nerve	Myenteric and submucosal plexus
Liver, gallbladder	(T7–T9)	Celiac ganglion	Dorsal motor nucleus of the vagus nerve (?)	Myenteric and submucosal plexus
Pancreas	T6–10	Celiac ganglion	Dorsal motor nucleus of the vagus nerve	Intrapancreatic ganglia[a]
Small intestine, ascending large intestine	T6–10 (T9–T10)	Celiac, superior and inferior mesenteric ganglia	Dorsal motor nucleus of the vagus nerve	Myenteric and submucosal plexus
Transverse large intestine	(T11–L1)	Celiac, superior and inferior mesenteric ganglia	Dorsal motor nucleus of the vagus nerve	Myenteric and submucosal plexus
Descending large intestine, sigmoid and rectum	T11–L2 (L1–L2)	Inferior mesenteric, hypogastric and pelvic ganglia	S2–S4	Pelvic ganglia, myenteric and submucosal plexus[b]

Ureter, urinary bladder	T11–L2	Hypogastric and pelvic ganglia	S2–S4	Pelvic ganglia
Internal sexual organs, male	T11–L2	Hypogastric and pelvic ganglia	S2–S4	Pelvic ganglia
Internal sexual organs, female	(T10–L1)	Hypogastric and pelvic ganglia	S2–S4	Pelvic ganglia
Head, neck (skin and skeletal muscle)	T1–4 (T1–T5)	Superior and middle cervical ganglia[c]	No parasympathetic innervation[d]	
Upper extremity	T3–6 (T2–T5)	Stellate and upper thoracic ganglia (projection to spinal nerves C5–C8)[e]	No parasympathetic innervation	
Lower extremity	T10–L2	Lumbar and upper sacral ganglia (ganglia L1–S1)[f]	No parasympathetic innervation	
Trunk (innervated by dorsal rami and intercostal nerves)	Most neurons in two segments corresp. to paravertebral ganglia	90% neurons in two paravertebral ganglia (corresp. to dorsal root ganglion and next caudal paravertebral ganglion)[g]	No parasympathetic innervation	

Modified from Brodal (1998) and from Gray's Anatomy (2016). Segmental locations in brackets from Gray's Anatomy (2016).

[a] Berthoud and Neuhuber (2019).

[b] Fukai and Fukuda (1985); Luckensmeyer and Keast (1998).

[c] The superior cervical ganglion projects to the spinal nerves C1 and C2 (possibly C3). The middle cervical ganglion projects inconstantly to the spinal nerves C3 to C6.

[d] Parasympathetic innervation of cerebral arteries, arteries of lower lip and other cutaneous and mucosal vessels.

[e] The stellate ganglion projects through the vertebral nerve to the spinal nerves C7 and C8 and frequently also to the spinal nerves (C4) C5 to C6.

[f] In the lumbar sympathetic chain the ganglia that are named by their white ramus (rami) project with their gray ramus (rami) to the next spinal nerve further caudal, i.e., the lumbar ganglion L1 to the spinal nerve L2, the lumbar ganglion L2 to the spinal nerve L3, etc. (see Pick 1970; Baron et al. 1985a).

[g] See Baron et al. (1995).

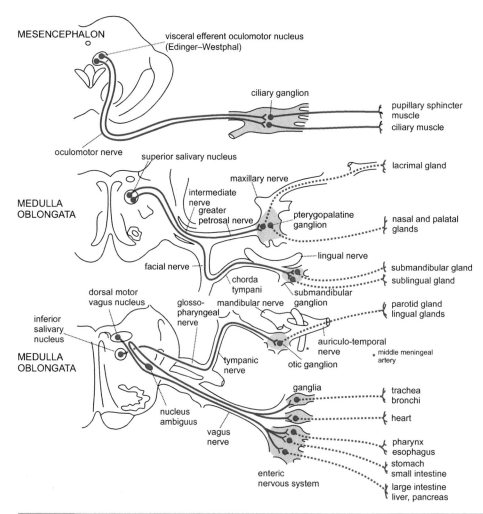

Figure 1.4 Location of cranial parasympathetic preganglionic neurons, the nerves through which the preganglionic axons project, the parasympathetic ganglia and the target organs. See also Table 9.1. Modified from Brodal (1998) with permission.

endocrine glands of the gastrointestinal tract (via the enteric nervous system), the heart (pacemaker cells and atria), the pelvic organs (lower urinary tract, hindgut, reproductive organs) and epithelia and mucosa throughout the body. Except for the helical arteries and sinusoids of the erectile tissues of the reproductive organs and some intracranial, uterine and facial blood vessels and blood vessels in the salivary glands, the parasympathetic system does not innervate blood vessels in somatic tissues and viscera. The parasympathetic supply to these vascular tissues is not involved in blood pressure regulation but is related to specific functions of each effector vessel.

1.3 Reactions of Autonomic Target Organs to Activation of Sympathetic and Parasympathetic Axons

Table 1.2 describes the overall reactions of the peripheral target organs and individual target tissues to activity in the sympathetic and parasympathetic neurons that innervate them. The responses have been defined by the reaction of the tissues to reflex activation or to electrical stimulation of the respective nerves, but not pharmacologically by their

Table 1.2 Effects of activation of sympathetic and parasympathetic neurons on autonomic target organs

Organ and organ system	Activation of parasympathetic nerves	Activation of sympathetic nerves	Adrenoceptor
Heart muscle	Decrease of heart rate	Increase of heart rate	β_1
	Decrease of contractility (only atria)	Increase of contractility (atria, ventricles)	β_1
Arteries[a]			
skin of trunk and limbs	0	Vasoconstriction	α_1
… skin and mucosa of face	Vasodilation	Vasoconstriction	α_1
… visceral domain (incl. kidney)	0	Vasoconstriction	α_1
… skeletal muscle	0	Vasodilation (cholinergic)[b]	α_1
… heart (coronary arteries)	?	Vasoconstriction	α_1
… intracranial tissues	Vasodilation	Vasoconstriction	α_1
… salivary glands	Vasodilation	Vasoconstriction	α_1
Veins	0	Vasoconstriction	α_1
Gastrointestinal tract			
longitudinal and circular muscle	Increase of motility	Decrease of motility (mostly indirect)	α_2, β_1
sphincters	Relaxation	Contraction	α_1
digestive glands	Secretion	Decrease of secretion or 0 (stomach, pancreas)	
… mucosa	Secretion	Decrease of secretion or 0 (small, large intestine) reabsorption[c]	
… endocrine cells (e.g., gastrin by G-cells)	Secretion	0	
Capsule of spleen	0	Contraction	
Kidney			
… juxtaglomerular cells	0	Renin release	β_1
… tubuli	0	Sodium reabsorption	α_1
Urinary bladder			
… detrusor vesicae	Contraction (micturition)	Relaxation (small)[d]	β_2
… trigone (internal sphincter)	0	Contraction (continence)	α_1
… urethra	Relaxation	Contraction (continence)	α_1

Table 1.2 (cont.)

Organ and organ system	Activation of parasympathetic nerves	Activation of sympathetic nerves	Adrenoceptor
Reproductive organs			
... seminal vesicle, prostate	0	Contraction	α_1
deferens.	0	Contraction	α_1
... uterus	Vasodilation	Contraction; relaxation[e]	α_1
... glands	Secretion	0	
... erectile tissue	Vasodilation (helical arteries and sinusoids in penis and clitoris)	Vasoconstriction; vasodilation	α_1
... vagina	Engorgement (vasodilation), transepithelial transudation of mucoid fluid	Vasoconstriction	
Eye			
dilator muscle of pupil	0 or inhibition of noradrenaline release[f]	Contraction (mydriasis)	α_1
... sphincter muscle of pupil	Contraction (miosis)	0 or inhibition[f]	
... ciliary muscle	Contraction (accommodation)	0 or inhibition[f]	
... blood vessels (chorioid)	Vasodilation	(Vasoconstriction?)	
... tarsal muscle	0	Contraction (lifting of lid)	
... orbital muscle	0	Contraction (protrusion of eye)	
Tracheobronchial muscles	Contraction	Relaxation (probably mainly by circulating catecholamines)	β_2
Piloerector muscles	0	Contraction	α_1
Exocrine glands[g,h]			
... salivary glands	Copious serous secretion	Weak mucous secretion (submandibular gland)	α_1
... lacrimal glands	Secretion	0	
... nasopharyngeal glands	Secretion	0	
... bronchial glands	Secretion	?	
... sweat glands	0	Secretion (cholinergic)	α_1

Pineal gland	Increase in synthesis of melatonin	β_2
Brown adipose tissue	Heat production	β_3
Metabolism		
... liver	Glycogenolysis, gluconeogenesis	β_2
	Inhibition of release of glucose and triglycerides	$?^j$
... white fat cells	Lipolysis (free fatty acids in blood increased)	β_2
... β-cells in islets of pancreas	Decrease of secretion of insulin	α_2
	Secretion of insulin	0
... α-cells in islets of pancreas	Secretion of glucagon	β
Adrenal medulla	Secretion of adrenaline and noradrenaline	0
Lymphoid tissue	Depression of activity (e.g., of natural killer cells)	β_2 ^{k}
		β_2, α_1 ^{i}

The right column shows the type of adrenoceptor in the membranes of the target cells mediating the effect of activation of sympathetic neurons (see Chapter 8).

0 indicates no effect.

a Other blood vessels see Eye and Reproductive organs.

b Only in some species (e.g., cat, see Bolme et al. [1970]). Circulating adrenaline may produce vasodilation via β_2-adrenoceptors.

c Mostly indirect by inhibiting secretomotor neurons; also indirectly following vasoconstriction?

d Very sparse innervation by noradrenergic fibers (Watanabe and Yamamoto 1979; Gosling et al. 1999).

e Relaxation (β_2) depends on species and hormonal state; only exogenously by noradrenaline?

f McDougal and Gamline (2015).

g Other glands see gastrointestinal tract and reproductive organs.

h Secretion of all exocrine glands generated by activation of secretomotor neurons is accompanied by vasodilation of the associated vasculature.

i Pineal gland innervated by parasympathetic neurons in sphenopalatine and otic ganglia (Moller and Baeres 2002).

k Adrenaline is a metabolic hormone and acts via β_2-adrenoceptors (see Subchapter 4.5).

reactions to adrenoceptor or cholinoceptor agonists. In some cases, the apparent effects of these nerves have been identified by changes in function after removing or blocking the nerve supply. The table shows that:

- Most target tissues are innervated by only one of the autonomic systems.
- A few target tissues are innervated by both autonomic systems (e.g., pacemaker cells and atria of the heart, detrusor vesicae and urethra, some blood vessels [erectile tissue, in salivary glands and oral mucosa, intracranial blood vessels]).
- Opposite reactions to the activation of sympathetic and parasympathetic neurons are more the exception than the rule (e.g., pacemaker and atria of the heart, erectile tissue of the reproductive organs, some exocrine digestive glands, insulin-producing islet cells of the pancreas).
- Most responses are excitatory, even when opposing actions of the organ result; inhibition (e.g., relaxation of muscle, decreased secretion) is rare.
- Adrenaline is a metabolic hormone. It is released by cells of the adrenal medulla in the blood during splanchnic nerve stimulation.

Table 1.2 clearly shows that the widely propagated idea of a universal antagonism between the parasympathetic and sympathetic nervous systems is a misconception. Where there is a reciprocal effect of the two autonomic systems on some target tissues, it can usually be shown either that the systems work synergistically or that they exert their influence under different functional conditions. For example, the opposite actions of sympathetic and parasympathetic systems on the size of the pupil are a consequence of the distinct target muscles (dilator pupillae for sympathetic, sphincter pupillae for parasympathetic) supplied by each system. Moreover, in larger mammals, fast changes in heart rate, e.g., during changes of body position or emotional stress, are generated via changes in activity in the parasympathetic cardiomotor neurons to the pacemaker cells; the sustained increase of heart rate during exercise is mainly generated by activation of sympathetic cardiomotor neurons supplying the heart. In addition, it is likely that some organs which can be affected by both systems under experimental conditions are primarily under the control of only one system in vivo (i.e., under physiological conditions).

It is evident from Table 1.2 that the two systems have some very specialized effects on particular organs but also generate functional effects that are similar in many tissues. For example, the parasympathetic innervation of mucosae and glands is almost always responsible for the generation of watery secretions, whereas at least part of the sympathetic innervation of most organs is associated with vasoconstriction.

In essence, Table 1.2 shows the macroscopic effects of activation of sympathetic and parasympathetic neurons on target organs; it does not show whether these responses have functional meaning nor how the autonomic systems work to regulate the behavior of these target organs. Finally, it is important to recognize that the effects of nerve activity on the autonomic target organs are not necessarily the same as the reactions of the effector organs to application of exogenous transmitter substances (see Subchapter 7.3) or to circulating adrenaline from the adrenal medulla (see Subchapter 4.5).

As already mentioned and as will be treated more extensively in Chapter 7, most sympathetic postganglionic neurons are noradrenergic (in mammals; and adrenergic in reptiles and amphibians) and all parasympathetic postganglionic neurons are cholinergic. Noradrenaline released by the postganglionic fibers reacts with adrenoceptors in the membranes of the effector cells. These adrenoceptors consist of two families, each being divided into several types (Alexander et al. 2011). Some of these types of adrenoceptors mediate the nerve-induced effector responses. The type of adrenoceptor responsible for responses elicited by nerve-released noradrenaline is listed in Table 1.2. Acetylcholine released by postganglionic neurons reacts in all effector cells with cholinergic muscarinic receptors. It is important to emphasize that it is a misconception to consider the sympathetic nervous system as a noradrenergic (autonomic) nervous system and the parasympathetic nervous system as a cholinergic (autonomic) nervous system, as is sometimes done.

1.4 Neuropeptides in Autonomic Neurons and the Idea of "Neurochemical Coding"

The presence of distinct functional subunits of the autonomic nervous system, in the sense of Langley and as outlined in this chapter, is supported by a substantial amount of histochemical evidence demonstrating that autonomic neurons may contain particular combinations of neuropeptides along with (and a few without) one of the classical transmitters, noradrenaline (NAd) or acetylcholine (ACh). The patterns of coexistence of one or more neuropeptides and a non-peptide transmitter within the same cell body in peripheral ganglia are correlated with combinations of the two coexisting substances in the nerve terminals associated with target tissues (see Furness et al. [1989]; Gibbins [1990, 1995, 2004]; Morris and Gibbins [1992]). Various combinations of substances are present in the innervation of various target organs. Furthermore, there are many examples of species-specific neuropeptide expression (see Nilsson and Holmgren [1994]).

Neuropeptides in Sympathetic Neurons

Examples of neuropeptide/neurotransmitter combinations in sympathetic postganglionic neurons in the cat are (Table 1.3):

Table 1.3 Neurochemical coding of different functional populations of postganglionic sympathetic neurons in the cat and guinea pig

Sympathetic system	Primary transmitter	Neuropeptide(s)
Cat		
Muscle vasoconstrictor	Noradrenaline	GAL/NPY
Muscle vasodilator	Acetylcholine	VIP
Visceral vasoconstrictor	Noradrenaline	GAL/NPY
Cutaneous vasoconstrictor	Noradrenaline	GAL/NPY
Pilomotor	Noradrenaline	GAL
Sudomotor	Acetylcholine	VIP/CGRP/SP
Salivary secretomotor	Noradrenaline	Ø
Motility-regulating (to ENS)[a]	Noradrenaline	SOM/?
Guinea pig		
Muscle vasoconstrictor	Noradrenaline	NPY
Muscle vasodilator	Acetylcholine	VIP/NPY/DYN
Visceral vasoconstrictor	Noradrenaline	NPY
Cutaneous vasoconstrictor	Noradrenaline	NPY, NPY/DYN, DYN
Pilomotor	Noradrenaline	DYN
Sudomotor	Acetylcholine	VIP/CGRP
Pupillodilator	Noradrenaline	NPY/DYN
Salivary secretomotor	Noradrenaline	Ø
Motility-regulating (to ENS)[a]	Noradrenaline	Ø
Secretomotor (to ENS)[b]	Noradrenaline	SOM
Visceromotor[c]	Noradrenaline	NPY, NPY/DYN

Ø, no colocalized neuropeptide; CGRP, calcitonin gene-related peptide; DYN, dynorphin; ENS, enteric nervous system; GAL, galanin; NPY, neuropeptide Y; SOM, somatostatin; SP, substance P; VIP, vasoactive intestinal peptide. From Gibbins (1995).
[a] Postganglionic neurons in the celiac ganglion innervating the myenteric plexus.
[b] Postganglionic neurons in the celiac ganglion innervating the submucous plexus.
[c] Sympathetic non-vasoconstrictor system which directly innervates visceral organs; this group does not include sympathetic postganglionic NAd/SOM and NAd/Ø neurons (see notes a and b).

- Many vasoconstrictor neurons to viscera, skin and skeletal muscle contain, in addition to NAd, neuropeptide Y (NPY) and galanin (GAL).
- Muscle vasodilator neurons have, in addition to ACh, vasoactive intestinal peptide (VIP) and many also have NPY (e.g., the uterine artery, which is a vasodilator).
- In addition to ACh, sudomotor neurons contain VIP, calcitonin gene-related peptide (CGRP) and substance P (SP).
- In addition to NAd, pilomotor neurons contain GAL.
- In addition to NAd, motility-regulating neurons contain somatostatin (SOM).
- In secretomotor neurons to the gastrointestinal tract or to the salivary glands no peptide has been detected so far.

Detailed investigation of the cutaneous vasoconstrictor neurons innervating the ear of the guinea pig has shown that different sections of the cutaneous vascular bed are innervated by neurochemically different groups of noradrenergic (NAd) neurons: (1) large distributing arteries are innervated by neurons containing NAd and NPY; (2) small arteries are innervated by neurons containing NAd, NPY and a prodynorphin-derived peptide; (3) arteriovenous anastomoses and precapillary resistance vessels are innervated by neurons containing NAd and a prodynorphin-derived peptide (but no NPY); (4) large veins are innervated by neurons containing NAd, NPY and a prodynorphin-derived peptide; (5) small veins are innervated by neurons containing NAd and a prodynorphin-derived peptide, but lack mostly NPY (Gibbins and Morris 1990; Morris 1995, 1999; Gibbins et al. 2003). These findings support (but do not prove!) the hypothesis that different sections of the cutaneous vascular bed are also innervated by functionally distinct cutaneous vasoconstrictor neurons and are consistent with the neurophysiological studies of cutaneous vasoconstrictor neurons in the cat (see Subchapter 4.1). Table 1.3 also demonstrates the difference, in neuropeptide content of functionally different types of postganglionic neurons, between cat and guinea pig to emphasize species differences.

For the guinea pig and the rat, more complete sets of data on the presence and absence of peptides in pre- and postganglionic neurons of some sympathetic pathways are available (e.g., Table 1.4). These

Table 1.4 Neurochemically identified preganglionic and postganglionic pathways in lumbar sympathetic ganglia of female guinea pig

Sympathetic system	Preganglionic neuron	Postganglionic neuron
Vasoconstrictor	ACh; Ø (most), CGRP, ENK, CGRP/ENK	NAd; NPY (most), NPY/DYN, Ø/DYN
Vasodilator	ACh; Ø, SP, ENK, SP/ENK	ACh; VIP/NPY/DYN
Pilomotor	ACh; Ø, ENK	NAd; DYN
Visceromotor[a]	ACh; ENK	NAd; NPY

Primary transmitters acetylcholine (*ACh*) or noradrenaline (*NAd*). The table shows with which neuropeptide or combinations of neuropeptides the primary transmitter may be colocalized. ENK, enkephalin; for further abbreviations see Table 1.3.

[a] Sympathetic non-vasoconstrictor system that directly innervates visceral organs; this group does not include sympathetic postganglionic NAd/SOM and NAd/Ø neurons that innervate the submucous plexus or the myenteric plexus of the enteric nervous system, and are involved in regulation of secretion and motility, respectively. From Gibbins (1995).

neurochemical codes are correlated with morphological data (geometry and size of soma and dendrites), electrophysiological data and anatomical data defining the projections of the sympathetic neurons. Unfortunately we do not have data about the discharge pattern of these neurons in vivo for the guinea pig and we have only limited data on the sympathetic innervation for the rat (see Chapter 4 for details).

Although only a few types of preganglionic neurons have been found to contain identified neuropeptides in the cat, neurochemical coding is also present to a certain extent in these pathways in this species (Lindh et al. 1989, 1993; Shafton et al. 1992; Anderson et al. 1995; Edwards et al. 1996; see Gibbins [1995, 1997]).

Neuropeptides in Parasympathetic Neurons
Data on neuropeptides in the parasympathetic neurons of humans and guinea pigs have been described in detail by Gibbins (2004). In the guinea

pig VIP is colocalized with acetylcholine in all types of postganglionic *parasympathetic neurons to cranial targets* except for those innervating the iris and ciliary muscle. Postganglionic neurons of the parasympathetic pathways to lacrimal, nasal, parotid, sublingual and submandibular glands and to the choroid, cerebral and facial blood vessels additionally contain nitric oxide (NO). The VIPergic parasympathetic postganglionic neurons to cranial targets are involved in secretion and vasodilation.

Postganglionic neurons of *vagal (parasympathetic) pathways* to airways (bronchomotor neurons), esophagus or gallbladder generating contraction have no known neuropeptide colocalized with acetylcholine. Postganglionic parasympathetic cardiomotor neurons (innervating the sinoatrial node, the atrioventricular node and the atrial musculature, and generating bradycardia and decrease of contractility) contain SOM (in addition to acetylcholine). All other types of postganglionic neurons that elicit relaxation of gastrointestinal muscles, vasodilation or secretion contain VIP and NO. These neurons are either cholinergic or non-cholinergic, some of the latter (to the esophagus) containing NPY.

Postganglionic neurons of *sacral parasympathetic pathways* to the distal colon and bladder body are cholinergic and do not contain a known neuropeptide. Other sacral postganglionic neurons contain VIP and NO (and some additionally NPY). These neurons are either cholinergic (urethra, male internal reproductive organs, erectile tissue) or non-cholinergic (ureter, detrusor vesicae, uterus, vagina, internal anal sphincter). They generate either vasodilation, relaxation of visceral smooth muscle or secretion.

The Concept of Neurochemical Coding

The term neurochemical coding has been coined for the coexistence of a classical transmitter and one or a set of neuropeptides in the autonomic neurons associated with a particular target tissue. The patterns of coding can often be used to identify different functional populations of autonomic neurons.

This concept is a powerful neuroanatomical and experimental tool in the analysis of the peripheral pathways of the autonomic nervous system, in particular the sympathetic one (Gibbins 1995, 1997). The functions of most neuropeptides are unknown, although they are beginning to be revealed for a few (Lundberg 1981; Furness et al. 1992; Ulman et al. 1992). In much of the literature it is assumed that

these neuropeptides act as transmitters, as the terms transmitter, cotransmitter, neuromodulator, etc. are generally applied to them. However, this assumption lacks experimental evidence and it may finally turn out that most neuropeptides do not have any obvious function as neurotransmitters in the adult organism. The principle of neurochemical coding has also been worked out and exploited to unravel the connectivity and function of the enteric nervous system in the guinea pig (Furness et al. 1992; Costa et al. 1996; see Subchapter 5.1 and Figure 5.2).

In *conclusion*: (1) neurochemical coding of autonomic neurons can be used as a tool to unravel the organization of the autonomic pathways, (2) neurochemical coding of many functionally distinct autonomic pathways is not straightforward, (3) the correlation between target tissue and neurochemistry is by no means absolute, (4) the function of the neuropeptides is mostly unclear and (5) neuropeptides expressed in particular functional pathways can differ markedly between species, even where a function has been demonstrated (Gibbins and Morris 1987; Potter 1991; Romano et al. 1991; Gibbins 1992, 1995; Ulman et al. 1992; Wanigasekava et al. 2003).

1.5 The Peripheral Autonomic Nervous System in Submammalian Vertebrates: A Comparative View

Knowledge about the autonomic nervous system (ANS) in non-mammalian vertebrates is largely restricted to the peripheral ANS and in particular to the anatomy. Neurobiological studies of central circuits associated with the peripheral autonomic systems and functional (neurophysiological) studies of peripheral autonomic neurons in vivo (see Chapter 4) are almost absent in non-mammalian vertebrates. However, the comparison of the anatomy of the peripheral ANS of the major vertebrate groups indicates that the principal organization of this system appears to be highly conserved in evolution over a time period of up to about 500 million years. This is further supported by studies of the principal transmitters acetylcholine, adrenaline and noradrenaline and of the neuropeptides in the neurons of the peripheral ANS (Nilsson 1983; Nilsson and Holmgren 1994; Holmgren and Olson 2011). Table 1.5 shows the autonomic innervation of the main target tissues (cardiovascular system, gastrointestinal tract, lung, spleen, urogenital tract, eye, chromaffin tissue) for the major non-mammalian vertebrate groups of animals, their reactions to stimulation of the (cranial) parasympathetic or of the spinal autonomic innervation, and the cholinergic receptors (nicotinic, muscarinic) or adrenoceptors involved. Common ancestors of these vertebrates cover an evolutionary time of about 500 to 200 million years from cyclostomes to birds:

- The peripheral ANS consists of the *cranial parasympathetic system* and the *spinal autonomic systems*. Spinal sympathetic and spinal parasympathetic systems cannot be distinguished in non-mammalian vertebrates (Nilsson 1983).
- The peripheral ANS consists of populations of cholinergic preganglionic neurons and populations of adrenergic or cholinergic postganglionic neurons which are synaptically connected. Adrenaline is the primary transmitter in some adrenergic neurons of teleosts, amphibians and birds. The receptors of these transmitters are cholinergic nicotinic (in the postganglionic cell bodies), cholinergic muscarinic (in the target tissues) or adrenergic (α-, β-adrenoceptors in the target tissues).
- Preganglionic neurons of the cranial parasympathetic system project through cranial nerves III (oculomotor), VII (facial), IX (glossopharyngeal) or X (vagal) to the postganglionic neurons located close to the target tissues (e.g., for the eye in the ciliary ganglia, for the gastrointestinal tract, neurons of the enteric nervous system).
- Preganglionic neurons of the spinal autonomic systems project through the ventral roots to the peripheral ganglia. In cyclostomes, elasmobranchs and amphibians they may also project through the dorsal roots. However, this is very much debated for elasmobranchs and amphibians.
- Sympathetic chains are present in dipnoans, teleost fish, amphibians, reptiles and birds. In cyclostomes these chains do not exist or consist of scattered ganglia along the aorta. In elasmobranchs they are incomplete.

Figure 1.5 depicts the sympathetic paravertebral chain, the sympathetic prevertebral systems, and the peripheral cranial parasympathetic system in an elasmobranch fish, a teleost fish and a reptile. These groups of vertebrates are about 100 million to more than 200 million years apart in their evolutionary origin.

- The enteric nervous system of the gastrointestinal tract is present in all groups of non-mammalian vertebrates and under the control of the brain via the (cranial) parasympathetic system (stomach and proximal gut) and via the spinal autonomic systems (small intestine and hindgut).
- Chromaffin tissues consist of cells that synthesize and release adrenaline or noradrenaline. With the exception of the cyclostomes, these tissues are innervated by spinal preganglionic neurons. In fish, these tissues are located within the heart (in cyclostomes) and close to the atria, posterior cardinal vein, intercostal arteries and ganglia of the paravertebral chain (in elasmobranchs, blue in Figure 1.5a). In amphibians, reptiles and birds this tissue is organized in adrenal glands. Adrenaline or noradrenaline released by the chromaffin tissue is probably primarily involved in cardiovascular regulation in cyclostomes, elasmobranchs and dipnoans, but not in teleosts, amphibians, reptiles and birds.

Overall we can conclude and hypothesize:

1. The general anatomical plan of the peripheral ANS (including the enteric nervous system) is strikingly similar in all vertebrate groups (except in cyclostomes).
2. The dominance of the brain in autonomic regulation is already present in the early evolution of vertebrates and this dominance of neural control by the brain increases with evolution.
3. The dominance of the control of autonomic functions by the brain is probably paralleled by an increasing complexity and functional differentiation of the autonomic regulation of target organs and tissues, particularly related to the adaptation of the vertebrates to terrestrial life.
4. The increased complexity of regulation may be reflected, e.g., in cardiovascular regulation in the field of gravity, in the regulation of body core temperature, in the regulation of fluid homeostasis (volume- and osmoregulation), in the regulation of metabolism (in relation to the terrestrial changes of climate), and in the regulation of body defenses (see Table 11.2).
5. The assumption of increased complexity of autonomic regulation with evolution does not imply that complex autonomic regulation has not already been developed relatively early in evolution, e.g., for the swim bladder (Campbell and McLean 1994, Nilsson and Holmgren 1994; Campbell and

Table 1.5 Peripheral autonomic systems in non-mammalian vertebrates (anatomy, neurotransmitters, effects of cranial parasympathetic and spinal autonomic systems)

	Cyclostome	Elasmobranch	Dipnoan	Teleost	Amphibian	Reptile/Bird
Time in evolution	~ 560 million years	~ 530 million years	~ 400 million years	~ 450 million years	~ 360 million years	~ 310–220 million years
Cranial nerves[a]	X (VII,IX)	III,X,(VII,IX)	X (III)	III,X	III,IX (VII,IX)	III,VII,IX,X
Sympathetic chain	no, scattered ganglia along dorsal aorta	incomplete	poorly developed	yes (continues into the head)	yes	yes, like in mammals
CVS heart	**P, S** Ø; CTβ+	**P** m−	**P** m−	**P** m−	**P** m−, **S** β+ anurans, **S** urodeles?	**P** m−, **S**β+
artery[b]	**S** Ø (H), **S**?(L); CT α	**S**Ø; via CT β+; **S** α+, β−	**S** Ø; via CTβ+; **S** α+, β−	**S** β−; via CTβ+; **S** α−, β−	**S** α+, β−	**S** α+, β−
vein[b]	**S** Ø(H),**S**?(L); CT α	Ø;CTα+, β−	**S** via CT?	**S** α+	**S** α+	**S** α+
GIT[c]	**ENS**[d]**(P, S)**	**ENS, P, S**	**ENS, P?, S?**	**ENS, P, S**	**ENS, P, S**	**ENS, P, S**
Lung		**P** m+	**P** m+		**P** +/−; **S** +/− (anurans), **P** − (urodeles?)	**P** m+ (birds), **P** m+; − (reptiles)
Spleen	embedded in gut wall	**S** α+	embedded in gut wall	**S** α+, m+	**S** α+	**S** α+ (birds), **S**? (reptiles)
Kidney	Ø	?[e]	**S**?	**S** adrenergic	**S** anurans, urodeles?	? reptiles, **S** birds
Urinary bladder/ ureter	?	?	?[e]	**S** ACh, adrenergic (osmoregulation)	**S** adrenergic? ACh? (osmoregulation)[f]	**S** ACh, adrenergic[f]
Gonads	?	**S** ♂ ♀	?	**S** ♂ ACh, **S** ♀ ACh, adrenergic	**S** ♂ ♀ adrenergic	**S** ♂ ♀? reptiles, **S** ♂ ♀ adrenergic, birds
Eye sphincter	Ø	Ø	not studied	**P** Ø, **S** α+[g]	**S** −β	**P** m+; also nicotinic+
dilator	**P** m+?	**P** m+	not studied	**P** m+[g]	Ø	**S** α+

Table 1.5 (cont.)

	Cyclostome	Elasmobranch	Dipnoan	Teleost	Amphibian	Reptile/Bird
Chromaffin tissue (CT)[h]	within heart, great veins; not innervated	paravertebral ganglia, axillary bodies	intercostal artery, atrium, posterior cardinal vein	intercostal artery, posterior cardinal vein, atrium	adrenal gland	adrenal gland

Abbreviations: ACh, acetylcholine; CT, chromaffin tissue; CVS, cardiovascular system; ENS, enteric nervous system; GIT, gastrointestinal tract; H, hagfish; L, lamprey; m, muscarinic cholinergic; P, parasympathetic (cranial autonomic); S, spinal autonomic; α, α-adrenoceptor; β, β-adrenoceptor; +, activation; −, inhibition/relaxation; $\varnothing$, innervation absent (or not found).

a   Cranial nerves with parasympathetic preganglionic fibers (III, oculomotor nerve; VII, facial nerve; IX, glossopharyngeal nerve; X vagal nerve).

b   Blood vessels involved in regulation of the CVS.

c   Stomach and proximal intestine vagally innervated, small intestine mainly spinally innervated.

d   No stomach (lack of acid-secreting mucosa).

e   Rectal gland secreting hypertonic NaCl under spinal autonomic control.

f   Cloacal bladder; β.

g   Only true for some species.

h   Chromaffin tissue (CT) innervated by spinal preganglionic neurons (except in cyclostomes).

Data from anatomy: Nilsson (1983, 2011); cardiovascular system (CVS): Morris and Nilsson (1994), Sandblom and Axelsson (2011); chromaffin tissue: Perry and Capaldo (2011); eye: Neuhuber and Schrödl (2011); gastrointestinal tract: Holmgren and Olsson (2011), Olsson and Holmgren (2011); kidney, urogenital tract, gonads: Jobling (2011); lung: Campbell and McLean (1994); spleen: Nilsson (1994); lungfish: Nilsson and Holmgren personal communication; time in evolution: Kumar and Hedges (1998).

Modified after Jänig (2013)

a

ELASMOBRANCH

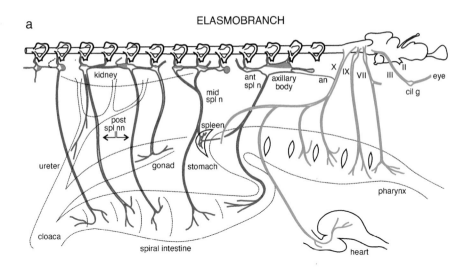

b

TELEOST

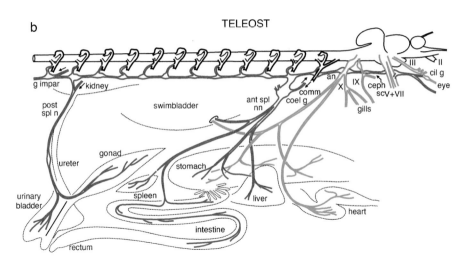

c

REPTILE

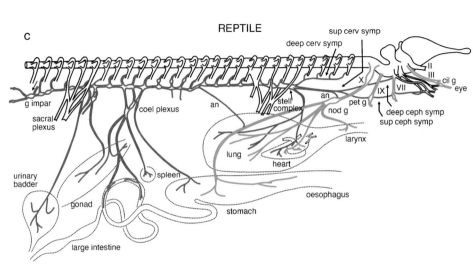

Figure 1.5 Arrangement and characteristics of the peripheral autonomic nervous system of (a) an elasmobranch, (b) a teleost and (c) a reptile. Cranial parasympathetic systems are in green; spinal autonomic systems in red. Note the chromaffin tissue associated with paravertebral ganglia in the elasmobranch (blue). Abbreviations: an, anastomosis between spinal autonomic and cranial nerves; ant spl n, anterior splanchnic nerve; ceph sc, cephalic sympathetic chain; cil g, ciliary ganglion; coel g, celiac ganglion; deep ceph symp, deep cephalic sympathetic; g imp, ganglion impar; mid splanchnic n, middle splanchnic nerve; nod g, nodose ganglion; pet g, petrous (glossopharyngeal) ganglion; post spl nn, posterior splanchnic nerves; sup cerv symp, superior cervical sympathetic; sup cerv g, superior cervical ganglion; stell g, stellate ganglion; Roman numerals refer to cranial nerves. Modified from Nilsson (1983, 2011). With permission.

McLean 1994; Nilsson 2009; Smith and Croll 2011) and for chromatophores in fish (Grove 1994).

6. The molecular mechanisms used by the peripheral autonomic neurons and their target cells in the regulation of autonomic target tissues are probably very similar or identical in all vertebrate groups (transmitters and their receptors, neuropeptides, intracellular pathways) (Hoyle 2011).

1.6 The Early Fascination with the Autonomic Nervous System: Little Brains and Sympathies

This short note on the detection of autonomic nerves and autonomic ganglia and their functions is based on Gaskell (1916), Langley (1921), Sheehan (1936, 1941), Pick (1970), Ackerknecht (1974), Spillane (1981) and Clarke and Jacyna (1987). The field was dominated almost up to the beginning of the nineteenth century without major changes by the concept of regulation of body functions formulated by *Aeilius Galen* (128 to 199 AC or 131 to 216 AC) about 1900 years ago. In short, the liver generates blood from nutritive substances taken up by the gastrointestinal tract. This blood is imbued by the *natural spirits* (spiritus naturalis) in the liver and transported by the right heart via the venous system to all tissues after being cleaned by a passage through the lung. Some of this venous blood gets into the left heart through pores in the cardiac septum and some link in the lung. The blood in the left heart is soaked with the *vital spirits* (spiritus vitalis) which derives from the external pneuma by a passage through the lung. The left heart pumps the blood with the vital spirits to all tissues, including the brain. In the brain the vital spirits are converted into the *animal spirits* (spiritus animalis). The animal spirits flow along peripheral nerves, which are considered to be hollow tubular structures, from the brain (including the spinal cord) to the peripheral tissues and from the peripheral tissues to the brain. The animal spirits are responsible for movements, sensations, thinking and feelings.

Galen described the vagosympathetic trunk as the sixth pair of cranial nerves (which included the glossopharyngeal nerve and the abducens nerve) whereby the vagus nerve and sympathetic trunk were not described as separate nerves. The sympathetic trunk, later called the intercostal nerve, was described together with the rami communicantes by Galen; its origin and central connection were assumed to be via the cerebellum. This was shown to be false by *Francois Pourfour du Petit* (1664–1741) in the first half of the eighteenth century, some 1500 years later. Du Petit described the Horner syndrome after section of the cervical vagosympathetic trunk in dogs, arguing that the origin of the sympathetic trunk is not the lower brain stem (cerebellum) but the spinal cord. The significance of this finding was only recognized more than 100 years later.

Galen described for the first time the ganglion cervicale superius (however without separating it from the ganglion nodosum), the ganglion stellatum and the ganglion celiacum. Galen believed that the interconnections between the ganglionated (sympathetic) nerves allow the animal spirits to travel from organ to organ leading to functional unity (physiological "sympathy") among internal organs innervated by these nerves. Galen's functional concept, including the functioning of the cardiovascular system (heart, veins, arteries) remained unchallenged for almost 1400 years. The functioning of the cardiovascular system was completely refuted in the seventeenth century by *William Harvey* (see his dissertation "Exercitatio anatomica de motu cordis et sanguinis in animalibus" [An anatomical exercise on the motion of the heart and blood in living beings], published by Wilhelm Fitzer, Frankfurt 1628). It took almost another 200 years to challenge Galen's concept related to the functioning of the autonomic nervous system being involved in regulation of visceral organs.

Thomas Willis (1621–1675) was still fully in Galen's tradition. He extended the action of the animal spirits into involuntary and voluntary actions. The voluntary actions are associated with movements generated by skeletal muscles and sensations. They act through the cerebrum and the spinal cord. The involuntary actions are associated with the vagosympathetic trunk acting on heart, breathing and movements of the gastrointestinal tract and lead to sympathy between visceral organs. Willis argued that the rami communicantes of the intercostal (sympathetic) nerve connecting to its ganglia bring together the involuntary animal spirits from the cerebellum and the voluntary animal spirits from the brain and spinal cord. The rami communicantes act as excretory channels of superfluous voluntary spirits in the brain and the ganglia serve as storehouse for the animal spirits. *Robert Whytt* (1714–1766) extended

Willis's concept on involuntary and voluntary movements.

Jacob Benignus Winslow (1669–1760) reasoned that the autonomic ganglia were small brains which have their own "nervous power" and function independently of the cerebrospinal system. He was the first to describe white and gray rami.

The English anatomist *James Johnstone* (1730?–1802) formulated the most extensive concept of the functioning of autonomic ganglia. He believed, as Winslow did, that these ganglia are small brains and consist of a mixture of cortical and medullary substances which are supplied with blood via blood vessels. The ganglia have their own nerves and are functionally independent of the cerebrospinal system (the "brain"), although they communicate with the latter system. The visceral ganglia control the involuntary movements of the visceral organs. They convert voluntary into involuntary messages and act as some sort of filter leading to the relative insensibility of the viscera. The ganglia are confined to nerves that are involved in the generation of involuntary motions of organs (e.g., heart, gastrointestinal tract). The work of Johnstone prepared the ground for the concept of the functioning of the body developed by *Marie Francois Xaver Bichat* (1771–1802).

Bichat divided life into animal life (vie animale) and organic life (vie organique). Animal life is related to the somatic tissues, brain and spinal cord, and the nerves originating from them. It is involved in volition, movement by skeletal muscles, sensory experience from the external world as well as free will and thoughts. Organic life is related to the visceral body domain and its innervation. The sympathetic chain is homologous to the spinal cord, and the celiac plexus to the brain. The autonomic ganglia act as nerve centers, are relatively independent and are small brains. The autonomic nerve centers of the ganglia are associated with regulation of the cardiovascular system, respiratory system, gastrointestinal tract, glands, etc. The ganglionated system and the cerebrospinal system are functionally separate systems. But the two systems are connected via the rami communicantes. In Bichat's view, these connections between spinal nerves and sympathetic ganglia remain obscure and have no function.

Bichat's concept of a functionally independent "ganglionic nervous system" being involved in regulation of visceral organs was well accepted in the scientific community in the first half of the nineteenth century. However, based on the experimental work of *Claude Bernard* (1813–1878) and particularly the systematic work of *Walter Holbrook Gaskell* (1847–1916) and *John Newport Langley* (1852–1925) over tens of years, Bichat's concept was practically entirely refuted. Gaskell and Langley laid the foundation for the structure and general functioning of the peripheral autonomic nervous system which stood the test of time. The essentials of their work are (Gaskell 1916, Langley 1921):

- Langley introduced the term "autonomic nervous system." He emphasized that the term "autonomic" expresses a much greater degree of independence than in fact exists, the exception being the enteric nervous system.
- The autonomic nervous system consists of the sympathetic (thoracolumbar) system, the parasympathetic (craniosacral) system and the enteric nervous system.
- Sympathetic and parasympathetic systems are purely motor systems.
- The sympathetic and parasympathetic systems consist of preganglionic and postganglionic neurons which are synaptically connected in autonomic ganglia.
- Sympathetic preganglionic neurons project with their myelinated axons through white rami. The communication between spinal cord and the peripheral sympathetic system occurs only via these rami. Sympathetic postganglionic neurons project to somatic tissues through gray rami with their unmyelinated axons (Gaskell was wrong to assume that all sympathetic preganglionic axons are thinly myelinated [Jänig 1985; Bahr et al. 1986; Boczek-Funcke et al. 1993]).
- Spinal sensory fibers from viscera traverse the sympathetic ganglia and project through the white rami. Their cell bodies are located in the dorsal root ganglia. (Many if not most spinal visceral afferent neurons have unmyelinated axons.)
- The sympathetic chain ganglia contain no reflex centers.
- Sympathetic and parasympathetic systems have antagonistic (excitatory or inhibitory) effects on the target organs. (This point was overdone, in particular by Gaskell [Gaskell 1916]).

Conclusions

1. The definition of the sympathetic and parasympathetic nervous systems is anatomical and based on the levels of outflow and therefore the developmental origin from the neuraxis. Visceral afferent neurons are not included in this definition, although they are indispensable to understanding the functioning of both autonomic systems (see Chapter 2).
2. The sympathetic system originates from the thoracic and upper lumbar spinal segments and is therefore called the thoracolumbar system.
3. The parasympathetic system originates from the brain stem (medulla oblongata, mesencephalon) and sacral spinal cord and is therefore called the craniosacral system.
4. Both systems are efferent and consist of a chain of preganglionic and postganglionic neurons, which are synaptically connected in peripheral autonomic ganglia.
5. Sympathetic ganglia are situated remotely from the target organs and organized bilaterally in the sympathetic chains and in the prevertebral ganglia. Parasympathetic ganglia are situated close to the target organs.
6. Stimulation of sympathetic neurons produces many distinct effector responses elicited from a variety of cell and tissue types, including blood vessels, heart, non-vascular smooth muscles, exocrine epithelia, endocrine cells (of the pancreas), adipocytes and lymphoid tissues.
7. The adrenal medulla is an endocrine gland made up of cells that release either adrenaline or noradrenaline during synaptic activation by sympathetic preganglionic neurons. Adrenaline is a metabolic hormone.
8. Stimulation of parasympathetic neurons leads to activation of most exocrine glands, non-vascular smooth muscles and some other target cells. The pacemaker and atria of the heart and a few specialized blood vessels are inhibited.
9. Most autonomic target tissues react under physiological conditions to only one of the autonomic systems. Only a few react to both. Opposite reactions to sympathetic and parasympathetic inputs are more the exception than the rule.
10. The widely propagated idea of the antagonism between sympathetic and parasympathetic nervous systems is misleading.
11. Postganglionic neurons (and to some degree also preganglionic neurons) of autonomic pathways contain combinations of neuropeptides in most cases colocalized with (but some without) the classical transmitters acetylcholine or noradrenaline. The peptide content may to some extent correlate with the function of the autonomic neurons. However, there are species and organ differences and the function of most peptides is unknown.
12. The principal organization of the peripheral autonomic nervous system in major submammalian vertebrate groups is highly conserved in evolution over a time period of about 500 million years.
13. Going back to Aeilius Galenus in the second century after Christ, the sympathetic nervous system was believed to consist of little brains and to generate sympathies between organ systems.

Suggested Reading

Gibbins, I. L., Jobling, P. and Morris, J. L. (2003) Functional organization of peripheral vasomotor pathways. *Acta Physiol Scand* **177**, 237–245.

Jänig, W., Keast, J. R., McLachlan, E. M., Neuhuber, W. L. and Southard-Smith, M. (2017) Renaming all spinal autonomic outflows as sympathetic is a mistake. *Auton Neurosci* **206**, 60–62.

Langley, J. N. (1903b) The autonomic nervous system. *Brain* **26**, 1–26.

Nilsson, S. and Holmgren, S. (eds.) (1994) *Comparative Physiology and Evolution of the Autonomic Nervous System*, Harwood Academic Publishers, Chur (Switzerland).

Sheehan, D. (1936) Discovery of the autonomic nervous system. *Arch Neurol Psychiat* **35**, 1081–1115.

Swanson, L. W. (2013) Basic plan of the nervous system. In *Fundamental Neuroscience*, 4th edn (Squire, L. R., Berg, D., Bloom, F. E., et al., eds) pp. 15–38, Elsevier Academic Press, Amsterdam.

All references cited in the text are available online at www.cambridge.org/janig.

Notes

1. A complete description of the gross anatomy of the peripheral sympathetic and parasympathetic nervous

system in vertebrates (including humans) has been done by Pick 1970. This book documents most variations of autonomic ganglia, white and gray rami, the sympathetic chain, and the splanchnic nerves in detail.

2. Choline acetyltransferase (ChAT) catalyzes the condensation of choline and acetyl-coenzyme A, forming acetylcholine and coenzyme A. Antibodies against ChAT or vesicular acetylcholine transporter (VAChT) are used to identify cholinergic postganglionic neurons and also preganglionic neurons immunohistochemically (Keast et al. 1995).

3. The nomenclatures used to describe the macroscopy of the peripheral sympathetic nervous system are sometimes confusing, not only for the beginner but also for the experienced experimenter. This is related to differences in species, to special emphasis on the human and probably also to differences in academic teaching by anatomists and by physiologists. For example, celiac ganglion (ganglia) and celiac plexus are equivalent; the inferior mesenteric ganglion (IMG) in the human is equivalent to the proximal IMG in the cat; the superior hypogastric plexus in the human is equivalent to the distal IMG in the cat; the abdominal aortic plexus or intermesenteric plexus in the human is equivalent to the intermesenteric nerve in the cat, rat, etc. Without discussing these differences further, the reader is referred to Pick (1970) [all laboratory animals, human], Baron et al. (1985a) [cat], Baron et al. (1988, 1995) [rat], Jänig and McLachlan (1987) [lumbar sympathetic outflow to viscera, all laboratory animals and human],

Gray's Anatomy (2016) [human] and Kraima et al. (2015) [human].

4. In books of anatomy the celiac ganglion is called celiac plexus and the inferior mesenteric ganglion superior hypogastric plexus (for details of nomenclature used in humans/primates and smaller animals see Jänig and McLachlan [1987] and Beveridge et al. [2015, 2016]).

5. White rami appear macroscopically white in cadavers of humans and other higher vertebrates because many sympathetic preganglionic axons are myelinated. Gray rami appear macroscopically gray because virtually all postganglionic axons are unmyelinated.

6. The vertebral nerve is a nerve in its own right. It contains postganglionic axons from the stellate ganglion and vertebral ganglion (small ganglion anterior to the vertebral artery). It gives branches with postganglionic axons to the cervical spinal nerves and is therefore interpreted as deep ramus communicans griseus (Tubbs et al. 2007). However, there exist additionally other rami communicantes grisei which branch from the cervical sympathetic trunk and pass between or through prevertebral muscles (e.g., musculi longus colli and capitis) to the spinal nerves.

7. Only in monkeys and birds are the preganglionic neurons located in the cytoarchitectonically defined Edinger–Westphal nucleus. In the rat, rabbit, cat and human, most cell bodies of parasympathetic preganglionic neurons to the eye are situated ventral to the cytoarchitectonically defined Edinger–Westphal nucleus (see Subchapter 8.2).

Chapter 2

Interoceptive Afferent Neurons and Autonomic Regulation with Special Emphasis on the Viscera[1]

In the following Chapter, I will describe functional aspects of spinal and vagal afferent neurons in relation to visceral sensations and autonomic regulation, with some emphasis on visceral pain and body protection. In Subchapter 2.6, I will generalize and transfer the concept of interoception to the somatic body domains. I will particularly concentrate on the representation of interoceptive systems in spinal cord, thalamus and dorsal posterior insular cortex. Anatomy and physiology of the afferent neurons for each organ is described in detail in the literature (see Note 1). Details about the regulation and the functional specificity of the afferent signals with respect to the autonomic regulation will be discussed in Part III of this book.

Sherrington (1906) made the functional distinction between interoception, exteroception and proprioception. Exteroceptive afferent neurons innervating the body surface are involved in the communication between environment and body. Proprioceptive afferent neurons monitor events in the deep somatic tissues, in particular skeletal muscle and joints. Both types of afferent neuron are mechanosensitive and have large-diameter myelinated ($A\alpha$, $A\beta$) axons. Interoceptive afferent neurons monitor events in the viscera (originally, events at the inner surface of the body, e.g., the gastrointestinal tract, that Sherrington termed the interoceptive surface of the body). These afferent neurons have small myelinated and unmyelinated axons. By the same token, processes in the brain are related to these functional classes of primary afferent neurons discussed in the framework of the concept of exteroception, proprioception and interoception. Sherrington (1900) also had a clear concept about thermoreception and nociception from skin, which can be regarded as the largest organ of the body. Would he have subsumed skin senses related to thermal stimuli and to tissue-damaging or potentially damaging stimuli and sensations elicited from deep somatic tissues that are related to the excitation of afferent $A\delta$- and C-fibers under the category interoception as proposed by Craig (2015)? From the discussion of the topic "The skin and common sensation" in his textbook chapter "Cutaneous sensations" (Sherrington 1900), I would say that the answer is in the affirmative. On p. 969 Sherrington says:

---

[1] This chapter is dedicated to my friend Arthur ("Bud") Craig. Bud introduced me into the scientific problems related to the representation of interoception in the central nervous system.

By common sensation is understood that sum of sensations referred, not to external agents, but to the processes of the animal body. Its "object" is the body itself – the material "me". Sensations derived from the body tissues and organs possess strong affective tone; while sensations of special sense are relatively free from affective tone.

Here I will subsume the sensory processes related to the activation of afferent neurons connected to Aδ- or C-axons under the category interoception meaning that these senses refer to the different body tissues. This view will become relevant in Subchapter 2.6. It is similar to that propagated by Craig. Craig has claimed that pain, thermal sensations, itch, muscular and visceral sensations (along with hunger, thirst, air hunger and other feelings from the body) are aspects of the representation of the physiological condition of the different body tissues and therefore belong to interoception (Craig 2003a, 2015, 2018; see below). I will fully follow his argumentation. Saper has claimed that nociceptive sensations are related to mechanical, thermal and metabolic stresses of deep somatic and visceral, and superficial, body tissues. These sensations monitor tissue integrity and are internally directed, i.e., they are concerned with that state of the body itself (Saper 2002).

2.1 | Visceral Primary Afferent Neurons: General Characteristics

2.1.1 Vagal and Spinal Visceral Afferent Neurons

Visceral organs in the thoracic, abdominal and pelvic cavities are innervated by vagal and spinal visceral afferent neurons that encode physical and chemical events in the visceral organs and convey this information to the spinal cord or lower brain stem. They are the interface between the visceral organs and the central nervous system. Most visceral afferent axons are unmyelinated, conducting at 1 m/s or less; some are myelinated, conducting at up to about 30 m/s. Visceral afferent neurons that convey information from the viscera to spinal cord or lower brain stem are distinguished from visceral afferent neurons of the enteric nervous system. These enteric neurons have their cell bodies in the wall of the gastrointestinal tract. They are called intrinsic primary afferent neurons (IPANs) of the enteric nervous system and encode mechanical and chemical events (see Chapter 5).

Visceral afferent neurons are involved in many functions (Figure 2.1):

- Organ regulation, organ reflexes, neuroendocrine regulation, related particularly to vagal afferents and sacral spinal afferents (see Chapter 10 and Subchapter 9.3).
- Multiple protective organ reflexes, particularly related to thoracolumbar spinal visceral afferents, but also to vagal afferents.
- Visceral non-painful sensations (see Table 2.1).
- Visceral discomfort and pain, related in particular to spinal visceral afferents.
- Visceral pain referred to deep somatic tissues, other visceral organs and skin. Referred visceral pain is associated with changes in the referred tissues that are mediated (or hypothesized to be mediated) by the sympathetic nervous system, such as changes in blood flow, edema and sweating as well as trophic changes (Jänig 2014, 2020a).
- Shaping of emotional feelings related to body states.
- Generation of sickness behavior, related particularly to the excitation of vagal afferents from the gastrointestinal tract (Watkins and Maier 1999; Jänig 2005; Dantzer et al. 2008; Jänig and Levine 2013).
- Neural and neuroendocrine regulation of hyperalgesia and inflammation, related particularly to the excitation of vagal afferents (Jänig 2005; Jänig and Levine 2013).

Figure 2.2 demonstrates the projections of spinal and vagal visceral afferent neurons from the organs in the thoracic, abdominal and pelvic cavities to the spinal cord or lower brain stem:

- Thoracolumbar spinal visceral afferents project from the viscera through splanchnic nerves (cardiac nerves; major, minor, lumbar splanchnic nerves; hypogastric nerve), which also contain pre- and postganglionic sympathetic axons, and the corresponding white rami to the thoracic or upper lumbar spinal cord. These afferent neurons have their cell bodies in the corresponding dorsal root ganglia (Figure 2.2 right side).
- Sacral spinal visceral afferent neurons innervating pelvic organs (ureter, urinary bladder and urethra; internal reproductive organs; distal colon, sigmoid and rectum, including anal canal) project through the pelvic nerves and have their cell bodies in the

**VISCERAL AFFERENT SYSTEMS
AUTONOMIC EFFERENT SYSTEMS**

FUNCTIONS

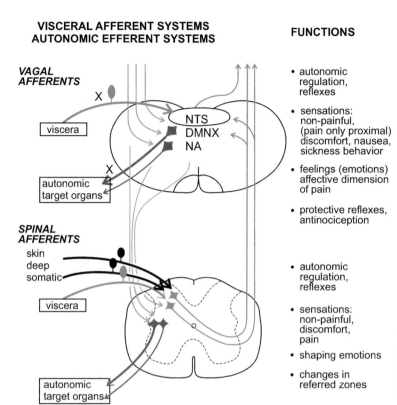

*VAGAL
AFFERENTS*

viscera

NTS
DMNX
NA

autonomic
target organs

*SPINAL
AFFERENTS*

skin
deep
somatic

viscera

autonomic
target organs

- autonomic
  regulation,
  reflexes

- sensations:
  non-painful,
  (pain only proximal)
  discomfort, nausea,
  sickness behavior

- feelings (emotions)
  affective dimension
  of pain

- protective reflexes,
  antinociception

- autonomic
  regulation,
  reflexes

- sensations:
  non-painful,
  discomfort,
  pain

- shaping emotions

- changes in
  referred zones

Figure 2.1 General scheme of visceral–autonomic relations. *Left*: visceral afferent inputs and efferent (autonomic) outputs of lower brain stem and spinal cord. *Right*: general functions of visceral afferent neurons. *Upper part*: medulla oblongata; cell bodies of preganglionic neurons that project to the vagus nerve are located in the dorsal motor nucleus of the vagus (DMNX) and in the nucleus ambiguus (NA, see Subchapters 8.4.2 and 10.7); X, vagus nerve; NTS, nucleus tractus solitarii. *Lower part*: spinal cord; spinal visceral afferents converge on viscero-somatic neurons with afferent input from skin and deep somatic tissues, including skeletal muscle, in laminae I and V of the dorsal horn and deeper laminae; visceral sensations are also referred to the segmentally corresponding parts of the three body domains (skin, deep somatic tissues, viscera). Note that all efferent autonomic systems and the transmission of impulses from visceral primary afferent neurons to second-order neurons (in the NTS and in the dorsal horn of the spinal cord) are under descending control from higher brain centers (green; see Jänig and Morrison [1986]; Jänig and Häbler [1995]). Modified from Jänig and Häbler (1995) with permission.

sacral dorsal root ganglia (in the rat, also in the sixth lumbar dorsal root ganglion) (Figure 2.2 lower left).
- Some afferent neurons projecting through the thoracolumbar white rami innervate the ventral compartment of the vertebral column (Bogduk 1983; Bahns et al. 1986b; Bogduk et al. 1988). These neurons are deep somatic afferent neurons.
- There is no evidence that spinal and trigeminal afferent neurons that innervate somatic tissues (skin, skeletal muscle, joints, etc.) project with their peripheral axons along the sympathetic chain and the major distributing arteries (e.g., the subclavian, iliac, carotid artery) to the extremities, the head or – with the exception of the ventral compartment of the afferent innervations of the vertebral column – to the body trunk (see Figure 1.2 for projections of sympathetic postganglionic neurons to targets in the extremities and the head). Large blood vessels of the body trunk (such as aorta, subclavian, iliac or carotid arteries) are surrounded by terminals of primary afferent neurons that form a plexus lying outside the perivascular noradrenergic plexus. These afferents

project to their target together with the visceral sympathetic innervation.
- About 1.5% to 2.5% of all spinal afferents that have their cell bodies in the dorsal root ganglia project to the viscera, the other spinal afferent neurons project to skin or deep somatic tissues (Jänig and Morrison 1986); in some dorsal root ganglia (e.g., sacral S2/S3, thoracic T8/T9 up to about 8% of all neural cell bodies may be visceral. In the cat, some 22 000 to 25 000 spinal primary afferent neurons project to the viscera. This number compares to the total number of about 1 to 1.5 million spinal afferent neurons (both sides; Jänig and Morrison 1986). This illustrates that visceral organs are much less densely innervated by spinal afferent neurons than the superficial and deep somatic body tissues.
- Vagal afferents innervating thoracic organs project through the superior and recurrent laryngeal branches, the aortic nerve, cardiac branches and branches from lung and esophagus to the NTS in the lower brain stem. Some afferents (from carotid arterial baro- and chemoreceptors) project through

the carotid sinus nerve or the glossopharyngeal nerve. Abdominal vagal afferents project through the common hepatic branch (from liver, upper duodenum and pylorus), two gastric branches (from the stomach) and two celiac branches (distal duodenum, small intestines, proximal colon) to the lower brain stem (Berthoud et al. 1997; Berthoud and Neuhuber 2000). The cell bodies of afferent neurons projecting to the vagus nerve lie in the inferior (nodose) ganglion of the vagus nerve (and some in the superior [jugular] ganglion); those projecting to the glossopharyngeal nerve (including afferents from arterial baro- and chemoreceptors) lie in the petrosal ganglion.

- In the cat, about 30 000 afferent neurons project through the abdominal vagal nerves. The number of vagal afferent neurons innervating thoracic visceral organs is in the range of 15 000 (Agostoni et al. 1957; Mei et al. 1980).

- Trigeminal afferent neurons innervating intracranial blood vessels and associated structures (e.g., the dura, trigemino-vascular afferents) may also be considered to be visceral. The same applies to afferents from the tongue (associated with taste), from the hard palate and the proximal part of the oropharynx that project through the facial or glossopharyngeal nerve to the NTS, taste afferents being a special class of visceral afferents.

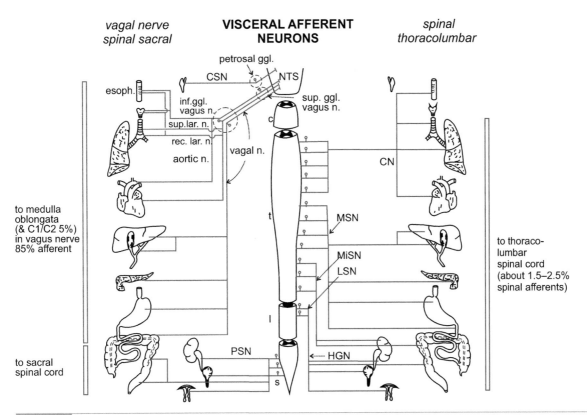

Figure 2.2 Projection of visceral afferent neurons. *Left side*: vagal visceral afferent neurons projecting to the nucleus tractus solitarii (NTS) and spinal visceral afferent neurons projecting through the pelvic splanchnic nerve (PSN) to the sacral spinal cord. Baroreceptor and chemoreceptor afferents from the carotid sinus and body project through the carotid sinus nerve (CSN) or the glossopharyngeal nerve to the NTS. *Right side*: spinal visceral afferent neurons projecting to the thoracic and upper lumbar spinal cord. Note that pelvic organs are supplied by both sacral and lumbar (some lower thoracic) spinal visceral afferent neurons. The number of spinal visceral afferent neurons is low compared to the number of spinal somatic afferent neurons (estimated from counting in the cat). CN, cardiac nerves; HGN, hypogastric nerve; inf. ggl. vagus n., inferior ganglion of the vagus nerve (nodose ganglion); LSN, lumbar splanchnic nerves; MaSN, major splanchnic nerve; MISN, minor splanchnic nerves; sup. ggl. vagus n., superior ganglion of the vagus nerve (jugular ganglion); sup./rec. lar. n., superior/recurrent laryngeal nerve; ggl., ganglion; c, cervical; t, thoracic; l, lumbar; s, sacral. Modified from Mei (1983), Berthoud and Neuhuber (2000), Neuhuber (1989), Wank and Neuhuber (2001) with permission, Neuhuber personal communication.

2.1.2 Visceral Afferent Neurons and Autonomic Nervous Systems

As described in Chapter 1, Langley defined the sympathetic and parasympathetic (cranio[bulbo-tectal]-sacral) systems on functional anatomical grounds, i.e., based on the reaction of autonomic target organs to electrical stimulation of preganglionic or postganglionic axons and on some other criteria. His definition of the two autonomic systems was not based on the functions and reflexes in which the autonomic neurons are involved. Thus, Langley never used the terms "sympathetic" and "parasympathetic" in a functional sense, as is sometimes done. He did not include in this definition the visceral afferent neurons projecting through the same nerves together with the preganglionic sympathetic and parasympathetic neurons (Langley 1900, 1903a, b, 1921). In fact, for good reasons he was extremely careful in his argumentation in his paper in *Brain* (Langley 1903b) as to why afferent fibers passing through "autonomic" nerves and innervating viscera should not be named sympathetic, parasympathetic or autonomic. For me the position of Langley on this issue was rather modern and is still, with some modifications, fully valid. This is best expressed in his own words:

In what I have said so far I have dealt with what seem to me facts about the afferent fibres accompanying the efferent autonomic nerves, but I have put on one side the fundamental difficulty with regard to them, and that is: Are there any afferent nerves which deserve to be separated from afferent somatic nerves, and if so, what are the characteristics of autonomic as opposed to somatic afferent nerves? I have above tried to show that the afferent nerves of the sympathetic system are indistinguishable in form and position from those of the somatic system, and it remains to consider what other distinguishing characters may be present . . .

It is clear that we cannot make a like division of afferent fibres according as they run to striated muscles or to other tissue; it would lead to nothing but confusion to consider the afferent fibres of the skin as autonomic fibres and the afferent fibres of striated muscle as the only somatic afferent fibres . . .

Since by hypothesis the one kind of fibre gives rise to sensation, and the other does not, there must be a difference in their central connection, such that in the one the upward path to the cerebral hemispheres is absent or very slightly developed. That, and that only, so far as we can say, distinguishes autonomic from somatic afferent fibres. Further progress waits for the discovery of some

distinguishing histological character. And in the meantime it is open to discussion whether the class of afferent fibres which are solely reflex in function can be properly considered as corresponding on the afferent side to the efferent fibres of the autonomic tissues.

Langley 1903b
(page 25–26)

Thus, the situation is still an open story, as expressed by Langley at the beginning of the twentieth century, and the putative classification of visceral (and other) afferent neurons as sympathetic or parasympathetic or autonomic awaits better, more stringent if not molecular-genetic, criteria.

Although visceral afferents are anatomically closely associated with either the sympathetic or parasympathetic parts of the autonomic nervous system I will call these afferent neurons *visceral* (qualified by spinal or vagal), fully in accordance with Langley. The terms *sympathetic afferent* and *parasympathetic afferent* neuron are misleading since they imply that the afferent neurons have functions that uniquely pertain to that particular part of the autonomic nervous system. There is an exception in that afferent neurons of the enteric nervous system are by definition *enteric afferent neurons* (intrinsic primary afferent neurons [IPANs], Chapter 5). No convincing functional, morphological, histochemical or other criteria exist to associate any type of visceral afferent neuron that projects to the spinal cord or brain stem with only one part of the autonomic system. The label *sympathetic* or *parasympathetic* would lead to complications as far as the understanding of the functions of these afferents is concerned. By the same token, spinal and vagal visceral afferent neurons should not be called autonomic.

This point is illustrated by two examples: (1) Pelvic organs are innervated by two sets of spinal visceral afferents, one entering the spinal cord at the rostral lumbar and most caudal thoracic segmental levels and the other at sacral segmental levels. Both are involved in visceral nociception. However, only the sacral visceral afferents, and not the visceral afferents projecting to the upper lumbar and lower thoracic spinal cord, are involved in regulation of the pelvic organs (and in corresponding sensations) (Jänig and Morrison 1986; Jänig and Koltzenburg 1990, 1993; Ritter et al. 1992; Cervero 1994; Jänig 1996). It makes no sense to speak of "sympathetic" and "parasympathetic" visceral nociception. (2) Arterial baro- and chemoreceptor afferents project through the aortic and glossopharyngeal nerves to the nucleus tractus solitarii. To label these afferents as parasympathetic is groundless.

Many visceral afferent neurons serve special functions related to distinct types of physiological control in which the autonomic nervous system is the efferent pathway, for example cardiovascular afferents, afferents from the respiratory tract and afferents from the gastrointestinal tract that project to the NTS or afferents from pelvic organs that project to the sacral spinal cord. These afferents monitor the inner state of the body and serve to adapt the internal milieu and organ functions to the behavior of the organism. *In this sense, these afferents belong functionally to the autonomic nervous system* (Note 2). However, the second-order neurons that the visceral afferents connect to synaptically are widespread and carry signals to higher levels of integration in the brain. The brain's "knowledge" of the body's inner state may influence behavior in the widest sense.

2.2 | Visceral Primary Afferent Neurons as Interface Between Visceral Organs and Brain

Many spinal afferent neurons and some vagal afferent neurons, in particular those with unmyelinated axons supplying viscera, seem to have general functions (Jänig 1996) that are related to impulse activity conducted orthodromically to spinal cord, brain stem or prevertebral sympathetic ganglia ("afferent" functions) and to the release of neuropeptides in the target tissues ("efferent" functions). Knowledge about some of these functions is well established, other concepts are at best hypothetical. These functions do not apply to every type of visceral afferent neuron and afferent neurons may not only be specialized with respect to their receptive properties, but also with respect to the putative efferent functions (de Groat 1987; Maggi and Meli 1988; Dockray et al. 1989; Holzer 1992, 1998a, 2002a, b, 2003; Holzer and Maggi 1998; Dockray 2013). Thus, spinal visceral afferents might further be differentiated for mediating preferentially peripheral extraspinal reflexes, local regulation or trophic influences (Figure 2.3).

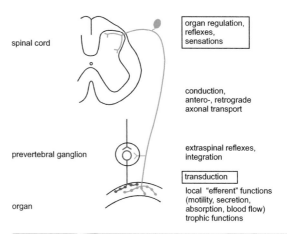

Figure 2.3 Spinal afferent neurons as interface between visceral organs and brain. Spinal primary afferent neurons supplying viscera have multiple functions. They contain neuropeptides, such as calcitonin gene-related peptide and substance P (de Groat 1989), that are transported from the soma to the central and peripheral terminals. (1) *Afferent functions*: the prime role is to send information to the central nervous system. They can also modify the regulation of viscera via extracentral reflexes mediated by prevertebral ganglia (see Subchapter 6.5). (2) *Local efferent (effector) functions*: they have local efferent functions by the release of neuropeptides from peripheral endings. (3) *Trophic functions*: the afferents can also signal events by slow transport of chemical substances rather than rapid electrical processes under normal conditions. These substances could have trophic effects on the peripheral tissues or might influence the synaptic connectivity between primary afferent neurons and second-order neurons in the spinal cord.

- The conventional function of visceral afferent neurons is to encode physical (distension, contraction) and chemical events and to signal these events by centripetal impulses to second-order neurons in the spinal cord or brain stem leading to organ regulation, reflexes and distinct sensations. The terminals of these afferents contain various molecules that enable the afferents to transduce and integrate the physical and chemical stimuli in their microenvironment, so as to generate impulse activity. Also involved in this transduction process are non-neural cells such as epithelia of the respiratory, gastrointestinal and urinary tracts, which contain the same molecules for sensing physical and chemical stimuli in the lumen of the organs as the afferent terminals (Apodaca 2004; Birder 2005, 2014).

- Collaterals of some spinal visceral afferent fibers form peptidergic synapses with noradrenergic neurons in prevertebral ganglia (celiac, mesenteric ganglia) that are particularly involved in gastro-intestinal functions (regulation of secretion and motility), establishing in this way extraspinal reflexes. The peptide transmitters are calcitonin gene-related peptide (CGRP) and substance P (Perry and Lawson 1998). These postganglionic neurons integrate activity in preganglionic neurons, peripheral intestinofugal neurons of the enteric nervous system and spinal visceral afferents (see Subchapter 6.5; de Groat, 1987; Furness and Costa 1987; Jänig 1988, 1995; Dockray et al. 1989; Szurszewski and King 1989; Furness et al. 2014).

- Visceral afferent neurons may participate in a variety of "efferent" functions (effector functions), by release of neuropeptides (such as CGRP and/or substance P) and other substances (e.g., ATP) within the viscera that are independent of the central nervous system and prevertebral ganglia. These functions consist of vasodilation, bronchoconstriction, secretory processes in the gastrointestinal tract, regulation of gut and urinary tract motility, and modulation of the protective function of epithelia against intraluminal and otherwise toxic substances. Thus, the afferents are involved in protection of the gastric mucosa against acid back-diffusion (Holzer 1992, 1995, 2002a, b, 2003; Maggi et al. 1995; Santicioli and Maggi 1998) and in the protective function of the urothelium of the urinary tract, keeping down its permeability to small molecules (water, ammonia, urea, proton ions) and toxins in the urine (Apodaca 2004; Birder 2005, 2014). Some visceral afferent neurons that have their cell bodies in the dorsal root ganglia may not project to the spinal cord at all (Häbler et al. 1990b). These afferent neurons may only have peripheral efferent functions (see also Holzer and Maggi 1998). The "efferent" functions of the afferent neurons may be particularly important under pathophysiological conditions, for example, inflammatory changes in the peripheral tissue (de Groat 1989; Dockray et al. 1989; Kumazawa 1990) (Note 3.)

- Visceral afferents may have trophic functions and could be important for the maintenance of the structure of visceral tissues (e.g., the mucosa of the urogenital tract [Apodaca 2004; Birder 2005] or of the stomach [Lundgren 1989]).

- Afferent neurons retrogradely transport neurotropic substances; this invites speculation that these substances might have long-term effects on

the synaptic connections formed by primary afferent terminals in the spinal cord with second-order neurons (cf. Lewin and McMahon 1993).

This cascade of functions of spinal visceral afferents may serve the same final general aim: protection and maintenance of the integrity of visceral tissues. For example, excitation of thoracolumbar spinal visceral afferent neurons may elicit pain and discomfort, protective supraspinal, spinal and extraspinal reflexes, and changes in target organ responses (such as increase of blood flow, change in motility and secretion). Thus, many visceral afferent neurons, in particular those with unmyelinated fibers, form an active interface between visceral organs and spinal cord as well as lower brain stem. Spinal visceral afferent neurons may be differentiated into those having only peripheral (efferent) functions, those having only central functions (i.e., signaling peripheral events to the spinal cord) and those having dual functions (see Figure 2.4; Holzer and Maggi 1998; Holzer 2002a, b, 2003).

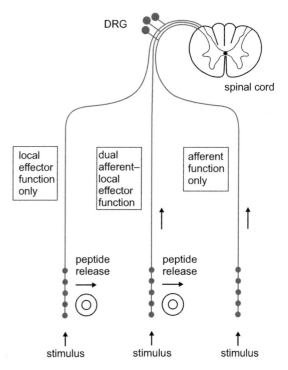

Figure 2.4 Spinal visceral afferent neurons having either afferent (central) functions (right), local effector ("efferent") functions (left) or dual functions (middle). This functional distinction of spinal visceral afferent neurons into three global types is a hypothesis. The cell bodies of each type of afferent neuron are located in the dorsal root ganglia (DRG). Modified from Holzer and Maggi (1998) with permission.

2.3 Receptive Functions of Visceral Afferent Neurons

The central nervous system receives information from the internal organs by two sets of visceral afferents (Figures 2.1, 2.2) and sends efferent impulses to the internal organs by two sets of autonomic efferents each consisting of many functionally distinct pathways (Chapter 4). Visceral afferent neurons being involved in visceral pain will be discussed separately (see Subchapter 2.4).

The degree of functional (physiological) specificity of afferent neurons is generally described by way of their quantitative responses to physical and chemical stimuli. If an afferent neuron responds preferentially to a particular physiological stimulus applied to its receptive endings at low stimulus energy, but not to other physiological stimuli, then this stimulus is considered to be an adequate stimulus and the receptive ending of the afferent neuron specific for this stimulus (see Cervero 1994). Many visceral receptors are specific with respect to the various adequate stimuli occurring in the visceral domain. Table 2.1 lists, separated for different organ systems, the physiologically distinct types of visceral afferent neurons and the sensations, organ functions and regulations that are associated with the activation of these afferent neurons.

In this context I want to emphasize that the activation of a functionally particular group of afferent neuron does not *cause* a particular sensation or regulation, and the afferent signals generated in the periphery are not "carried through" to the cortical representations of these sensations and regulations in the form of a labeled-line system. We have to distinguish three classes of events involved that are not interchangeable, but correlate with each other: (1) The anatomy, histochemistry and pharmacology of the primary afferent neurons. (2) The physiology of the primary afferent neurons and the regulation and reflexes associated with them. (3) The sensations and emotional feelings elicited by their activity, both being mental events (Table 2.1).

2.3.1 Vagal Afferent Neurons

About 85% of the nerve fibers in the *vagus nerve* are *afferent*. Their cell bodies are located in the jugular ganglion (superior ganglion nervi vagi) which originates from the neural crest (25%) or in the nodose ganglion (inferior ganglion nervi vagi), which is of placodal origin. Most of these afferents are unmyelinated, some are thinly myelinated, but this varies between organs and between species. The fibers project viscerotopically to the NTS (Loewy and Spyer 1990; Ritter et al. 1992; Barraco 1994; Paton and Kasparov 2000; see Subchapters 8.3 and 10.7). The second-order neurons in the NTS project to various sites in the lower brain stem, upper brain stem, hypothalamus and amygdala, establishing well-organized neural pathways that are the basis for distinct organ regulation and associated body perceptions (see Subchapters 2.6 and 8.3).

Using single-cell RNA (ribonucleic acid) sequencing in the mouse, the molecular characteristics of vagal afferent neurons have been extensively studied (Egerod et al. 2018, 2019; Kupari et al. 2019). The studies used the transcriptome of the neurons to classify them. The neurons in the jugular ganglion were divided into six molecular types, which were similar to the neural cells in the dorsal root ganglia (Usoskin et al. 2015; Emery and Ernfors 2018). The neurons in the nodose ganglion were divided into 18 types by way of molecular criteria. The studies show a seemingly unexpected molecular diversity of vagal afferent neurons. However, this molecular diversity is in principle not surprising given the complexity of the neural regulation of the cardiovascular system, the respiratory system and the gastrointestinal tract. The molecular studies will open the door for new experimental strategies to study the morphology and physiology of the peripheral and central connectivity of the vagal afferent neurons. The combination of transcriptional, anatomical and neurophysiological characteristics of the vagal afferent neurons will lead to much deeper understanding of the autonomic regulation represented in the lower brain stem. In my understanding, these elegant molecular studies will not replace studies of single afferent neurons in vivo in showing how the vagal afferent neurons function in the different types of organ regulation. In fact, the molecular and the in vivo studies will complement each other.

Receptive Properties and Organ Regulation

Vagal afferents monitor mechanical and chemical events related to the respiratory tract, cardiovascular organs and gastrointestinal tract and therefore related to the regulation and reflexes associated with these organ systems. Neurophysiological recordings have shown that these afferent neurons exhibit specificity or relative (preferential) specificity with respect to adequate mechanical (distension, contraction, shearing stimuli) and chemical stimuli (changes in blood gases, osmotic stimuli, changes in glucose, proton ions, protein products, lipids in duodenum and small intestines). This specificity is brought about by the anatomical arrangement of the receptive endings and by the transduction mechanisms. The main functional types of vagal afferents are listed in Table 2.1 (Undem and Weinreich 2005):

- The *respiratory tract* is innervated by various functionally specific types of vagal afferents with myelinated and unmyelinated fibers (Widdicombe 1986, 2001, 2003; Coleridge and Coleridge 1997; Lee and Pisarri 2001; Schelegle and Green 2001).
- The *cardiovascular system* (heart, ascending aorta, carotid artery) is innervated by afferents encoding in their activity arterial blood pressure and its changes (arterial baroreceptors), arterial blood gases (in particular oxygen tension, arterial chemoreceptors), right atrial pressure (volume receptors in the right atrium and large intrathoracic veins) and ventricular contraction (Thorén 1979; Chapleau and Abboud 2001).
- In the *gastrointestinal tract*, vagal afferents monitor mechanical and chemical events in the intestine (for review see Grundy and Scratcherd [1989]). Intramural endings consist of intraganglionic laminar endings (IGLEs) in the myenteric plexus with functional characteristics of tension receptors or intramuscular arrays (IMAs) that probably have properties of stretch receptors (Page and Blackshaw 1998; Lynn and Blackshaw 1999; Phillips and Powley 2000; Zagorodnyuk and Brookes 2000; Zagorodnyuk et al. 2001; Page et al. 2002; Lynn et al. 2003). Mucosal afferent endings are situated in the lamina propria but do not penetrate the basal lamina (i.e., they are not located juxtaepithelially) and do not directly come into contact with the luminal content. Exceptions are afferents innervating the squamous epithelium of the esophagus and anal canal. Responses of vagal afferents to maltose, glucose and intraluminal osmotic stimuli are mediated by enterochromaffin cells releasing 5-hydroxytryptamine

(5-HT, serotonin) and by 5-HT$_3$ receptors in the terminals of the vagal afferents (Zhu et al. 2001). Responses of vagal afferents to protein products of long-chain lipids are mediated by enteroendocrine cells releasing cholecystokinin (CCK) and the CCK$_A$ receptor in the terminals of the vagal afferent neurons. These afferents do not seem to be mechanosensitive (Richards et al. 1996; Lal et al. 2001; Beyak and Grundy 2005; Brookes et al. 2013; Spencer et al. 2016c).

Vagal Afferent Neurons and Body Protection

Experiments on animals show that vagal afferents play an important role in general body protection (see Jänig 2005, 2020b):

- Vagal afferent neurons may be associated with the gut-associated lymphoid tissue (GALT) and excited by inflammatory and toxic processes. This excitation is probably mediated by enterochromaffin cells releasing 5-HT, by enteroendocrine cells releasing CCK and by mast cells releasing histamine and other compounds (Williams et al. 1997; Kirkup et al. 2001; Kreis et al. 2002). The functional specificity of these afferents, with respect to the different types of intraluminal stimuli, is unknown (see Subchapter 5.6 and Figure 5.13).
- Excitation of vagal afferents, innervating the liver and upper gastrointestinal tract (proximal duodenum and distal stomach) and projecting through the hepatic branch of the abdominal vagus nerve, triggers during inflammation in the viscera (e.g., generated experimentally by intraperitoneal injection of the bacterial cell wall endotoxin, lipopolysaccharide) so-called *illness or sickness responses* (which includes immobility, decrease of social interaction, decrease in food intake, formation of taste aversion to novel food, decrease of digestion, loss of weight [anorexia], fever, increase of sleep, change in endocrine functions, malaise, hyperalgesic behavior) (Dantzer et al. 1998, 2000, 2008; Maier and Watkins 1998; Watkins and Maier 1999, 2000; Goehler et al. 2000). Based on lesion experiments, it is hypothesized that vagal afferents innervating the liver are activated by proinflammatory cytokines (interleukin 1 [IL-1β], IL-6, tumor necrosis factor α [TNFα]) released by activated macrophages (Kupffer cells), dendritic cells and leukocytes and signal these events to the brain

Table 2.1 Visceral afferent neurons, sensations, regulations and reflexes

Organ[a]		Afferent neuron[b]	Sensation[c]	Regulation/reflex[d]
Respiratory tract				
Pharynx, larynx	Vagal	Mechanoreceptor (pressure), irritant receptors, cold receptors, flow receptors	Rawness, irritation, desire to cough, pain, nausea	Aspiration reflex, cough reflex, swallowing, bronchodilatation, etc.
Trachea, bronchi, lung	Vagal	Irritant receptors, C-fiber (epithelial) receptors	Substernal rawness, irritation, urge to cough, tightness	Burn–cough reflex, laryngoconstriction, bronchoconstriction, mucus secretion, hyperpnea
	Vagal	Slowly adapting receptors	?/no	Hering–Breuer reflex
	Vagal	J-receptor	Irritation in throat, breathlessness, discomfort, pain	Respiratory-protective reflexes
	Spinal	Yes (function?)	?/no	?
Cardiovascular organs				
Large blood vessels	Vagal	Baroreceptors, chemoreceptors	No	Cardiovascular regulation, reflexes
	Spinal	Mechanoreceptors	Discomfort, pain	Spinal reflexes
Heart	Vagal	Mechanoreceptors (atrial, ventricular)	No	Cardiovascular regulation, reflexes
	Spinal	Atrial receptors	No	Cardiovascular reflexes
	Spinal	Ventricular, coronary	Discomfort, pain, other sensations ?	Cardio-cardiac reflexes, other cardiovascular reflexes
Gastrointestinal tract				
Esophagus	Vagal	Mechanoreceptors (tension)	Fullness, thermal sensations, heartburn	Propulsive peristalsis, vomiting
	Spinal	Mechanoreceptors	Discomfort, (tension) pain	?
Stomach	Vagal	Mechanoreceptors (tension)[e]	Fullness/emptiness	Storage, relaxation
	Vagal	Mucosal receptors (mechano-, chemo-, thermo-)[f]	Satiety/hunger thermal sensations (?)	Secretion, peristalsis, vomiting

Table 2.1 (cont.)

Organ[a]		Afferent neuron[b]	Sensation[c]	Regulation/reflex[d]
Duodenum	Spinal	Mechanoreceptors (serosal)[g]	Discomfort, pain	Intestino-intestinal reflexes
	Vagal	Mechanoreceptors (tension)[e]	?	Secretion, peristalsis
Ileum, jejunum	Vagal	Mucosal receptors[f] (mechano-, chemo-, thermo-)	?	Secretion (?), peristalsis (?)
Liver	Spinal	Mechanoreceptors (serosal)[g]	Discomfort, pain	Intestino-intestinal reflexes
	Vagal	Osmoreceptors	Thirst	Osmoregulation (?)
Gallbladder	Spinal	Mechanoreceptors	Discomfort, pain	?
Pancreas	Spinal	Mechanoreceptors	Discomfort, pain	
Colon, rectum	Spinal-sacral[h]	Mechanoreceptors (wall)	Fullness, call to defecate, discomfort, pain	Defecation, continence reflexes
	Spinal-ThL[h]	Mechanoreceptors (serosal)[g]	Discomfort, pain	?
Anal canal	Spinal-sacral[h]	Mechanoreceptors, thermoreceptors, nociceptors (?)	Shearing sensation, thermal sensation (?), pain	Ano-rectal, ano-vesical reflexes
Urinary tract				
Kidney	Spinal-ThL	Mechanoreceptors, chemoreceptors	Pain	Reno-renal reflexes, other reflexes
Ureter	Spinal-sacral/ThL[h]	Mechanoreceptors	Pain	?
Urinary bladder, urethra	Spinal-sacral[h]	Mechanoreceptors	Fullness, urge to micturate, discomfort, pain	Micturition, continence reflexes
	Spinal-ThL[h]	Mechanoreceptors	Discomfort, pain	?
Spleen	Spinal	Mechanoreceptors	Discomfort, pain	?
General				

Table 2.1 (cont.)

Organ[a]	Afferent neuron[b]	Sensation[c]	Regulation/reflex[d]
All organs, inclusive of blood vessels etc.	Spinal	Mechanoreceptors (high-threshold) chemoreceptors (?) (mechanoinsensitive afferents)	?; Pain under pathophysiological conditions	Defensive reactions/reflexes (?), trophic functions (?)

Spinal: Spinal afferent neurons projecting through the splanchnic nerves to the thoracic, upper lumbar or sacral spinal cord. The cell bodies of these afferents lie in the thoracic, upper lumbar or sacral dorsal root ganglia.

Vagal: Visceral afferent neurons projecting through the vagal or glossopharyngeal nerves to the nucleus of the solitary tract in the medulla oblongata. The cell bodies of these afferent neurons lie in the inferior (nodose) or superior (jugular) ganglion of the vagal nerve or in the petrosal ganglion.

Data from Hertz (1911), Paintal (1973, 1986), Malliani (1982), Mei (1983, 1985), Coleridge and Coleridge (1984), Andrews (1986), Jänig and Morrison (1986), Widdicombe (1986), Grundy (1988), Jänig and Koltzenburg (1993), Undem and Weinreich (2005). Modified from Jänig (1996).

a Organ or organ system.
b Functional type of afferent neuron.
c Type of sensation(s) elicited when the respective afferent neuron(s) is (are) stimulated.
d Type(s) of regulation and reflexes associated with the afferent neurons.
e Receptors lying in the muscular wall of the gastrointestinal tract, responding to distension and contraction.
f Stimulus specificity unclear.
g Receptors lying particularly at the insertion of the mesenteries and responding to mechanical and chemical stimuli.
h Spinal-sacral, sacral visceral afferent neurons; Spinal-ThL thoracolumbar visceral afferent neurons.

resulting in illness responses (Figure 2.5). The proinflammatory cytokines are suggested to activate the vagal afferents. The physiological properties of these vagal afferents are rather unknown. Some vagal afferents innervating the hepatoportal system are excited by IL-1β (Niijima 1996). The central mechanisms underlying the sickness responses are also not established but likely involve ascending visceral afferent input to the ventrolateral hypothalamus and especially the bed nucleus of the stria terminalis (BNST) by way of the A1 noradrenergic cell group in the caudal ventrolateral medulla (see Craig 2018).

- Activity in vagal afferents innervating the small intestine (i.e., projecting through the celiac branches of the abdominal vagus nerves) is important in reflex modulation of inflammatory processes (e.g., in the knee joint) and mechanical hyperalgesic behavior (by sensitization of nociceptors) in remote body tissues involving the sympatho-adrenal system and possibly the hypothalamo–pituitary–adrenal system (Green et al. 1995, 1997; Miao et al., 1997a, b, 2000, 2001, 2003a, b; Khasar et al. 1998a, b, 2003; Jänig et al. 2000; Jänig and Green 2014; Jänig 2020a).

- Electrical stimulation of abdominal vagal afferents inhibits nociceptive impulse transmission in the spinal dorsal horn and depresses nociceptive behavior, showing that these afferents have antinociceptive function (Gebhart and Randich 1992; Randich and Gebhart 1992). Electrical stimulation of cervical vagal afferents in monkeys suppresses transmission of impulse activity in spinothalamic relay neurons with nociceptive function at all levels of the spinal cord, whereas electrical stimulation of subdiaphragmatic vagal afferents has no effect on spinothalamic relay neurons in this species, arguing that (particularly cardiopulmonary) vagal afferents are involved in this inhibitory control in monkeys. In the rat, indirect evidence shows that some ongoing central inhibition of nociceptive impulse transmission (occurring probably in the dorsal horn) is normally maintained by spontaneous activity in vagal afferents (Khasar et al. 1998a, b). The central pathways mediating the inhibitory effect are neurons in the subceruleus–parabrachial complex (noradrenergic) and neurons in the nucleus raphe magnus of the rostral ventromedial medulla (serotonergic) that project to the spinal cord (see Foreman [1989]). The functional types of vagal afferents involved in this antinociception are unknown.

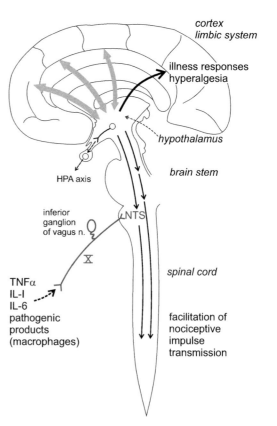

Figure 2.5 Illness responses (including hyperalgesia and pain) elicited by pathogenic stimuli in the viscera. Pathogens (bacteria, viruses, others) activate phagocytic immune cells (macrophages; Kupffer cells in the liver). These activated immune cells release proinflammatory cytokines (interleukin 1 [IL-1], IL-6, tumor necrosis factor α [TNFα]). The cytokines activate vagal afferents projecting through the hepatic branch of the abdominal vagus nerves. Stimulation of vagal afferents activates second-order neurons in the nucleus tractus solitarii (NTS) in the medulla oblongata. This leads to activation of pathways creating illness responses, which include hyperalgesia and pain. Illness responses are generated by activation of the paraventricular nucleus of the hypothalamus and structures in the limbic system (e.g., the hippocampus). Specifically, pain and hyperalgesia are generated by facilitation of nociceptive impulse transmission in the spinal cord (and probably elsewhere). This facilitation is mediated by descending pathways from the NTS (via the nucleus raphe magnus) and probably from the hypothalamus. HPA axis, hypothalamo–pituitary–adrenal axis; X, vagus nerve. After Goehler et al. (2000).

In *conclusion*, the animal experiments clearly indicate that cardiopulmonary and abdominal vagal afferent neurons are not only important in the context of regulation of respiratory, cardiovascular and gastro-intestinal functions but also in the context of protection of the body. This latter function involves the spinal cord, brain stem, hypothalamus and limbic system structures and, as efferent pathways, neuro-endocrine systems to the effector cells, such as the sympatho-adrenal system and the hypothalamo–pituitary–adrenal system (Jänig 2005, 2020a). Thus, vagal afferents seem to sense activity related to injurious events in the visceral body domain, including microorganisms and toxic substances invading the body via the largest defense barrier of the body, the gut-associated lymphoid tissue (GALT; Mowat 2003) in the small intestine, and via the liver. The physiological response properties of these vagal afferents are unknown; however, it is not far-fetched to predict that several different types of vagal afferents are involved (see also Subchapter 5.6 and Figure 5.13).

2.3.2 Spinal Visceral Afferent Neurons

The projections of visceral afferent neurons to the spinal cord from different organs are segmentally organized, the projection from each organ exhibiting a wide segmental distribution (Jänig and Morrison 1986). No distinct organotopic organization of this projection is present in the dorsal horn. The afferents project to laminae I (including outer lamina II) and V of the dorsal horn and to deeper laminae (laminae VI, VII and X), sparing largely lamina II (substantia gelatinosa Rolandi; see Figure 2.6) and laminae III and IV (nucleus proprius). Occasionally they project to the contralateral laminae V and X. Single visceral afferent neurons with unmyelinated fibers project over four to five segments and over the whole mediolateral width of the dorsal horn (Figure 2.6). This projection pattern is similar to that of small-diameter afferents from deep body structures (skeletal muscle and joints [Craig and Mense 1983; Craig et al. 1988; Mense and Craig 1988]) and contrasts with that of single cutaneous afferent neurons with unmyelinated fibers, which is spatially much more restricted (Cervero and Connell 1984; Sugiura et al. 1989; for review of spinal projection of visceral and other afferents see Willis and Coggeshall [2004a]).

The low density of the spinal visceral afferent innervation, the broad segmental projection of spinal afferents from different organs, and the broad spinal segmental projection of individual visceral afferent neurons are consistent with the poor localization and graduation of visceral sensations mediated by spinal visceral afferent neurons.

Thoracolumbar Visceral Afferent Neurons

The sensory receptors of *thoracolumbar visceral afferents* are situated in the serosa, at the attachment sites of the mesenteries, in the walls of some

SPINAL PROJECTIONS OF AFFERENT C-FIBERS

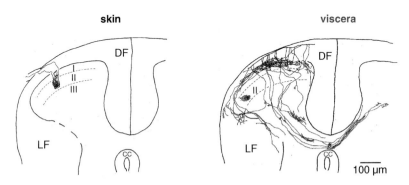

Figure 2.6 Camera lucida drawing of the central termination patterns of single unmyelinated afferent fibers innervating somatic (left) or visceral tissues (right) in the guinea pig. The tracer (*Phaseolus vulgaris* leuco-agglutinin) was injected intracellularly through a micropipette into the cell bodies of afferent neurons of the dorsal root ganglion Th13 in anesthetized animals. The afferent neurons were recorded through the same micropipette and identified as somatic or visceral by their responses to electrical stimulation of a somatic (subcostal nerve) or visceral nerve (stimulation of celiac ganglion) and the receptive fields were stimulated by noxious stimuli (pinch, heat, cold). The animals recovered from this experimental procedure. Two to four days later the animals were fixed under anesthesia and the spinal cord removed and cut into transverse 50 μm-thick parasagittal sections. The tracer was visualized in the spinal cord sections and the axon ramifications of the labeled neurons reconstructed. I, II, III indicate the laminae of the gray matter according to Rexed (1954). Transverse sections. cc, central canal; DF, dorsal funiculus; LF, lateral funiculus. For details see text. From Sugiura et al. (1989) with permission.

organs and in the mucosa. It is unclear whether afferents supplying hollow organs (e.g., the gastrointestinal tract or the urinary bladder) innervate the mucosa as well as serosa and wall of the organs, or whether afferents innervating the mucosa are separate from those innervating the serosa and wall of the organs. Furthermore, the density of visceral afferent neurons innervating serosa, musculature or mucosa is unknown (Note 4). Most of these afferents seem to be mechanosensitive and react to distension and contraction of the organs. But they are also activated by chemical stimuli as occurs during inflammation and ischemia of the organs. Thus, these afferents are polymodal and probably do not signal specific events to the spinal cord, except that they are associated with a particular organ; they trigger protective reflexes and regulations, pain, discomfort and local protective responses when excited (Haupt et al. 1983; Longhurst 1995; Pan and Longhurst 1996; Pan et al. 1999).

Thoracolumbar spinal visceral afferent neurons are involved in extraspinal and spinal intestino-intestinal reflexes and probably also in specific organ reflexes, for example to the heart (cardio-cardiac reflexes), the kidney (reno-renal reflexes) or bronchopulmonary system (see Malliani 1982; Jänig 1988; DiBona and Kopp 1997; Hummel et al. 1997; Kopp and DiBona 2000). However, this has not been thoroughly studied (see Subchapter 9.2). Activity in these visceral afferent neurons may be related mainly to visceral nociception, visceral pain and discomfort (see next Subchapter) in addition to the peripheral ("effector") functions (see Subchapter 2.2).

Sacral Visceral Afferent Neurons

Pelvic organs are innervated by sacral as well as thoracolumbar visceral afferent neurons. The density of innervation by sacral visceral afferent neurons is higher than that by thoracolumbar ones. This is related to the precise control of the pelvic organs by the central nervous system (see Subchapter 9.3). The sacral component of this visceral afferent innervation is essential for the regulation of evacuation and storage functions and of the reproductive organs, as well as for the generation of non-painful and most painful sensations associated with the pelvic organs. Thoracolumbar visceral afferents are not essential for the regulation of the pelvic organs and the associated non-painful sensations but may be important for the generation of

pain (see Jänig and Morrison [1986]; Jänig and McLachlan [1987]; Jänig and Koltzenburg [1993]; Jänig and Häbler [2002]).

2.4 Role of Visceral Afferent Neurons in Visceral Nociception and Pain

2.4.1 Vagal Afferent Neurons

Vagal Afferent Neurons Innervating Abdominal Organs

The general contention is that visceral pain elicited from pelvic and most abdominal organs is triggered by excitation of spinal visceral afferent neurons and not by excitation of vagal afferent neurons (Cervero 1994). This is supported by studies of behavioral responses in animals and clinical studies of patients using stimulation and blocking techniques (Foerster 1927; Cannon 1933). However, the situation is not entirely clear for the gastroduodenal section of the gastrointestinal tract. Whether patients with complete interruption of spinal ascending impulse transmission at the thoracic level T1 or at a more rostral segmental level can experience pain from the gastroduodenal section of the gastrointestinal tract (e.g., during gastritis, a peptic ulcer or distension of the stomach) has never been systematically investigated. Patients with complete lesion of the cervical spinal cord may experience abdominal hunger, dread and nausea (Crawford and Frankel 1971). Furthermore, these patients may experience vague sensations of fullness after a hot meal, but usually acid reflux or an obstructed or distended visceral organ does not generate discomfort and pain (Juler and Eltorai 1985; Strauther et al. 1999). There are occasional observations in these patients showing that gastric distension may generate pain and discomfort (Dietz, personal communication) and that an acute perforation of a duodenal ulcer is accompanied by violent pain in the right or left shoulder (page 284 in Guttmann [1976]), indicating that vagal afferents may be involved or possibly phrenic afferents projecting through the phrenico-abdominal ramus to the cervical segments C3 to C5.

Activation of vagal afferents innervating the stomach elicits emesis, bloating and nausea, all three being protective reactions. In the rat, acute gastric inflammation generated by acid triggers aversive responses, which are dependent on activity in vagal afferents (Lamb et al. 2003). Experiments on rats show that influx of acid into, or other chemical insults of, the gastroduodenal mucosa lead to a host of locally and centrally organized protective reactions that are mediated by spinal visceral and vagal afferent neurons. Activation of vagal afferents by these chemical stimuli leads to activation of neurons in the NTS, area postrema, lateral parabrachial nucleus, thalamic and hypothalamic paraventricular nuclei, supraoptic nucleus and central amygdala, but not in the insular cortex (the major central representation area of the stomach; see Subchapter 2.6) (Michl et al. 2001). Holzer has put forward the idea that vagal afferents innervating the mucosa of the gastroduodenal section of the gastrointestinal tract are involved in chemonociception and mediate autonomic, endocrine and behavioral protective reactions.

Vagal afferents are not involved in pain perception, but in the emotional aspect of pain and therefore indirectly in upper abdominal hyperalgesia (Holzer and Maggi 1998; Holzer 2002a, b, 2003). This fascinating idea needs verification by further experimentation. For example, it is unclear how activity in spinal visceral afferents and vagal afferents is centrally integrated in vivo so as to elicit the protective reflexes, protective behavior and pain sensations, including visceral hyperalgesia. Furthermore, it is also unclear how activity in vagal afferents is responsible for the emotional aspects of visceral pain, whereas activity in spinal visceral afferents is responsible for the conscious perception of visceral pain (see Subchapter 2.6).

Vagal Afferents Innervating Thoracic Visceral Organs

The situation is at least as complex for the thoracic visceral organs. Pain elicited from the proximal esophagus and proximal airways is probably mediated by vagal afferents innervating the mucosa of these organs. These afferents are peptidergic (i.e., they contain CGRP and/or substance P); their cell bodies are probably located in the superior (jugular) ganglion of the vagus nerve (see Berthoud and Neuhuber [2000] [cells in the inferior (nodose) ganglion of the vagus nerve are almost exclusively peptide-negative, whereas many neurons in the jugular ganglion contain peptides]). Activation of these afferents generates neurogenic inflammation in the mucosa, which has been extensively studied in the mucosa of the airways (venular plasma extravasation and vasodilation; McDonald et al. 1988; McDonald

1990, 1997). Pain elicited from the more distal sections of esophagus and airways, as well as from the bronchi, may be produced by stimulation of spinal visceral afferent neurons and not of vagal afferents. However, this situation is unclear and needs further experimentation (see Hummel et al. 1997).

Cardiac pain (e.g., during ischemic heart disease) is generally considered to be mediated by spinal visceral afferents having their cell bodies in the dorsal root ganglia C8 to T9 (mainly T2 to T6). However, attempts to relieve pain associated with cardiac angina by surgical manipulations (cervico-thoracic sympathectomy, dorsal rhizotomy, injection of alcohol into the sympathetic chain) consistently showed that only 50% to 60% of patients report complete relief from angina following these interventions, while the remaining patients report either partial relief or no relief at all. With the caveat that some failures to relieve pain were attributed to incomplete spinal denervation of the heart, it is concluded that vagal afferents innervating particularly the inferior-posterior part of the heart may also mediate cardiac pain (for review and references see Meller and Gebhart [1992]).

This conclusion is supported by neurophysiological investigations in monkeys and rats showing that some spinothalamic tract (STT) neurons in the superficial dorsal horn and deeper laminae of the cervical segments C1 to C2 (C3) can be synaptically activated by electrical stimulation of cardiopulmonary spinal and vagal afferents or by injection of algogenic chemicals in the pericardial sac via both afferent pathways. The activation of the STT neurons by vagal afferents is relayed through the NTS. These STT neurons can also be activated synaptically by mechanical stimulation of the somatic receptive fields in the corresponding segments from the head, jaw, neck and shoulder (dermatomes, myotomes). These results are fully in line with clinical observations showing that cardiac pain may be referred to neck, shoulder and jaw (Lindgren and Olivecrona 1947; White and Bland 1948; Meller and Gebhart 1992). Finally, it must be taken into account that some phrenic afferents innervate the pericardium. These afferents are independent of vagal afferents and thoracic spinal afferents and project to the cervical segments C3 to C5. The same high cervical spinal segments contain neurons with similar convergent synaptic inputs from vagal, spinal visceral and somatic afferents that project to more caudal spinal thoracic, lumbar and sacral segments. These neurons are involved in the inhibitory control of nociceptive impulse transmission (for discussion and literature see Foreman [1989, 1999]; Qin et al. [2001]; Chandler et al. [2002]).

2.4.2 Spinal Visceral Afferent Neurons

Visceral Afferent Neurons and Peripheral Mechanisms of Visceral Nociception

Spinal visceral afferents are involved in neural regulation of visceral organs (in particular, sacral visceral afferents), reflexes and sensations. The messages that trigger these activities must be derived entirely from the activity in the spinal visceral afferent neurons. How do central neurons decode the afferent messages in order to produce appropriate regulation, reflexes and sensations? Does the decoding process of the afferent activity depend on different types of visceral afferent neurons with respect to the different (adequate) stimuli? In other words, are there distinct functional types of spinal visceral afferent neurons that can be characterized with respect to particular functions, such as painful and non-painful sensations and organ reactions (Cervero and Jänig, 1992; Cervero 1994, 1996)? These questions have been systematically addressed for the lumbar and sacral afferent supply of the urinary bladder and colon in the cat (Blumberg et al. 1983; Haupt et al. 1983; Bahns et al. 1986a, 1987; Jänig and Koltzenburg 1990, 1991) and rat (Sengupta and Gebhart 1994a, b, 1995; Su and Gebhart 1998), for the thoracic afferent supply of the rat stomach (Ozaki and Gebhart 2001), the heart of the cat (Lombardi et al. 1981; Malliani 1982; Malliani and Lombardi 1982), the biliary system of the ferret (Cervero, 1982) and the esophagus of the opossum (Sengupta et al. 1990), for the afferent supply of the ureter in the guinea pig (Cervero and Sann 1989), for the hypogastric and pelvic afferents innervating the female reproductive organs (Berkley et al. 1988, 1990, 1993) and for the afferent innervation of the testis (Kumazawa 1986; Kumazawa et al. 1987).

Spinal visceral afferents can be distinguished according to the visceral organs or organ components they innervate (a visceral afferent neuron innervates only one organ or part of an organ) and to the spatial arrangement of their terminals (e.g., in the smooth musculature, in the mucosa, in the serosa, in the myenteric plexus). These spatial arrangements also determine the adequate stimuli that excite the visceral afferents (such as distension, contraction, shearing and intraluminal chemical stimuli). Morphologically,

the peripheral terminals of spinal visceral afferent neurons appear rather uniform. However, this uniformity does not necessarily apply to the transduction mechanisms for physical and chemical stimuli.

Most spinal visceral afferents are polymodal and can be excited by mechanical and chemical stimuli and possibly also by thermal stimuli. In the cat, sacral visceral afferents innervating the urinary bladder or colon have no spontaneous activity, but about 50% of the thoracolumbar visceral afferents innervating the two organs do (about 0.2 to 1 imp/s). In the rat, both populations of spinal visceral afferents may have spontaneous activity under physiological conditions. The classification of spinal visceral afferent neurons as nociceptive or non-nociceptive is difficult, in view of the different types of visceral organs. Based on the experimental investigations of mechanosensitive spinal visceral afferents innervating urinary bladder, hindgut, stomach, gallbladder and ureter, most investigators believe that the afferent neurons can be divided into low-threshold and high-threshold afferents and that the low-threshold afferents are involved in organ regulation and non-painful sensations, whereas the high-threshold afferents are involved in visceral pain and protective reflexes. Figure 2.7 demonstrates a representative example for sacral afferents innervating the urinary bladder in the cat. The afferents respond in a graded way to distension of the urinary bladder (generated by slow filling or intraluminal pressure steps). Two populations of sacral visceral spinal afferents can be discriminated: a low-threshold population with high maximal discharge rates and a smaller high-threshold population with relatively low maximal discharge rates (marked by crosses [unmyelinated] and asterisks [myelinated]). Similar results have been obtained in the rat urinary bladder, rat and cat colon, and rat stomach (Cervero 1994, 1996; Gebhart 1996; Su and Gebhart 1998; Su et al. 1997a, b; Coutinho et al. 2000; Ozaki and Gebhart 2001).

The distinction between two groups of spinal visceral afferents that has been reported particularly for hollow organs, a high- and a low-threshold group associated with nociceptive and non-nociceptive functions, respectively, must be considered with caution. It is probably too simple:

• Low-threshold spinal visceral afferents encode in their activity a large range of intraluminal pressures during distension and contraction, covering the non-noxious as well as the noxious range

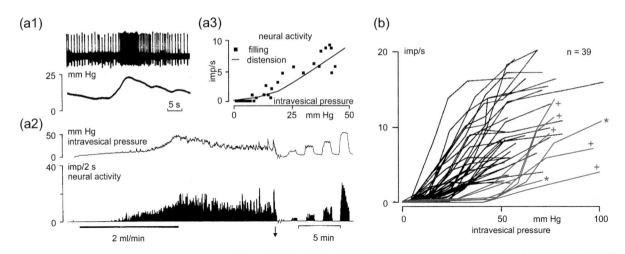

Figure 2.7 Activation of sacral visceral afferents innervating the urinary bladder by distension. (a) Activation of a single myelinated (Aδ) low-threshold afferent fiber during slow filling and to intravesical pressure steps. (a$_1$) Activity during filling (2 ml/min) through a urethral catheter. Lower record, intravesical pressure with isovolumetric contractions. (a$_2$) Activity during slow filling (bar) and during a series of intravesical pressure steps (right). Arrow, release of bladder content. The afferent fiber had no spontaneous activity when the bladder was empty. (a$_3$) Stimulus–response functions of the afferent fiber during slow filling (squares) and during intravesical pressure steps (solid-line curve). (b) Stimulus–response functions of sacral afferents innervating the urinary bladder to bladder distension by slow filling (n = 39 fibers). All low-threshold afferents were small-diameter (Aδ) fibers. Five of the seven high-threshold afferents (+) were C-fibers and two Aδ-fibers (*). After Häbler et al. (1990a, 1993a).

(Bahns et al. 1987; Häbler et al. 1993a; Su et al. 1997a, b; Coutinho et al. 2000).

- High-threshold spinal visceral afferents are relatively rare and exhibit lower rates of activity to maximal stimuli (Häbler et al. 1990a; Su et al. 1997a, b; Coutinho et al. 2000).

- Many thoracolumbar spinal visceral afferents (Blumberg et al. 1983; Bahns et al. 1986a) and (in the rat) sacral visceral afferents are spontaneously active (Su et al. 1997a, b; Ozaki and Gebhart 2001).

- Low- and high-threshold afferents are polymodal and can be activated and sensitized by chemical stimuli and experimental inflammation, as well as by distortion and ischemia (Haupt et al. 1983; Häbler et al. 1993a, b; Su et al. 1997a, b; Coutinho et al. 2000).

- Low- and high-threshold spinal visceral afferents cannot be distinguished by independent physiological (transduction mechanisms), anatomical (e.g., projection patterns to the spinal cord), histochemical (e.g., peptide content) or pharmacological criteria (e.g., receptors for inflammatory mediators, opioids etc.; Sengupta et al. 1996; Su et al. 1997a, b).

These results may imply that, *under biological conditions*, the same populations of afferents may well encode processes that lead to organ regulation, non-painful sensations as well as painful sensations. Pain from these organs would then be associated with a high intensity of discharge in the visceral afferent neurons, with the degree of their recruitment, and with the recruitment of high-threshold afferents at intraluminal pressures of >50 mmHg, which are frankly painful (Häbler et al. 1993b; Jänig and Häbler 1995), but which contribute relatively little to the impulse activity from the urinary bladder. Also, for the heart, the same spinal cardiac afferent neurons may be involved in regulation of the cardiovascular system (e.g., during exercise) as well as cardiac pain (Malliani 1982; Malliani and Lombardi 1982).

As already mentioned, this interpretation is not generally accepted and cannot necessarily be generalized for other organs. (1) Neurophysiological investigations of the spinal afferents supplying the biliary system in the ferret (Cervero 1982) or the ureter in the guinea pig in vitro (Cervero and Sann 1989) have shown that most spinal visceral afferents can only be activated at high intraluminal pressures that are normally associated with pain and an equivalent behavior in animals. These afferents probably have only nociceptive function. (2) Baker et al. (1980) have analyzed the spinal afferent supply of the heart and claimed to have found a small separate group of afferent neurons that respond preferentially to bradykinin (a pain-producing substance) and have rather high thresholds to mechanical stimuli.

It is possible that noxious stimuli, damage and impending damage in the visceral domain are encoded in different ways by spinal afferents for different organs. Therefore care must be taken when generalizing from the investigation of one organ to the others (Cervero and Jänig 1992). It is, however, also possible that some of the investigations just mentioned concentrated on populations of spinal visceral afferents that are activated only under pathophysiological conditions and are normally silent (see below).

Recruitment of Normally Mechanoinsensitive Afferent Neurons

It has been shown for the sacral afferent innervation of the urinary bladder and colon of the cat that about 90% of the visceral afferent neurons with unmyelinated fibers projecting through the pelvic splanchnic nerve are silent under normal conditions and cannot be activated at intraluminal pressures of up to 70 mmHg (Bahns et al. 1987; Häbler et al. 1990a; Jänig and Koltzenburg 1991), i.e., at pressures that elicit pain in humans. Some of these silent sacral visceral afferent neurons with unmyelinated fibers may innervate the internal reproductive organs, urethra or anal canal and some may innervate the mucosa of the colon or the urothelium of the urinary bladder, and distension and contraction of the hollow organs may not be adequate stimuli for them. When the urinary bladder is inflamed, some of these silent afferent neurons may develop resting activity and can be activated during normal non-noxious stimulation of the organ. The afferent neurons that are activated during evacuation under healthy conditions may develop ongoing activity after inflammation, even when the organ is empty, and may exhibit increased responses to adequate stimulation. Thus, under pathophysiological conditions such as inflammation, the visceral afferent supply of the urinary bladder is sensitized and novel types of visceral afferent neurons with chemo- and mechanosensitivity are recruited (Häbler et al. 1990a; Jänig and Koltzenburg 1990).

Recruitment of normally mechanoinsensitive spinal visceral afferents under pathophysiological conditions (e.g., during inflammation) may occur in all visceral organs. For example, various structures in the retroperitoneal space, such as blood vessels, nerves, lymph nodes, etc., are innervated by afferents that are normally not activated, but are recruited in pathophysiological states (Bahns et al. 1986b). During angina pectoris, afferents may be sensitized and recruited, although Malliani believed that this is not the case (Lombardi et al. 1981). It is a matter of debate whether these silent and normally mechanoinsensitive visceral afferents constitute a distinct category of spinal visceral afferents that is recruited under inflammation and other pathophysiological conditions or whether these afferents are simply extremely high-threshold nociceptive fibers (for discussion see Cervero [1996]).

The idea that tissues are innervated by silent and mechanoinsensitive afferent neurons with unmyelinated fibers that are activated in diseased states (Michaelis et al. 1996) was first demonstrated for the afferent innervation of the joint capsule in the cat (Grigg et al. 1986; Schaible and Schmidt 1988). It probably applies to *all tissues* (for the skin in rat and monkey see Meyer et al. [1991], Simone et al. [1991], Kress et al. [1992], Davis et al. [1993], for the vein in cats see Michaelis et al. [1994], for the skin in humans see Schmidt et al. [1995, 2002]). These silent and normally mechanoinsensitive (or mechanically extremely high-threshold) spinal visceral afferent neurons may overlap with the spinal visceral afferent neurons that have only peripheral (efferent) functions under physiological conditions (Figure 2.4; Holzer and Maggi 1998; Holzer 2002a, b, 2003).

2.5 Relation Between Functional Types of Visceral Afferent Neurons, Organ Regulation and Sensations

2.5.1 General Considerations

Events in the visceral organs are encoded in the activity of visceral afferent neurons and in the activity of central neurons in the neuraxis, which then leads to appropriate organ regulation, reflexes and sensations. Several points need to be emphasized:

1. In healthy conditions, afferent activity elicited during regulation of visceral organs is usually *not* accompanied by distinct visceral sensations and aversive feelings. This is quite obvious for the regulation of the cardiovascular system, of the respiratory system and of most parts of the gastro-intestinal tract.

2. Visceral sensations are dependent on the representations of the visceral organs in the rostral part of the dorsal posterior insular cortex (see Subchapter 2.6 and Figure 2.15). Distinct non-painful sensations can be elicited particularly from those organs that are precisely regulated in the social context of human and animal behavior, such as the entrance organs and the evacuative organs (trachea, esophagus, stomach, hindgut, lower urinary tract). These sensations are integral components of the neural regulation of the organs, leading to appropriate behavior and suppression or enhancement of organ activity (e.g., continence and evacuation).

3. Events that endanger visceral organs and therefore also the organism may lead to discomfort and pain. These sensations can be elicited from all visceral organs or their capsules. Activity in spinal visceral afferent neurons and in vagal afferent neurons innervating the proximal esophagus and the proximal trachea is correlated with these sensations. They are integral components of protective behavior (which includes autonomic protective reflexes).

4. Emotional feelings and their expression (by the somatomotor system, e.g., in facial expression, and by the autonomic systems, e.g. in the adaptive responses of the cardiovascular system, gastrointestinal tract, evacuative organs, etc.) are represented in the telencephalon. Both are generated *in parallel* by the brain without needing to be triggered by the peripheral afferent input from the visceral and deep somatic body domains (see Figure 11.1 and Subchapter 11.3). However, activity in visceral afferent neurons (and in afferent neurons from superficial and deep somatic tissues) shapes the centrally generated emotional feelings. It is virtually impossible to disprove that emotions (feelings and expression) are evoked ("caused") by afferent activity from viscera and deep somatic structures during bodily changes, as originally proposed by James and Lange (James 1884, 1994; Meyers 1986).

2.5.2 Encoding of Visceral Events in the Activity of Afferent and Central Neurons: A Concept

Are the different qualities of sensation (including visceral discomfort and pain), organ regulation and reflexes that originate from a visceral organ elicited by the excitation of different types of afferents, or are they all subserved by a single category of afferent? Theoretically, there are several ways in which different peripheral stimuli in the visceral domain could be encoded by primary afferent and central neurons so as to elicit these sensations, reactions and reflexes:

1. Primary afferents from an organ react specifically to certain stimuli and not to others. These afferents are more or less specifically connected to second-order neurons in the spinal cord and brain stem, leading, when excited, to characteristic sensations and reflexes. This concept is compatible with the specificity theory and with the idea of an "adequate stimulus" as originally described by Sherrington (1900, 1906). According to this idea, non-painful sensations, organ reflexes and regulation would be elicited by low-threshold afferents, and painful sensations, as well as protective reflexes, by high-threshold afferents (Figure 2.8a).

2. Primary afferents from an organ are homogeneous and encode the whole stimulus range in their activity but may have different thresholds (Figure 2.8b). This is described by the "intensity theory" or "summation hypothesis" and some physiologists believe that it may apply to the sensations associated with some visceral organs (Malliani and Lombardi 1982; Jänig and Morrison 1986).

3. The way in which the afferent activity is decoded in the spinal cord is unknown. Different classes of interneuron linked to the autonomic pathways supplying the visceral organs and other target organs and to neural pathways ascending to the brain stem and thalamus (which are concerned with organ regulations and sensations) must be postulated (see Chapter 9). Each of these types of interneurons must decode the afferent messages from these visceral organs in a different way and must have different stimulus–response functions for their activity. Otherwise it would be very difficult to understand in which way the distinct regulations, sensations and reflexes are brought about by stimulation of a rather homogeneous population of visceral afferents, such as the afferents from the urinary bladder (see Subchapter 9.3) or colon. We need to know how the different populations of interneurons, or networks of

interneurons, involved in organ regulation, protective reflexes and various types of sensations, behave during physiological activation of distinct groups of visceral afferents (see Chapter 9).

This point of view is somewhat simplistic. Specificity is brought about by a molecular specialization of the peripheral receptors with respect to the adequate (physical and chemical) stimuli and by the central synaptic connectivity of the central projections of the afferent neurons. The specificity applies certainly to cutaneous sensations elicited by stimulation of mechanosensitive myelinated and nociceptive

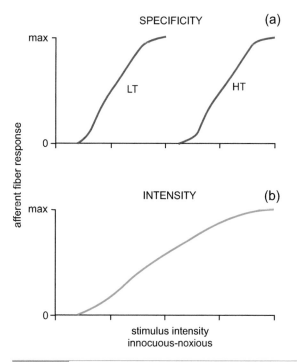

unmyelinated cutaneous afferents from the distal parts of the extremities in humans. Repetitive intraneural electrical microstimulation of *single* large-diameter myelinated afferents from Pacinian corpuscles, rapidly adapting receptors or slowly adapting type I receptors in the hand elicits distinct elementary vibration, touch or pressure sensations, respectively. These elementary sensations are projected to the receptive fields of the stimulated afferent fibers. Electrical microstimulation of microbundles of cutaneous C polymodal nociceptive afferents elicits dull or burning pain sensations, which are in most cases projected to skin areas lying within 10 mm of the C nociceptor receptive fields. Thus, for cutaneous mechanical and painful sensations the "stimulus specificity" of the cutaneous afferent neurons is connected to their "modality specificity" (Ochoa and Torebjörk 1983, 1989; Vallbo et al. 1984). This specificity applies to many autonomic reflexes too (see Chapters 4, 9 and 10).

2.5.3 A General Model of Central Encoding

The perception of non-painful and painful sensations and the complex regulation of visceral organs cannot be explained by reference to the encoding of peripheral events in afferent activity. We do not know the actual neuronal mechanisms of central decoding of the activity in most visceral afferent neurons, and in particular of spinal visceral afferent neurons. Practically all second-order neurons in the spinal cord (laminae V and deeper laminae; a few lamina I) with synaptic input from visceral afferents are viscerosomatic convergent neurons that receive additional synaptic input from skin and probably deep somatic tissues (see Subchapter 2.6). Traditionally the answer to the problem is that separate populations of afferent and central neurons are involved in the generation of painful and non-painful visceral sensations and regulatory visceral reflexes. Models explaining the mechanisms of normal painful and other sensations under biological and pathological conditions have been developed from studies of cutaneous sensations in animal models and humans (Baumann et al. 1991; Simone et al. 1991; LaMotte et al. 1992; Torebjörk et al. 1992; Willis and Coggeshall 2004a; Ringkamp et al. 2013). In analogy to these models, a model has been proposed that may explain how the different sensations (including pain) and regulations are triggered from hollow viscera (such as the urinary bladder or colon) in physiological and pathophysiological conditions. This model includes low-threshold, high-threshold as well as normally silent visceral afferents (Figure 2.9):

1. Normal distension and contraction of an organ activate low-threshold visceral afferents. Spinal neurons (interneurons, propriospinal neurons, tract neurons projecting to the brain stem and thalamus), which are involved in organ regulation (e.g., micturition, defecation and continence) and/or non-painful sensations, are activated (neuron R in Figure 2.9a).

2. Short intense distensions or contractions of the organ with an increase of intraluminal pressure above 40 to 50 mm Hg (a pressure that elicits discomfort and pain) generate high-frequency bursts in these low-threshold visceral afferents and activate some high-threshold afferents. This afferent excitation also activates other spinal second-order neurons (neuron P in Figure 2.9b), the excitation of which leads to a transient pain sensation. This situation may occasionally occur in everyday life.

3. Continuous or intermittent high-frequency activation of low- and high-threshold visceral afferents and recruitment of silent normally mechanoinsensitive afferents from the visceral organs (e.g., by inflammation of the organ) sensitizes the second-order neurons of the spinal nociceptive pathways (neuron P in Figure 2.9c; high-threshold ["nociceptive-specific"] neurons, wide dynamic range [convergent] neurons). This sensitization is either generated by all (high- and low-threshold) visceral afferents or only by high-threshold and normally silent visceral afferents. Now, activity in low-threshold afferents during normal regulation of the organs activates central sensitized neurons, resulting in enhanced pain perception (Figure 2.9c).

4. For visceral organs whose spinal afferent innervation consists largely of high-threshold afferents (e.g., the ureter or the biliary system), only pathway P may be excited when these afferents are activated (Figure 2.9c).

A component, which is possibly important in the generation of pain and other sensations elicited from visceral organs and which has not been explored so far, is the dual autonomic – parasympathetic and sympathetic – innervation of the organs. Neurons of these autonomic pathways exhibit distinct reflexes to

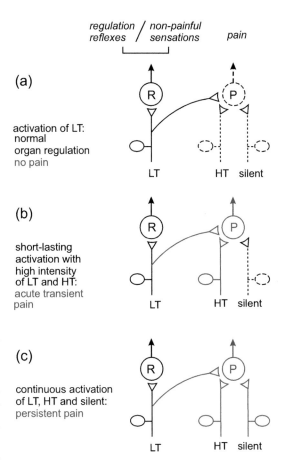

Figure 2.9 Diagrammatic representation of possible neuronal mechanisms of pain, other sensations and regulatory reflexes elicited from visceral organs. Visceral afferent neurons are shown to activate different central mechanisms, those mediating regulatory reflexes and non-painful sensations (left, pathway R) and those mediating pain (right, pathway P). (a) During normal organ regulation, low-threshold (LT) intensity encoding afferents are active. This activity is associated with the activation of pathway R. (b) Short transient, high-intensity stimuli evoke large responses in the low-threshold afferents. These responses may be grouped and burst-like. This afferent activity now activates pathway P and leads to brief periods of pain. The activation of pathway P may be supported by the recruitment of some high-threshold visceral afferents (HT), which may be present in variable percentages according to the visceral organ. (c) During prolonged forms of activation, including activation during inflammation, normally mechanoinsensitive nociceptors may be recruited and sensitized and high-threshold receptors sensitized. The afferent barrages in both of these may now increase the excitability of central neurons of the pathway P for input from low-threshold afferents (central sensitization). As a result, normal regulatory activity in the viscera could now be perceived as painful. Pathways involved in regulatory reflexes may also be sensitized. Modified from Cervero and Jänig (1992) with permission.

physiological stimuli (see Chapter 4). It is possible that these autonomic neurons exhibit abnormal reflexes when spinal visceral afferents are continuously activated, sensitized and recruited, and spinal second-order neurons are sensitized. These abnormal autonomic reflex activities may in turn enhance the impulse traffic in visceral afferent neurons and establish positive feedback loops consisting of visceral afferents, spinal cord neurons and autonomic output systems to the viscera. This type of feedback loop may be important for the understanding of mechanisms of visceral pain and of other sensations in coronary ischemia and myocardial infarction, non-cardiac chest pain, non-ulcer dyspepsia, irritable bowel syndrome, interstitial cystitis and other functional diseases of the viscera (Mayer and Raybould 1993; Mayer et al. 1995; Jänig 2009; Mayer and Bushnell 2009).

2.6 Central Ascending Pathways Associated with Autonomic Regulation and Body Interoception: A Generalization

Central pathways mediating the activity of spinal visceral and vagal visceral afferent neurons are related to autonomic and endocrine regulation, non-painful and painful visceral sensations and the shaping of emotions (see Figure 2.1). The physiology and anatomy of these pathways are only incompletely understood. This is due to: (1) difficulties in dissecting out central pathways conveying information in spinal visceral afferent neurons compared to information in primary afferent neurons with small-diameter axons (Aδ, C) from skin and deep somatic tissues; (2) difficulties in dissecting out central pathways related to vagal afferent neurons projecting to the NTS (see Subchapter 8.3) and (3) species differences between primates and non-primates (in particular the mouse and the rat).

Autonomic reflex pathways in spinal cord and lower brain stem linked to spinal visceral or vagal afferent neurons will be described in more detail in Chapters 8 to 10. In this subchapter I will generalize and concentrate on central ascending pathways mediating and representing interoceptive body sensations, including those related to the viscera and mediated by spinal and vagal visceral afferent neurons. Knowledge about these central pathways is based on anatomical and physiological studies conducted on animals (rat, cat, monkey), on recording and stimulation experiments conducted on patients undergoing brain surgery and on studies using brain imaging methods in humans (for review and literature see Cechetto and Saper [1990]; Cechetto [1995]; Saper [1995, 2002]; Craig [1996, 2002, 2003a, b, c, 2015]; Bernard and Bandler [1998]; Gauriau and Bernard [2002]; Willis and Coggeshall [2004a, b]). Here I will summarize what is known about ascending spinal and trigeminal tract neurons projecting to autonomic centers in the brain stem and (indirectly) hypothalamus and to thalamocortical systems, and about ascending pathways from the NTS related to specific and general visceral sensations. This short summary does not imply that information in primary afferent neurons is relayed to the autonomic centers and thalamocortical systems in passive ascending labeled-line systems. Probably every synapse in these ascending systems is subject to powerful multiple descending control by the forebrain. This descending ("efferent") control is exerted by pathways that are, in number of neurons, hypothesized to be up to five times more powerful than the ascending pathways. This expresses the importance of the control of ascending pathways by the forebrain.

2.6.1 Ascending Spinal Pathways Conveying Information From Interoceptive Afferents

Spinal interoceptive afferent neurons connect synaptically with second-order neurons in laminae I, V, VII, VIII and X of the spinal gray matter. They largely spare laminae II, III and IV. Some projections of spinal visceral afferents go to the contralateral side (Figure 2.6). The second-order neurons (excitatory or inhibitory) are either segmental or propriospinal interneurons or tract neurons projecting to supraspinal centers (i.e. to the lower and upper brain stem, and indirectly to the hypothalamus and thalamus). Interneurons have multiple functions mediating the effects of supraspinal centers on spinal circuits and being involved in autonomic regulation and reflexes (see Chapter 9), in regulation of movements as well as in regulation of synaptic transmission from primary afferent neurons to second-order neurons by acting pre- or postsynaptically.

In the rat, by far the most common second-order neurons in the superficial and deep spinal dorsal horn are segmental interneurons or propriospinal neurons, and only a few neurons project to supraspinal centers. For example, lamina I of the lumbar segment L_4 contains about 7500 to 8000 neurons. Only 5% of these neurons are tract neurons projecting to supraspinal centers and the rest are interneurons (Spike et al. 2003; Polgar et al. 2004). These proportions most likely also apply to the deeper laminae of the spinal gray matter of the rat and to primates, although quantitative data are not available. In primates, the number of spinothalamic neurons is significantly higher than in the rat (Willis and Coggeshall 2004b; Dostrovsky and Craig 2013, 2020).

Functions and Projections of Lamina I Neurons
Lamina I projection neurons of the spinal and trigeminal dorsal horn receive *monosynaptic input* from primary afferent neurons with small-diameter axons (Aδ, C) innervating skin, deep somatic tissues or viscera. Neurophysiological investigations of the lamina I neurons show that they consist of several functionally and to some extent morphologically distinct types. They are excited from the skin by noxious mechanical stimulation (mechanosensitive nociceptive-specific neurons) or heating, pinch and noxious cooling (polymodal nociceptive-specific neurons [called HPC neurons by Craig]) or histamine ("itch" receptors) or innocuous cooling or warming, or sensual touch (Figure 2.10a, b) (Bester et al. 2000; Craig et al. 2001; Andrew and Craig 2001a, b, 2002a, b; Craig 2004a; see Craig [2003a, 2015] for discussion and references). A few lamina I projection neurons are multireceptive (wide dynamic range, WDR) neurons responding to rapid brushing, pinch and noxious heat. However, these neurons are not spinothalamic but rather propriospinal and/or spinomedullary projection neurons (Willis and Coggeshall 2004a; Andrew 2010) (Note 5).

The differentiation of lamina I projection neurons with respect to afferent inputs from deep somatic structures and from viscera has not been extensively studied. However, a few lamina I neurons excited from the skin may also receive additional convergent synaptic input from small-diameter primary afferent neurons innervating deep somatic tissues (such as skeletal muscle, joints) and/or viscera. A few lamina I neurons are activated by small-diameter muscle afferents only (Craig and Kniffki 1985; Wilson et al. 2002). However, no class of lamina I projection neurons receiving synaptic input from visceral afferent neurons only has so far been detected, possibly because the right experiment has not yet been performed. Almost all neurons being activated by stimulation of visceral afferents are *viscero-somatic convergent (WDR) neurons*, i.e., they can be activated by stimulation of small-diameter (Aδ, C) afferents of skin, deep somatic tissues (skeletal muscle, joint, bone, fascia) and/or viscera (Cervero and Tattersal 1986; Cervero 1994, 1995; Katter et al. 1996) and by large-diameter afferents from skin. Cutaneous high-threshold (nociceptive-specific) dorsal horn neurons receiving visceral afferent input seem to be rare. Thus, the neurons of the ascending pathways from lamina I are functionally not specific for the viscera (Note 6). This is probably not very surprising since non-painful visceral sensations, temperature sensations, sensations related to deep body tissues and pain sensations elicited from all body domains have the commonality to be directed towards the *body* (Craig 2002, 2003b, c; Saper 2002). Furthermore, sensations projected to visceral organs have a poor spatial resolution and are referred to skin, deep somatic tissues and other visceral organs (Giamberardino 1999; Jänig 2020a). Sensations elicited by noxious, temperature or chemical stimuli and projected to the body surface (skin) are graded and have a high spatial resolution, showing that the sensory-discriminative component is marked for these sensory submodalities (for review see Gauriau and Bernard [2002]; Craig [2003a]; Dostrovsky and Craig [2013, 2020]).

It is debated whether the uniformity of the convergent viscero-somatic lamina I neurons is an experimental artifact and related to the anesthesia and experimental surgery, i.e. whether these neurons exhibit functional specificity under more physiological conditions. The functional specificity of viscero-somatic lamina I neurons may, e.g., be preferentially dependent on the control of synaptic transmission from primary afferent neurons to second-order neurons by descending systems. These descending control systems are represented in the rostral ventromedial medulla (nucleus raphe magnus, paragigantocellular medial nucleus, parapyramidal nucleus), dorsolateral pontomesencephalic tegmentum (area A5, area A7, nucleus ceruleus, parabrachial nucleus, cuneiform nucleus [lateral to the periaqueductal gray]) and the periaqueductal gray (Heinricher and Fields 2013; Heinricher and Ingram 2020).

The functional characteristics of lamina I projection neurons indicate that these neurons mediate information on the state of body tissues to

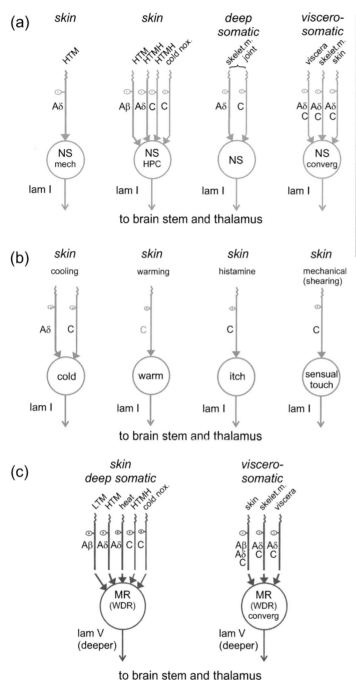

Figure 2.10 Functional classes of neurons in laminae I and V of the spinal dorsal horn that can be excited by stimulation of afferent neurons with $A\delta$- and/or C-axons and project to brain stem and thalamus. (a) Nociceptive-specific (NS) neurons in lamina I. (b) Non-nociceptive neurons in lamina I. (c) Multireceptive neurons (MR) neurons (WDR neurons) in lamina V and deeper laminae (a few in lamina I). Synaptic connections from afferent neurons to most lamina I neurons are monosynaptic, those to lamina V neurons are polysynaptic (interrupted synaptic inputs). Cold nox., cold noxious; HTM, high-threshold mechanical; HPC, heat pinch noxious cold; HTMH, high-threshold mechanical heat (polymodal nociceptive); skelet.m., skeletal muscle; $A\beta$, $A\delta$, C, neurons with large-diameter myelinated, small-diameter myelinated or unmyelinated axons; WDR, wide dynamic range. After Craig (2003a).

supraspinal centers. Most of them project through the contralateral lateral spinothalamic tract to supraspinal centers in primates and some through the ipsilateral lateral spinothalamic tract (Figure 2.11a). In the rat, these neurons project through the lateral and dorsolateral tracts. This difference between primates and rat is related to the large pyramidal tract in primates (in particular the human) that occupies most of the lateral and dorsolateral spinal funiculus. Propriospinal lamina

I neurons project ipsilaterally to the sympathetic pre-ganglionic neurons in the intermediate zone. The main supraspinal projections of lamina I neurons are (Figure 2.11a; Craig 1996; Villanueva and Nathan 2000; Gauriau and Bernard 2002; Dostrovsky and Craig 2013, 2020):

- In the medulla oblongata, lamina I neurons project to the ventrolateral medulla (rostral and caudal, see Figure 10.2), to the subnucleus reticularis dorsalis and to the caudal NTS. These projections are weak. The nuclei are involved in autonomic regulation.
- In the pons and mesencephalon, lamina I neurons have a powerful projection to the lateral parabrachial area (Figure 2.12). This will be discussed below. Furthermore, they project to the lateral and ventrolateral periaqueductal gray and to the deep layers of the superior colliculus (see Subchapter 11.3.3 and Figure 11.6).
- Lamina I neurons project to various nuclei of the thalamus. This will be discussed further below (Figure 2.13). Some lamina I neurons project to the hypothalamus, most of them via the posterior thalamus (Dado et al. 1994) but only in rat and very weakly in monkey.

We do not know whether lamina I neurons are specialized to project to particular nuclei only. However, as it is likely that every tract neuron projects to several sites (Zhang et al. 1995; Kostarczyk et al. 1997; Spike et al. 2003), there may exist subgroups of ascending tract neurons that project to specific groups of target nuclei (e.g., nuclei of the posterior thalamus; Zhang and Giesler 2005; Wercberger and Basbaum 2019).

Functions and Projections of Deep Dorsal Horn Neurons

Other ascending projection neurons that transmit information are afferent neurons with small-diameter (Aδ, C) fibers from skin, deep somatic tissues and viscera located in lamina V (a few in lamina IV) and deeper laminae of the spinal gray matter (laminae VII, VIII, X). The projection neurons in lamina V have been most extensively studied, those in the other deep spinal laminae have not; therefore the latter projection neurons are functionally poorly characterized (Note 7). Most lamina V projection neurons are activated by physiological stimulation of large- and small-diameter myelinated (Aβ, Aδ) and unmyelinated (C) afferent fibers from skin, deep somatic tissues and viscera, the latter synaptic connections being polysynaptic. Most of these neurons are therefore multireceptive (MR; see Note 5) neurons; a few are nociceptive-specific (NS) neurons and a few low-threshold neurons (Figure 2.10c) (Craig 2003a; Dostrovsky and Craig 2013, 2020). Projection neurons in deeper laminae probably have similar functional properties.

Most ascending tract neurons in lamina V and deeper laminae have large receptive fields and relatively high ongoing discharge rates. They encode in their activity the intensity of stimuli applied to the peripheral tissue spanning the innocuous and noxious range. They are somatotopically organized; however, this organization is relatively poor. They are modality-ambiguous, i.e., they poorly differentiate the modality of innocuous or noxious stimulation or the tissue of origin. However, they can have their strongest activation to noxious stimuli and weak activation to innocuous stimuli, or strong activation to visceral stimuli and weak activation to cutaneous or deep somatic stimuli. Whether they are involved in the generation of pain and visceral sensations is a matter of controversial discussions as far as primates are concerned (Craig and Blomqvist 2002; Willis et al. 2002; Craig 2003a). To clarify this important question it is necessary to look at the physiology of *populations* of deep spinal tract neurons.

Ascending tract neurons in spinal lamina V and deeper laminae preferentially project through the anterior spinothalamic tract (Craig 1996; Villanueva and Nathan 2000; Gauriau and Bernard 2002; Dostrovsky and Craig 2013; Figure 2.11b):

- bilaterally to the caudal medulla oblongata (subnucleus reticularis dorsalis, lateral reticular nucleus);
- bilaterally to the rostral medulla (gigantocellular reticular area), to pons and mesencephalon (internal lateral nucleus of the parabrachial area [which does not receive synaptic input from lamina I neurons], pontine reticular area); and
- contralaterally to various nuclei of the thalamus (see below). This projection to the thalamus is strong in primates (about 25% each of the spinothalamic neurons are located in lamina V and deeper laminae in primates; the remaining 50% are located in lamina I) (Willis et al. 2001, 2002;

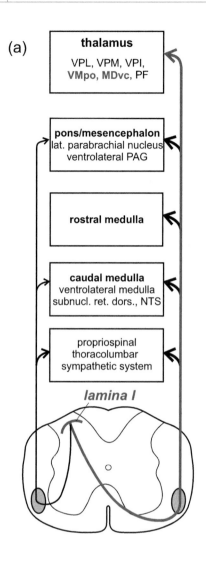

(a)

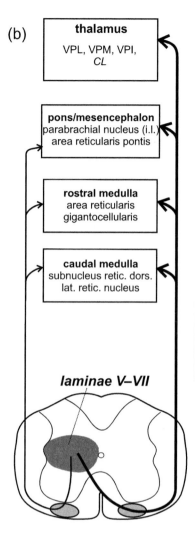

(b)

Figure 2.11 Supraspinal and spinal projections of neurons in lamina I (a) or laminae V to VII (b) of the dorsal horn in primates. (a) Projection of lamina I neurons through the lateral spinothalamic tract. (b) Projection of neurons in laminae V to VII through the anterior spinothalamic tract. CL, centrolateral nucleus; i.l., internal lateral nucleus in the parabrachial complex; lat. retic. nucleus, lateral reticular nucleus; NTS, nucleus tractus solitarii; MDvc, ventrocaudal part of medial dorsal nucleus; PF, parafascicular nucleus; subnucl. ret. dors., subnucleus reticularis dorsalis; VMpo, posterior part of the ventromedial nucleus; VPI/VPL/VPM, ventral posterior inferior/lateral/medial nucleus. For details see text. Modified after Villanueva and Nathan (2000).

Craig 2006; Craig and Zhang 2006; Dostrovsky and Craig 2013, 2020) but weak in the rat (Gauriau and Bernard 2004b).

Projections Through the Postsynaptic Dorsal Column Pathways

Based on clinical and experimental investigations conducted on rats or monkeys there is discussion as to whether an ascending tract in the dorsal columns conveys information about visceral nociception in the pelvic, abdominal and thoracic viscera to the thalamocortical system. Myelotomy in the midline of the dorsal columns relieves or significantly attenuates chronic visceral pain in some patients (e.g., of the colon due to cancer [Hirshberg et al. 1996]). Dorsal horn neurons in the sacral spinal cord, which are located close to the central canal and can be activated by colon distension or inflammation, project through the dorsal columns close to the septum to the gracile nucleus (postsynaptic dorsal column [PSDC] tract). In the gracile nucleus, these neurons synapse with neurons that project to the ventral posterior lateral nucleus of the thalamus (VPL). Activation of neurons in the VPL by colon distension is largely reduced after interruption of the PSDC tract, but not when the lateral spinothalamic tracts are interrupted bilaterally. Activation of these thalamic neurons by cutaneous noxious stimuli is not affected when the PSDCs are lesioned. For the thoracic and abdominal visceral organs, a corresponding PSDC pathway seems to exist that has its origin in the thoracolumbar spinal

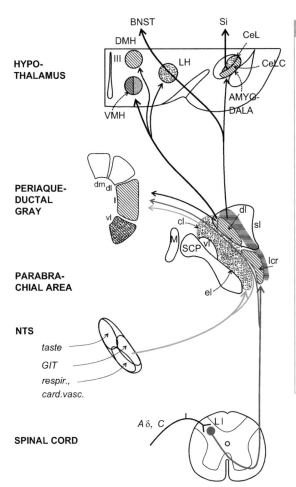

Figure 2.12 Projection of lamina I neurons and second-order neurons of the nucleus tractus solitarii (NTS) to the parabrachial nucleus and projection of parabrachial subnuclei to nuclei involved in autonomic and endocrine regulation. Spinal lamina I neurons project to the dorsolateral (dl) and the lateral crescent (lcr) nuclei (hatched) and to sites lateral to these nuclei (shaded) in the parabrachial area. Second-order neurons in the NTS receiving synaptic input from cardiovascular, respiratory or gastrointestinal vagal afferents project to the centrolateral (cl) and external lateral (el) nuclei (dotted) of the lateral parabrachial area (for details see Herbert et al. [1990]). The parabrachial nuclei project to the lateral (l) and ventrolateral (vl) periaqueductal gray (PAG), to the dorsomedial, ventromedial and lateral hypothalamus (DMH, VMH, LH), to the central amygdala (lateral capsular division [CeLC] and lateral division [CeL]) and to the lateral part of the bed nucleus of the stria terminalis (BNST). Parabrachial nuclei receiving synaptic input from lamina I neurons or NTS neurons exhibit differential projections to the hypothalamus (see hatched [lamina I], shaded [lamina I], dotted [NTS] areas). Not included is the NTS projection to the external medial parabrachial nucleus that projects to the basal part of the ventromedial nucleus (VMb) of the thalamus (see Figure 2.14). card.vasc., cardiovascular system; dl, dm, dorsolateral, dorsomedial PAG; GIT, gastrointestinal tract; M, mesencephalic trigeminal tract; respir., respiratory system; SCP, superior cerebellar peduncle; Si, substantia innominata; sl, vl, superior lateral nucleus, ventrolateral nucleus of the parabrachial area; III, third ventricle.
Modified from Bernard and Bandler (1998) and Gauriau and Bernard (2002) with permission.

segments and projects through the dorsal columns to the cuneate nuclei (Al-Chaer et al. 1996a, b, 1997, 1999; Hirshberg et al. 1996; Willis et al. 1999).

Projection to the Parabrachial Nuclei
Spinal and trigeminal lamina I neurons strongly project to the lateral parabrachial area. Spinal lamina I neurons project mainly contralateral to the dorsolateral (dl) and lateral crescent (lcr) parabrachial nuclei and less intensely to areas lateral to these nuclei (shaded; e.g., the superior lateral [sl] nucleus) (Figure 2.12). Trigeminal lamina I neurons project mainly ipsilateral to the external medial parabrachial nucleus (not shown in Figure 2.12). The spinal projections to the parabrachial nuclei are largely separate from the projections of the second-order neurons in the NTS that are related to taste, cardiovascular, respiratory or gastrointestinal afferent neurons. The dotted area in Figure 2.12 demonstrates that the NTS mainly projects ipsilaterally, which includes the central lateral (cl) and external lateral (el) nuclei.

The neurons in the dorsolateral, lateral crescent and external medial parabrachial nuclei have the same functional characteristics as nociceptive lamina I neurons, although their receptive fields are significantly larger than those in lamina I. In the rat, these neurons are excited by either cutaneous noxious mechanical and/or heat stimuli or by cutaneous noxious cold stimuli or by both. About two-thirds of these neurons are also excited by noxious visceral stimuli (e.g., colorectal distension), i.e. they are viscero-somatic convergent neurons. Neurons excited by visceral stimuli only are absent. Furthermore, neurons specifically excited by innocuous cold or innocuous mechanical stimuli are absent (Bernard and Besson 1990; Bernard et al. 1994; Menendez et al. 1996).

Neurons in the parabrachial nuclei receiving synaptic input from lamina I neurons project to the lateral and ventrolateral periaqueductal gray, heavily to the ventromedial nucleus of the hypothalamus (VMH, dorsomedial part), to the dorsomedial hypothalamus (DMH) and to a lesser extent to other hypothalamic nuclei. Furthermore, they project to the amygdala (central nucleus), to the lateral division of the bed nucleus of the stria terminalis (Figure 2.12), and (via the medial thalamus) to the anterior cingulate cortex (the *limbic motor cortex* representing homeostatic autonomic and endocrine regulations [not shown in Figure 2.12]). It is hypothesized that the spino(trigemino)-parabrachial system and its projection areas are involved in pain (nociception)-related autonomic and emotional reactions (see Subchapter 11.3).

Projection to the Thalamocortical System
Figure 2.13 summarizes the organization of the thalamocortical systems that receive their synaptic input from spinothalamic (and trigeminothalamic) neurons in lamina I, lamina V and deeper laminae, and are involved in different types of interoceptive body sensation, including pain. Traditionally the thalamic nuclei involved in nociception (and probably other body sensations) are divided into nuclei located in the lateral thalamus and nuclei located in the medial thalamus (the two groups of nuclei are divided in Figure 2.13 by a vertical dotted line). This division into lateral and medial thalamic systems probably also applies to the cortical areas to which these thalamic nuclei project: the primary (SI) and secondary somatosensory (SII) cortex belong to the lateral system, the anterior and middle cingulate cortex (ACC, MCC) to the medial system and the insula would take an intermediate position. The lateral system would represent somatosensory exteroception and the medial and intermediate system interoception (Treede et al. 1999, 2000; Craig 2003a; Gauriau and Bernard 2004b; Vogt 2005):

- In *primates*, lamina I neurons project primarily to an area in the postero-lateral thalamus named by Craig as the posterior part of the ventromedial nucleus (VMpo) (Craig et al. 1994; Craig 2004b; Craig 2006) and to a lesser extent to the ventral posterior inferior nucleus

(VPI), as well as to the ventral portion of the medial dorsal nucleus (MDvc) and to the parafascicular nucleus (Pf) (Craig 2004b). Evidence from small iontophoretic injections of retrograde tracers in the thalamus demonstrates that lamina I projections to ventral posterior nuclei (to the VPL [from the spinal cord], to the ventroposterior medial nucleus [VPM; from the spinal trigeminus nucleus]) are at best very sparse (Craig and Zhang, 2006; Craig, 2008). In the *rat*, the lamina I neurons project particularly to the triangular posterior nucleus (which has been compared to the VMpo in primates [Gauriau and Bernard 2004a] but actually also receives deep spinal lamina projections and projects mainly to the amygdala [Craig, 2015 p. 147]), to the VPL/VPM, to the posterior nucleus (PO; which is large in rat but small in monkey) and to the MDvc and Pf nuclei.

- In *primates*, lamina V neurons project to the VPL/VPM (Zhang et al. 2000a, b) and VPI and heavily to the centrolateral (CL) nucleus. In the *rat*, the projections of lamina V neurons to the VPL/VPM and VPI are weak.

- Spinothalamic neurons in deeper laminae project to the CL.

- Neurons in VPL/VPM project heavily to SI and less strongly to SII. Neurons in VPI project to the SI and SII. These cortical areas are involved in exteroception and possibly in discriminative aspects of body sensations, including pain, thermal sensations and visceral sensations (although this is very much doubted by Craig; see below).

- Neurons in the region called the VMpo project preferentially to the dorsal posterior insula (Figure 2.14), possibly including parts of SII and the adjacent orbitofrontal cortex. A small projection from VMpo exists to area 3a in the SI.

- Neurons in the MDvc, Pf and CL project mainly to the ACC and to the MCC. The neurons in the MDvc project to area 24c in the ACC that is located anterior to the visceral cingulate motor areas (Craig and Blomqvist 2002; Vogt 2005; Dostrovsky and Craig 2013, 2020).

It has been proposed by Bud Craig that the layer of spinal and trigeminal lamina I neurons represents an interface between body tissues and thalamocortical systems that consists of various functionally distinct neural channels related to skin, deep somatic tissues

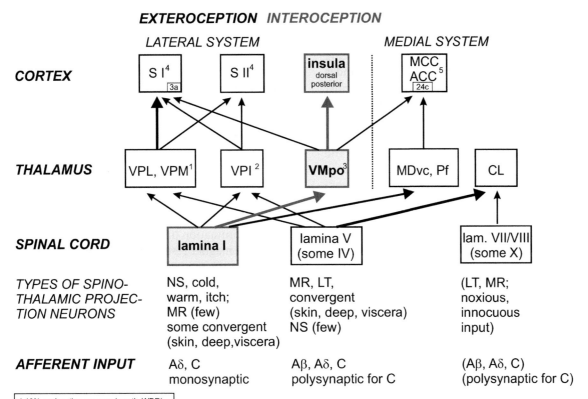

Figure 2.13 The spino-thalamo-cortical systems involved in body sensations including pain in primates. Systems connected to the primary (SI) and secondary (SII) somatosensory cortex are involved in exteroception (and proprioception) and systems connected to the insula cortex and the anterior and middle cingulate cortex (ACC, MCC) are involved in interoception. The pathway from lamina I neurons to the posterior part of the ventromedial nucleus of the thalamus (VMpo) and the dorsal posterior insula, emphasized in red, is mainly involved in the generation of pain in skin, deep somatic tissues or viscera, cold, warm or itch sensations, and non-painful sensations from deep somatic tissues and viscera. Pathways from lamina I to SI and SII via the thalamic nuclei VPL (spinal), VPM (trigeminal) and VPI may be involved in discriminative aspects of these sensations. Pathways from lamina V to VPL/VPM and VPI may also be involved in discriminative aspects of these sensations but this is a controversial issue. Pathways to the ACC via the thalamic nuclei MDvc and Pf are involved in the affective aspects of these sensations. The pathway via the thalamic nucleus PO which is large in rat is not included. The vertical dotted line divides lateral and medial thalamic nuclei. The lower part of the figure shows the afferent inputs to the spinothalamic neurons (afferent neurons with Aβ-axons from low-threshold [LT] receptors; with Aδ-axons from nociceptors and cold receptors; with C-fibers from nociceptors, cold receptors, warm receptors or itch receptors) and the functional types of spinothalamic neurons (NS [nociceptive-specific], cold [non-noxious], MR [multireceptive] neurons). For details see text. ACC, anterior cingulate cortex; CL, centrolateral nucleus; Pf, parafascicular nucleus; MDvc, ventrocaudal part of medial dorsal nucleus; VMpo, posterior part of ventromedial nucleus; VPI, ventral posterior inferior nucleus; VPL, ventral posterior lateral nucleus (spinal input); VPM, ventral posterior medial nucleus (trigeminal input); WDR, wide dynamic range. Based on Vogt et al. (1979), Apkarian and Shi (1994), Craig (1996, 2003a). References for notes in box lower left: 1. Dostrovsky and Craig (2013, 2020); 2. Apkarian and Shi (1994), Dostrovsky and Craig (2013); 3. Gauriau and Bernard (2004a); 4. Dostrovsky and Craig (2013, 2020). Changed from Treede et al. (1999).

and viscera, and that is topographically organized (mediolaterally, craniocaudally) (Figure 2.14; Craig 2003a, b, c):

- The projections of the lamina I neurons to the VMpo, together with projections of the NTS to the basal part of the ventromedial nucleus (VMb;

see below), are considered to be essential for the generation of sensations related to the states of the body tissues (including viscera), such as mechanical, thermal, chemical and metabolic states. Craig argues that the VMpo only exists in primates and is particularly large in humans (Strigo and Craig, 2016). Its size is about half the size of the ventral posterior nuclei (VPL, VPM) that receive their main ascending synaptic input from the medial lemniscal system. The VMpo is located caudally to the VMb, which receives viscerotopic synaptic input from vagal afferents via the NTS and the external medial parabrachial nucleus (see below). In the rat, the posterior triangular nucleus may correspond to the VMpo in primates (Gauriau and Bernard 2004a, b); however, it is unclear whether this nucleus is just a part of the posterior thalamic nuclei.

- The lamina I neurons project *topographically* to the VMpo, the lumbar segments being represented posteriorly in the VMpo and the cervical segments and trigeminal part anteriorly. The anterior part of the VMpo is continuous with the representation of taste and internal organs in the VMb related to the NTS, taste afferents and vagal afferents (see below). This would imply: (1) that *interoception of the body* (including pain and thermal sensations) is represented in the anterior–posterior axis of the VMb/VMpo and (2) that this thalamic representation of interoception is perpendicularly organized to the mediolateral axis of the VPM/VPL system representing *exteroception and proprioception of the body* (Craig 2004b).

- Studies in humans (microstimulation, functional imaging studies) suggest that the VMpo is important to mediate body sensations related to the tissue states (pain, temperature, itch, muscle sensations, visceral sensations) (Dostrovsky and Craig 2013, 2020; Craig 2015).

- The thalamic nucleus VMpo projects to the posterior part of the dorsal insula. This projection is topographically organized (Hua et al. 2005). The posterior part of the dorsal insula is, together with the more rostrally located part, which receives the NTS projections via the thalamic nucleus VMb, the primary sensory representation of the state of the body tissues and therefore the *primary interoceptive cortex* (Figure 2.15).

- The idea that the system consisting of lamina I, VMpo and dorsal posterior insula is the primary

cortical representation of painful, thermal, deep somatic and visceral body sensations in primates is fully supported for the cortical primary representation of interoception by studies in humans: (1) Low intensity electrical stimulation of the insular cortex in patients undergoing presurgical evaluation of epilepsy shows that pain can be elicited only from the dorsal posterior insula (and the adjacent medial parietal operculum). This pain representation is somatotopically organized (Mazzola et al. 2009, 2012). (2) Using intracerebral electroencephalographic recording, it has been shown in the same type of patients that the dorsal posterior insula can be specifically activated during thermal noxious stimulation (Liberati et al. 2019). (3) Using functional magnet resonance imaging, it has been shown that the dorsal posterior insula exhibits an anteroposterior somatotopic organization for cool sensation, muscle pain, cutaneous heat pain and sensual (affective) touch (Craig 2015).

- Craig proposes that the system consisting of lamina I, VMpo and dorsal posterior insula is responsible for the generation of body sensations in primates such as sharp and burning pain, itch, sensual touch, muscle burn and pain, and different types of visceral sensation including visceral pain. This includes the sensory-discriminative component (intensity coding, spatial resolution) as well as the affective component.

- The organization of the pathways underlying visceral sensations (and also muscle sensations) has not been as well explored compared to those underlying cutaneous sensations.

2.6.2 Vagal Afferents and the Thalamocortical System

As will be described in Chapter 8 in more detail, taste afferents and vagal afferents from the gastrointestinal tract, respiratory system and cardiovascular system project viscerotopically to the NTS. The rostrocaudal and mediolateral projection pattern of vagal afferents is transformed into the viscerotopic organization of the second-order neurons in the NTS and preserved in the ascending pathways to the dorsal posterior insular cortex. The anterior part of the dorsal posterior insular cortex represents the sensations related to the organ systems and is hypothesized to mediate the information from the viscera to the *autonomic motor cortices* (e.g., in the *anterior*

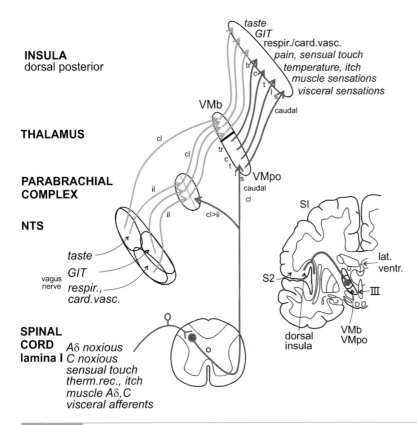

INSULA
dorsal posterior

taste
GIT
respir./card.vasc.
pain, sensual touch
temperature, itch
muscle sensations
visceral sensations

VMb

caudal

THALAMUS

cl

cl

tr
c
t

VMpo
caudal
cl

SI

cl

il

il

cl>il

PARABRACHIAL COMPLEX

NTS

taste
GIT
vagus nerve *respir., card.vasc.*

S2

lat. ventr.

III

dorsal insula

VMb VMpo

SPINAL CORD lamina I

Aδ noxious
C noxious
sensual touch
therm.rec., itch
muscle Aδ,C
visceral afferents

Figure 2.14 Neural pathways responsible for eliciting somatic body and visceral sensations (including taste) to stimulation of small-diameter spinal somatic or visceral afferents or of vagal afferents in primates. Vagal and taste afferents project viscerotopically to the nucleus tractus solitarii (NTS) (see Figures 8.11, 8.12). Second-order neurons in the NTS project viscerotopically, via the parabrachial nucleus and the basal part of the ventromedial nucleus of the thalamus (VMb), to the anterior part of the dorsal posterior insula, taste being represented probably more caudally and visceral organ systems probably more rostrally (see Figure 2.15b). In primates, neurons in the rostral NTS (taste) may also project directly to the contralateral VMb (Beckstead et al. 1980). NTS neurons and lamina I neurons project to separate subnuclei in the parabrachial nucleus (see Figure 2.12). Lamina I (LI) neurons encode activity from various afferents in somatic tissues (thermoreceptors, nociceptors, ergoreceptors, etc.) and visceral afferents (see Figure 2.10); they project via the posterior part of the ventromedial nucleus of the thalamus (VMpo located caudally to the VMb) to the dorsal posterior insula caudal to the projection from the VMb. The inset on the right illustrates on a frontal section the location of the dorsal insula and the VMb/VMpo. cl, il contralateral, ipsilateral; tr, c, t, l, s, trigeminal, cervical, thoracic, lumbar, sacral; SI, SII, primary and secondary somatosensory cortex; III, third ventricle; lat. ventr., lateral ventricle; card.vasc., cardiovascular system; GIT, gastrointestinal tract; respir., respiratory system. For details see text. Figure designed after Saper (2002) and Craig (2003a). Inset on the right from Craig (2003a).

cingulate cortex) and to other cortices that are responsible for the emotional feelings accompanying the organ sensations. Also for these reasons the dorsal posterior insular cortex is the primary interoceptive cortex.

As described in Subchapter 2.3, excitation of vagal afferents does not generate visceral pain sensations, with a few exceptions related to the rather proximal esophagus and trachea, but is related to hunger, satiety, thirst, nausea, fullness, desire to cough and other

pleasurable or uncomfortable body sensations (see Table 2.1). The pathway believed to be essential to elicit non-painful visceral sensations associated with the excitation of vagal afferents innervating thoracic or abdominal organs includes the thalamic nucleus VMb (basal part of the ventromedial nucleus of the thalamus). This nucleus is called the most medial part of the parvicellular part of the ventroposterior nucleus (VPpc or VPMpc) in rats (Cechetto 1995; Saper 1995, 2002).

In primates (but not in rats), second-order neurons in the taste area of the NTS (rostral part of the NTS) project directly to the ipsilateral VMb; these projections are stronger than those to the contralateral VMb (Beckstead et al. 1980). Whether the caudal part of the NTS that represents the afferent (vagal) input areas from the respiratory tract, the cardiovascular system and the gastrointestinal tract projects directly to the contralateral VMb in primates is unexplored. The main projection from the NTS to the VMb occurs via the medial external nucleus of the parabrachial complex in rats and probably in primates as well (Herbert et al. 1990). This projection via the parabrachial external nucleus is suggested to be important for sensations generated by activation of vagal afferents. Neurons in the VMb probably project viscerotopically to the anterior portion of the dorsal insula. Whether this applies to humans too is unclear (Craig, Evrard personal communication). The pathways transmitting information in taste, gastrointestinal, respiratory or cardiovascular afferents are viscerotopically organized. This viscerotopy is probably preserved in the parabrachial external medial nucleus, in the VMb of the thalamus and in the anterior part of the dorsal posterior insula, taste being represented caudally to the sensations related to the respiratory, cardiovascular and gastrointestinal systems (Figures 2.14 and 2.15).

The organization of the primary interoceptive cortex in the dorsal posterior insula and the interoceptive afferent inputs from skin, deep somatic tissues and viscera is demonstrated and summarized in simplified form in Figure 2.15: (a) demonstrates the insula cortex in humans and (b) the functional aspects of the primary interoceptive cortex in the macaque monkey.

Conclusions

1. Visceral organs are innervated by vagal and spinal visceral afferent neurons. Most of these afferent neurons have unmyelinated axons and some have thinly myelinated axons. The visceral afferent neurons encode in their activity mechanical and chemical events. They are involved in peripheral ("efferent" or effector) functions and central (afferent) functions. These functions are closely associated with autonomic and neuroendocrine regulation of body tissues.

2. 85% of the axons in the vagal nerves are afferents innervating the respiratory tract, the cardiovascular system and the gastrointestinal tract. They have their cell bodies in the inferior (nodose) ganglion of the vagus nerve (75%) or in the superior (jugular) ganglion.

3. Vagal afferents innervating each visceral organ system are differentiated into several functional types. They are involved in autonomic reflexes and regulation (see Chapters 8 to 11) as well as in visceral sensations such as hunger, satiety, thirst, nausea and respiratory sensations. They are (with some exceptions related to the proximal esophagus, proximal trachea and oral cavity) not involved in visceral pain. Vagal afferents innervating the mucosa of the gastroduodenal region are involved in nociceptive (protective) reflexes.

4. Subgroups of vagal afferents (in particular those innervating the gastrointestinal tract) are involved in general body protection. They are activated by inflammatory processes involving the immune system and activated by proinflammatory cytokines. Their activation generates illness responses, one component being hyperalgesia. Vagal afferents are also involved in inhibitory control of transmission of nociceptive impulses in the spinal and trigeminal dorsal horn.

5. Vagal afferents project viscerotopically to the nucleus tractus solitarii (NTS) in the medulla oblongata (see Subchapter 8.3). Sensations generated by activation of vagal afferents (or taste afferents) are represented in the dorsal posterior insula (dpINS; interoceptive cortex). In primates the sensations elicited by vagal afferent neurons are mediated by a viscerotopically organized pathway consisting of the NTS, the external medial nucleus of the parabrachial nucleus and the basal part of the ventromedial thalamus (VMb) and from here to the dpINS. Respiratory, cardiovascular and gastrointestinal organ systems are represented most rostrally and taste somewhat more caudally.

6. Spinal visceral afferent neurons have their cell bodies in the thoracic, upper lumbar and sacral dorsal root ganglia. They project through splanchnic nerves to visceral organs. The number of spinal visceral afferent neurons is low compared to the total number of spinal afferent neurons, being in the range of 1.5% to 2.5% (in some dorsal root ganglia up to 8%). Many spinal visceral afferent

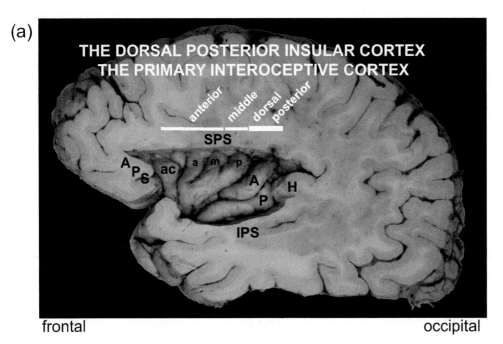

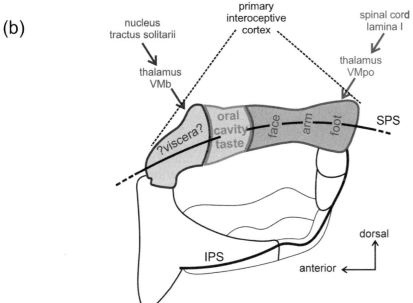

Figure 2.15 (a) Anatomy of the insula cortex in the human. Lateral view after removal of the operculum. APS/IPS/SPS, anterior/inferior/ superior periinsular sulcus; ac/a/m/p accessory/anterior/middle/posterior short insular gyrus; A/P anterior/posterior long gyrus; H, Heschl gyrus. Modified from Thomas Naidich with permission. (b) Simplified working model of the functional organization of the macaque monkey insula. On the left, topical organization of taste and visceral organs via the nucleus tractus solitarii (NTS) and the basal part of the ventromedial nucleus of the thalamus (VMb). On the right, topical organization of the interoception of the body tissues via spinal and trigeminal lamina I neurons and the posterior ventromedial nucleus of the thalamus (VMpo). Modified and simplified from Evrard (2018, 2019).

neurons are peptidergic, containing substance P and/or calcitonin gene-related peptide.

7. Spinal visceral afferent neurons are involved in multiple organ reflexes, organ regulation (pelvic organs), extraspinal "peripheral" reflexes (mediated by prevertebral sympathetic ganglia [see Subchapter 6.5.2]), protective "axon reflex"-mediated effector reactions, non-painful visceral sensations (particularly sacral visceral afferents) and visceral pain.

8. Many spinal visceral afferent neurons (in particular thoracolumbar ones) have peripheral "efferent" effector functions. Their activation generates local increase in blood flow, change in motility, secretion, absorption and other changes by release of peptides. In addition, these afferents may have trophic functions (e.g., maintenance of the barrier function of the urothelium). Spinal visceral afferents may be specialized with respect to the peripheral "efferent" (effector) functions or to the central (afferent) functions (reflexes, sensations).

9. Most thoracolumbar spinal visceral afferent neurons are polymodal and activated by mechanical (distension, contraction) and chemical stimuli (occurring during ischemia and inflammation). They do not seem to signal specific organ events to the spinal cord. The distinction between nociceptive and non-nociceptive thoracolumbar spinal visceral afferents is difficult.

10. Sacral visceral afferent neurons are specialized with respect to the pelvic organs (urinary bladder, hindgut, internal reproductive organs) and are involved in specific organ regulation, lumbar-sacral and sacro-lumbar reflexes, and visceral sensations, including pain. They are mechano- and chemosensitive. Several types can be distinguished: low threshold, a few high-threshold and some mechanoinsensitive (extremely high-threshold or silent) afferents. All types of sacral visceral afferents can be sensitized. The distinction of nociceptive and non-nociceptive sacral afferents by different criteria is problematic.

11. Spinal visceral afferents project to lamina I, lamina V and deeper laminae of the spinal gray matter (sparing laminae II to IV). Single thoracolumbar visceral afferent neurons project over the whole mediolateral width of laminae I and V and over several segments rostral and caudal to their spinal cord entry.

12. Sensations related to spinal visceral afferent neurons are probably triggered by ascending tract neurons in lamina I, together with thermal sensations, pain and other sensations related to the state of somatic body tissues. All spinal neurons receiving synaptic input from spinal visceral afferents are convergent viscerosomatic neurons. The decoding of activity in spinal visceral afferent neurons by second-order neurons in the dorsal horn leading to distinct organ regulations, organ reflexes and sensations (including visceral pain) is poorly understood.

13. Spinal lamina I neurons represent an interface between somatic and visceral body tissues and supraspinal autonomic centers in the brain stem, hypothalamus and limbic system on one side and thalamocortical systems on the other. This interface is composed of functionally distinct neural channels that are activated by afferent neurons with small-diameter myelinated and unmyelinated (Aδ, C) axons innervating skin (noxious, temperature, itch), deep somatic tissues or viscera.

14. Lamina I tract neurons project via various nuclei in the medulla oblongata and the lateral parabrachial nucleus to autonomic and neuroendocrine centers in the brain stem, hypothalamus and limbic system.

15. In primates, lamina I neurons project topographically to the posterior part of the ventromedial nucleus of the thalamus (VMpo). The VMpo projects topographically to the dpINS caudal to the projection field of the VMb.

16. The dpINS is the primary interoceptive cortex and represents sensations related to the states of the tissues of the body, including the visceral organs. It is synaptically connected to limbic centers that are involved in autonomic regulation, emotional feelings and conscious experience.

Suggested Reading

Bielefeld, T. K. and Gebhart, G. F. (2013) Visceral pain: basic mechanisms. In *Wall and Melzack's Textbook of Pain*, 6th edn (McMahon, S. B., Koltzenburg, M., Tracy, I. and Turk, D.C., eds.) pp. 703–717, Elsevier Saunders, Philadelphia.

Cervero, F. (1994) Sensory innervation of the viscera: peripheral basis of visceral pain. *Physiol Rev* **74**, 95–138.

Craig, A. D. (2015) *How Do You Feel? An Interoceptive Moment with Your Neurobiological Self*, Princeton University Press, Princeton, Oxford.

Craig, A. D. (2018) Central neural substrates involved in temperature discrimination, thermal pain, thermal comfort, and thermoregulatory behavior. In *Thermoregulation: From Basic Neuroscience to Clinical Neurology. Part I. Handbook of Clinical Neurology*, Vol 156 (Romanovsky, A. A., ed.) pp. 317–338, Elsevier, Amsterdam.

Dostrovsky, J. O. and Craig, A. D. (2013) Ascending projection systems. In *Wall and Melzack's Textbook of Pain, 6th edn* (McMahon, S. B., Koltzenburg, M., Tracey, I., and Turk, D. C., eds.) pp. 182–197, Elsevier Saunders, Philadelphia.

Evrard, H. C. (2019) The organization of the primate insular cortex. *Front Neuroanat* **13**, 43.

Jänig, W. (2014) [Neurobiology of visceral pain]. *Schmerz* **28**, 233–251.

Jänig, W. (2020a) Sympathetic nervous system and pain. In *The Senses: A Comprehensive Reference, Vol 5 – Pain, 2nd edn* (Pogatzki-Zahn, E. and Schaible, H. G., eds.) pp. 349–378, Elsevier Academic Press, Amsterdam.

Jänig, W. and Morrison, J. F. B. (1986) Functional properties of spinal visceral afferents supplying abdominal and pelvic organs, with special emphasis on visceral nociception. *Prog Brain Res* **67**, 87–114.

All references cited in the text are available online at www.cambridge.org/janig.

Notes

1. Thorén [1979]; Coleridge and Coleridge [1980, 1984]; Malliani [1982]; Mei [1983, 1985]; Cervero and Morrison [1986]; Grundy [1988]; Grundy and Scratcherd [1989]; Jänig and Koltzenburg [1990, 1993]; Ritter et al. [1992]; Cervero [1994]; Gebhart [1995]; Jänig [1996]; Bielefeld and Gebhart [2013]; Undem and Weinreich [2005]; Brookes et al. [2013]; Dockrey [2013]; Lee and Yu [2014]; Mazzone and Undem [2016]; Spencer et al. [2016a, b, c]; Williams et al. [2016]; Powley et al. [2019].

2. This applies in principle also to primary afferent neurons with small-diameter myelinated and unmyelinated fibers that have nociceptive function or monitor the metabolic, inflammatory or thermal state of the tissues. The cell bodies of primary afferent neurons consist by histological criteria of large light neurons (A-afferent neurons) and small dark neurons (B-afferent neurons). The two groups of afferent neurons are distinguished by several criteria (ontogeny, cell phenotype, functional characteristics). Thus, nociceptors, thermoreceptors and metaboreceptors of skeletal muscle would belong to the class of B-afferent neurons across the three body domains (skin, deep somatic tissues, viscera). Prechtl and Powley (1990) have put forward the idea that B-afferent neurons innervating skin, deep somatic tissues or viscera are particularly associated with the autonomic nervous system. They proposed grouping these primary afferent neurons together as part of a common system involved in homeostatic regulations and labeling these afferents "autonomic." This has met quite some criticism (see Open Peer Commentary in Prechtl and Powley [1990]) and overall was not accepted. However, this idea resembles the concept of a general body sense of interoception propagated by Craig (2002, 2003c). The opinion, to label afferents innervating viscera neutrally as spinal visceral or vagal visceral, does not clash with the view that these afferents, together with small-diameter afferents innervating deep somatic tissues or skin, are important in the generation of body feelings that are related to the states of body tissues and to homeostatic body regulation. These body feelings include pain elicited from all tissues, all visceral sensations, thermal sensations, sensations from skeletal muscle during vigorous exercise, etc. and belong to interoception "as the sense of the physiological conditions of the entire body." They have distinct cortical representations in the insular cortex (Craig 2002, 2003a, b, c; see Subchapter 2.6).

3. Axon reflex, neurogenic inflammation: some primary afferent neurons with unmyelinated nerve fibers (and a few with small-diameter myelinated ones) have dual functions: (1) *Afferent function*: They encode physical and chemical stimuli in their activity by specific transduction mechanisms in their peripheral terminals. The activity is transmitted by action potentials to the central terminals and then synaptically transmitted to the second-order neurons. The transmitter involved is glutamate and possibly one or two neuropeptides (such as substance P and calcitonin gene-related peptide, CGRP). (2) *Efferent function*: During excitation, peptidergic afferents release one or two neuropeptides (such as neurokinins [substance P and neurokinin A] and CGRP) at their peripheral terminals and induce precapillary arteriolar vasodilation and postcapillary venular plasma extravasation. The afferent-induced vasodilation was originally called "axon reflex" (Bayliss 1901; Bruce 1910, 1913). This is in the narrower sense not a reflex since no synapse is involved and since the afferent terminal excited by physical or chemical stimuli releases the neuropeptide(s). The afferent-induced plasma extravasation is called "neurogenic inflammation," a concept introduced by the Hungarian Jancsó (Jancsó 1960; Jancsó et al. 1967, 1968). Sometimes the afferent-induced vasodilation and plasma extravasation (together

with other afferent-induced peripheral changes, see Figures 2.2 and 2.3) are collectively called neurogenic inflammation. The peptides released act either directly on the effector cells (smooth muscle cells, endothelial cells) or via other cells (e.g., mast cells). Arteriolar vasodilation is primarily generated by release of CGRP and enhanced in some tissues by neurokinins such as substance P (Häbler et al. 1999). Plasma extravasation is induced by release of neurokinins. Afferent-induced vasodilation and plasma extravasation are present in many tissues, such as skin (human glabrous skin does not exhibit afferent-induced plasma extravasation); mucosal tissues of the oronasal cavities, of the proximal esophagus, of trachea and bronchi, of the urinary tract (urinary bladder, urethra) and of the anus; serosa and mesenteries of intestinal organs; deep somatic tissues (fascia, joint capsule, synovia); dura and pia mater. Only subpopulations of small-diameter primary afferent fibers are involved in afferent-induced vasodilation, most of them probably having nociceptive function. In the rat, a small subpopulation of polymodal nociceptors with C-fibers is involved in afferent-induced vasodilation, but most of them in plasma extravasation. In the pig, only heat nociceptors with C-fibers but no polymodal nociceptors are involved in vasodilation (Lynn 1996a, b; Lynn et al. 1996). In humans, chemonociceptors with C-fibers are involved in vasodilation but polymodal nociceptors are not (Schmelz et al. 2000; Schmidt et al. 2000). Cutaneous small-diameter myelinated (Aδ) fibers in the rat are involved in vasodilation but not in plasma extravasation (Jänig and Lisney 1989) (for review see McDonald [1997]; Holzer [1998b]; Siiskonen and Harvima [2019]).

4. Figures of spinal visceral afferents are normally drawn as if the same afferent fiber innervates all three structures (see Figures 2.3 and 2.4). However, there is no experimental basis supporting this.

5. Dorsal horn neurons that process nociceptive afferent information are functionally divided as follows: (1) *Nociceptive-specific neurons* that can only be excited by noxious stimuli. They are synaptically excited by stimulation of afferent neurons with Aδ- or C-axons. Lamina I tract neurons activated by heat, pinch and noxious cold stimuli of the skin (Figure 2.10a) are one prominent example. (2) *Multireceptive neurons* are excited by noxious and non-noxious stimuli. They are synaptically activated by stimulation of afferent neurons with Aβ-, Aδ- and C-axons. These neurons are also called wide dynamic range (WDR) neurons. (3) *Convergent nociceptive neurons* are activated from skin, deep somatic tissues and/or viscera. These neurons can be nociceptive-specific or multireceptive (Willis and Coggeshall 2004a).

6. In view of the rather small number of spinothalamic neurons in lamina I and deeper laminae that are involved in painful and non-painful somatic and visceral sensations in relation to the number of spinal interneurons and propriospinal neurons, it is theoretically possible that spinal tract neurons that receive selective or relatively selective synaptic input from visceral afferent neurons are difficult to detect and have been overlooked. For example, it is conceivable that there exist ascending tract neurons in the sacral gray matter that are functionally relatively specific for the urinary tract, the hindgut or the sexual organs. Otherwise it would be difficult to understand the distinct regulation of these organ systems and the distinct sensations elicited from them.

7. Many lamina V projection neurons have dendrites that project into laminae I and II. The functional significance of this projection is unknown.

Part II

Functional Organization of the Peripheral Autonomic Nervous System

In Chapter 1, I described the anatomical and physiological characteristics of the peripheral autonomic nervous system on the macroscopic level. The overall conclusion from this conservative approach is that the autonomic neurons are integrated into the neural regulation of many target tissues of the body (see Table 1.2). In other words, autonomic pathways that transmit signals from the spinal cord and brain stem to the peripheral effector cells must have some functional specificity with respect to these effector tissues. Otherwise it would be impossible to understand how the precise autonomic regulation that is the basis for the continuous adaptation of the body during various demands occurs. Implicit in this idea is that these autonomic pathways are connected to distinct neuronal circuits in the spinal cord, brain stem, hypothalamus and telencephalon.

In Chapters 3 and 4, I will give arguments, and describe, that principally each type of target tissue that is innervated by autonomic neurons is influenced by one or two autonomic pathways and that these pathways transmit distinct messages to the periphery and are connected to distinct central circuits. Chapter 3 describes the final autonomic pathway and its analysis using particularly neurophysiological methods.

In Chapter 4 I will describe in some detail the functional characteristics of the pre- and postganglionic autonomic neurons. I will focus on the discharge reflex patterns to physiological stimulation of afferent neurons innervating various tissues. These reflex patterns of the autonomic neurons, as recorded under standardized experimental conditions in vivo, are the cornerstone of the book; they are the functional labels of the neurons and clearly show that the parasympathetic and sympathetic systems consist of subsystems that are defined by the target tissues and their functions. The structure of the reflex patterns is a function of the respective neuronal circuits in the spinal cord, brain stem and hypothalamus. For the sympathetic and parasympathetic systems in which this has not yet been shown, I will make conclusions based on indirect evidence. Morphological analysis of the parasympathetic and sympathetic systems will be described in Chapter 8 and elsewhere in the book.

Chapter 5 describes the enteric nervous system. This system is functionally and morphologically a nervous system in itself, with specific afferent neurons, interneurons and motoneurons that can function independently of the central nervous system.

Chapter 3

The Final Autonomic Pathway and its Analysis

3.1 | The Final Autonomic Pathway

The concept that the motoneurons are the "final common motor paths" (Sherrington 1906), which are shared by segmental and propriospinal reflex pathways and descending systems from the brain stem and cortex, has dominated the analytical approach to the somatomotor system for a long time. This concept will also be applied to the autonomic nervous system in the description of the functional properties of autonomic neurons (Chapters 4, 9 and 10). The sympathetic and parasympathetic systems consist of several functionally distinct subsystems, each associated with a different type of target tissue (Table 1.2). Each autonomic pathway consists of a set of preganglionic and postganglionic neurons that are synaptically connected in the autonomic ganglia; each transmits the central message to its target tissue. I will call this pathway the "*final autonomic pathway*" (Jänig 1986).

The *final autonomic pathways* are the building blocks of the peripheral autonomic nervous system and the concept described by this term applies to all sympathetic and parasympathetic pathways. With the exception of the vagal pathways to the gastrointestinal tract (see Furness and Costa [1987]; Furness [2006]; Subchapters 5.6 and 10.7), the parasympathetic

pathways appear to be more distinct and simpler in organization than the sympathetic ones. This is probably true for the parasympathetic pathways to some target organs or tissues, such as the sphincter pupillae and ciliary muscle (concerned with the pupillary light reflex and accommodation via the ciliary ganglion), the salivary and lacrimal glands (controlling fluid secretion via the pterygopalatine, otic and submandibular ganglia) or the helical arteries of the penis (responsible for erection via neurons in the pelvic ganglia). However, it is unlikely to apply to the parasympathetic pathways of other target organs, such as the urinary bladder and colon (that are responsible for evacuation and continence via neurons in the pelvic ganglia), the heart (decreasing heart rate and atrial contractility via neurons in the cardiac plexus) or smooth muscle and glands of the trachea and bronchi (producing constriction via neurons of the paratracheal ganglia). For these organs, the parasympathetic postganglionic neurons lie in ganglia or plexi within or near the organs; these ganglia contain afferent neurons and, in some cases, interneurons as well as the final postganglionic neurons and there is evidence of integration within them (see Subchapter 6.5). Thus, the simplicity results more from the relatively small size and simple anatomy of the former group of target organs compared to the latter group. Similarly, the

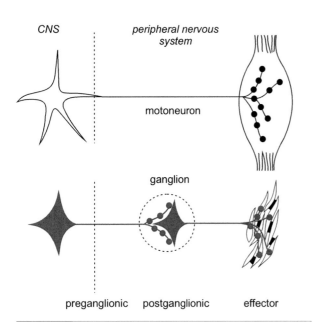

CNS   peripheral nervous
       system

motoneuron

ganglion

preganglionic   postganglionic   effector

Figure 3.1 The "final autonomic pathway" (lower part) in comparison to the "final common motor path" (upper part) of the somatomotor system. CNS, central nervous system.

organization of sympathetic pathways to organs like the pineal gland and dilator pupillae is probably just as simple.

As far as transmission of the central message to the target organs is concerned, the concept of the "final autonomic pathway" is for most autonomic systems similar to that of the "final common motor path" in the somatomotor system, in the sense that it corresponds to the innervation of a skeletal muscle or group of muscles with the same function by a pool of α-motoneurons (Figure 3.1).

The main differences between the somatomotor and autonomic systems are:

- The same autonomic target organ can be innervated by more than one "final autonomic pathway." The component tissues are either independently innervated (e.g., in the eye) or the same tissues are innervated by both final autonomic pathways (e.g., pacemaker cells, atria of the heart). However, the latter is more the exception than the rule (see Chapter 1 and Table 1.2).
- The central message may undergo quantitative changes within autonomic ganglia because of convergence and divergence, and the variable effectiveness of different preganglionic inputs (see Subchapters 6.2 and 6.5).

- In prevertebral ganglia and in some other ganglia (e.g., cardiac ganglia), synaptic inputs from the periphery may summate with those from preganglionic neurons. Intestinofugal cholinergic neurons (of the enteric nervous system) and collateral branches of spinal peptidergic visceral afferent neurons may establish peripheral autonomic circuits that modulate the firing of postganglionic neurons, which are integrated in the final autonomic pathways (see Subchapter 6.5; Jänig 1995).
- The neurally derived signals may interact with other parameters in the target organ or in the ganglion. These include local neural influences (e.g., peptides released from activated afferent terminals), remote and local hormones, local metabolites and the endogenous activity of the target organ (e.g., myogenic activity), including substances released from local cells (e.g., from the endothelium). Such factors vary for neuroeffector transmission in functionally different autonomic pathways (see Subchapter 7.4).

3.2 Functions of the Autonomic Nervous System and Levels of Integration

The autonomic nervous system is a nervous system in its own right and regulates body functions in order to enable the body to act in a coordinated way under various challenging conditions. It consists of subsystems that are hierarchically organized and represented in both the peripheral and central nervous systems. Figure 3.2 shows, in a schematic and simplified form, the different levels of functioning of the autonomic nervous system:

- The lowest level occurs at the *target tissue*. The effector responses of the target cells may depend on several classes of signals, which potentially impinge on them. The target cells are under the control of autonomic neurons and some individual tissues are supplied by more than one type of autonomic nerve terminal (e.g., pacemaker cells of the heart, some blood vessels; see Table 1.2). The effectiveness of the signals of postganglionic autonomic neurons in generating an effector response may also depend on signals arising from other sources (e.g., spontaneous myogenic activity of

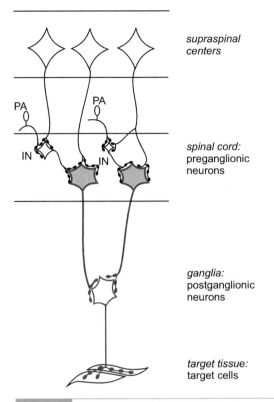

supraspinal
centers

PA   PA

IN   IN

spinal cord:
preganglionic
neurons

ganglia:
postganglionic
neurons

target tissue:
target cells

Figure 3.2 Principal levels of integration of the autonomic nervous system. IN, interneuron; PA, primary afferent neuron.

some smooth muscle cells; local physical factors, e.g., P_{CO2}, pH, temperature), other neurons (e.g., nociceptive primary afferent terminals; see Subchapter 2.2), remotely derived hormones (e.g., circulating angiotensin, adrenaline, vasopressin), endothelium-derived factors in blood vessels (e.g., nitric oxide) or local paracrine signals (e.g., cytokines) (see Subchapter 6.5).

- The next level of integration occurs in some *autonomic ganglia*. Postganglionic neurons may integrate signals derived from several convergent preganglionic neurons. Some postganglionic neurons in prevertebral and possibly in some parasympathetic ganglia also integrate signals from other peripheral neurons. These might be interneurons of the enteric nervous system (intestinofugal neurons) or collateral branches of spinal visceral primary afferent neurons. These neurons establish reflex pathways that are completely organized outside of the spinal cord (see Subchapter 6.5.2).

- *Preganglionic neurons* are situated in the spinal cord and brain stem. These neurons integrate a diverse range of synaptic activity from interneurons, primary afferent neurons (via interneurons) and systems in higher levels in the central nervous system. This level of organization is associated with reflexes and regulating systems that are represented in the spinal cord and lower brain stem (e.g., cardiovascular system, gastrointestinal tract, evacuative systems) (see Chapters 9 and 10).

- *Central pathways* in the upper brain stem and hypothalamus are antecedent to the spinal and lower brain stem reflex centers. They integrate activity from several sources concerned with autonomic homeostatic regulation, neuroendocrine regulation and regulation of the somatomotor system (see Chapter 11).

- *Pathways in the telencephalon* (limbic system and neocortex) adapt the complex homeostatic regulation to the needs of the organism, according to the environmental conditions, and, through memory processes, according to previous experiences.

While generally applicable, this type of functional hierarchical organization is of course a simplification, since the afferent and efferent communication between levels of central integration does not only occur between adjacent levels but also across levels. For example, some neurons from the hypothalamus project directly to preganglionic neurons or autonomic interneurons in the spinal cord (see Figure 8.15) and second-order neurons in lamina I of the spinal cord may project directly to the hypothalamus. Second-order neurons in the nucleus tractus solitarii (NTS) project to nuclei in the brain stem, hypothalamus and limbic system (see Figure 8.13). Furthermore, the functional hierarchical organization is not uniform across the different autonomic pathways. In some systems, the hypothalamus is the main integrative structure that determines the firing characteristics of the peripheral autonomic neurons, while in others the lower brain stem or even the spinal cord serves this function (see Chapters 4, 9 and 10 for extensive description). In essence, the preganglionic neurons are the final arbiter of the autonomic discharge. Although patterns of responses arise at different central sites, the discharge of the final outflow neuron can be modified by other inputs before the signals are sent out to the postganglionic neurons.

3.3 Activity in Peripheral Autonomic Neurons Reflects the Central Organization

The discharge reflex patterns recorded from the peripheral autonomic neurons are the result of integrative processes in the central representations of the respective autonomic system. The circuits of these central representations are located in the spinal cord, brain stem, hypothalamus and telencephalon. Although details about many of these circuits are still missing, we can forward the hypothesis that the organization of these central circuits is specific for each autonomic system. The evidence comes from the following sets of observations:

1. Neural regulation of all autonomic effector organs is amazingly precise. This observation, though apparently trivial and a universally accepted fact, has to be emphasized and remembered. The mechanisms behind most of these precise regulations under various behavioral conditions are still unknown and are to be found in the central integration of autonomic systems. Walter Bradford Cannon probably had this in mind when he wrote his book *The Wisdom of the Body* with the emphasis on "wisdom" (Cannon 1939).

2. Recordings from single peripheral autonomic neurons show a bewildering variety of distinct discharge patterns related to peripheral afferent and centrally generated events. This aspect is extensively discussed in Chapter 4.

3. At least some neurophysiological studies of neurons of central circuits that are related to peripheral autonomic pathways demonstrate rather specific reflexes that are typical for the neurons of the peripheral autonomic pathways. Most of these studies have concentrated on central autonomic circuits related to peripheral autonomic pathways innervating resistance vessels or heart (such as muscle and visceral vasoconstrictor neurons, sympathetic and parasympathetic cardiomotor neurons) (see Spyer 1981, 1994; Guyenet 1990, 2000; Dampney 1994; Guyenet et al. 1996; Blessing 1997). However, other studies have concentrated on central circuits that are involved in regulation of activity in cutaneous vasoconstrictor neurons (Kanosue et al. 1998; Rathner et al. 2001), neurons innervating the adrenal medulla (Morrison and Cao 2000; Morrison 2001a) or neurons innervating the brown adipose tissue (lipomotor neurons; Morrison 1999, 2001a, b). These aspects will be discussed extensively in Chapters 9 and 10.

4. A breakthrough in unraveling aspects of the microanatomy of the central organization of autonomic systems came: (1) with the introduction of axon tracer methods in the 1970s and (2) with the introduction of transneuronal labeling of neuron populations using neurotropic viruses at the end of the 1980s by Arthur Loewy's group. The first method allows labeling of cell bodies of autonomic pre- and postganglionic neurons and of central autonomic neurons (e.g. sympathetic and parasympathetic premotor neurons) and also the field of termination of their axons. The second method in principle allows labeling of whole networks of neurons in the neuraxis that are connected with a specific autonomic output system. Using these morphological techniques, new ideas about the various neuronal networks in the spinal cord, brain stem, hypothalamus and telencephalon, which are involved in the regulation of the final autonomic pathways, were obtained. In this way the groundwork for future physiological studies on the central organization of the different autonomic systems was laid down (Strack et al. 1989; Jansen et al. 1993, 1995; Saper 1995). Results obtained with these techniques, although somewhat disappointing as far as the second method is concerned, will be discussed in Chapter 8.

5. Further progress was made in the last 30 years in research on the mechanisms of integrative action of autonomic systems by combining various techniques. Examples are:

- The development of working-heart-brainstem (WHBP) preparations in mouse and in rat in which the isolated lower brain stem attached to the thorax is continuously perfused. In this preparation, the efferent (parasympathetic) connections to the heart and the afferent (vagal) connections from heart, arterial baroreceptors and chemoreceptors are intact. This in vitro preparation allows detailed intracellular studies in neurons *in situ* related to cardiovascular regulation (e.g., in the NTS, caudal and rostral ventrolateral medulla, etc.) (see Chapter 10; Paton 1996a, b, 1999; Paton and Kasparov 2000).

- The WHBP preparation can be combined with an attached (and perfused) spinal cord, allowing the study of sympathetic neurons *in situ* and with intact cardiovascular centers (Chizh et al. 1998; Stalbovskiy et al., 2014).
- Labeling of functionally (neurophysiologically) identified neurons. Markers are injected into the neurons, using intracellular or juxtacellular injection techniques (see Note 3 in Chapter 10). In this way neurons with distinct function can be visualized.
- Neurophysiological recording from central neurons that have been labeled by a marker beforehand (e.g., preganglionic neurons projecting to distinct ganglia; sympathetic premotor neurons projecting to the spinal cord).
- Intracellular markers of neurons that are activated when the neurons are activated can be used to label populations of central neurons following physiological stimulation of afferent neurons (e.g., arterial baroreceptors or chemoreceptors; distinct classes of afferent neurons from the gastrointestinal tract or pelvic organs; nociceptive afferent neurons in various tissues). One cellular marker used is the immediate early gene *c-fos* and its protein (see Note 1 in Chapter 10).
- Optogenetic techniques that enable specific neuron populations to be (de)activated in vivo (e.g., Farmer et al. 2019).

These points strongly support the methodological approach, as outlined in Figure 3.3, in the neurophysiological analysis of the organization of the sympathetic (and principally also the parasympathetic) systems in the periphery and in the central nervous system (see Subchapter 3.5).

Three further points strengthen the idea of the functional differentiation of the autonomic nervous system:

1. Histochemical investigations of sympathetic pre- and postganglionic neurons show that functionally different types of neurons (as defined by their target tissue) can often be characterized by neuropeptides, enzymes or intrinsic genetic markers (e.g., Niu et al. 2020) colocalized with the "classical" transmitter (*neurochemical coding*). It is irrelevant in this context that we do not know the function of most of these peptides in the autonomic neurons

and that there are species differences (see Gibbins [1995]) (see Subchapters 1.4 and 5.1).
2. Activity is transmitted function-specifically from preganglionic to postganglionic neurons in the autonomic ganglia (McLachlan 1995; see Chapter 6).
3. Where investigated with morphological, neurophysiological and pharmacological techniques, it has been shown that the activity in sympathetic and parasympathetic postganglionic axons is transmitted by distinct neuroeffector junctions to the target cells (see Chapter 7).

3.4 Reflexes in Autonomic Neurons as Functional Markers

Physiologists have always known that autonomic involvement in the regulation of organ function is marked by the precision with which this occurs in relation to the overall behavior of the organism. This is the basis of homeostasis and of the ability to adapt to various external and internal perturbations (allostasis; McEwen 1998, 2000, 2001; Goldstein and Kopin 2017; Goldstein 2019; Schulkin and Sterling 2019; see Chapter 11). Such precise control implies that there are subgroups of pre- and postganglionic autonomic neurons that are discrete with respect to the function they control in their target organs and tissues. Differences in the subgroups of pre- and postganglionic neurons are reflected in the discharge patterns elicited by physiological afferent stimuli and can be measured in neurophysiological experiments.

This addresses the question of whether individual autonomic neurons can be recognized in vivo to belong to one of the autonomic subsystems listed in Table 1.2 by particular reflex discharge patterns. If this is possible, we would have *functional markers* for different systems of neurons that are independent of recorded responses from target organs. Such functional markers should be sufficiently characteristic to allow them to be recognized wherever they are recorded, for example in the preganglionic cervical or lumbar sympathetic trunks. The functional markers might be correlated with other characteristics of the neurons such as passive and active biophysical properties (determining the firing of action potentials in response to synaptic inputs), projection and geometry of dendrites and axons, histochemical characteristics (neuropeptide content, genetic markers) and synaptic transmission in the autonomic ganglia and at the neuroeffector junctions. The strategy used to define such functional markers in experiments on animals and human beings has been:

1. to select appropriate nerves in which the autonomic pre- or postganglionic axons to be recorded from project only to known targets,
2. to use natural (adequate) stimuli to excite afferent neurons, which are appropriate to elicit reflex changes in activity in the pathways to those targets and consequently in the autonomic neurons to be analyzed, and
3. to record the target organ/cell responses.

The types of reflexes elicited in autonomic neurons by afferent stimuli and the correlation between this activity and other centrally generated parameters (e.g., the centrally generated respiratory cycle and the cycle of sleep and wakefulness) depend on the organization of the different control systems in the spinal cord, brain stem, hypothalamus or higher centers, and therefore reflect this organization. Thus, this approach may be applied in future studies of the central organization of the autonomic nervous system by recording autonomic reflexes under appropriate conditions (e.g., experiments on animals or human subjects with transected spinal cords or central disruptions, such as focal lesions or focal activation of known populations of neurons). However, knowing the function of the stimulated afferents, the function of the efferent neurons from which recordings are made, and even the organization of the central reflex pathways, does not necessarily reveal how the autonomic neurons behave under closed-loop conditions (Note 1; i.e., during ongoing regulation of the target organs). For example, the neural elements of the arterial baroreceptor and chemoreceptor reflexes, their projections and the transmitters involved at each synapse are essentially known (Guyenet 1990, 2000; Guyenet et al. 1996; see Chapter 10). However, the functions of these reflex pathways during normal regulation can only be studied under closed-loop conditions. Therefore experiments in the intact, non-anesthetized (awake) organism are important to investigate autonomic regulation under closed-loop conditions and to record the activity of autonomic neurons (see Kirchheim et al. [1998]).

3.5 Some Methodological Details About Recording From Peripheral Autonomic Neurons In Vivo

3.5.1 Neurophysiological Recordings in Animals

Recording from autonomically innervated target organs under closed-loop conditions in anesthetized and awake animals gives valuable insight into the overall capacity and efficiency of the autonomic systems and their target organs in the maintenance of homeostasis and in regulating the inner milieu during various physiological behaviors (e.g., regulation of arterial blood pressure, organ and tissue blood flow, micturition and defecation, body temperature, sexual organ function, etc.) (Folkow and Neil 1971; Randall 1984; Eckberg and Sleight 1992; Rowell 1993; Korner 1995; Dampney 2016; see articles in Robertsen et al. [2012], Mathias and Bannister [2013], Buijs and Swaab [2013]). However, in such studies, the central and peripheral nervous systems are treated like a black box. This approach has given only limited insight into the organization of the peripheral autonomic nervous system and its central control mechanisms. Therefore, it has been necessary to record from single autonomic neurons or small groups of neurons in vivo or in vitro and to combine these (mostly neurophysiological) recordings with other techniques for recording target organ function (see Loewy and Spyer [1990]).

The neurophysiological approach in vivo has been applied extensively in studies of the activity of some groups of autonomic neurons in cats, rats and some other species, using extracellular recording from peripheral autonomic axons. This approach has concentrated on pre- and postganglionic neurons of the lumbar sympathetic system supplying skeletal muscle, skin or pelvic organs, and on preganglionic neurons of the thoracic sympathetic system innervating postganglionic neurons in the superior cervical ganglion, which are destined for target organs in the head and upper neck (Jänig, 1985, 1986, 1988, 1996; Jänig and McLachlan 1987; Jänig et al. 1991; Boczek-Funcke et al. 1992a, b, c, 1993; Häbler et al. 1992, 1993, 1994a, b, 1996, 1999; Grewe et al. 1995; Bartsch et al. 1996, 1999; Kirillova-Woytke et al. 2014). The advantage of this experimental approach is that the activity in the neurons of the final sympathetic pathways reflect the central organization of the respective system and can be correlated with the effector responses under controlled experimental conditions. The limitations are clearly to be seen in the technical difficulties in isolating signals from single neurons routinely.

Results obtained with the neurophysiological techniques in vivo are combined with results obtained with other experimental approaches to the autonomic nervous system. This includes electrophysiological techniques in vitro, as well as morphological, immunohistochemical, pharmacological, molecular-genetic, behavioral and psychobiological techniques.

A few in vivo experiments of a similar type have been performed on parasympathetic systems in which spontaneous and reflex activity was recorded in vivo from preganglionic neurons (e.g., to the heart, the respiratory tract and the upper gastrointestinal tract) or postganglionic neurons (e.g., in the ciliary ganglion; see Jänig [1995]). There are limitations to the application of the method if exposure of the nerve of interest involves intrusive or extensive surgery that may compromise the responses of the autonomic neurons.

Figure 3.3 illustrates the arrangement of the recording from peripheral sympathetic neurons in both animals and humans. As mentioned, the discharge patterns recorded from the peripheral neurons in this way are the result of integrative processes in the central representations of the respective sympathetic system.

The methodological approach as outlined in Figure 3.3 in the analysis of the functional organization of the sympathetic (and principally also the parasympathetic) systems in the periphery and in the central nervous system is to record from bundles with few autonomic axons or, if possible, from single autonomic axons. In view of the thousands of postganglionic neurons projecting into individual peripheral somatic or visceral nerves (McLachlan and Jänig 1983; Baron et al. 1985a, b), and in view of the fact that as many as thousands of postganglionic neurons may innervate the same type of target tissue and therefore have the same function (e.g., muscle, visceral or cutaneous vasoconstrictor neurons), critics sometimes say that conclusions made from single unit recordings are not representative of the whole population of sympathetic neurons with the same function. This has turned out not to be true and has

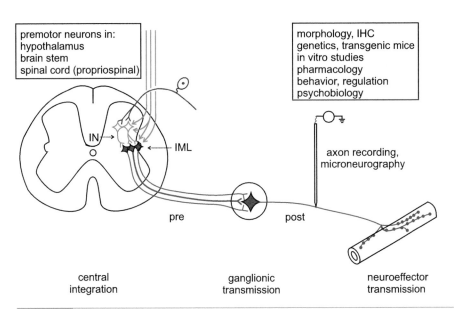

Figure 3.3 Arrangement of recording situation using microneurography from bundles with postganglionic axons in human subjects or from fiber strands isolated from peripheral nerves in anesthetized animals in vivo. Note that signals recorded from the postganglionic axons in both experimental situations reflect the result of central integrative processes in the respective sympathetic system; the impulses in the sympathetic pathways are specifically transmitted through the sympathetic ganglia and to the target cells by the neuroeffector junctions (see Chapters 6 and 7). Other techniques used are listed in the upper right box. IHC, immunohistochemistry; IML, intermediolateral nucleus; IN, interneuron; pre, preganglionic neuron; post, postganglionic neuron. Modified from Jänig and Häbler (2003) with permission.

clearly been refuted in experiments in which activity from two bundles containing sympathetic postganglionic axons with the same function was recorded simultaneously (e.g., muscle vasoconstrictor axons in humans, see Sundlöf and Wallin [1977]) or from functionally different types of sympathetic postganglionic or preganglionic axons in the same bundle (see Subchapters 4.2 and 4.3). In fact, experiments using this type of recording from sympathetic neurons have enabled us to provide the ultimate underpinning for the differential organization of the sympathetic nervous system, in the periphery and in the central nervous system.

Recording of multiunit activity in autonomic axons from whole nerves or large bundles isolated from peripheral nerves may be favorable in certain experimental situations. For example, spontaneous activity and reflex patterns elicited in sympathetic axons of the major splanchnic nerve by stimulation of arterial baroreceptors, arterial chemoreceptors, nociceptors, etc. probably occur exclusively in visceral vasoconstrictor neurons. Activity in other types of sympathetic neuron that project in the major splanchnic nerve and that is related to regulation of the motility or secretion of the gastrointestinal tract or to other non-vasoconstrictor functions cannot be recognized in the recordings of multiunit activity from the major splanchnic nerve in anesthetized animals. Therefore, splanchnic nerve recording can be used as reference recording for vasoconstrictor neurons innervating resistance blood vessels of the viscera in the analysis of central circuits that are connected with this sympathetic pathway (see Figures 10.12, 10.15). The same applies in the rat to the nerve innervating the adrenal medulla (in rats and humans most preganglionic neurons projecting to the adrenal medulla innervate cells that synthesize and release adrenaline), to the nerves innervating the interscapular brown adipose tissue in rats (most postganglionic axons innervate the adipocytes of the brown adipose tissue; see Figure 10.17) or to nerves innervating the rat tail (most sympathetic postganglionic axons in these nerves innervate blood vessels involved in thermoregulation).

3.5.2 Representative Examples of Recordings From Sympathetic Neurons In Vivo in Animals

Most data shown in Chapter 4 were obtained in recordings from post- or preganglionic axons made with metal electrodes in anesthetized animals; some were done with microelectrode recordings from the cell bodies of the autonomic neurons (see McLachlan et al. [1997]; Bratton et al. [2010]). Recordings from the axons are stable (once one succeeds in isolating the axons from the respective nerve and obtaining a sufficient signal-to-noise ratio between the extracellularly recorded action potentials and the recording noise) and can last for hours from the same axon or axon bundle. These long-term recordings from the same neurons in vivo enable the measurement of the complete functional characteristics of the neurons (see examples in Chapter 4).

Figures 3.4 and 3.5 illustrate three examples showing how sympathetic post- and preganglionic neurons are identified and how activity is recorded from the axons of these neurons that were isolated in bundles under a microscope from the respective nerves. The bundles were positioned on recording platinum electrodes and the activity in the axons was recorded and amplified by a high-impedance amplifier. The size of the signals recorded from unmyelinated or small-diameter myelinated nerve fibers is normally in the range of 20 to 100 µV (sometimes larger) and the recording noise is in the range of 10 to 20 µV.

- In the first example (Figure 3.4b), the activity was recorded from a bundle isolated from a nerve innervating hairy skin of the cat hindlimb. The bundle contained three unmyelinated fibers conducting at less than 1 m/s, as shown by the responses to electrical single pulse stimulation of the peripheral nerve (stim. nerve in Figure 3.4a). The responses in axons 1 to 3 appeared at latencies of about 75 to 90 ms (Figure 3.4b, lower trace), showing that the action potentials traveled at 0.66 to 0.8 m/s over the distance between stimulation and recording electrodes. Axons 1 and 2 were also activated by electrical stimulation of the preganglionic axons in the lumbar sympathetic trunk (stim LST) with single pulses (Figure 3.4b, upper trace). Axon 1 responded with three action potentials to stimulation of the LST because there is a synapse between pre- and postganglionic neurons and there is convergence of more than one preganglionic axon on one postganglionic cell body. This leads, in some postganglionic neurons, to repetitive responses upon preganglionic single pulse stimulation (for details see

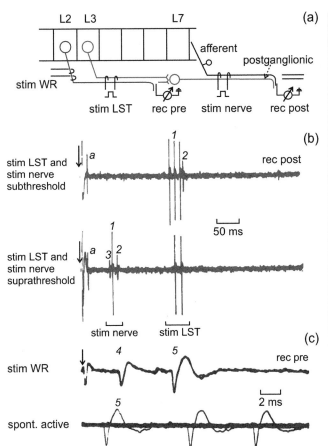

Figure 3.4 Identification of pre- and postganglionic sympathetic neurons in the cat. (a) Arrangement of stimulation (*stim. WR, LST, nerve*) and recording electrodes at the pre- and postganglionic sides (*rec. pre, rec. post*). (b) Recording from a bundle isolated from the superficial peroneal nerve (skin nerve) with two (unmyelinated) postganglionic fibers (*1, 2*) and one unmyelinated afferent fiber (*3*). Simultaneous electrical stimulation of the LST (suprathreshold) and of the peripheral nerve subthreshold for unmyelinated fibers (*upper trace*) or suprathreshold for unmyelinated fibers (*lower trace*). Postganglionic fiber *1* was activated with three spikes by electrical stimulation of the LST; the first of these three action potentials collided with the antidromic signal when the postganglionic axon was stimulated directly. The LST-evoked action potential in postganglionic axon *2* collided with the antidromic signal after suprathreshold peripheral stimulation. Note that one afferent Aδ-fiber [*a*] was activated. (c) Recording from a bundle with two axons dissected from the LST. Electrical stimulation of the WRL2 (stim. WR) excited the two axons. Axon *5* had ongoing activity and was therefore preganglionic (see "spont. active" lower trace). Axon *4* was silent (it was either a visceral afferent axon or a silent preganglionic axon). Recordings in (c) several times superimposed. LST, lumbar sympathetic trunk; WR, white ramus. Modified from Jänig and Szulczyk (1981) and Blumberg and Jänig (1982) with permission.

Chapter 6). The latencies of the responses elicited from the LST were long (here about 200 to 250 ms) because the conduction distance between the stimulation site at the LST and the peripheral recording site was long and the postganglionic fibers were unmyelinated. The lower trace of Figure 3.4b shows what happens when both the LST and the peripheral nerve are stimulated *simultaneously suprathreshold* for both postganglionic fibers with single pulses. Now the first action potential in postganglionic axon *1* and the action potential in postganglionic axon *2* elicited from the LST are no longer present because these action potentials collided with antidromically traveling action potentials generated in the same axons by peripheral nerve stimulation. This example clearly demonstrates that axons *1* and *2* were postganglionic and axon *3* was (by exclusion) afferent (because it could not be activated from the LST

and because afferent neurons that project to the extremities do not do so through the LST (McLachlan and Jänig [1983]; see Chapter 2).

• In the second example in Figure 3.4, activity was recorded from a bundle that was isolated from the lumbar sympathetic trunk (LST in Figure 3.4a) and that contained two axons (axons *4* and *5* in Figure 3.4c). Electrical stimulation of the lumbar white ramus L2 (stim WR) with single pulses elicited responses in these axons at short latencies (upper trace in Figure 3.4c), demonstrating that these axons were myelinated. Axon *5* had spontaneous activity that was centrally generated (lower trace in Figure 3.4c; note the characteristic shape of the extracellularly recorded action potentials recorded from axon *5* [spontaneously active and after stim WR]). Axon *4* had no spontaneous activity (and could not be reflexly activated). Thus, this axon was either a preganglionic axon that was

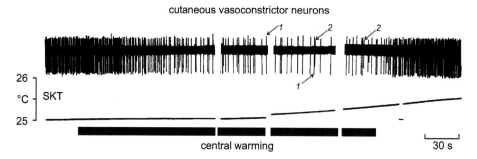

cutaneous vasoconstrictor neurons

Figure 3.5 Decrease of activity in postganglionic cutaneous vasoconstrictor axons innervating the plantar skin of the cat hindpaw during central warming in relation to change in skin temperature. Activity was recorded from a fine nerve fiber bundle, isolated from the medial plantar nerve of the cat paw, which contained two postganglionic vasoconstrictor fibers with resting activity at about 38 °C body core temperature which could be discriminated by the size of their action potentials (fiber 1 and fiber 2). Skin temperature (SKT) was recorded from the surface of the central pad. The black bar indicates simultaneous warming of the spinal cord (by warm water flowing through a U-shaped tubing positioned epidurally dorsal to the spinal cord) and hypothalamus (by warm water perfused through a thermode positioned into the anterior hypothalamus). Note the strong inhibitory effect on the vasoconstrictor activity during central warming and its reversal after termination of warming. As a consequence of this decrease of activity in the cutaneous vasoconstrictor neurons, the cutaneous blood vessels dilated, the blood flow through skin increased and the SKT increased. Increase and decrease in SKT were delayed with respect to neural activity because of the thermal capacity of the skin. Modified from Grewe et al. (1995) with permission.

silent under the experimental conditions or an axon of an afferent neuron that projected through the white ramus L2 to the viscera.

- The third example demonstrates the recording of spontaneous activity from two postganglionic axons in one bundle innervating hairless skin of the cat hindpaw (the bundle was isolated from the medial plantar nerve of the hindpaw) and of the temperature on the surface of the hairless skin (Figure 3.5). Warming of the hypothalamus and the spinal cord (which occurs in vivo when the body is overheated) decreases the activity in the postganglionic neurons, which is then followed by dilatation of the cutaneous blood vessels, increase in blood flow and heat transfer through the skin, and a subsequent increase in skin temperature (SKT). Thus the postganglionic neurons recorded from in Figure 3.5 were most likely cutaneous vasoconstrictor neurons (for details see Chapter 4).

The size and shape of extracellularly recorded signals from pre- or postganglionic axons are the basis for discriminating signals from different axons using window discriminators and template (shape) analysis. In this way, several simultaneously recorded signals in the same microbundle can be analyzed separately.

3.5.3 Neurophysiological Recordings in Humans

The introduction of microneurography at the Department of Clinical Neurophysiology in Uppsala under the guidance of the Swedish neurologist Karl-Erik Hagbarth in the 1960s (Vallbo et al. 2004) has made it possible to study the activity of sympathetic postganglionic axons in peripheral nerves of conscious human beings. Insulated tungsten microelectrodes, with fine uninsulated tips having diameters of 1 to 5 µm, are inserted manually through the intact skin into fascicles of underlying skin or muscle nerves (see Figure 3.6a). The situation is conceptually and methodologically comparable to the analysis of the neuronal control of skeletal muscle during movement. This field initially obtained its impetus (starting with Sherrington in 1906, see Sherrington [1906]) from the application of the reflex concept and the subsequent formulation of hypotheses that can be tested during ongoing movements in animals and human beings, such as locomotion, target reaching, ballistic movements and manipulation (Baldissera et al. 1981; Granit 1981; Jankowska and Lundberg 1981). This technique allows activity in peripheral afferent and efferent axons in skin and muscle nerves to be studied in conscious subjects who can communicate freely with the experimenters. Activity in

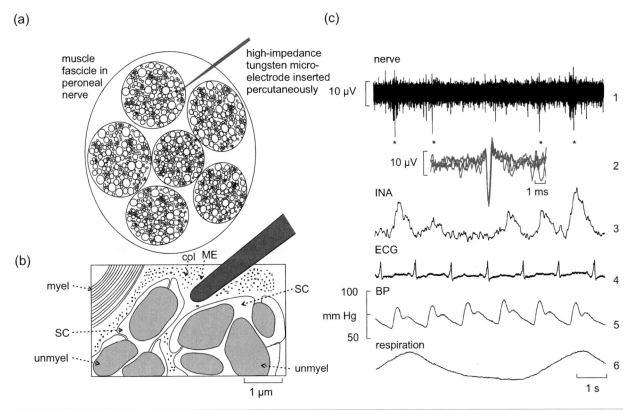

Figure 3.6 Microneurographic recording of activity from postganglionic muscle vasoconstrictor axons in an awake human being. (a) Schematic representation of a tungsten microelectrode inserted percutaneously into a human peroneal nerve. (b) The bundles of unmyelinated fibers recorded from in (c) can only be seen at high magnification. col., collagen bundles; ME, tip of tungsten microelectrode; myel., myelinated nerve fiber; SC, Schwann cell cytoplasm; unmyel., profiles of unmyelinated nerve fibers (pink). (c) Recording from a bundle with several postganglionic axons (multiunit activity) in the deep peroneal (muscle) nerve. *Traces 1 and 2*: one single unit was identified by the size and shape of the extracellularly recorded action potential (see asterisk and superimposed spikes on expanded time scale in the second trace to demonstrate that these spikes have exactly the same shape). *Trace 3*: integrated nerve activity (INA) representing the activity in several postganglionic axons (see large and small spikes in trace *1*). *Traces 4 to 6*: electrocardiogram (ECG), arterial blood pressure (BP) and respiration parameter. This record was made from a patient with heart failure. Modified from Macefield et al. (2002) with permission.

these neurons can be correlated with sensory perceptions, somatomotor responses, autonomic effector responses (e.g., blood pressure, heart rate, electrocardiogram [ECG], respiration, blood flows, galvanic skin responses [sweat gland activity]) and central commands (Vallbo et al. 1979; Wallin and Fagius 1988).

The advantages of this technique are obvious. However, the signals recorded from unmyelinated axons have limited resolution when recording from postganglionic axons with relatively low-impedance electrodes. The signals usually consist of multiunit ongoing activity (because several unmyelinated fibers usually run together in one Schwann cell bundle and

the bare tip of a tungsten electrode is large when compared to the diameter of the unmyelinated axons [Figure 3.6b]). Finally, microneurography can only be applied in human beings to nerves that are located relatively superficially but not to visceral nerves and other deeply located nerves.

Using metal electrodes with a very small bare tip for recording, i.e., electrodes with high impedance, recording from single postganglionic axons is possible, although this single unit recording cannot be used routinely. To find single postganglionic axons generating signals with sufficiently large signal-to-noise ratio for discrimination (see single unit marked by asterisk and the shape of its action potential [signals in red] in Figure 3.6c, upper two records) is much more difficult since the "seeing distance" of the fine-tipped high-impedance electrodes is short when compared to the "seeing distance" of the low-impedance electrodes (see Vallbo et al. 1979; Macefield and Wallin 1996; Macefield et al. 2002).

Figure 3.6c shows a microneurographic recording from a bundle containing muscle vasoconstrictor axons in a human subject. To obtain this recording, a tungsten microelectrode was inserted percutaneously into the deep peroneal (muscle) nerve of a human subject. The original record (trace c1) shows multiunit activity, which could be discriminated from the recorded noise, and the activity in a single postganglionic axon identified (marked by asterisks). The electronic discrimination of the single unit is demonstrated in the trace c2. This type of "clean" discrimination of activity in single postganglionic axons is more the exception than the rule (Macefield et al. 2002). The multiunit activity has a relatively poor signal-to-noise ratio. The third to sixth recording traces in Figure 3.6c show the integrated neural activity (INA) (Note 2), the electrocardiogram (ECG), the arterial blood pressure (BP) and a parameter of inspiration and expiration, respectively. These traces show that the activity in the postganglionic axons is correlated with the ECG and the pulse pressure wave. This type of microneurographic recording is the basis of all data obtained in human beings from postganglionic neurons innervating skin or skeletal muscle (see Subchapters 4.1 and 4.2).

3.6 Confounding Effects of Anesthesia in Animal Experiments

Other than anesthesia (see Jänig and Räth [1980]; Häbler et al. [1994b]), the conditions under which discharges in post- and preganglionic neurons have been measured are probably close to normal for the autonomic systems under investigation. This can be judged from the rate of spontaneous activity in single autonomic neurons and the reactions of the effector organs, such as skin temperature, systemic blood pressure and blood flow through skeletal muscle, skin or viscera. All vital parameters, such as rate of ventilation, end-tidal CO_2, acid–base balance, body core temperature, can be kept as close to normal as possible. Consequently, it is not surprising that both the level and the pattern of discharge recorded from single sympathetic axons in anesthetized animals are comparable to those observed in equivalent sympathetic systems in conscious human beings (Jänig et al. 1983; Wallin and Fagius 1988; Wallin and Elam 1994; Jänig and Häbler 2003; Wallin 2013). It seems likely then that they are also similar to those in the awake animal. For example, the cardiac and respiratory patterns of discharge in the muscle vasoconstrictor neurons of an anesthetized cat and that of human subjects resting in a prone position are almost indistinguishable, except that cats have a higher heart rate and a higher frequency of respiration (Häbler et al. 1994a; Jänig and Häbler 2003; see Figure 10.24). In anesthetized rats and mice, heart rate and respiratory rate are higher again.

The central effect of the anesthesia used, of course, produces quantitative and sometimes even qualitative distortions of some reflexes and regulatory outflow. This has been demonstrated for thermoregulation and baro- and chemoreceptor regulation of cardiovascular parameters (Hensel 1981, 1982; Eckberg and Sleight 1992; Kirchheim et al. 1998). Any anesthetic will affect brain functions that are dependent on the cortex and limbic system and many also affect glutamatergic synapses at the spinal level. These confounding effects on the discharges of autonomic neurons have to be taken into account when comparing results obtained in different animal species (including human beings) under different conditions (see Jänig and Räth [1980]). Thus, anesthesia is not a major problem in the analysis of the neural organization of autonomic systems in the periphery and in the neuraxis, but it should always be taken into account in the interpretation of the data. It certainly is a major problem in the analysis of the regulation of autonomic circuits by the forebrain.

Conclusions

1. The spinal cord and brain stem are connected to the autonomic target cells by two neuron chains of the peripheral sympathetic and parasympathetic nervous systems. These chains consist of populations of preganglionic neurons and postganglionic neurons that are synaptically connected in the autonomic ganglia. They transmit

messages from the central nervous system to the target cells. By analogy to motoneurons, these pathways are "final autonomic pathways."

2. The final autonomic pathways are the building blocks of the peripheral autonomic nervous system. The main difference between the final somatomotor pathways and the final autonomic pathways is that the central messages may undergo quantitative changes in the autonomic ganglia, and that some effector cells are innervated by more than one type of functional autonomic pathway.

3. The impulse pattern transmitted by these peripheral autonomic pathways to the target cells is the result of central integration in the spinal cord, brain stem, hypothalamus and telencephalon. Reflex patterns that are generated by afferent stimuli in peripheral autonomic neurons may serve as physiological markers to analyze the functional structure of the autonomic circuits in the neuraxis.

4. Using this approach of neurophysiological recording from single autonomic neurons in vivo, detailed knowledge has accumulated about the organization of the autonomic nervous system in animals and the human being.

Suggested Reading

Häbler, H. J., Hilbers, K., Jänig, W., et al. (1992) Viscerosympathetic reflexes responses to mechanical stimulation of pelvic viscera in the cat. *J Auton Nerv Syst* **38**, 147–158.

Jänig, W. (1985) Organization of the lumbar sympathetic outflow to skeletal muscle and skin of the cat hindlimb and tail. *Rev Physiol Biochem Pharmacol* **102**, 119–213.

Jänig, W. and Häbler, H. J. (2003) Neurophysiological analysis of target-related sympathetic pathways: – from animal to human: similarities and differences. *Acta Physiol Scand* **177**, 255–274.

Jänig, W., Sundlöf, G. and Wallin, B. G. (1983) Discharge patterns of sympathetic neurons supplying skeletal muscle and skin in man and cat. *J Auton Nerv Syst* **7**, 239–256.

Paton, J. F. (1996b) A working heart-brainstem preparation of the mouse. *J Neurosci Methods* **65**, 63–68.

Wallin, B. G. (2013) Intraneural recordings of normal and abnormal sympathetic activity in humans. In *Autonomic Failure, 5th edn* (Mathias, C. J., and Bannister, R., eds.) pp. 323–331, Oxford University Press, Oxford.

All references cited in the text are available online at www.cambridge.org/janig.

Notes

1. In *closed-loop conditions,* neurons are studied when all afferent and efferent systems, including the afferent feedback from these effector systems, are intact. An example is given in Figure 4.6, which demonstrates the activity in muscle vasoconstrictor neurons in a conscious human subject under resting conditions. In *open-loop conditions*, the responses of neurons to experimental afferent or other stimuli are studied in vivo or in vitro. Examples are demonstrated in Chapter 4, showing the responses of neurons to well-defined afferent stimuli (e.g., applied to skin, arterial baroreceptors, arterial chemoreceptors, urinary bladder, etc.).

2. The original signal is recorded at a 700 to 2000 Hz bandpass filter, amplified and fed through an amplitude discriminator (in order to improve the signal-to-noise ratio). A resistance-capacitance (RC) integrator network with a time constant of 0.1 seconds is used to obtain the integrated nerve activity of the multiunit neural activity (INA integrated neural activity [mean voltage display] in Figure 3.6).

Chapter 4

The Peripheral Sympathetic and Parasympathetic Pathways

In this chapter I describe the reflex patterns for different groups of autonomic neurons, in particular sympathetic ones. For autonomic neurons that have not yet been investigated using neurophysiological techniques in vivo on the single neuron level, I will draw indirect conclusions by analogy to those that have been investigated. We gather information about the functional specificity of different autonomic neurons, about the relation between activity in certain types of neurons and the responses of the target tissue, as well as information about the main organization of the central circuits that determine the discharge reflex pattern of these neurons (see Chapters 8 to 11). The experimental data described in this chapter are an important cornerstone of this book; they show that neurons of each autonomic pathway exhibit a characteristic pattern of discharge and that this is dependent on the structure of the central circuits in the spinal cord, brain stem and hypothalamus, and the synaptic connections of these circuits with the different groups of afferent input to the neuraxis. This type of analysis provides the ultimate underpinning for the concept that the autonomic nervous system consists of functionally distinct

building blocks (Jänig and McLachlan 1992a, b). As I have emphasized in Chapter 3, this description does not show how these autonomic systems function during ongoing regulation of autonomic function. This will be discussed in Chapters 6 to 10.

A similar conceptual and technical approach has been used in the analysis of the somatomotor system. Here too, detailed analyses of the spinal and supraspinal reflex loops linked to the Ia, Ib, joint, cutaneous and other primary afferent neurons gave valuable insight into the system, which then became the basis for further analysis in order to understand how length and strength of skeletal muscle and the coordination of muscles are regulated by the brain, so as to understand how movements are brought about by the brain and their underlying mechanisms. To unravel the central circuits, this systematic analysis of the somatomotor system used functionally distinct afferent inputs and efferent outputs (motoneurons) (Baldissera et al. 1981). By analogy, the autonomic reflex loops have been analyzed with respect to the various afferent signals from the target organs and tissues in the somatic and visceral body domains, and from the extracellular fluid matrix of the body. Thus, these afferent feedbacks include neural, hormonal and humoral (e.g., glucose concentration) signals (see Figure 0.1 in the introduction).

4.1 | Sympathetic Vasoconstrictor Pathways

Large and small arteries, arterioles and most veins are innervated by sympathetic noradrenergic neurons. Capillaries (exchange vessels) and most venules are not innervated. The density of the anatomical innervation varies considerably between vascular beds in different tissues, between different sections of the same vascular tree, between different functional types of blood vessel and, to some extent, between mammalian species. Activation of noradrenergic vasoconstrictor neurons generates vasoconstriction leading to increased resistance to blood flow and decreased capacitance of veins. These neurons are therefore called *vasoconstrictor neurons*. Large numbers of sympathetic neurons originating at the thoracolumbar spinal levels innervate blood vessels in tissues throughout the body. These pathways have been studied in detail in the anesthetized cat at both pre- and postganglionic levels, in conscious human subjects at the postganglionic level and to a lesser extent in the anesthetized rabbit and rat. Some functional properties for different types of vasoconstrictor neurons in the *cat* (and some in the rabbit) are listed in Table 4.1.

4.1.1 Vasoconstrictor Neurons in Animals

Reflex patterns in vasoconstrictor neurons in cat and rat are similar. However, those in the rat appear to be less differentiated. Furthermore, the respiratory patterns in the activity of the vasoconstrictor neurons of the two species are different (Häbler et al. 1993, 1994a, b, 1996, 1999, 2000; Bartsch et al. 1996, 1999, 2000; see Subchapter 10.6).

Muscle Vasoconstrictor Neurons

About 90% of the postganglionic axons in the muscle nerves of the hindlimb consist of vasoconstrictor axons; these noradrenergic axons are associated with small and large arterial blood vessels, but not with veins in skeletal muscle. A few postganglionic axons in muscle nerves may have vasodilator and other functions (see Subchapter 4.2.2). The vast majority of muscle sympathetic neurons are spontaneously active; a few appear to be silent under experimental conditions. The rate of spontaneous activity is in the range of 0.5 to 3 imp/s in the anesthetized cat (Jänig 1985, 1988) and 1.4 ± 0.5 imp/s (range 0.3 to 2.4 imp/s) in the anesthetized rat (Häbler et al. 1994a) (see Table 6.2). The proportion of spontaneously active and silent neurons may vary between individual animals. However, it is safe to say that the ongoing activity recorded from bundles containing postganglionic axons isolated from muscle nerves arises only from muscle vasoconstrictor axons.

Muscle vasoconstrictor neurons have the following key functional properties, some of which are demonstrated in Figure 4.1:

1. They are under powerful inhibitory control by the arterial baroreceptors. This generates rhythmic firing due to periods of inhibition resulting from the rhythmic activation of the arterial baroreceptors by the increase of blood pressure during each cardiac cycle (Figure 4.1c).

2. They are excited by most inputs from the body surface (e.g., nociceptors, Figure 4.1a), from the viscera (e.g., distension-sensitive receptors in the urinary bladder and colon), from arterial chemoreceptors (Figure 4.1b) and from high-threshold trigeminal receptors (Figure 4.2). Stimulation of low-threshold mechanoreceptive afferents from cutaneous hair follicles on one of the limbs leads to inhibition of the activity in muscle vasoconstrictor neurons (Figure 4.1d; Horeyseck and Jänig 1974a).

3. They are inhibited by stimulation of muscle nociceptors of the same extremity (Kirillova-Woitke et al. 2014), but mostly excited by stimulation of other nociceptors (see Box 4.1).

4. Stimulation of central thermoreceptors (by hypothalamic and/or spinal cord warming) does not influence muscle vasoconstrictor neurons (Grewe et al. 1995).

5. The activity of muscle vasoconstrictor neurons is modulated during the respiratory cycle in a characteristic way in the cat. They are excited during central inspiration (particularly when the respiratory drive is high), with a period of decreased activity in postinspiration and sometimes with a period of decreased activity in early inspiration. This profile of respiratory modulation of activity in muscle vasoconstrictor neurons interacts with the inhibitory effects of arterial baroreceptors and possibly other cardiovascular afferents, which are stimulated rhythmically

Table 4.1 Functional types of sympathetic vasoconstrictor neurons in the cat based on reflex behavior in vivo

Likely function	Location	Target organ	Likely target blood vessel	Major identifying stimulus	Ongoing activity[a]
Muscle vasoconstrictor	Lumbar	Hindlimb muscles	Resistance vessels	Baro-inhibition	Yes
	Cervical	Head and neck muscles	Resistance vessels	Baro-inhibition	Yes
Cutaneous vasoconstrictor	Lumbar	Hindlimb skin	Thermoregulatory blood vessels	Inhibited by CNS warming	Yes
	Cervical	Head and neck skin	Thermoregulatory blood vessels	Inhibited by CNS warming	Yes
Visceral vasoconstrictor	Lumbar splanchnic	Pelvic viscera	Resistance vessels	Baro-inhibition	Yes
Renal vasoconstrictor	Thoracic splanchnic	Kidney	Resistance vessels	Baro-inhibition	Yes

For details about rates of ongoing activity in pre- and postganglionic neurons, reflexes to various afferent stimuli, spinal and supraspinal reflex pathways, coupling to regulation of respiration and conduction velocities of pre- and postganglionic axons see Table 6.2 and Jänig (1985, 1988), Jänig and McLachlan (1987), Jänig et al. (1991), Boczek-Funcke et al. (1992b, c, 1993), Häbler et al. (1994b), Grewe et al. (1995), Kirillova-Woytke et al. (2014).

CNS, central nervous system.

Modified from Jänig and Häbler (1999).

[a] Some neurons do not have spontaneous activity and are recruited under special functional conditions.

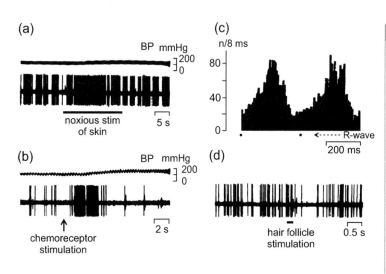

(a)

BP mmHg

noxious stim of skin — 5 s

(b)

BP mmHg

↑ chemoreceptor stimulation — 2 s

(c)

n/8 ms

R-wave

200 ms

(d)

hair follicle stimulation — 0.5 s

Figure 4.1 Reflexes in a sympathetic postganglionic neuron projecting to the peroneal muscle with putative muscle vasoconstrictor function in the anesthetized cat. (a) Excitation in response to mechanical noxious stimulation of a toe of the ipsilateral hindpaw. (b) Excitation in response to stimulation of arterial chemoreceptors projecting through the carotid sinus nerve by retrograde bolus injection of 0.8 ml CO_2-enriched Ringer solution into the left lingual artery. (c) Strong rhythmic changes in activity with respect to phasic stimulation of arterial baroreceptors by pulsatile blood pressure (and therefore phasic inhibition of activity; "cardiac rhythmicity" of the activity, 2000 periods of activity superimposed, triggered by the R-wave of the electrocardiogram [indicated by dots]). (d) Inhibition in response to short-lasting stimulation of hair follicle receptors on the trunk of the cat by air jets (ten trials superimposed). From Blumberg et al. (1980) and unpublished.

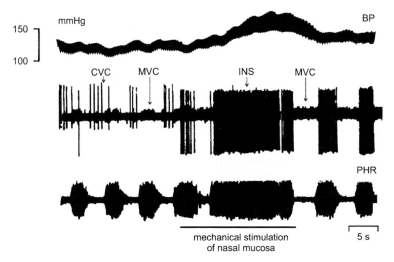

Figure 4.2 Reflexes in sympathetic preganglionic neurons elicited by mechanical stimulation of the nasal mucosa. Simultaneous recording of the activity in a cutaneous vasoconstrictor (CVC) neuron, an inspiratory (INS) neuron and a muscle vasoconstrictor (MVC) neuron in an anesthetized cat. The activity was recorded from a strand of nerve fibers isolated from the cervical sympathetic trunk and from the phrenic nerve (PHR). Before stimulation, the CVC neuron was active in expiration, the MVC neuron in inspiration and expiration and the INS neuron was almost silent. Mechanical (probably noxious) stimulation of the nasal mucosa with a small tooth brush inhibited the CVC neuron, activated the MVC neuron and activated the INS neuron in inspiration. Note that the reflex activation and inhibition in the neurons outlasted the stimulus and that the increase in blood pressure (BP) was correlated with the continuous MVC discharge. Modified from Boczek-Funcke et al. (1992b).

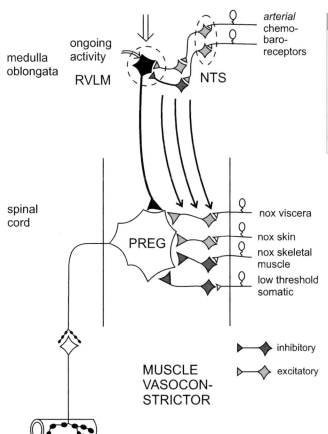

Figure 4.3 Simplified schematic diagram of the central pathways involved in the reflexes in muscle vasoconstrictor neurons elicited by physiological stimulation of spinal afferents, arterial baroreceptor afferents or arterial chemoreceptor afferents. The reflex pattern in the neurons is generated by spinal and supraspinal circuits. Excitatory interneurons gray. Inhibitory interneurons red. Sympathetic premotor neuron in medulla oblongata black. PREG, preganglionic; NTS, nucleus tractus solitarii; RVLM, rostral ventrolateral medulla. See Subchapters 9.2, 10.2 and 10.3.

when the arterial blood pressure rises and falls with inspiration and expiration (for details see Subchapter 10.6 and MVC in Figure 4.2; Häbler et al. 1993, 1994b, 1999).

The distinctive functional properties of muscle vasoconstrictor neurons are determined by reflex pathways in the spinal cord (Jänig 1996a) and by supraspinal reflex pathways through the medulla oblongata and higher central structures, as demonstrated schematically for some of these pathways in Figure 4.3. These reflex pathways will be discussed in

more detail in Chapters 9 and 10. The respiratory modulation of activity in muscle vasoconstrictor neurons is determined by the coupling between cardiovascular sympathetic premotor neurons in the medulla oblongata (e.g., in the rostral ventrolateral medulla [RVLM], see Figure 4.3) and neurons of the ponto-medullary respiratory network (see Häbler et al. [1994b]). This has been worked out in experiments on anesthetized animals in which respiratory parameters (activity in phrenic nerve) were recorded in parallel with the activity of muscle vasoconstrictor neurons (see Subchapter 10.6).

Box 4.1 | The Inhibitory Nociceptive Reflexes in Vasoconstrictor Neurons: The Lovén Reflexes

In anesthetized rats and cats, noxious stimulation of the hindpaw skin leads to inhibition of the activity in most cutaneous vasoconstrictor (CVC) neurons innervating the same hindpaw, but not to inhibition (or even to weak excitation) of most CVC neurons innervating the contralateral hindpaw. Most muscle vasoconstrictor (MVC) neurons innervating the ipsilateral or contralateral hindlimb are not affected or excited by these noxious cutaneous stimuli. Noxious stimulation of skeletal muscle leads to strong inhibition of activity in most MVC neurons of the same extremity; CVC neurons are not inhibited by these noxious muscle stimuli but weakly excited [1] (Figure 4.4). These functionally distinct inhibitory nociceptive reflexes in vasoconstrictor neurons demonstrate the close integration between nociceptive and vasoconstrictor systems at the spinal cord level.

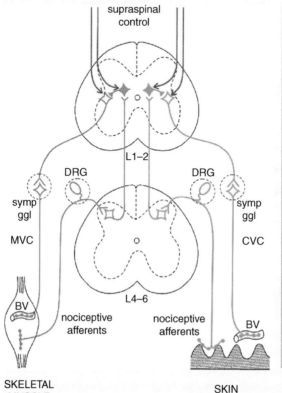

Figure 4.4 Organization of the inhibitory nociceptive reflexes in the cutaneous vasoconstrictor (CVC) system (right) and the muscle vasoconstrictor (MVC) system (left): a hypothesis. Stimulation of cutaneous nociceptive afferent neurons leads to inhibition of ipsilaterally projecting CVC neurons, but not of MVC neurons. Stimulation of muscle nociceptive afferent neurons leads to inhibition of ipsilaterally projecting MVC neurons but not of CVC neurons. The inhibitory reflexes are organized within the spinal cord (here between different lumbar segmental levels). The inhibitory interneurons are possibly located in the same spinal segments as the preganglionic vasoconstrictor neurons. The spinal nociceptive inhibitory reflex pathways are largely, but not entirely, lateralized. It is hypothesized that they are under differential supraspinal modulation. BV, blood vessel; DRG, dorsal root ganglion; L, lumbar; symp ggl, sympathetic ganglion. Modified from [1].

Based on indirect observations, the inhibitory reflex in CVC neurons was first described by Christian Lovén (Jänig 2021) in the skin of rabbits while working in Carl Ludwig's laboratory in Leipzig [2]. He found that electrical stimulation of the central stump of the dorsal nerve of the hindpaw, a branch of the superficial peroneal nerve (the nervus dorsalis pedis, which is a skin nerve), leads to dilation of the saphenous artery of the same extremity, no vasodilation but sometimes vasoconstriction in the ear skin and an increase in blood pressure. Stimulation of the central stump of the posterior branch of the auricular nerve generates vasodilation in the ear skin, no vasodilation but sometimes vasoconstriction of the saphenous artery and an increase in blood pressure. Lovén concluded that vasodilation of skin vessels is generated reflexly by stimulation of afferents which innervate either the same skin territory that is innervated by the cutaneous vasomotor fibers or a nearby territory of skin. Lovén concluded furthermore that vasomotor fibers innervating the saphenous artery or ear blood vessels must be different from the vasomotor fibers responsible for the increase in blood pressure [2]. Lovén did not use terms like "vasoconstrictor fibers" and "vasodilator fibers." Therefore he did not describe his results as being generated by decrease of activity in vasoconstrictor neurons or activation of vasodilator neurons. Bayliss [3] reproduced the Lovén reflex indirectly for skeletal muscle in dogs by measuring plethysmographically the volume change of the hindlimb, which is largely dependent on blood flow through skeletal muscle. Electrical stimulation of the distally cut lumbar dorsal root L6 elicited a vasodilation and electrical stimulation of the median nerve and a vasoconstriction in the hindlimb. Bayliss and various authors of textbook chapters describing the Lovén reflex [4,5,6,7] believed that the reflex vasodilation resulting from stimulation of (probably nociceptive) afferents supplying the same tissues as the efferent sympathetic vasomotor fibers is likely to be a general phenomenon everywhere in the body. Thus, the results of Lovén were generalized to apply to other organs or tissues than the skin, although Lovén never investigated the reflex inhibition in other organs.

The Lovén reflex was only described in Anglo-American textbooks but not in German textbooks. It was almost forgotten after the 1950s. The Lovén reflex in CVC neurons was redetected in my laboratory in Heidelberg [8,9] and in Kiel [10,11, 12,13,14] and extended to the skeletal muscle in rats [1]. There is some indirect experimental evidence that the Lovén reflex also exists in the skin of humans (see Figure 4.9 [15]). I hypothesize that this prominent inhibitory nociceptive spinal reflex is a basic building block of various reflexes involving the sympathetic vasoconstrictor system (see Subchapters 9.1 and 9.2).*

References

1. Kirillova-Woytke I, Baron R and Jänig W. Reflex inhibition of cutaneous and muscle vasoconstrictor neurons during stimulation of cutaneous and muscle nociceptors. *J Neurophysiol* 111: 1833–1845, 2014.
2. Lovén C. Über die Erweiterung von Arterien in Folge einer Nervenerregung [On the vasodilation of arteries as a consequence of a nerve stimulation]. *Ber Verh Königl-sächs Ges Wiss: Math-phys Classe* 18: 85–110, 1866.
3. Bayliss WM. On reciprocal innervation in vaso-motor reflexes and the action of strychnine and of chloroform thereon. *Proc Roy Soc B* 80: 339–375, 1908.
4. Bard P. Regulation of the systemic circulation. In Mountcastle VB (ed.): *Medical Physiology Vol I, 12th edn.* The C.V. Mosby Company, p. 194, 1968.
5. Bell GH, Davidson JN and Scarborough H. *Textbook of Physiology and Biochemistry, 6th edn.* Edinburgh and London: E. & S. Livingstone Ltd, p. 520, 1950.

---

* Lovén conducted his experiments on rabbits in an unethical way by present-day standards. The rabbits were unanesthetized and curarized in a way that the animals could still breath. These types of unethically conducted experiments should not normally be discussed in the international literature. In addition it usually remains unclear whether results obtained in this way represent the real functioning of the investigated system under physiological conditions.

6. Detweiler DK. Control mechanisms of the circulatory system. In Brobeck JR (ed). *Best & Taylor's Physiological Basis of Medical Practice*, 10th edn. Baltimore: The Williams & Wilkins Company, p. 3–178, 1979.

7. Hamilton W. Circulation through special regions. In Fulton J (ed). *A Textbook of Physiology*, 16th edn, Philadelphia, London: WB Saunders Company, 1950, p. 760–765.

8. Horeyseck G and Jänig W. Reflexes in postganglionic fibres within skin and muscle nerves after noxious stimulation of skin. *Exp Brain Res* 20: 125–134, 1974b.

9. Horeyseck G and Jänig W. Reflex activity in postganglionic fibres within skin and muscle nerves elicited by somatic stimuli in chronic spinal cats. *Exp Brain Res* 21: 155–168, 1974c.

10. Grosse M and Jänig W. Vasoconstrictor and pilomotor fibres in skin nerves to the cat's tail. *Pflügers Arch* 361: 221–229, 1976.

11. Häbler HJ, Jänig W, Krummel M and Peters OA. Reflex patterns in postganglionic neurons supplying skin and skeletal muscle of the rat hindlimb. *J Neurophysiol* 72: 2222–2236, 1994a.

12. Jänig W and Kümmel H. Functional discrimination of postganglionic neurones to the cat's hindpaw with respect to the skin potentials recorded from the hairless skin. *Pflügers Arch* 371: 217–225, 1977.

13. Jänig W and Kümmel H. Organization of the sympathetic innervation supplying the hairless skin of the cat's paw. *J Auton Nerv Syst* 3: 215–230, 1981.

14. Jänig W and Spilok N. Functional organization of the sympathetic innervation supplying the hairless skin of the hindpaws in chronic spinal cats. *Pflügers Arch* 377: 25–31, 1978.

15. Blumberg H and Wallin BG. Direct evidence of neurally mediated vasodilatation in hairy skin of the human foot. *J Physiol* 382: 105–121, 1987.

The observed responses in *postganglionic* muscle vasoconstrictor neurons are typical of what would be expected for vasoconstrictor neurons that determine peripheral vascular resistance. These neurons terminate virtually exclusively on resistance vessels (arterioles and small arteries 20 to 250 μm in diameter). Activation of these neurons is followed by an increase in arterial blood pressure. An identical discharge pattern has been observed in lumbar *preganglionic* neurons in pathways that project to the hindlimb (Jänig and Szulczyk 1980, 1981) and in thoracic *preganglionic* neurons that project to the head and neck via the superior cervical ganglion (Boczek-Funcke et al. 1992a, b). Thus, in the cat, about 20% of the preganglionic neurons projecting through the cervical sympathetic trunk to the superior cervical ganglion (targets in head and neck; Boczek-Funcke et al. 1992a, 1993) and 10% of the preganglionic neurons projecting to paravertebral ganglia distal to the lumbar ganglion L5 (targets in hindlimb and tail; Jänig and Szulczyk 1980) have functional properties of muscle vasoconstrictor neurons (see Table 4.5 and Subchapter 4.7).

Visceral Vasoconstrictor Neurons

A discharge pattern that is very similar to that of muscle vasoconstrictor neurons, i.e., showing spontaneous activity, strong inhibitory control of activity by arterial baroreceptors, activation during stimulation of arterial chemoreceptors and rhythmic changes in activity with central respiration, has been found in three separate groups of sympathetic neurons: (1) in a subpopulation of sympathetic *preganglionic* neurons in the upper lumbar segments that project in the lumbar splanchnic nerves to the inferior mesenteric ganglion, (2) in a subpopulation of sympathetic *postganglionic* neurons in the inferior mesenteric ganglion that project to the colon or pelvic viscera and (3) in a subpopulation of spontaneously active *postganglionic* neurons in the renal nerves. It is likely that pre- and postganglionic visceral vasoconstrictor neurons, projecting through the major and minor splanchnic nerves to the celiac and superior mesenteric ganglia and from there through mesenteric and other nerves to blood vessels in the viscera, also have the same functional discharge pattern. In the cat, about 15% of the preganglionic neurons projecting in the lumbar splanchnic nerves (target vessels in the pelvic organs and colon; Bahr et al. 1986c) have functional properties of visceral vasoconstrictor neurons (see Table 4.5 and Subchapter 4.7).

There are quantitative differences between the reflex patterns in visceral and muscle vasoconstrictor neurons indicating that the central outputs to these two sets of vasoconstrictor pathways are not identical. Furthermore, renal vasoconstrictor neurons may differ functionally from vasoconstrictor neurons innervating other viscera and from sympathetic neurons controlling non-vascular functions in the kidney (see Subchapter 4.4; Bahr et al. 1986b; Dorward et al. 1987; Jänig 1988; Jänig et al. 1991; Kopp and DiBona 1992; DiBona and Kopp 1997; Johns et al. 2011).

The pattern of activity present in muscle and visceral vasoconstrictor neurons is found in peripheral pathways throughout the body. Because of the ubiquity of small-resistance vessels, the constriction of which is the primary determinant of the level of arterial blood pressure, discharge patterns in sympathetic neurons with predominantly cardiac and respiratory rhythms dominate almost all recordings from the cervical and lumbar sympathetic trunks, the renal nerves and the splanchnic nerves (Häbler et al. 1994b).

Cutaneous Vasoconstrictor Neurons

Most postganglionic axons in skin nerves supply blood vessels, sweat glands or piloerector muscles. The sympathetic innervation of the blood vessels is largely vasoconstrictor but in some parts of the skin there may also be sympathetic vasodilator axons (see Subchapter 4.2). The cutaneous vasoconstrictor axons probably differ according to the section of the vascular bed they innervate (small muscular artery, arteriole, arteriovenous anastomosis, vein) and according to the type of skin (hairless [glabrous] skin of the distal extremities, hairy skin, skin of the trunk and proximal extremities, skin of the face). This is reflected in a differential colocalization of neuropeptides in noradrenergic neurons to the cutaneous vasculature of the guinea pig where different sections of the cutaneous arterial tree are supplied by postganglionic axons with different peptide content (Gibbins and Morris 1990; Morris 1995; see Subchapter 1.4). It is also reflected in the finding that vasomotor control of rat tail and proximal hairy skin is independent (Tanaka et al. 2007). These studies suggest different functions for different types of cutaneous vasoconstrictor neurons. Thus, it would not be unexpected that the activity pattern in cutaneous vasoconstrictor neurons is not as uniform as that in muscle vasoconstrictor neurons. Further, the functional identification of cutaneous vasoconstrictor neurons innervating different sections of the cutaneous vascular bed remains to be elucidated.

Many cutaneous vasoconstrictor neurons are spontaneously active in the anesthetized cat and rat. However, the exact percentage of spontaneously active postganglionic cutaneous vasoconstrictor neurons under thermoneutral conditions is unknown. The rate of spontaneous activity in these active postganglionic neurons is 1.2 ± 0.7 imp/s (mean ± SD; range 0.1 to 4 imp/s) in the cat (hairy and hairless skin; Jänig 1985, 1988), 1.2 ± 0.6 imp/s (range 0.3 to 2.4 imp/s) in cutaneous vasoconstrictor neurons innervating the hairy skin of the rat hindlimb (Häbler et al. 1994a) and 1.1 ± 0.7 imp/s (range 0.23 to 2.6 imp/s) in those innervating the rat tail (Häbler et al. 1999) (see Table 6.2).

Most cutaneous vasoconstrictor neurons that innervate the hairy or hairless skin of the cat and rat hindpaw or tail (i.e., the distal skin of the extremities or tail) have complex discharge patterns that differ from those of muscle vasoconstrictor neurons (Figure 4.5) in the following ways (data taken from Jänig and Kümmel [1981]; Jänig [1985, 1988]; Häbler et al. [1992, 1994a]; Grewe et al. [1995] [cat hindpaw, tail]):

1. Inhibition of activity elicited by stimulation of arterial baroreceptors is weak or absent in about 80% of cutaneous vasoconstrictor neurons innervating hairy skin and probably in all cutaneous vasoconstrictor neurons innervating hairless skin of the paw. In these neurons, the phasic bursts of discharge in parallel with the pulse pressure wave, which are typical of muscle vasoconstrictor activity, are absent or weak (Figure 4.5c).
2. Warming the hypothalamus and/or the spinal cord inhibits activity in almost all cutaneous vasoconstrictor neurons (both hairy and hairless skin). This also applies to neurons that are responsive to arterial baroreceptor stimulation. Decreased activity in the cutaneous vasoconstrictor neurons is followed by increased skin temperature (Figure 3.5).
3. Stimulation of cutaneous nociceptors in the ipsilateral paw inhibits most cutaneous vasoconstrictor neurons innervating the stimulated paw, whereas stimulation of cutaneous nociceptors at more remote body sites has weaker inhibitory effects or is even excitatory (Horeyseck and Jänig 1974b). This type of reflex pattern is also very pronounced for cutaneous vasoconstrictor neurons innervating the cat tail (Figure 4.5a) (Grosse and Jänig 1976). This unique inhibitory nociceptor reflex is described in Box 4.1 for cutaneous and muscle vasoconstrictor neurons in animals.

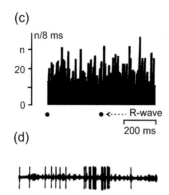

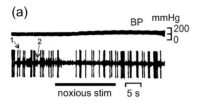

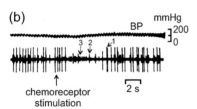

(a)

BP mmHg

noxious stim   5 s

(b)

BP mmHg

chemoreceptor stimulation   2 s

(c)

n/8 ms

n

R-wave
200 ms

(d)

hair follicle stimulation   0.5 s

Figure 4.5 Reflexes in a sympathetic postganglionic neuron with putative cutaneous vasoconstrictor function in an anesthetized cat. Postganglionic neuron (large action potential 1) innervating hairy skin of the hindlimb (innervation territory of the superficial peroneal nerve). (a) Inhibition in response to mechanical noxious stimulation of a toe of the ipsilateral hindpaw. (b) Inhibition in response to stimulation of arterial chemoreceptors projecting through the carotid sinus nerve (see legend Figure 4.1b). (c) No rhythmic changes in activity with respect to phasic stimulation of arterial baroreceptors by pulsatile blood pressure (1000 periods of activity superimposed, triggered by the R-wave of the electrocardiogram [indicated by dots]). See Figure 4.1c. (d) Excitation in response to short-lasting stimulation of hair follicle receptors on the trunk by air jets (10 trials superimposed). Note that the bundle recorded from contained two other postganglionic axons, one behaving like a cutaneous vasoconstrictor neuron (axon 2) and the other like a muscle vasoconstrictor neuron (axon 3). From Blumberg et al. (1980) and unpublished.

4. Stimulation of low-threshold mechanoreceptive afferents from the skin of one of the limbs (e.g., hair follicle receptors) leads to excitation of the activity in cutaneous vasoconstrictor neurons (Figure 4.5d; Horeyseck and Jänig 1974a).

5. Stimulation of other afferent inputs (from pelvic organs, from arterial chemoreceptors, from trigeminal nasal afferents) also inhibits cutaneous vasoconstrictor neurons in the cat (Figures 4.2, 4.5b).

6. Cutaneous vasoconstrictor neurons exhibit either no respiratory rhythm in their activity, or activity decreases during inspiration and increases during expiration or, alternatively, only increases during inspiration. These various distinct respiratory patterns in the activity of cutaneous vasoconstrictor neurons show that the ponto-medullary respiratory network in the lower brain stem and the circuits regulating activity in cutaneous vasoconstrictor neurons are coupled and that this coupling is different from that to the vasoconstrictor pathways innervating resistance vessels in skeletal muscle or viscera (see Subchapters 10.6.4 and 10.6.5; see CVC in Figure 4.2).

Cutaneous vasoconstrictor neurons innervating the hairy skin of the rat hindpaw (Häbler et al. 1994b) or the rat tail (Häbler et al. 1999, 2000; Owens et al. 2002) have discharge patterns similar to those in the cat; however, the reflexes are not as pronounced as in the cat.

There are quantitative differences in functional properties between the populations of postganglionic cutaneous vasoconstrictor neurons innervating hairy skin and those supplying hairless skin. A small group of cutaneous vasoconstrictor neurons innervating hairy skin (<20%) behaves at least qualitatively like muscle and visceral vasoconstrictor neurons, i.e., they are under strong inhibitory reflex control from arterial baroreceptors and are excited by both stimulation of arterial chemoreceptors and of cutaneous nociceptors (Blumberg et al. 1980). This group of cutaneous vasoconstrictor neurons has not been found among vasoconstrictor neurons to hairless skin of the cat paw (Jänig and Kümmel 1977; Figures 4.11, 4.12). This is consistent with the existence of functional subgroups of cutaneous vasoconstrictor neurons innervating different sections of the vascular bed (nutritive blood vessels, arteriovenous anastomoses, capacitance vessels). All or most cutaneous vasoconstrictor neurons innervating skin of the distal extremity are likely to be involved in thermoregulation (Grewe et al. 1995; Morrison 2018).

The typical reflex pattern seen in *postganglionic* cutaneous vasoconstrictor neurons has also been identified in lumbar *preganglionic* neurons projecting to the hindlimb and in thoracic preganglionic neurons projecting to the superior cervical ganglion. About 12% to 13% of the preganglionic neurons projecting in the lumbar sympathetic trunk distal to the paravertebral ganglion L5 (target vessels in hindlimb and tail; Jänig and Szulczyk 1980) or in the cervical sympathetic trunk (target vessels in head and neck; Boczek-Funcke et al. 1992a, 1993) exhibit functional properties of cutaneous vasoconstrictor neurons (see Table 4.5 and Subchapter 4.7).

The complex reflex patterns in cutaneous vasoconstrictor neurons are most likely not the result of integration of functionally different synaptic inputs in sympathetic paravertebral ganglia. We have, however, no absolute experimental proof that preganglionic neurons with muscle vasoconstrictor-like discharge patterns and preganglionic neurons with cutaneous vasoconstrictor-like discharge patterns converge on the same postganglionic neurons (see Chapter 6). The functional properties of cutaneous vasoconstrictor neurons are determined by reflex pathways in the spinal cord, lower brain stem and hypothalamus. Experiments in cats with chronically transected spinal cords show that there are several spinal reflex pathways that are specific for the cutaneous vasoconstrictor system (Figure 4.6; see Subchapter 9.2). In essence, these reflex pathways seem to be more complex than those of muscle and visceral vasoconstrictor neurons (Jänig 1985, 1996a). They are under complex control of the lower brain stem and hypothalamus largely related to thermoregulation (Morrison 2018; Romanovsky 2018), but available information is limited (see Chapters 9 and 10).

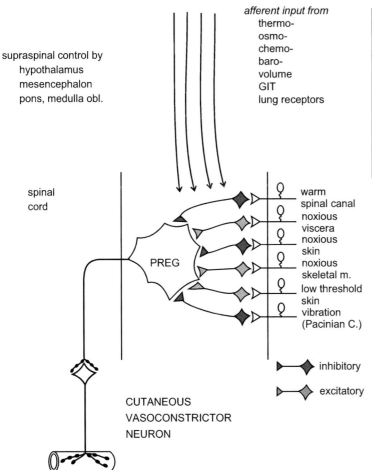

afferent input from
thermo-
osmo-
chemo-
baro-
volume
GIT
lung receptors

supraspinal control by
hypothalamus
mesencephalon
pons, medulla obl.

spinal
cord

PREG

warm
spinal canal
noxious
viscera
noxious
skin
noxious
skeletal m.
low threshold
skin
vibration
(Pacinian C.)

inhibitory

excitatory

CUTANEOUS
VASOCONSTRICTOR
NEURON

Figure 4.6 Schematic diagram of the central pathways involved in the reflexes in cutaneous vasoconstrictor neurons elicited by physiological stimulation of spinal afferents, vagal afferents or thermosensitive neurons. The reflex pattern in the neurons is generated by spinal and supraspinal circuits. The supraspinal components are related to the hypothalamus, and upper and lower brain stem. Inhibitory interneurons in red; excitatory interneurons in gray. See Subchapters 9.2 and 10.5. GIT, gastrointestinal tract; PREG, preganglionic neuron.

4.1.2 Vasoconstrictor Neurons in Human Subjects

Muscle Vasoconstrictor Neurons

Healthy humans and anesthetized cats and rats (with intact vagus and baroreceptor nerves) have very similar discharge patterns in muscle vasoconstrictor neurons but in resting recumbent humans the rate of spontaneous activity is significantly lower than in the anesthetized cat and rat (0.33 ± 0.04 imp/s, mean ± SD, range 0.09 to 0.69 imp/s, n = 33; Macefield and Wallin 1999a). In humans there are considerable interindividual differences in the rate of resting activity in muscle vasoconstrictor neurons, which are reproducible in an individual over weeks, months and years (Sundlöf and Wallin 1977; Fagius and Wallin 1993); the reason for these interindividual differences is unclear, but homozygotic twins have similar levels of activity in muscle vasoconstrictor neurons (Lundblad et al. 2017). Overall, the resting activity increases with age (Mano 1999); however, it is unclear if the percentage of active muscle vasoconstrictor neurons is higher or if individual postganglionic neurons have a higher rate of resting activity or both.

The activity in muscle vasoconstrictor neurons exhibits rhythmic changes that are correlated with the pulse pressure wave (Figure 4.8b) and with respiration (Figure 4.7). The pulse-synchronous bursts of activity are triggered by rhythmic unloading of the arterial baroreceptors and are clearly equivalent to the cardiac rhythmicity of the activity in muscle vasoconstrictor neurons of animals (see Figure 4.1; Hagbarth and Vallbo 1968; Delius et al. 1972; Sundlöf and Wallin 1978; Eckberg et al. 1985; Wallin and Fagius 1988). The "respiratory" rhythmicity of the activity in the muscle vasoconstrictor neurons is mostly closely linked to the respiratory fluctuations of the arterial blood pressure, suggesting that both rhythmic changes are generated by activation of arterial baroreceptors during each increase in arterial blood pressure. However, there is also a respiratory rhythmicity that is independent of the arterial baroreceptors (for details see Subchapter 10.6).

Any procedure that leads to changes in arterial blood pressure or changes in volume in the venous capacitance system generates reflex changes of activity in the muscle vasoconstrictor neurons ("sympathetic bursts") via stimulation or unloading of arterial baroreceptors or of intrathoracic low-pressure receptors in

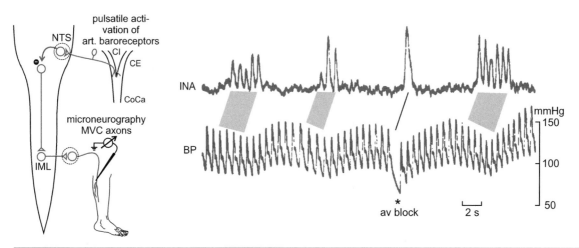

Figure 4.7 Pulsatile unloading and activation of arterial baroreceptors leads to pulsatile excitation and inhibition of muscle vasoconstrictor (MVC) neurons in an awake human subject. Integrated multiunit neural activity (INA) in postganglionic MVC axons recorded microneurographically (see Figure 3.6) from the deep peroneal nerve. Lower trace, arterial blood pressure (BP). Respiration-related increase in BP is followed by inhibition of MVC activity. Note that during respiration-related decrease of BP the MVC neurons are activated in a pulsatile manner. This is generated by pulsatile decrease of arterial baroreceptor activity. An atrioventricular (av) block is followed by a large decrease of BP (asterisk) and subsequently by a strong activation of the MVC neurons (due to unloading of arterial baroreceptors). Left: arterial baroreceptor circuit in simplified form. Θ, inhibition; CoCa, common carotid artery; CE, external carotid artery; CI, internal carotid artery; IML, intermediolateral nucleus; NTS, nucleus tractus solitarii. Modified from Wallin and Fagius (1986) with permission.

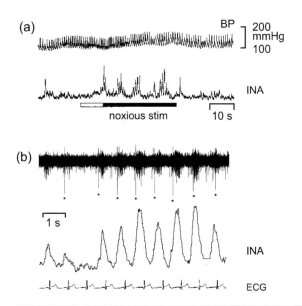

Figure 4.8 Microneurographic recordings in awake human subjects from nerve fiber bundles containing several muscle vasoconstrictor axons in the deep peroneal nerve. (a) Activation by mechanical noxious stimulation (black bar); non-noxious mechanical stimulation (open bar). Note pulsatile and respiratory modulation of neural bursts. (b) Activation during apnea (cessation of respiration). Note rhythmic multiunit and single unit (*) activity with respect to electrocardiogram (ECG). BP, blood pressure; INA, integrated neural activity. Modified from Nordin and Fagius (1995) and Macefield and Wallin (1999a) with permission.

the right atrium and large veins (Sundlöf and Wallin 1978; Vissing et al. 1994). For example, a short transient block of atrioventricular conduction in the pacemaker system of the heart is followed by a transient drop in arterial blood pressure (because the ventricle fails to pump one stroke volume into the arterial system) and a decrease in activity of arterial baroreceptors; this is then followed by a reflex activation of muscle vasoconstrictor neurons (see asterisk in Figure 4.7). Noxious stimuli (e.g., excitation of cutaneous nociceptors by mechanical stimulation [Figure 4.8a] or by radiant heat or with iced water [the cold pressor test] [Victor et al. 1987]), stimulation of trigeminal receptors (e.g., by immersion of the face in water [Fagius and Sundlöf 1986]) or apnea (arrest of respiration) activate muscle vasoconstrictor neurons in human subjects, as they do in the cat.

Cutaneous Vasoconstrictor Neurons

In humans, cutaneous vasoconstrictor neurons projecting to the distal parts of the extremities have ongoing activity at neutral ambient temperatures. They discharge at rates that are lower than those in anesthetized cats and rats. The rates (measured in cooled subjects) are 0.53 ± 0.11 imp/s (mean ± SEM; range 0.08 to 2.04, n = 17; Macefield and Wallin 1999b). Most cutaneous vasoconstrictor neurons that supply proximal skin areas in human subjects seem to be silent at neutral ambient temperatures (Bini et al. 1980b; see Johnson and Kellogg [2018]). The same may be true for cutaneous vasoconstrictor neurons innervating the trunk.

Thermal stimuli are the most specific stimuli that change the activity in these cutaneous vasoconstrictor neurons: exposure to warm or cold environments is followed by a decrease or increase, respectively, in activity of vasoconstrictor neurons innervating the distal skin of the extremities (Figure 4.9a; Bini et al. 1980a). The ongoing activity in groups of cutaneous vasoconstrictor neurons innervating hairless skin of the palm in human subjects is not, or is only weakly, under the control of either arterial baroreceptors (Bini et al. 1981; Fagius et al. 1985) or low-pressure baroreceptors in the right atrium (Vissing et al. 1994). Therefore, in human subjects, changes of activity in cutaneous vasoconstrictor neurons with the pulse pressure wave are absent or small. However, human subjects undergoing whole-body cooling exhibit cardiac rhythmicity in the activity recorded microneurographically from bundles in the superficial peroneal nerve which innervate hairy skin (Macefield and Wallin 1999b). Thus, as in the cat, there is a difference between cutaneous vasoconstrictor neurons innervating hairy skin and cutaneous vasoconstrictor neurons innervating hairless skin: those innervating hairless (glabrous) skin are under weak or no control of the baroreceptor reflexes, whereas those innervating hairy skin are under some baroreceptor control.

It is unclear whether cutaneous vasoconstrictor neurons in humans are reflexly inhibited during noxious stimulation of the skin. The absence of the inhibitory nociceptive reflexes in cutaneous vasoconstrictor neurons in humans may have a simple explanation: noxious cutaneous stimuli in conscious humans excite cortical centers which then lead to activation of the cutaneous vasoconstrictor system and a complete masking of the inhibitory reflexes. Blumberg and Wallin (1987) may have overcome this masking by electrical microstimulation of nociceptive Aδ-afferents

Table 4.2 Functional classification of sympathetic neurons innervating skeletal muscle and skin in human subjects based on microneurographic studies

Likely function	Target organ	Likely target tissue	Major identifying stimulus	Ongoing activity[a]
Muscle vasoconstr.	Leg, arm distal	Resistance vessels	Baro-inhibition	Yes
Cutaneous vasoconstr.	Leg, arm	Thermoregul. blood vessels	Excited by general cooling	Yes
Sudomotor	Leg, arm	Sweat glands	Excited by whole-body warming	Yes
Cutaneous vasodilator	Proximal extremities and trunk; face	Blood vessels	Excited by whole-body warming	No (?)
Pilomotor	Hairy skin	Piloerector muscles	?	No (?)

All data are obtained from postganglionic neurons in awake humans. For details about rates of ongoing activity, reflexes to various stimuli and maneuvers, coupling to respiration and conduction velocity of postganglionic axons see Hagbarth et al. (1972), Bini et al. (1980a, b), Nordin (1990), Macefield et al. (1994), Noll et al. (1994), Nordin and Fagius (1995), Macefield and Wallin (1996, 1999a, b, 2018), Wallin et al. (1998).

[a] Some neurons do not have spontaneous activity and are recruited under particular functional conditions. Modified from Jänig and Häbler (1999).

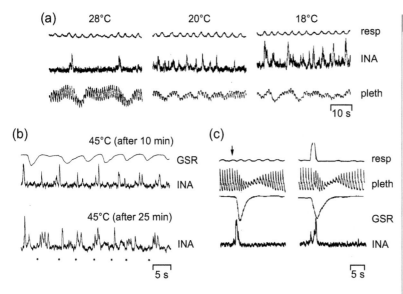

(a) 28°C 20°C 18°C resp INA pleth 10 s

(b) 45°C (after 10 min) GSR INA 45°C (after 25 min) INA 5 s

(c) resp pleth GSR INA 5 s

Figure 4.9 Microneurographic recordings of activity in cutaneous vasoconstrictor neurons and sudomotor neurons in awake human subjects. (a) Integrated cutaneous vasoconstrictor activity (median nerve) at three different ambient temperatures in relation to a finger pulse plethymogram (pleth, vasoconstriction downward and reduction of pulsatile amplitude) (Note 1). Note increase of neural activity and decrease of finger pulse amplitude during decrease of ambient temperature and relation of neural bursts to phasic vasoconstriction. Upper record, respiration (resp). (b) Integrated sudomotor activity at high central (and ambient) temperature in relation to palmar skin resistance change (GSR; galvanic skin response; reduction of skin resistance downward during activation of sudomotor neurons). Activation of sudomotor neurons is accompanied by perception of heat waves (indicated by *). (c) Activation of both cutaneous vasoconstrictor neurons and sudomotor neurons by arousal stimulus (sudden shout, arrow left) or by deep inspiration (right). INA, integrated neural activity (mean voltage neurogram). Modified from Wallin and Fagius (1986) and Bini et al. (1980a) with permission.

(Figure 4.10). Painful intraneural electrical microstimulation in the superficial peroneal nerve at the ankle, which probably excites thinly myelinated nociceptive afferents, elicits reflex dilation (increased blood flow) in skin areas lying adjacent to, as well as in, the territory of the stimulated nerve (Blumberg and Wallin 1987) (Note 2). The dilation is larger in the skin of the stimulated hindlimb than in the skin of the hindlimb contralateral to the noxious stimulus. The dilation in the ipsi- and contralateral skin is abolished by local anesthesia of the nerve proximal to the stimulation site and the dilation

is enhanced by body cooling (i.e., when the activity in cutaneous vasoconstrictor neurons is high). Thus, this reflex in human subjects appears to be very similar to the inhibitory reflex in cutaneous vasoconstrictor neurons elicited by cutaneous noxious stimuli in anesthetized cats and rats (Figure 4.10; see above and also Figure 4.5a; see Box 4.1 on Lovén reflexes, and Figure 4.4 and Note 3).

Cutaneous vasoconstrictor neurons in human subjects are inhibited during stimulation of trigeminal receptors by immersion of the face in water

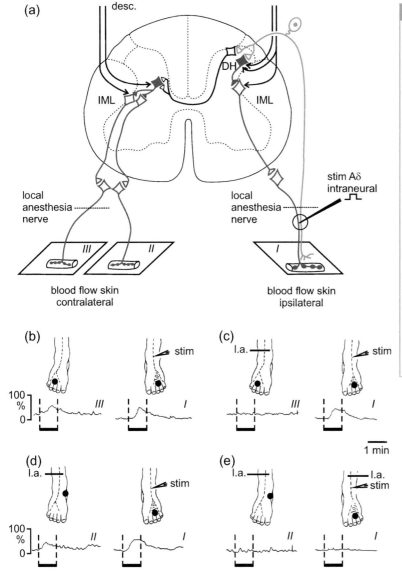

Figure 4.10 Reflex vasodilation in hairy skin generated by intraneural microstimulation of afferent Aδ-fibers in the superficial peroneal (SP) nerve in an awake human subject. The stimulation parameters were 1.1 V, 0.2 ms pulse duration and 5 Hz for 1 min. Blood flow was measured by laser Doppler flowmetry in the innervation territory of the stimulated SP nerve (territory *I*), in the innervation territory of the contralateral SP nerve (territory *III*), and outside the SP nerve innervation territory of the contralateral foot (territory *II*). Electrical intraneural stimulation elicited vasodilation in the three skin territories (b, d). Local anesthesia (l.a.) of the contralateral SP nerve prevented the vasodilation in territory *III* but not in territory *II* (c, d). Local anesthesia of the ipsilateral SP nerve proximal to the stimulation electrode prevented the contra- and ipsilateral vasodilation (e). Possible mechanisms underlying this reflex vasodilation are inhibition of activity in cutaneous vasoconstrictor neurons (a) or activation of cutaneous vasodilator neurons. DH, dorsal horn; IML, intermediolateral nucleus. Modified from Blumberg and Wallin (1987) with permission.

(Fagius and Sundlöf 1986) and during hypoglycemia (Berne and Fagius 1986). The same stimuli simultaneously excite muscle vasoconstrictor neurons. Arousal, emotional stimuli, deep breaths and hyperventilation do activate cutaneous vasoconstrictor neurons in human subjects (Figure 4.9c) (Note 2). This is typical of the conscious subject and largely depends on activity in the cerebral cortex and limbic system. Thus, excitatory and inhibitory reflexes to somatic and visceral stimuli evoked, in the anesthetized cat, in cutaneous vasoconstrictor neurons that are organized at the spinal cord level are probably masked in conscious human beings.

The data from human subjects show that cutaneous vasoconstrictor neurons are very similar in their discharge patterns to those in the anesthetized cat. The differences probably result because any change of mental state in human subjects (which certainly occurs during noxious or other uncomfortable stimuli) is reflected in the cutaneous vasoconstrictor activity, as it is in the sudomotor system in human subjects (see Subchapter 4.2).

In *summary*, the behavior of muscle and cutaneous vasoconstrictor neurons is at least as distinctive in human subjects as in anesthetized animals, indicating that the activity in the two populations of neurons is regulated by different central mechanisms. It is also important to remember that cutaneous vasoconstrictor neurons are likely to include functionally heterogeneous subtypes that are related to the type of cutaneous blood vessel and to the type of skin area (e.g. distal hairless [acral] skin and proximal hairy skin) they innervate (Johnson and Kellogg 2010, 2018; Johnson et al. 2014).

4.2 Sympathetic Non-Vasoconstrictor Pathways Innervating Somatic Tissues

Skin and deep somatic tissues are also innervated by sympathetic neurons that have other functions than vasoconstrictor neurons. So far, sudomotor neurons, pilomotor neurons and vasodilator neurons supplying target organs in skin or skeletal muscle have been studied. Some functional properties of these types of sympathetic neurons in the cat are listed in Table 4.3. Functional properties of neurons innervating the

skin of human subjects are listed in Table 4.2. From physiological studies, it is evident that other types of neurons must also exist, for example pupillodilator neurons, neurons supplying the pineal gland, sympathetic neurons supplying fat cells, etc. These neurons are likely to be activated by quite distinct central control mechanisms (see Subchapter 4.4).

4.2.1 Sympathetic Postganglionic Neurons Innervating Skin

Sudomotor Neurons

STUDIES ON ANIMALS
Postganglionic cholinergic sudomotor neurons innervate eccrine sweat glands in the hairless skin of the paw pads of the *cat* and other mammals (for review of autonomic regulation of eccrine sweat glands see Gibbins [1997]). In the cat, sweat glands are confined to the hairless skin and do not appear to be involved in thermoregulation (Grewe et al. 1995).

Sudomotor neurons have a low rate of spontaneous activity (up to 0.4 Hz under chloralose anesthesia; Figure 4.11c), or they are silent. Activity in sudomotor neurons generates changes of potential on the surface of the hairless skin of the paw pad (Figures 4.11, 4.12). The spontaneous and evoked skin potential changes can be as large as 30 mV in amplitude and are blocked by atropine, indicating that they are generated by the muscarinic action of acetylcholine released from the sudomotor axons. The potential changes are generated by synaptic activation of secretory cells and most likely extracellularly recorded secretory potentials. They are negative with respect to the extraglandular tissue, because synaptic activation of the glandular cells by the cholinergic sudomotor fibers increases the potassium conductance of the extraluminal membrane, leading to hyperpolarization of the extraluminal membrane (Note 4). Discharges in single sudomotor axons innervating the cat paw pad are followed by transient skin potentials, at constant latencies of about 600 to 800 ms (see large extracellularly recorded action potentials recorded from SM axons in Figure 4.11b,c). Simultaneously recorded activity in cutaneous vasoconstrictor neurons innervating the same hairless skin area is not followed by transient skin potential changes (see small extracellularly recorded action potentials *CVC* in Figure 4.11c). The observation that single action potentials in individual postganglionic sudomotor neurons are followed by fast transient

Table 4.3 Functional classification of sympathetic non-vasoconstrictor neurons in the cat based on reflex behavior in vivo

Likely function	Location	Target organ	Likely target tissue	Major identifying stimulus	Ongoing activity
Muscle vasodilator	Lumbar	Hindlimb muscles	Muscle arteries, feeding vessels	Hypothalamic stim., emotional stim.	No
Cutaneous vasodilator	Lumbar	Hindlimb skin	Skin blood vessels	Excited by CNS warming	No
Sudomotor	Lumbar	Paw pads	Eccrine sweat glands	Vibration (in cat)	Yes
Pilomotor	Lumbar	Skin tail, back	Piloerector muscles	Hypothalamic stim., emotional stim.	No
Inspiratory	Cervical	Airways?	Nasal mucosal vasculature	Inspiration	Yes
Pupillo-motor	Cervical	Iris	Dilator pupillae muscle	Inhibition by light	Yes
Motility-regulating					
Type 1	Lumbar splanchnic	Hindgut, urinary tract	Visceral smooth muscle	Bladder distension	Yes
Type 2	Lumbar splanchnic	Hindgut, urinary tract	Visceral smooth muscle	Inhibited by bladder distension	Yes
Reproduction	Lumbar splanchnic	Reproductive organs	Visceral smooth muscle	Central stim (?)	No

For details see Footnotes of Table 4.1.
Modified from Jänig and Häbler (1999).

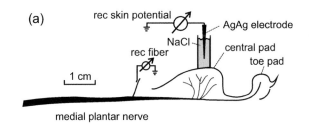

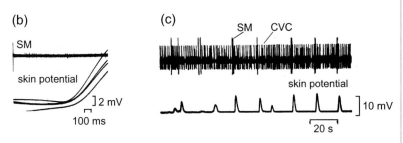

Figure 4.11 Activity in postganglionic sudomotor (SM) and cutaneous vasoconstrictor (CVC) axons innervating hairless skin in the anesthetized cat. (a) Experimental setup. Skin potential (negative transient potential changes) was recorded from the surface of the central pad with Ag/AgCl electrodes via a fluid bridge of physiological saline (0.9% sodium chloride [NaCl] solution). Recordings of activity in filaments isolated from fascicles of the medial plantar nerve innervating the hairless skin of the hindpaw. (b) Ongoing discharges in an SM axon are followed by deflections of the skin potential at about 600 ms latency (four traces superimposed). (c) Ongoing activity in a single SM axon and several CVC axons and skin potential. Most SM discharges are followed by transient skin potential changes; activity in CVC neurons is not correlated with the skin potential. Modified from Jänig and Kümmel (1977) with permission.

skin potential changes (Figure 4.11b, c) indicates that many sudomotor neurons must discharge synchronously. This might be explained by a large divergence of preganglionic sudomotor axons in paravertebral ganglia (Chapter 6) and/or by central synchronizing processes.

The most unique stimulus that leads to reflex activation of sudomotor neurons in the cat hindpaw is vibration that excites Pacinian corpuscles (largely in the hindpaw) (Figure 4.12a). Individual deflections of the skin potential elicited during this type of afferent stimulation may be preceded by individual sudomotor discharges. This excitatory reflex is a definitive functional marker for sudomotor neurons in the *cat*: no other type of sympathetic neuron can be activated in this way and stimulation of other cutaneous mechanoreceptors with large-diameter Aβ-fibers (e.g., from hair follicles) does not lead to reflex activation of sudomotor neurons. The discharge rate of sudomotor neurons

during vibrational stimuli, which elicit large skin potentials of 10 to 20 mV, ranges from 0.2 to 2.1 Hz, implying that the sudomotor neurons work in a low-frequency range under physiological conditions. Interestingly, in some experiments, cutaneous vasoconstrictor neurons innervating the same hairless skin were inhibited during the vibration stimulation (Figure 4.12a; Jänig and Kümmel 1977; Jänig and Räth 1977; see Figure 9.5).

Excitatory reflexes are also elicited in sudomotor neurons by noxious cutaneous stimuli (Figure 4.12b), by stimulation of visceral receptors in the pelvic organs (e.g., by distension and contraction of the urinary bladder [Häbler et al. 1992]) and by stimulation of arterial chemoreceptors (Figure 4.12c; Jänig and Kümmel 1981). Stimulation of arterial baroreceptors has no effect on the activity of sudomotor neurons. Warming the hypothalamus or the spinal cord does not activate sudomotor neurons in the cat

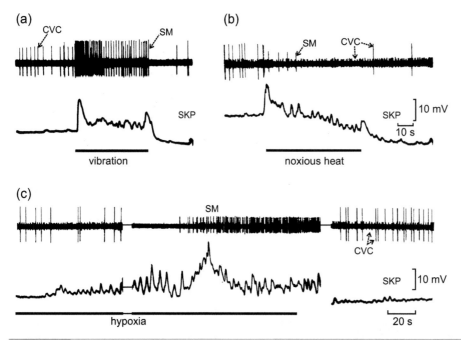

Figure 4.12 Reflex patterns, recorded simultaneously in the anesthetized cat, in sudomotor (SM) neurons and cutaneous vasoconstrictor (CVC) neurons innervating hairless skin. Upper records, activity in postganglionic neurons; lower records, skin potential (SKP; negativity up). (a) Reflex activation of a single SM neuron and reflex inhibition of a single CVC neuron during a vibration stimulus (stimulation of Pacinian corpuscles in the paws). (b) Excitation of a single SM neuron and inhibition of CVC neurons (large signal: single CVC axon; small signals: several CVC axons) to noxious stimulation of a toe of the ipsilateral hindpaw by radiant heat (55 °C). For the slow positive deflection of skin potential after activation of the SM neurons see Note 4. (c) Excitation of a single SM neuron and inhibition of CVC neurons during stimulation of arterial chemoreceptors by ventilating the cat with a gas mixture of 8% O_2 in N_2 (hypoxic ventilation started about 1 min before the record). Note complete inhibition in CVC neurons. Same preparation as in (b). Modified from Jänig and Kümmel (1977) with permission.

(Grewe et al. 1995). Activity in sudomotor neurons is modulated by central respiration (Boczek-Funcke et al. 1992c; Häbler et al. 1994b). The discharge pattern of this respiratory modulation is different from that in muscle and most cutaneous vasoconstrictor neurons, indicating a distinct coupling between the respiratory network in the medulla oblongata and sudomotor premotor neurons (see Subchapter 10.6).

The reflex pattern in sudomotor neurons is organized reciprocally to that in the cutaneous vasoconstrictor neurons innervating the cat paw: sudomotor neurons are excited by afferent stimuli that inhibit cutaneous vasoconstrictor neurons. For example, the nerve fiber bundle recorded from in Figure 4.12b,c contained one sudomotor axon (*SM*) and two cutaneous vasoconstrictor axons (*CVC*) innervating the hairless skin of the cat hindpaw. Noxious heat stimulation of skin and stimulation of arterial chemoreceptors by hypoxia inhibited the activity in the cutaneous vasoconstrictor neurons and activated the sudomotor neuron. This reciprocal reflex pattern is largely based on spinal circuits and supraspinal control mechanisms (Jänig and Kümmel 1981; Jänig 1996a; see Subchapter 9.2). The consequence of the reciprocal organization is that neural activation of sweat glands is accompanied by increased blood flow through the skin and probably subcutaneous tissue.

The function of the "vibration reflex" in the sudomotor neurons is to hydrate the epithelium of the skin in order to keep the surface of the hairless skin soft and flexible, by secretion of sweat, which diffuses into the epithelium. This increases friction during contact and creates optimal conditions for somatosensory discrimination, since any contact of the paws with surfaces during movements and manipulations always excites the Pacinian corpuscles in the paw skin. I presume that this reflex activation of sweat glands could be an ideal way to mark territory in felines and it has been speculated that the secretion is important for scent marking of walking trails (Matthews 1969).

STUDIES ON HUMAN SUBJECTS

In contrast to the cat and many other hairy mammals (not horse), sweat glands are present in skin all over the body surface in *humans*. Sudomotor neurons in human subjects are active at high ambient temperatures (Figure 4.9b) and silent at low ambient temperatures (Figure 4.9a). Some sudomotor neurons show rhythmic discharges with the arterial pressure wave at high temperatures (Bini et al. 1981). This may be because of rhythmic activation of low-pressure cardiovascular receptors: it has been shown that lower body negative pressure and head tilted up leads to a reduction in activity in sudomotor neurons (Dodt et al. 1995). Sudomotor neurons supplying sweat glands in proximal hairy skin of the extremities have a lower threshold for activation in response to warming of the body surface than sudomotor neurons supplying hairless (acral) skin, which are only activated at relatively high and unpleasant ambient temperatures. This suggests that sudomotor activity dominates the sympathetic activity in the skin nerves to, for example, the proximal forearm skin, because there is almost no activity in cutaneous vasoconstrictor neurons at ambient temperatures, whereas cutaneous vasoconstrictor activity dominates in nerves to the glabrous skin of the hand (Bini et al. 1980b). This may indicate that the primary function of sudomotor neurons destined to human glabrous skin (Note 5) is again to keep the skin flexible for optimal sensory discrimination. This function is fully consistent with the function of the vibration reflex in sudomotor neurons in the cat (see Note 6).

Like cutaneous vasoconstrictor neurons, subsets of sudomotor neurons are activated by arousal and mental (emotional) stimuli, as well as by deep breathing (Figure 4.9c; Bini et al. 1980a); these include sudomotor pathways to the glabrous skin of the hands and feet, to the armpits and to some parts of the face. The simultaneous activation of both sympathetic pathways to skin of the extremities is initiated from the forebrain and shows that the neural circuits in the neuraxis that are responsible for the reciprocal activation of the two systems are inhibited by the central signals initiated in the forebrain.

Activity of the sudomotor system is monitored by measuring electrodermal activity (either change in skin potential or change in skin resistance upon activation of the sudomotor neurons). Electrodermal activity has been used for more than 100 years by psychophysiologists to monitor intrapsychic processes (Boucsein 2012) and is the basis of the lie detector test (Lykken 1998). Any change in mental state in human subjects (e.g., generated by arousal or emotional stimuli) will activate these subsets of the sudomotor system (Note 6), depending on the thermal condition of the body (Bini et al. 1980a).

Pilomotor Neurons

Piloerector muscles exist in the hairy skin of the *cat* all over the body surface. These smooth muscles are strongly developed in the hairy skin of the tail, back, dorsal part of the upper hindleg and dorsal part of the head, but not in other parts of hairy skin (Strickland and Calhoun 1963). Repetitive electrical stimulation of the sympathetic chain is followed by piloerection on the tail, back and dorsal parts of the head, and weak piloerection on the dorsal part of the hindlimb, but no piloerection in other parts of the hairy skin (Langley and Sherrington 1891; Langley 1894). Piloerection with this distribution can be observed in the cat and other mammals during different behavioral states (e.g., defense behavior). It is unclear whether only piloerector muscles in those parts of the hairy skin that exhibit piloerection on nerve stimulation are innervated or whether the putative innervation of the small piloerector muscles is functionally ineffective in eliciting piloerection.

The pilomotor neurons supplying the tail are silent in anesthetized (and probably also in awake) cats under thermoneutral and emotionally neutral conditions. In the anesthetized cat, the central pilomotor circuits cannot be activated by any physiological stimulus except asphyxia (Grosse and Jänig 1976). It is unknown whether pilomotor neurons are activated by body cooling. It could well be that piloerection observed in cats in cold environments is produced by an increase in sensitivity of erector pili muscles to circulating adrenaline and noradrenaline (Hellmann 1963). It is likely that pilomotor neurons are activated specifically during certain species-specific behaviors. They may be controlled predominantly by the hypothalamus and the limbic system and normally not influenced by stimuli applied to the body surface (Figure 4.13). However in cats, in which cortex and large parts of the limbic system have been removed ("hypothalamic cats"), noxious and non-noxious stimuli may lead to piloerection (Bard 1928; Bard and Rioch 1937; Ectors 1941; Bard and Macht 1957).

Pilomotor neurons also innervate piloerector muscles in *human subjects*. They are activated during exposure to a cold environment during central cooling, fever, strong emotional stimuli and paradoxical cold sensations (e.g., during a hot bath after strong exercise). All these stimuli may lead to piloerection and to "goose bumps" on the skin.

Vasodilator Neurons Supplying Skin

STUDIES ON ANIMALS

When noradrenergic neuroeffector transmission to blood vessels is blocked by guanethidine (Note 7), electrical stimulation of preganglionic axons in the lumbar sympathetic trunk leads to vasodilation in both hairless and hairy skin of the cat paw. This vasodilation is resistant to atropine (an antagonist of muscarinic cholinergic transmission, which blocks sweat gland activation), but is abolished by blockade of impulse transmission in autonomic ganglia with hexamethonium (Note 8) (Bell et al. 1985). Thus, blood vessels of the cat paw are supplied by cutaneous vasodilator neurons that are neither noradrenergic nor cholinergic (Note 9).

Using a thermoregulatory paradigm (warming of the spinal cord or hypothalamus), and assuming that sympathetic cutaneous vasodilator neurons are involved in thermoregulation, an attempt was made to recognize directly putative cutaneous vasodilator neurons that project to the skin of the cat hindlimb. Warming of spinal cord and/or hypothalamus inhibits activity in cutaneous vasoconstrictor neurons and increases blood flow through skin, and therefore increases skin temperature. Under the same conditions, some normally silent unmyelinated fibers are activated in nerves to hairless and hairy skin (Gregor et al. 1976; Jänig and Kümmel 1981; Grewe et al. 1995). The responses elicited by spinal cord warming are graded. Interestingly, the neurons exhibiting these responses to spinal cord warming did not project through the sympathetic chain. They could neither be activated by electrical stimulation of the sympathetic chain nor could their activity, generated by spinal cord warming, be prevented by blockade of synaptic transmission in sympathetic ganglia using hexamethonium. This indicates that these neurons activated by spinal cord warming are either not sympathetic postganglionic or that the impulse transmission through the sympathetic ganglia is not nicotinic for this system (Jänig and Kümmel 1981). I hypothesize that we recorded antidromically conducted impulses in unmyelinated axons of spinal afferent neurons and that their cell bodies in the dorsal root ganglia or the axons projecting in the dorsal roots were excited by central warming. If these afferent neurons were peptidergic they could generate arteriolar vasodilation and increased blood flow in the skin (see Häbler et al. 1997). It has been suggested that this neurogenic mechanism may contribute to inflammation (Willis 1999). An afferent-induced vasodilation of this type could be a protective mechanism against central overheating (Jänig 2018).

STUDIES ON HUMAN SUBJECTS

In human subjects, body heating increases blood flow through the skin, which is closely paralleled by increased sweating. This increase in cutaneous blood flow during heat load is extremely powerful and can reach 8 L/min of cardiac output. Blocking conduction in the nerves to the forearm and hand abolishes sweating at the peak of the vasodilator response in the corresponding skin areas. It also abolishes most of the vasodilation in the forearm skin but it does *not* abolish the vasodilation in the glabrous skin of the hand and foot (Roddie et al. 1957). This observation suggests that increased blood flow through acral (glabrous) skin (hand and foot) occurs due to release from activity in cutaneous vasoconstrictor neurons. In contrast, increased blood flow through the forearm (and other) hairy skin areas is elicited largely by *cutaneous active vasodilation*. Several arguments support the idea that increased blood flow in human hairy skin during heat load is generated by a sympathetically mediated vasodilation mechanism (Joyner and Halliwill 2000): (1) In patients with a surgically sympathectomized extremity, vasodilation can no longer be produced by whole-body heating (Roddie et al. 1957). (2) In patients with autonomic neuropathy (Note 10), whole-body-heating-induced vasodilation is absent. (3) The magnitude of vasodilation in forearm skin during increase of body core temperature is far greater than that achieved by removal of vasoconstrictor activity (Roddie et al. 1957; Kellogg et al. 1989). (4) Atropine (which abolishes sweat production by blocking muscarinic cholinergic transmission) does not abolish vasodilation during heat load, but only weakly attenuates it (Roddie et al. 1957; Kellogg et al. 1995). (5) Local injection of botulinum toxin into the skin (which prevents the release of acetylcholine by blocking prejunctionally the fusion of the secretory vesicles in the cholinergic terminals with the plasma membrane) prevents active vasodilation in skin as well as sweating during heat load (Kellogg et al. 1995). These results would argue that the vasodilation is dependent on the activation of the sweat glands. (6) Cutaneous

vasoconstrictor neurons supplying forearm skin are nearly silent at neutral ambient temperatures (Bini et al. 1980b).

These points were fully supported by quantitative investigations in humans, using more advanced techniques to analyze the putative mechanisms underlying the cutaneous active vasodilation during hyperthermia (Johnson et al. 2014; Smith and Johnson 2016; Francisco and Minson 2018). These investigations support the idea that the active vasodilation in human hairy skin during hyperthermia is not directly generated by a cholinergic mechanism, but that cholinergic (e.g., sudomotor) neurons may be indirectly involved. Thus, whether the active vasodilation seen in proximal skin of human extremities during heat load is generated by a distinct population of cutaneous vasodilator neurons, which are different from sudomotor neurons, or is generated in association with the activation of sweat glands by sudomotor neurons remains unclear. The peripheral mechanisms of cutaneous active vasodilation are also still poorly understood. They involve acetylcholine, nitric oxide (NO) and possibly peptides such as vasoactive intestinal peptide (VIP) and/or pituitary adenylate cyclase-activating peptide (PACAP). However, how these substances interact with effector cells (vascular smooth muscle, vascular endothelium) so as to generate powerful cutaneous vasodilation during hyperthermia remains a puzzle (Kellogg et al. 1995; Johnson et al. 2014; Francisco and Minson 2018).

Further evidence that human skin is innervated by cutaneous vasodilator neurons is largely indirect because direct recordings from putative postganglionic vasodilator axons with microneurography in skin nerves of human subjects have not been done (Bini et al. 1980a; Wallin 1990; Wallin et al. 1998). Specifically, during non-REM (rapid eye movement) sleep in human subjects, single skin sympathetic activity bursts and short periods of increased skin sympathetic activity are sometimes followed by increased skin blood flow, with and without skin resistance changes (which indicates activity in sudomotor fibers) (Noll et al. 1994). During mild body heating, bursts of skin sympathetic activity in the superficial peroneal nerve are mostly followed by sweat expulsion and vasodilation in skin, and very rarely by vasodilation only (Sugenoya et al. 1998). Furthermore, Nordin (1990) has shown that sympathetic multiunit bursts of activity in the supraorbital nerve, elicited by mental stress, arousal or whole-body warming, are followed by vasodilation in the forehead skin and decreased skin resistance (activation of sweat glands). Again it is unclear whether the cutaneous vasodilation is generated by activation of cutaneous vasodilator neurons or mediated via activation of sweat glands. The results of both groups indicate indirectly that cutaneous blood vessels of the extremities and forehead in humans may be innervated by sympathetic vasodilator neurons and that these neurons may be activated under various circumstances.

There is indirect evidence that parasympathetic vasodilator neurons innervate the skin of the face and oral mucosa of humans (Drummond 1995) and rats and cats (Izumi 1999). However, this issue is rather controversial and unsolved (for discussion see Jänig [1985, 1990]; Rowell [1993]).

Sympathetic Postganglionic Neurons Supplying Sensory Receptors in Skin

Some cutaneous mechanoreceptors with myelinated afferents seem to be supplied by unmyelinated fibers. It is believed that this innervation is sympathetic postganglionic. Studies using catecholamine fluorescence have shown that catecholaminergic axons are present but, in most cases, direct proof is missing (see Akoev [1981]). Similarly, electrical stimulation of the sympathetic supply at unphysiological frequencies may excite primary afferent fibers in normal somatic tissues. However, there is no functional evidence that a distinct group of sympathetic neurons innervates cutaneous sensory receptors and regulates their sensitivity under physiological conditions (for extensive discussion see Jänig and Koltzenburg [1991b]) (Note 11).

The situation appears to be different under pathophysiological conditions after nerve lesions, in which case stimulation of sympathetic neurons may lead to excitation and sensitization of somatic afferent terminals (see Jänig and McLachlan [1994]; Jänig et al. [1996]; Jänig and Häbler [2000b]; Jänig and Baron [2001, 2002, 2003]; Jänig [2013, 2020]).

4.2.2 Sympathetic Postganglionic Neurons Innervating Deep Somatic Structures, Including Skeletal Muscle, Joints, Bone, etc.

All deep somatic structures are innervated by sympathetic noradrenergic postganglionic neurons. It is commonly believed that these are vasoconstrictor in function and that their reflex patterns are similar to those of muscle vasoconstrictor neurons. However: (1) there is no evidence that the reflex patterns in these neurons are identical to those of muscle vasoconstrictor neurons and (2) it is unclear whether all sympathetic postganglionic neurons projecting to these tissues have vasoconstrictor function (see Elefteriou [2018]). There is evidence that the bone is innervated by sympathetic neurons that contain vasoactive intestinal peptide and are presumably not noradrenergic, but cholinergic. This sympathetic innervation has no vascular function and is probably involved in bone mineralization (Hohmann et al. 1986). Here I will only concentrate on muscle vasodilator neurons and on sympathetic postganglionic neurons that appear to supply skeletal muscle cells and muscle spindles.

Vasodilator Neurons Supplying Skeletal Muscle

STUDIES ON ANIMALS

Integral components of the defense reaction in animals are: (a) increased blood flow through skeletal muscle with concomitant decreased blood flow through viscera and skin; (b) increased blood pressure and heart rate; (c) pupil dilation; (d) sweat gland activation; (e) activation of piloerector muscles and (f) activation of the adrenal medulla and adrenal cortex (see Subchapter 11.3.3). This type of behavior is organized at the hypothalamic and mesencephalic levels and under the control of the limbic system and cortex. The defense reaction has puzzled and fascinated physiologists and psychologists since Darwin published his famous book *The Expression of the Emotions in Man and Animals* (Darwin 1872). Figure 4.13 illustrates a cat in rage, as originally shown in Darwin's book, which should have all the autonomic responses mentioned above. Today we know that this behavior consists of three behaviors: confrontational defense, flight and quiescence, which are differentiated according to their somatomotor, autonomic, neuroendocrine and endogenously generated analgesic responses. They are organized in rostrocaudal cell columns of the dorsolateral and ventrolateral mesencephalon. These defensive behaviors are displayed by animals (and probably humans) under stress and pain and are archetypal integrated protective responses of the body (Bandler et al. 1991; Bandler and Shipley 1994; Bandler and Keay 1996; see also Akert [1981]; Jänig, [2020]) (see Subchapter 11.3.3 and Table 11.1).

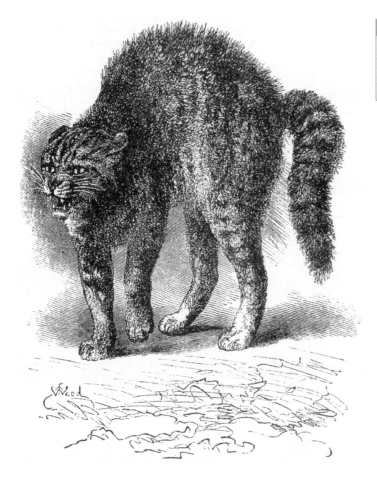

Figure 4.13 A cat in rage. Note the piloerection and dilation of the pupil. Muscle vasodilator neurons innervating the left extremity that is going to strike are activated during this behavioral state. From Darwin (1872) with permission.

When the defense reaction is elicited by "emotional stimuli" in an awake cat (e.g., by confrontation with a dog or another cat), an initial rapid increase in blood flow occurs in the skeletal muscle of the limb that strikes or is going to strike (Mancia et al. 1972; Ellison and Zanchetti 1973). This vasodilation is blocked by atropine, suggesting that it is mediated by cholinergic postganglionic sympathetic neurons. Repetitive electrical stimulation of the hypothalamic defense area in anesthetized cats also elicits an atropine-sensitive vasodilation in skeletal muscles of the hindlimbs in conjunction with the other characteristic cardiovascular responses (Eliasson et al. 1951; Uvnäs 1954, 1960; for references see Jänig [1985]).

During atropine-sensitive vasodilation in the hindlimb of anesthetized cats, elicited by local electrical stimulation of the hypothalamic defense area (perifornical area), about 10% of the postganglionic neurons supplying skeletal muscle that probably have vasodilator functions are activated (Figure 4.14b right side). Electrical stimulation of a nearby hypothalamic site that leads to vasoconstriction in the skeletal muscle does not or only weakly activate(s) the putative vasodilator neurons (Figure 4.14b left side) but activates muscle vasoconstrictor neurons. These putative vasodilator neurons are not spontaneously active and do not exhibit reflex activation in response to stimulation of somatic or cardiovascular afferents. They innervate only large resistance vessels in skeletal muscle upstream of the small resistance vessels, which are densely innervated by vasoconstrictor fibers (Bolme and Fuxe 1970; Anderson et al. 1996). Thus, by acting at this strategically favorable vascular site, activation of only relatively few sympathetic cholinergic postganglionic vasodilator neurons will generate a rapid increase in blood flow through the muscle vascular bed. Cutaneous vasoconstrictor neurons are activated (leading to decreased blood flow through skin) and muscle

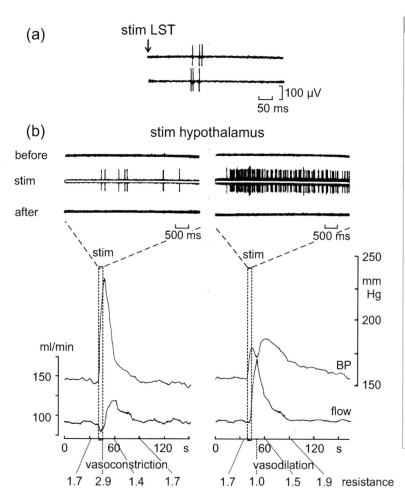

Figure 4.14 Reaction of a postganglionic muscle vasodilator neuron to electrical stimulation of the hypothalamus, inducing atropine-sensitive vasodilation (right) or vasoconstriction (left) in the hindlimbs of an anesthetized artificially ventilated cat. Postganglionic axon isolated from the gastrocnemius–soleus nerve. Blood flow was measured 1 cm proximal to the aortic bifurcation using an electromagnetic flow probe. (a) Stimulation of the preganglionic axons in the lumbar sympathetic trunk (LST) between paravertebral ganglia L4 and L5 with single pulses (5 V, 0.2 ms pulse duration) excited the postganglionic neuron with three action potentials because of synaptic impulse transmission in a lumbar paravertebral ganglion (see Figure 3.4). (b) Upper: Neural activity before, during (middle traces) and after bipolar stimulation at two hypothalamic sites close by generating vasoconstriction (left) or vasodilation (right, hypothalamic defense area). Stimulation parameters, 8 to 10 V (pulse duration 1 ms) at 100 Hz for 5 s. (b) Lower: Measurement of arterial blood flow (flow, left ordinate scale) and blood pressure (BP, right ordinate scale). Change in blood flow resistance indicated by numbers. Modified from Horeyseck et al. (1976) with permission.

vasoconstrictor neurons (at least those supplying the striking extremity) are inhibited during active vasodilation in skeletal muscle (Horeyseck et al. 1976). Therefore it is believed that the cholinergically mediated vasodilation in skeletal muscle of the cat is brought about by activation of a specific sympathetic muscle vasodilator pathway. Although all animal species display typical defense behaviors, only some of them seem to have an active muscle vasodilator system (e.g., cat and dog, Bolme et al. [1970]; Guidry and Landis [2000]).

STUDIES ON HUMAN SUBJECTS

It is controversial whether the muscle vasodilator system exists in human beings. During mental stress, blood flow through skeletal muscle of the forearms increases rapidly. This increase in blood flow is absent after block of the stellate ganglion with a local anesthetic or after sympathectomy. Thus, it is neurogenically mediated. However, it is difficult to explain the blood flow increase by withdrawal of activity in muscle vasoconstrictor neurons because it remains when adrenoceptors are blocked; furthermore, cholinoceptor-blocking drugs have ambiguous effects (Blair et al. 1959; Barcroft et al. 1960; Anderson et al. 1987; see Greenfield [1966]; Roddie [1977]). It has been shown that increased blood flow through skeletal muscle of the human forearm during mental stress is reduced by atropine, as well as by a nitric oxide (NO) synthase inhibitor (Dietz et al. 1994). However, it remains entirely unclear whether a neuronally mediated active mechanism exists in human skeletal muscle that is responsible for increased blood flow through skeletal muscle during mental stress. Other experimental evidence suggests that this vascular dilation is generated by circulating adrenaline released by the adrenal medulla acting via β_2-adrenoceptors on vascular smooth muscles and endothelial cells (here leading to release of NO) (see Joyner and Halliwill [2000]; Joyner and Dietz [2003]).

Sympathetic Postganglionic Neurons Supplying Muscle Spindles

The number of postganglionic neurons innervating non-vascular structures in skeletal muscle is very small when compared to the number of vasomotor neurons. Some muscle spindles (but no tendon organs) are anatomically associated with postganglionic axons (Barker and Saito 1981; see Akoev [1981] for literature). Occasional postganglionic fibers seem to have terminals near skeletal muscle fibers.

Electrical stimulation of the sympathetic supply of skeletal muscle may activate some Ia-fibers from muscle spindles (Note 12), but not the Ib-fibers from tendon organs. This activation is usually small and can only be elicited at stimulation frequencies that are supraphysiological (for discussion see Jänig and Koltzenburg [1991b]). In humans, resting discharge in muscle spindles is not modulated by increased activity in sympathetic neurons to skeletal muscle (Macefield et al. 2003). Therefore it is debatable whether these few sympathetic fibers have any function or whether the sensitivity of muscle spindles and therefore muscle afferents can be changed by activity in sympathetic neurons. If the latter, the effect appears to be small.

4.3 | Sympathetic Non-Vasoconstrictor Neurons Innervating Pelvic Viscera and Colon

In Subchapters 4.1 and 4.2, I have discussed the functional properties of sympathetic neurons innervating target cells in the skin and skeletal muscle and of visceral vasoconstrictor neurons. Here I will discuss the functional properties of sympathetic neurons that innervate viscera and have no vasoconstrictor function.

Viscera receive abundant sympathetic innervation and most of these neurons are not involved in regulation of vascular resistance, but rather in regulation of motility and secretion/reabsorption in the gastrointestinal tract or regulation of motility and secretion in pelvic organs. Others are probably involved in regulation of immune function (e.g., spleen and Peyer's patches; see Subchapter 4.6) and possibly in other functions (Figures 5.13 and 5.15). The cell bodies of the postganglionic neurons of the visceral sympathetic pathways are largely located in the prevertebral ganglia. Some that are associated with pelvic organs are located in the pelvic ganglia (Keast 1995a, b, 1999). Using neurophysiological and morphological techniques, the sympathetic innervation of pelvic organs and distal colon is the most systematically studied part of this innervation in the cat. The organ systems in the pelvic region have storage and evacuation as major functions. The lower urinary tract (urinary bladder and urethra) retains and evacuates urine (continence and micturition; Jänig 1996b; de Groat 2013; de Groat et al. 2015). The distal part of the large bowel (distal colon, rectum, anus) stores and evacuates feces and also reabsorbs water and sodium ions. The internal reproductive organs and erectile tissues of the external reproductive organs are more specialized but have basically similar functions related to retention and transport of semen and ova. In the female, this includes implantation of fertilized ova, storage and development of the fetus, and subsequently birth of the new individual (Jänig and McLachlan 1987; Jänig 1996c; see Subchapter 9.3). Finally, a sympathetic vasodilator pathway innervates the erectile tissue of the reproductive organs. This pathway may duplicate the sacral parasympathetic vasodilator pathway. Its functioning under physiological conditions is unknown (see Subchapter 9.3; Jänig 1996c).

In the cat, the sympathetic innervation of pelvic organs and the colon has its main preganglionic representation in the lumbar spinal segments L3 to L5 (see Chapter 8, Figures 8.6 and 8.8). Although there are vasoconstrictor axons, the sympathetic supply to the pelvic organs is primarily non-vascular. Activity in these neurons is involved in inhibition of motility and mucosal secretion, excitation of sphincteric muscles and excitation of smooth muscles of male reproductive organs. The instances in which these neurons are excited or inhibited at the same time as the vasoconstrictor neurons are rare. Many sympathetic neurons (both pre- and postganglionic) in nerves projecting to the pelvic viscera (e.g., through the lumbar splanchnic and hypogastric nerves) (Bahr et al. 1986a, b, c; Bartel et al. 1986; Jänig and McLachlan 1987; Jänig et al. 1991) have the following functional characteristics:

- They do not respond to stimulation of typical cardiovascular afferents (i.e., of arterial baroreceptors or arterial chemoreceptors).
- Almost all of them do not display respiratory rhythmicity in their activity (Boczek-Funcke et al. 1992c).
- They exhibit distinct reflexes in response to activation of *sacral* visceral afferents from the lower urinary tract, colon or anal canal by innocuous stimuli, which do not affect the visceral vasoconstrictor neurons (Note 13). These reflexes fall into the following categories: excitation or inhibition from the urinary bladder, from the colon and from the anal canal. Most of these neurons are spontaneously active (0.8 ± 0.7 imp/s for preganglionic neurons and 0.7 ± 0.5 imp/s for postganglionic neurons; Table 6.2; Bahr et al. 1986c; Jänig et al. 1991).
- At least three functional types of sympathetic non-vasoconstrictor neuron that innervate pelvic organs have been identified. These neurons have been called motility-regulating (MR) neurons although they may also be involved in secretory processes (see Table 4.3). Two types of MR neurons exhibit reciprocal reflex patterns to physiological stimulation of sacral afferents of the urinary bladder and colon. MR neurons type 1 are excited during contraction and/or distension of the urinary bladder, and inhibited (or not affected) during contraction and/or distension of the colon (Figure 4.15a). Type 2 MR neurons are inhibited during contraction or distension of the urinary bladder and excited (or not affected) by contraction or distension of the colon (Figure 4.15b). There are other types of MR neuron, which are either only excited by stimulation of the mechanoreceptors in the anal canal, or not excited by any stimulus so far tested under standardized experimental conditions, but have resting activity, or are entirely silent. These MR neurons have not been further characterized. A small group (about 3% to 4%) of pre- and postganglionic sympathetic visceral neurons projecting into the lumbar splanchnic and hypogastric nerves has functional properties of both visceral vasoconstrictor neurons and of MR neurons (Bahr et al. 1986a, b; Jänig et al. 1991).
- Some of the most prominent and unique reflexes in sympathetic neurons are those generated during excitation of visceral sacral afferents from the anal canal by mechanical shearing stimuli. These stimuli excite a specific class of myelinated low-threshold afferent neuron (Bahns et al. 1987; Jänig and Koltzenburg 1991a). Physiological activation of these afferents for 10 to 20 seconds by mechanical shearing stimuli generates excitatory reflexes in about 80% of the identifiable lumbar MR neurons (Figure 4.16) and inhibition in 8% of them. In 60% of these neurons the excitation is followed by afterdischarges lasting for 1 to 12 minutes (mean 4.8 minutes). This unique reflex activity can only be elicited from the anal canal, not from the colon–rectum and only rarely or not at all from the perianal hairy skin. The long-lasting afterdischarge is a property of the spinal sacro-lumbar reflex pathway and is not due to afterdischarges in the sacral visceral afferent neurons (Bahns et al. 1987; Jänig and Koltzenburg 1991a).
- Most excitatory and inhibitory reflexes elicited in the MR neurons from pelvic organs are preserved after *acute* thoracic spinalization, but those in visceral vasoconstrictor neurons are abolished. Similar to the other vasoconstrictor systems, the visceral vasoconstrictor system is dependent on supraspinal centers for its resting activity and cardiovascular, respiratory and other reflexes (Figure 4.3). In contrast, activity in the MR sympathetic systems is less dependent on supraspinal centers. The vasoconstrictor systems (and the sudomotor system) therefore exhibit "spinal shock" (total areflexia) after transection of the spinal cord, but the sympathetic systems regulating motility and probably other non-vascular parameters do not (for details see Subchapter 9.2). This shows: (1) that multiple sacro-lumbar reflex circuits connected to the sympathetic non-vasoconstrictor systems do not require the descending influence from supraspinal centers in order to function (Figure 4.17) and (2) that spinal reflex circuits to vasoconstrictor neurons require the descending excitatory influence from supraspinal centers (Figure 4.3; see Subchapter 9.2).
- The functional distinction between vasoconstrictor neurons and non-vasoconstrictor neurons of the lumbar sympathetic visceral outflow is supported by differences in some other characteristics, including the conduction velocity of the preganglionic axons (vasoconstrictor vs. motility-regulating 2.8 vs. 8.1 m/s), segmental distribution of preganglionic neurons (L1 to L4 vs. L3/L4),

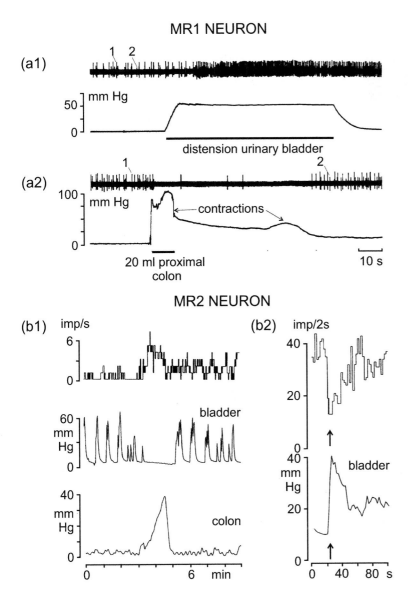

MR1 NEURON

(a1)

50 / 0 mm Hg

distension urinary bladder

(a2)

100 / 0 mm Hg

contractions

20 ml proximal colon

10 s

MR2 NEURON

(b1) imp/s

6 / 0

60 mm Hg / 0 — bladder

40 mm Hg / 0 — colon

0   6   min

(b2) imp/2s

40 / 20 / 0

40 mm Hg / 20 / 0 — bladder

0   40   80 s

Figure 4.15 Reflexes in motility-regulating (MR) neurons in response to stimulation of the urinary bladder or colon in the cat. Recording from postganglionic axons isolated from the hypogastric nerve. (a) Two MR neurons type 1: activation during distension of the urinary bladder ([a1], filling with 20 ml saline) and inhibition during distension/contraction of the colon ([a2], filling with 20 ml saline); during filling of the colon (black bar) and afterwards the colon contracted. (b) MR neuron type 2: activation during contraction of the colon (b1) and inhibition during contraction of the urinary bladder (b1,b2). In (b2) responses to 20 contractions are superimposed. Ordinate scales, intraluminal pressure or impulse rate (upper records in [b1] and [b2]). (a), Jänig, Schmidt, Schnitzler and Wesselmann, unpublished; (b), modified from Jänig et al. (1991).

ongoing activity (1.6 vs. 0.8 imp/s), segmental and suprasegmental reflexes upon electrical stimulation of somatic or visceral afferents (see Figure 9.2) and neurochemistry of the neurons (see Subchapter 1.4).

It is still unclear how individual sympathetic non-vasoconstrictor pathways are linked to the different target cells in the pelvic viscera and colon. However, the results of the analysis reported above demonstrate beyond any doubt that this system is highly differentiated. In the cat, about 40% of the preganglionic neurons projecting in the lumbar splanchnic nerves have the functional properties of MR neurons (Bahr et al. 1986c). The functional differentiation between different sympathetic visceral pathways is further detailed in Subchapter 1.4 on neuropeptides and "neurochemical coding" of autonomic neurons and in Subchapter 6.5 on transmission of impulses in autonomic ganglia.

The lumbar sympathetic outflow to the pelvic organs and colon is entirely separate from the lumbar sympathetic outflow to the hindlimbs and the tail of the cat. Otherwise all sympathetic systems to skin, skeletal muscle and pelvic viscera are represented in lumbar segment L3 in the cat. I will discuss in

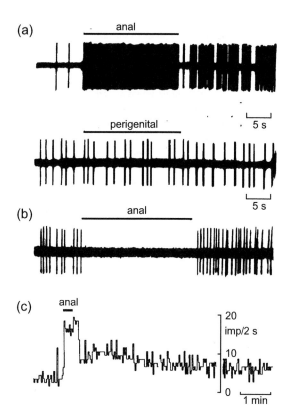

Reactions of preganglionic motility-regulating neurons in response to mechanical stimulation of the mucosa of the anal canal. Preganglionic axons were isolated from a lumbar splanchnic nerve in the cat. Anal stimulation consisted of a light shearing stimulus applied at a moving frequency of about 0.5 to 1 Hz with a spatula to the anal mucosa for 20 s. (a) Activation and afterdischarge in response to anal stimulation. No activation in response to perigenital mechanical stimulation. (b) Inhibition in response to anal stimulation. (c) Long-lasting afterdischarge after reflex activation in response to anal stimulation. Modified from Bahr et al. (1986a) with permission.

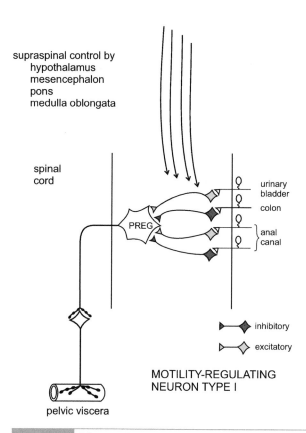

Figure 4.17 Schematic diagram of the pathways involved in the reflexes elicited in MR neurons type 1 by stimulation of sacral visceral afferents from pelvic organs. The reflex pattern in the neurons can be fully explained by sacro-lumbar spinal reflex pathways. Little is known about the supraspinal pathways which are probably associated with the hypothalamus, upper and lower brain stem. See Subchapter 9.2.

Subchapter 8.2 viscerotopic aspects of the lumbar preganglionic neurons being involved in regulation of the pelvic organs, colon or autonomic targets in somatic tissues.

The sympathetic non-vasoconstrictor outflow projecting via the celiac and superior mesenteric ganglia to the gastrointestinal tract has not been studied at the single neuron level using neurophysiological methods. However, based on functional, morphological and other studies it can be inferred that this sympathetic outflow is also differentiated into the categories of MR and secretomotor neurons, both major pathways probably consisting of several subtypes.

4.4 | Other Types of Sympathetic Neuron

So far, functional properties of sympathetic neurons have been described, which have been explicitly investigated using neurophysiological and morphological methods. There are other target organs that are most likely also innervated by functionally distinct groups of sympathetic neurons; however, they have not been studied systematically or not at all on the single neuron level (see Table 1.2):

- The heart is innervated by a large group of sympathetic cardiomotor neurons, which are probably similar to muscle and visceral vasoconstrictor neurons in their reflex discharge pattern. These cardiomotor neurons may consist of functional subgroups as far as the innervation of ventricles, atria and the pacemaker system is concerned (Jänig 2016).

- Indirect experimental evidence obtained in the guinea pig shows that the airway smooth muscle cells are innervated by a sympathetic pathway that is functionally distinct from the sympathetic innervation of the vasculature of the airways. Noxious stimulation of the airway mucosa (e.g., by capsaicin) activates this sympathetic broncho-motor pathway leading to relaxation of the air-ways mediated by β_1- and β_2-adrenoceptors (Oh et al. 2006). It is unknown whether this type of sympathetic pathway exists in other species, including primates. Also, mucus secretion of the airways may be under control of sympathetic neurons. However, there are considerable species differences in the sympathetic control of smooth muscle and glands of airways and in some species (including humans and non-human primates) cir-culating catecholamines are the main component influencing airway resistance via β_2-adrenoceptors (Undem and Potenzieri 2012).

- The sympathetic innervation of the kidney modi-fies glomerular filtration, renin release from the juxtaglomerular cells and tubular Na^+ reabsorp-tion, as well as vascular resistance (DiBona and Kopp 1997; Kopp and DiBona 2000; Johns 2013). Activation of these sympathetic neurons leads to vasoconstriction, renin secretion and increase of tubular sodium (and water) reabsorption. Physiological studies indicate that the glomerular filtration rate is differentially controlled by separ-ate sympathetic vasoconstrictor neurons (Denton et al. 2004; Eppel et al. 2004). However, whether renin release or tubular Na^+ reabsorption is con-trolled by functionally different types of sympa-thetic neuron and by anatomically separate sympathetic pathways is unclear (Luff et al. 1992).

- In rodents, lipocytes of the brown adipose tissues are innervated by a group of functionally distinct sympathetic neurons involved in thermoregula-tion. These neurons may be called lipomotor neurons. Compared to cutaneous vasoconstrictor neurons involved in thermoregulation, lipomotor neurons exhibit differential sensitivity to changes in skin or core temperature, different premotor neurons in the rostral raphe pallidus and different

descending central pathways between the preop-tic area of the hypothalamus and the raphe nuclei (Himms-Hagen 1991; Morrison 1999, 2001a, b, 2018; Cao et al. 2010; McAllen et al. 2010).

- Sympathetic neurons may be directly involved in glycogenolysis and gluconeogenesis of liver cells and in lipolysis of fat cells of the white adipose tissue (Rosell and Belfrage 1979; Rosell 1980; Frayn and MacDonald 1996; Bartness and Bamshad 1998; Dodt et al. 1999; Bartness and Song 2007a,b).

- The dilator muscle of the pupil is innervated by a distinct sympathetic pathway (see Boczek-Funcke et al. [1992a]). This corresponds to a dense innervation of the iris dilator muscle and a sparse innervation of the iris sphincter muscle and ciliary muscle by noradrenergic fibers.

- Salivary glands are innervated by sympathetic neurons that are involved in secretion. Stimulation of the sympathetic supply to salivary glands leads to mucus secretion. In the rat and mouse, 15% to 25% of the neurons in the superior cervical ganglion are estimated to innervate saliv-ary glands (Gibbins 1991). These sympathetic neurons are involved in regulation of blood flow (vasoconstrictor neurons), secretion of mucus sal-iva and activation of myoepithelial cells (Bartsch et al. 1996). The main function of the sympathetic innervation of the salivary glands seems to be to modify the composition of the saliva as to its pro-tein and mucus content (Garrett et al. 1999).

- In the cat, some 10% of the thoracic preganglionic neurons projecting through the cervical sympa-thetic trunk to the superior cervical ganglion are active only during inspiration ("inspiration"-type neurons). Most of these neurons are not under the control of arterial baroreceptors. They decrease their activity during hyperventilation and increase their activity during hypoventilation (increase in arterial P_{CO2}), and are activated by stimulation of nociceptors, arterial chemoreceptors, nasopha-ryngeal receptors and other receptors (Figure 4.2). Most of their cell bodies are located in the thoracic segments T1 or T2 and their axons conduct significantly faster than those of preganglionic muscle and cutaneous vasoconstrictor neurons (Boczek-Funcke et al. 1992a, 1993). Thus this class of sympathetic preganglionic neuron is function-ally distinct from the other main classes of pregan-glionic neurons. Their target cells are unknown, but may be related to the respiratory tract.

- The pineal gland is innervated by a group of sympathetic neurons, which are dependent in their activity on the suprachiasmatic nucleus in the hypothalamus. These neurons are involved in the circadian induction of melatonin synthesis (Moore 1996; Moller and Baeres 2002; Aulinas 2019).
- Cells of the adrenal medulla synthesizing adrenaline or noradrenaline are innervated by two separate groups of sympathetic preganglionic neurons (Morrison and Cao 2000; Morrison 2001b; see Subchapter 4.5).
- The immune tissues may be innervated by a functionally distinct sympathetic pathway. This will be discussed in Subchapter 4.6.

4.5 | Adrenal Medulla

4.5.1 Circulating Adrenaline and Noradrenaline

The adrenal medulla, when activated, releases both adrenaline and noradrenaline (in addition to other substances, which, in the present context, are functionally unimportant [Winkler 1988]). There are considerable species differences in the proportion of each catecholamine that is released. For example, the adrenal medulla of the rabbit releases 100% adrenaline, the whale up to 100% noradrenaline, the cat 50% of each and the human subject, as well as the rat, 80% adrenaline and 20% noradrenaline. The reason for these differences between species remains unclear (von Euler 1956).

The release of the two catecholamines from the adrenal medulla is regulated by activity in preganglionic sympathetic neurons that project from the thoracic spinal cord through the splanchnic nerves to the adrenal medulla (Holman et al. 1994). These neurons form synapses with adrenal medulla cells (Coupland 1965). Histological and immunohistochemical studies show that adrenaline and noradrenaline are synthesized by different cells, which are also innervated by different groups of preganglionic neurons (Edwards et al. 1996). These data suggest that there are two separate sympathetic pathways to the adrenal medulla, one mediating the release of adrenaline and the other noradrenaline (see Vollmer [1996]). This idea is supported by functional studies that show that the release of adrenaline and noradrenaline from the adrenal medulla can be regulated differentially in

animals (Folkow and von Euler 1954; see Folkow [1955] [for early studies]; Vollmer [1996]).

Morrison and Cao (2000) have shown in the rat that preganglionic neurons that innervate adrenergic cells of the adrenal medulla are not affected by arterial baroreceptor reflexes and respiratory reflexes, but are strongly excited by hypoglycemia. In contrast, preganglionic neurons that innervate noradrenergic cells of the adrenal medulla behave like muscle vasoconstrictor neurons (i.e., they are not excited by hypoglycemia and they are under strong arterial baroreceptor reflex control). These results are consistent with the idea that the two groups of adrenal medullary cells are differentially regulated by the brain. However, the context in which this occurs, its functional meaning, as well as the central pathways involved, are only incompletely understood (Morrison 2001b).

In humans, under resting conditions, the concentration of noradrenaline in the blood plasma is 1 to 1.5 pmol/mL (0.17 to 0.25 µg/L) and of adrenaline about 0.25 pmol/mL (0.05 µg/L; see Kopin [1989]). Furthermore, under almost all physiological conditions, the concentration of circulating noradrenaline is three to five times higher than the concentration of adrenaline (Figure 4.18; Cryer 1980; Kopin 1989). In humans, only about 2% to 8% of the circulating noradrenaline is released by the adrenal medulla and the rest is released by sympathetic nerve endings in the peripheral tissues (overflow of noradrenaline; Cryer 1980; Esler et al. 1990). Systematic studies of various effector organs in the cat (Celander 1954) have shown that adrenaline, released from the adrenal medulla by electrical stimulation of the preganglionic axons innervating the adrenal medulla, has almost no effect on peripheral effector organs, which are under the control of sympathetic noradrenergic neurons. The only important exception, which is supported by experimental investigations, is that circulating adrenaline may generate a vasodilation in skeletal muscle by acting on β_2-adrenoceptors, e.g., during defense behavior in animals or emotional excitation in humans (see Note 14). Steady state intravenous (i.v.) infusion of adrenaline moderately increases heart rate and systolic blood pressure and decreases diastolic blood pressure at plasma concentrations of ≥ 100 ng/L and mobilization of glucose and lactate at plasma concentrations of ≥ 200 ng/L (Figure 4.18a; Clutter et al. 1980).

In essence, adrenaline in the plasma released from the adrenal medulla under physiological

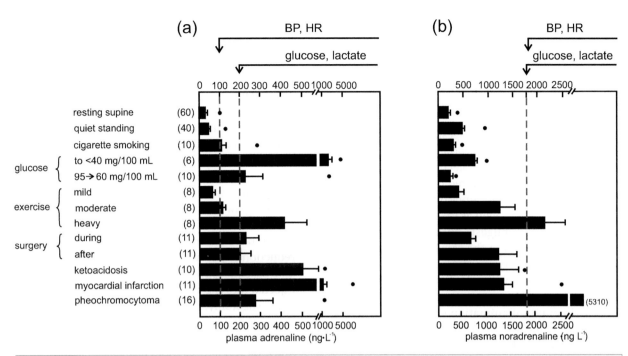

Figure 4.18 Relative changes in plasma concentrations of adrenaline and noradrenaline in various physiological and some pathophysiological conditions in humans. The horizontal bars represent mean (+1 S.E.M. [standard error of mean]) of adrenaline (a) or noradrenaline (b) in ng per liter. The numbers of subjects tested are given in brackets. The highest values measured are indicated by the solid circles. The vertical red dashed lines indicate the steady-state plasma concentrations of adrenaline or noradrenaline that elicit cardiovascular changes (BP, blood pressure; HR, heart rate) or metabolic changes (glucose, lactate) when adrenaline or noradrenaline are continuously intravenously infused. Adrenaline is released by the adrenal medulla. Most noradrenaline in the blood is released by nerve endings of sympathetic postganglionic noradrenergic neurons. About 2% to 8% is released by the adrenal medullae. Note that hypoglycemia (low glucose concentration in plasma) relatively selectively stimulates the release of adrenaline and that, during other conditions, both catecholamines increase, the concentration of noradrenaline being three to five times higher than the concentration of adrenaline. From Cryer (1980) with permission. Infusion experiments (see vertical lines) from Clutter et al. (1980) and Silverberg et al. (1978) with permission.

conditions is primarily a *metabolic hormone*, which chiefly serves to catalyze the mobilization of glucose and lactic acid from glycogen in the liver and skeletal muscle, and of free fatty acids from adipose tissue. In addition, it has moderate cardiovascular effects in humans (Kopin 1989). Overall, it seems that adrenaline secretion by the adrenal medulla is unimportant in the maintenance of circulatory homeostasis in everyday life (Young and Landsberg 2001).

Noradrenaline infused i.v. at concentrations of ≤1800 ng/L has neither hemodynamic nor metabolic effects in human subjects. These plasma concentrations may occur in human subjects only under extreme conditions (Silverberg et al. 1978; Cryer 1980). Noradrenaline, infused in physiological concentrations i.v. in the cat, has only negligible effects on peripheral effector organs when compared with the

effects of sympathetic nerve stimulation (Celander 1954). Thus, plasma noradrenaline, spilled over from the varicosities of activated sympathetic fibers and released to a minor degree by the adrenal medulla, has no known function in practically all physiological conditions; it primarily reflects activity in sympathetic postganglionic neurons (Kopin 1989; Esler et al. 1990).

Taken together, the available data challenge Cannon's concept that the sympathico-adrenal system is a unitary system (see Folkow [1955]). In fact, the data clearly support indirectly the general idea that the sympathetic nervous system consists of functionally distinct pathways. One of these pathways regulates the release of adrenaline from the adrenal medulla. However, the situation may change dramatically under *pathophysiological conditions*, for example when peripheral organs (blood vessels, heart) are denervated and become sensitive to circulating catecholamines (Kopin 1989) (Note 15).

4.5.2 Previously Unrecognized Functions of Circulating Adrenaline

Role of Adrenaline in Mechanical Hyperalgesia and Inflammation

Inflammation and hyperalgesia following tissue trauma are *protective body reactions.* They occur in all tissues and support *healing.* Mechanisms of inflammation are commonly considered to be confined to the periphery, involving immune-competent and related inflammatory cells as well as vascular cells. The main mechanism of hyperalgesia during inflammation in this view is confined to the sensitization of nociceptors by inflammatory mediators leading to central changes (central sensitization) and appropriate protective behavior. However, using animal (rat) models of experimental inflammation of the knee joint synovia or mechanical hyperalgesic behavior to intradermal injection of the inflammatory mediator bradykinin, it can be shown that both types of protective body reactions (Note 16), namely inflammation and nociceptor sensitization, are potentially under the control of the sympatho-adrenal system. More specifically, adrenaline released by the adrenal medulla may have a previously unknown function. Both animal models (bradykinin-induced plasma extravasation in the synovia of the knee joint; bradykinin-induced mechanical hyperalgesic behavior) may appear rather artificial. Furthermore, there exist, up to now, no human models and no clinical situation that correspond to these animal models. However, I am convinced that we can learn from these animal models how the brain can regulate peripheral mechanisms of inflammation and nociceptor sensitization via the sympatho-adrenal system. This is a biological territory that is almost entirely unexplored:

- Noxious stimulation (of skin or viscera) depresses bradykinin-induced venular plasma extravasation in the synovia of the rat knee. This depression is mediated by reflex activation of the adrenal medulla involving spinal cord and lower brain stem and most likely by the release of adrenaline. The reflex circuits are under powerful control of abdominal viscera via vagal afferent neurons. The released adrenaline does not inhibit plasma extravasation by vasoconstriction in the synovia. Instead it prevents the increased permeability of the synovial endothelium for plasma proteins generated by the inflammatory mediator bradykinin (probably by acting on β_2-adrenoceptors). The cellular mechanisms of this fascinating effect of adrenaline on the experimental inflammatory process are unknown (Miao et al. 2000, 2001; Jänig and Green 2014; Jänig 2020).

- In rats, injection of the inflammatory mediator bradykinin into the dermis of the dorsal skin of the hindpaw reduces the paw-withdrawal threshold to mechanical stimulation of the dorsum of the ipsilateral rat hindpaw. This bradykinin-induced reduction of paw-withdrawal threshold is enhanced and baseline paw-withdrawal threshold (to saline injected into the skin) is reduced after subdiaphragmatic vagotomy. The vagotomy-induced decrease of paw-withdrawal threshold is prevented by prior denervation or removal of the adrenal medulla. The interpretation of these results is that adrenaline released by the adrenal medulla sensitizes nociceptors in the skin to mechanical stimulation. The time course of the development and reversal of this sensitization is slow, taking days to about two weeks. The mechanism underlying this sensitization of nociceptors to mechanical stimulation is unknown, but it is mediated by β_2-adrenoceptors and may involve inflammatory cells in the skin (Khasar et al. 1998a, b, 2003; Jänig et al. 2000; Jänig 2020).

In *conclusion* (Figure 4.19), the release of adrenaline by the adrenal medulla is controlled by central circuits that are distinct from those linked to other sympathetic pathways. Under physiological conditions, adrenaline released by the adrenal medulla has the following functions:

1. regulation of metabolism such as catalyzing the mobilization of glucose and lactic acid from glycogen in the liver and probably of fatty acids from adipose tissue;
2. modulation of sensitivity of nociceptors;
3. modulation of inflammation and
4. not supporting responses of target organs elicited by activation of other sympathetic pathways (with the possible exception of β_2-adrenoceptor-mediated vasodilation in skeletal muscle), except possibly under strong emergency conditions.

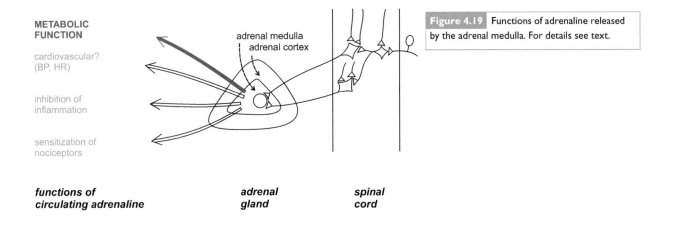

METABOLIC FUNCTION

cardiovascular? (BP, HR)

inhibition of inflammation

sensitization of nociceptors

functions of circulating adrenaline

adrenal gland

spinal cord

adrenal medulla
adrenal cortex

Figure 4.19 Functions of adrenaline released by the adrenal medulla. For details see text.

Functions 2 and 3, as fascinating they are, need independent reproduction and extension. Furthermore, in view of the fact that: (1) the concentration of circulating noradrenaline is three to five times higher than the concentration of circulating adrenaline in humans and (2) there exist considerable differences between species in the proportions of the two catecholamines released by the adrenal medulla, it is debatable how important the different functions of the adrenal medulla are in humans.

4.6 | Sympathetic Neurons Innervating Immune Tissues

Anatomical, physiological, pharmacological and behavioral experiments on animals support the notion that the sympathetic nervous system can influence the immune system and therefore control protective mechanisms of the body at the cellular level (Hori et al. 1995; Madden and Felten 1995; Madden et al. 1995). Control of the immune system by the sympathetic nervous system would mean that the brain is, in principle, able to influence immune responses, probably via the hypothalamus. This attractive idea is based on clinical and experimental observations (Jänig and Häbler 2000b). The mechanisms of this influence remain largely unsolved (Besedovsky and del Rey 1992, 1995; Ader and Cohen 1993; Saphier 1993) for conceptual and methodical reasons. In view of the functional specificity of the sympathetic pathways, as outlined in this chapter, the key question to be asked is: Does a specific sympathetic subsystem exist which communicates signals from the brain to the immune system or is this efferent communication a general function of the sympathetic system? In other words, is the immune system supplied by a sympathetic pathway that is functionally distinct from other sympathetic pathways (see Subchapters 4.1–4.4) and mediates immunomodulatory effects (Figure 4.20)?

Several observations support the idea that the efferent communication from the brain to the immune system occurs via the sympathetic nervous system and that this sympathetic channel *is functionally distinct from all other sympathetic channels* (Bellinger and Lorton 2014; Jänig 2014).

1. Primary and secondary lymphoid tissues are innervated by postganglionic noradrenergic sympathetic neurons. Varicosities of the sympathetic terminals can be found in close proximity to T lymphocytes and macrophages, as described for other sympathetic target cells (Bellinger and Lorton 2014).

2. The spleen of the cat is innervated by sympathetic postganglionic neurons that are numerically, relative to the weight of the organs, three times as large as the sympathetic innervation of the kidneys (Baron and Jänig 1988). The sympathetic innervation of the spleen is functionally different from that of the kidney: sympathetic neurons innervating the kidney behave like "classical" vasoconstrictor neurons (Meckler and Weaver 1988; DiBona and Kopp 1997; Kopp and DiBona 2000). Many sympathetic neurons innervating the spleen are not under the control of the arterial baroreceptors and show distinct reflexes to stimulation of

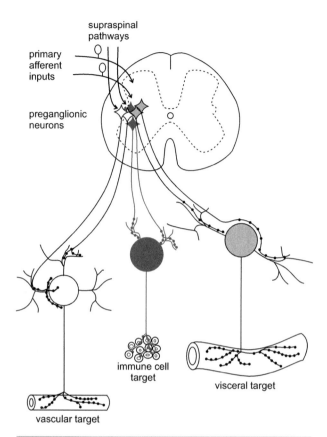

Figure 4.20 A separate sympathetic pathway to the immune tissue: a hypothesis. For details see text. Modified from Jänig (2014)

afferents from the spleen and the gastrointestinal tract, which differ from those of vasoconstrictor neurons (Meckler and Weaver 1988; Stein and Weaver 1988). These results, as incomplete as they are, suggest that many sympathetic neurons innervating the spleen have a function other than to elicit vasoconstriction. This function may be related to the immune system.

3. The activity in the sympathetic postganglionic neurons is transmitted to the cells of the primary or secondary lymphoid organs via release of noradrenaline that activates β_2- and α_1-adrenoceptors expressed by the immune cells. Bellinger and others have shown that most types of cells of the immune tissue express adrenoceptors (see Bellinger and Lorton 2014). Are all adrenoceptor-expressing immune cells involved in the transmission of the central message to the immune tissue?

4. The skin is a powerful defense barrier for the body against invading microorganisms, toxins and injury, and is permanently exposed to exogenous and endogenous stressors. It contains various cell types, which interact and are associated with cells of the immune system such as mast cells, keratinocytes, macrophages and Langerhans cells. Furthermore, the number of T-cells in the skin is almost twice as high as the total number of T-cells in the circulation (Clark et al. 2006). It is believed that the immune cells and the skin cells associated with them are very important in the normal (physiological) defense processes operating in skin and, under pathophysiological conditions, in the development and maintenance of various skin diseases (e.g., atopic dermatitis, psoriasis, seborrheic eczema, prurigo nodularis, lichen planus, chronic urticaria, alopecia areata). Dermatologists have coined the term "skin immune system" (SIS) or "skin-associated lymphoid tissue" (SALT) to describe the role of immune cells and their interaction conditions (Williams and Kupper 1996; Kupper 2000; Kupper and Fulbridge 2004; Arck and Paus 2006; Arck et al. 2006; Bos and Luiten 2009; Peters et al. 2012). The skin is densely innervated by primary afferent neurons with unmyelinated axons, most of them being peptidergic and having nociceptive functions, and by sympathetic postganglionic neurons. These postganglionic neurons have – depending on the type of skin – vasoconstrictor, sudomotor, pilomotor or possibly vasodilator functions. They form separate, functionally distinct sympathetic pathways as described in Subchapters 4.1 and 4.2. The integrated cellular activity at the cutaneous defense line is under neuroendocrine control involving the hypothalamus–pituitary–adrenal (HPA) axis and possibly the sympathetic nervous system (Arck and Paus 2006; Buske-Kirschbaum 2007). Is the skin innervated by sympathetic neurons which are normally silent and the function of which is not to regulate the "classical" sympathetic target cells but to modulate defense processes in skin involving the SIS? Or is the sympatho-adrenal system releasing adrenaline primarily involved? Reviews on the SIS neither mention nor discuss this possibility, but remain rather vague about the function of the efferent sympathetic pathways in the "brain-skin axis," the reason probably being the erroneous belief that the sympathetic nervous system functions as a unitary neurohumoral system and

not in a functionally differentiated way (see Subchapter 4.2) (Williams and Kupper 1996; Kupper 2000; Kupper and Fulbridge 2004; Bos and Luiten 2009).

5. Functional studies performed on the spleen of rodents have shown (for review see Hori et al. [1995] and references herein):

   a. Surgical or chemical sympathectomy alters the splenic immune responses (e.g., generating increase of natural killer cell cytotoxicity, lymphocyte proliferation responses to mitogen stimulation and production of interleukin-1β).

   b. Electrical stimulation of the splenic nerve reduces the splenic immune responses.

   c. Lesions or stimulation of distinct hypothalamic sites or microinjection of cytokines at distinct hypothalamic sites activates some splenic immune responses. These changes are no longer present after denervation of the spleen.

   d. The interventions in the hypothalamus lead to changes of activity in the splenic nerve and changes of this activity are correlated with the changes in the splenic immune responses. For example, activity in sympathetic neurons to the spleen elicited by interventions at the hypothalamus (in particular the ventromedial nucleus of the hypothalamus) is significantly correlated with suppression of natural killer cell cytotoxicity in the spleen. This suppression is mediated by β-adrenoceptors (Katafuchi et al. 1993a, b; Okamoto et al. 1996). A *hypothalamo-sympathetic neural system which controls the immune system* has been postulated (Hori et al. 1995).

6. In rats experimental generation of abdominal inflammation by an immune challenge with intravenous injection of the bacterial wall substance lipopolysaccharide (LPS) is followed by an increase in plasma levels of the key inflammatory tumor necrosis factor α (TNFα) and an increase of activity in sympathetic neurons projecting through the greater splanchnic nerve. The level of plasma TNFα is strongly enhanced if the greater splanchnic nerve is interrupted. This experiment demonstrates that the immune challenge with LPS activates a sympathetic reflex in the viscera which powerfully suppresses the acute systemic inflammatory response. The efferent arm of this reflex is sympathetic neurons projecting through the splanchnic nerves. Activation of these neurons leads to suppression of the immune response (via β$_2$-adrenoceptors), and interruption of the axons of these neurons in the greater splanchnic nerves to enhancement of the immune response. The afferent arm of this reflex is unknown, but presumably humoral (Martelli et al. 2014, 2019).

Using classical neurophysiological recordings in vivo from sympathetic neurons, it should be possible to discriminate and recognize neurons innervating the immune tissue from other functional types of sympathetic neuron (e.g. vasoconstrictor neurons to skin, skeletal muscle, kidney or spleen). This is exemplified in Table 4.4, showing the target cells in particular organs that are innervated and possibly controlled by sympathetic neurons. One sympathetic channel in three of these organs potentially projects to the immune tissue and possibly regulates the immune response.

Thus, it should, in principle, be possible to characterize the sympathetic neurons innervating lymphoid tissues functionally by using stimuli that are adequate to elicit immune responses and to assign to these sympathetic neurons characteristic functional markers (see Hori et al. [1995]). This idea leads to the formulation of *two alternative testable hypotheses* (Jänig 2014):

1. Hypothesis 1: Peripheral sympathetic neurons are functionally specific for the immune tissues. These neurons show distinct reflex patterns generated by physiological (peripheral and central) stimuli that are related to the immune system

Table 4.4 | Examples of function-specific sympathetic pathways to different targets within some organs with emphasis on immune tissue

Organ	Target cells	Function
Spleen	BV, *IC*	VC, *IR*
Hairy skin	BV$_{skin}$, *IC*	VC (VD), *IR*
Hairless skin	BV$_{skin}$, SG, *IC*	VC (VD?), SM, *IR*
Kidney	BV, JGA	VC, renin release
Skeletal muscle	BV$_{muscle}$	VC (VD)

Abbreviations: BV, blood vessel; VC, vasoconstriction; VD, vasodilation; *IC*, immune cells; *IR*, immune response; JGA, juxtaglomerular apparatus; SG, sweat gland; SM, sudomotor response.

and not to other functionally irrelevant afferent inputs. These sympathetic pre- and postganglionic neurons constitute a distinct sympathetic pathway to the immune tissue that is connected to special central circuits. This neural immune-regulatory system is active during defense and protection of the body tissues.

2. Hypothesis 2: The alternative hypothesis is that reflex responses in sympathetic neurons that modulate immune responses are found indiscriminately in all populations of sympathetic neurons. These responses would therefore not be functionally specific for the lymphoid tissue. This could mean that more or less *all* sympathetic noradrenergic pathways have, in addition to their specific target-organ-related functions, a general function, which is related to defense and protection of the tissues. This hypothesis does not clash with the idea that regulation of defense and protection of body tissues by the CNS is based on special circuits in the brain stem and hypothalamus (Bellinger and Lorton 2014).

4.7 Proportions of Preganglionic Neurons in Major Sympathetic Nerves

The discussion in this chapter and Table 1.2 show that the peripheral sympathetic system is composed of many functionally different types of pathways that are defined by their target cells. For some of these pathways it has clearly been shown that the pre- and postganglionic neurons exhibit characteristic reflex patterns ("functional fingerprints"), indicating that these pathways are linked with distinct reflex pathways in the neuraxis. For other sympathetic pathways, this has not been shown yet or it has been demonstrated that they exhibit no reflexes and no spontaneous activity under the experimental conditions in which they were studied. This applies, for example, to pilomotor neurons and to vasodilator neurons. To show how many different types of preganglionic neurons there are, it is of interest to look at some numerical data about *preganglionic* neurons, projecting in major "sympathetic" nerves of the cat, that have been investigated neurophysiologically and morphologically. These nerves are the lumbar sympathetic

trunk (LST) distal to the paravertebral ganglion L5 (innervation territory mainly hindlimb and tail), the cervical sympathetic trunk (CST; innervation territory head and upper neck) and the lumbar splanchnic nerves (LSN; innervation territory pelvic organs and distal colon) (Table 4.5).

Based on neurophysiological investigations (Table 4.5) it can be estimated that:

- About 10% to 20% of the preganglionic neurons in the three nerves have vasoconstrictor function innervating resistance vessels and are involved in blood pressure regulation (muscle and visceral vasoconstrictor neurons).
- About 12% to 13% of the preganglionic neurons projecting in the CST or LST participate in regulation of cutaneous blood flow and thermoregulation (cutaneous vasoconstrictor neurons). This percentage may be somewhat higher, since some 20% of the postganglionic cutaneous vasoconstrictor neurons exhibit a reflex pattern similar to that in muscle vasoconstrictor neurons.
- About 10% of the preganglionic neurons projecting in the CST are neurons with the discharge pattern of inspiratory neurons (INS). The target of these neurons may be the respiratory tract (see Figure 4.2 and Subchapter 4.4).
- About 40% of the preganglionic neurons projecting in the LSN are involved in regulation of visceral organ functions (MR neurons).
- Varying between the "sympathetic" nerves (CST, LST, LSN), about 40% to 70% of the preganglionic neurons exhibit no spontaneous activity and no reflexes under the experimental conditions. It is unlikely that this high proportion of silent preganglionic neurons is mainly related to the anesthesia under which the experiments were conducted:
  - Some of the silent preganglionic neurons have distinct functions and are only activated during specific behavioral conditions (e.g., pilomotor neurons, vasodilator neurons supplying skin or skeletal muscle, neurons supplying internal reproductive organs).
  - Silent preganglionic neurons may have vasoconstrictor function and are only recruited under extreme conditions (e.g., emergency such as during severe blood loss, extreme exposure to cold).
  - Most cutaneous vasoconstrictor neurons innervating skin of the proximal extremities

Table 4.5 Numbers and proportions of major classes of preganglionic neurons projecting in major "sympathetic" nerves in the cat[a]

	CST[b]	LST[c]	LSN[d]
Location of neurons	T1–T5	L1–L4	L1–L5
Target tissues	Head, upper neck	Hindlimb, tail[e]	Pelvic organs, colon
Number of neurons	6200	4500	2300
MVC/VVC neurons	20%	10%	15%
CVC neurons[f]	12%	13%	zero
MR neurons[g]	zero	zero	41%
INS neurons[h]	10%	zero	zero
Silent neurons[i]	45%	70%	40%

Abbreviations: CVC, cutaneous vasoconstrictor; INS, inspiratory type; MR, motility-regulating; MVC, muscle vasoconstrictor; VVC, visceral vasoconstrictor.

[a] The percentages are estimates and do not add up to 100% since some preganglionic neurons have spontaneous activity but exhibit no known reflexes or have characteristics of sudomotor neurons (LST).

[b] Cervical sympathetic trunk (CST); Boczek-Funcke et al. (1992a, 1993), Wesselmann and McLachlan (1984).

[c] Lumbar sympathetic trunk (LST) distal to lumbar paravertebral ganglion L5; Jänig and Szulczyk (1980), Jänig and McLachlan (1986a, b).

[d] Lumbar splanchnic nerves (LSN); Bahr et al. (1986c), Baron et al. (1985).

[e] A few preganglionic fibers in the distal LST synapse with postganglionic neurons in the sacral paravertebral ganglia which project through the pelvic splanchnic nerves to pelvic organs and probably innervate blood vessels (for references see Jänig and McLachlan 1987).

[f] CVC neurons innervating the distal parts of the extremities and the tail. Some 20% of the postganglionic CVC neurons innervating hairy skin have a reflex pattern similar to that in MVC neurons (excitation to the stimulation of arterial chemoreceptors, strong baroreceptor control, excitation during stimulation of cutaneous nociceptors; see Subchapter 4.1). These CVC neurons cannot be recognized by way of their reflex pattern in the population of preganglionic neurons. Thus, the neurons are hidden in the population of preganglionic MVC neurons.

[g] MR neurons project in the LSN and are activated or inhibited by at least one of the following stimuli: distension/contraction of the urinary bladder or colon, mechanical stimulation of anal or perianal skin. A few MR neurons have no ongoing activity.

[h] INS neurons are only active during inspiration (see Subchapter 4.4).

[i] Silent neurons have no ongoing activity and no reflex activity under the experimental conditions tested. A few silent neurons can be recruited (e.g. by hypercapnia or hypoxia).

and trunk are silent under thermoneutral conditions in humans (see Subchapter 4.2.1).

■ Silent preganglionic neurons may be involved in the regulation of metabolism (e.g., white adipose tissue), immune tissue (see Subchapter 4.6), bone metabolism (Elefteriou 2018), or others.

The numerical estimates of the four major groups of functionally identified sympathetic preganglionic neurons clearly show that only small fractions of the total number of preganglionic neurons are involved in cardiovascular regulation or regulation of cutaneous blood flow (MVC/VVC neurons, CVC neurons in Table 4.5). However, recordings of multiunit activity from "sympathetic" nerves (e.g., lumbar or major splanchnic nerves, renal nerve, sympathetic trunk) show that the discharge patterns are rather uniform and always dominated by the discharge pattern in neurons that are involved in cardiovascular regulation, as shown by the cardiac and respiratory rhythmicity of their activity. This is important to know once the central pathways in the spinal cord, brain stem and hypothalamus that are linked to the functionally different types of cardiovascular and non-cardiovascular preganglionic neurons are worked out (see Chapters 8 to 10). It implies, as expected, that the other neurons do not exhibit cardiac and respiratory rhythmicity of their activity or are silent.

4.8 | Parasympathetic Systems

Pre- and postganglionic parasympathetic neurons have always been presumed to constitute distinct peripheral pathways which transmit centrally derived signals to their target organs and exhibit distinct reflexes to afferent stimuli that are appropriate for their function. Compared to the amount of experimentation on the reflex discharge conducted in single sympathetic pre- and postganglionic neurons, corresponding studies of the functional properties of parasympathetic neurons are relatively few (Table 4.6). The lack of systematic studies is probably because:

- Many parasympathetic ganglia are located close to or on the wall of their target organs, often in small groups, and are therefore less well defined than the sympathetic ganglia. A consequence is that the postganglionic axons are very short and difficult to visualize for dissection.
- Parasympathetic preganglionic neurons are relatively difficult to record from and to separate with respect to their target organs. This applies to recordings from cell bodies of the neurons (e.g., in the dorsal motor nucleus of the vagus [DMNX], in the nucleus ambiguus [see Subchapter 4.8.1], in the sacral spinal cord [see Subchapters 4.8.2 and 9.3]) as well as to recordings from their axons.
- Functionally and anatomically, peripheral parasympathetic neurons constitute more discrete pathways to the target organs than sympathetic neurons. It is widely accepted that most parasympathetic ganglia act as simple relay stations (i.e. without integration; see Subchapter 6.5.3). However, this may not be entirely true for some parasympathetic ganglia (e.g., cardiac parasympathetic ganglia [McAllen et al. 2011] [see Subchapters 6.5.3 and 6.5.4; Figures 6.12 and 6.13] and some pelvic ganglia [see Keast 1995a, 1999]).

A main difference between sympathetic and parasympathetic systems is that each type of target organ of the parasympathetic system is spatially restricted (such as sphincter pupillae and ciliary body, salivary and other exocrine glands of the head, the heart, the blood vessels of the erectile tissue, and the smooth muscle cells of the urinary tract and hindgut).

In contrast, some types of target organs of the sympathetic nervous system are widely distributed (e.g., blood vessels in skeletal muscle, in hairy skin, in viscera; sweat glands, erector pili muscles, etc.). This has consequences for the organization of the autonomic ganglia in each system. However, some target organs of the sympathetic nervous system are as restricted as those of the parasympathetic pathways (e.g., cardiac pacemaker and atria, dilator pupillae muscle, pineal gland). Furthermore, the sympathetic innervation of vascular beds of skeletal muscle or skin may be subdivided according to the anatomical region (e.g., distal or proximal skin of the extremities, skin of trunk; skeletal muscle of extremities or of trunk).

4.8.1 Parasympathetic Pathways to Pelvic Organs

Pelvic organs (which include the rectum–sigmoid of the descending colon) are innervated by and regulated via sacral (in the rat sacral and caudal lumbar [L_6]) spinal autonomic (parasympathetic) systems (Figure 4.21). Cranial parasympathetic (vagal) systems are not involved in their regulation. Some details about the anatomy and neural regulation of these systems are described in Chapter 8 and Subchapter 9.3 and in the literature (see below, Hindgut, Lower Urinary Tract and Reproductive Organs).

Hindgut

The sacral parasympathetic pathways to the hindgut are rather complex and little understood in their physiology. They largely consist of (pre-postganglionic) neuron chains that innervate enteric neurons in the myenteric plexus (but not in the submucosal plexus), or neurons in the serosal plexus, similar to the sympathetic non-vasoconstrictor pathways to the gastrointestinal tract. Thus, the neural connection between the sacral spinal cord and target cells in the rectum–sigmoid consists of chains of at least three neurons connected synaptically. Only a few postganglionic neurons in pelvic splanchnic ganglia innervate targets (e.g., circular smooth muscle) directly. No projections exist to mucosa, submucosa, longitudinal muscle and submucosal blood vessels (Fukai and Fukuda 1985; Luckensmeyer and Keast 1998a, b).

It appears as if the sacral parasympathetic innervation of the hindgut is only involved in the regulation of its motility and above all in the control of its

Table 4.6 Functional classification of parasympathetic neurons in animals based on reflex behavior in vivo

Likely function	Location	Target organ	Likely target tissue	Major identifying stimulus	Ongoing activity[a]
Pupillo-constrictor	Ciliary ganglion, postggl.[b]	Iris	Constrictor pupillae muscle	Excitation/ inhibition by light	Yes
	EW lateral, preggl. [c]	Iris	Constrictor pupillae muscle	Excitation by light	Yes
Accommodation[d]	EW lateral, preggl.	Ciliary body	Ciliary muscle	Excitation by target moving	Yes
Cardiomotor [e]	N. ambiguus preggl.	Heart	Pacemaker cells, atrial muscle cells	Excited by stimulation of baroreceptors	Yes
Bronchomotor[f]	N. ambiguus preggl., trachea, bronchial ganglia	Trachea, bronchi	Smooth muscle cells	Stim. of tracheal mucosa, excitation in inspiration	Yes
Bronchosecreto-motor[f]	Tracheobronchial ganglia	Trachea, bronchi	Glands	Excited in expiration	Yes
Gastromotor excitatory[g]	DMNX preggl.	Stomach	Smooth muscle	Inhibition of response to duodenal distension	Yes
Gastromotor inhibitory[g]	DMNX preggl.	Stomach	Smooth muscle	Excitation of response to duodenal distension	Yes
Urinary bladder[h]	Sacral spinal cord, preggl.	Urinary bladder	Smooth muscle	Excitation of response to bladder distension	No
Colon[h]	Sacral spinal cord, preggl.	Colon	Smooth muscle	Excitation of response to colon distension	Yes

Abbreviations: EW, Edinger–Westphal nucleus; DMNX, dorsal motor nucleus of the vagus; N. ambig., nucleus ambiguus; preggl., preganglionic; postggl., postganglionic; tracheobronch. ggl., tracheobronchial ganglia. Modified from Jänig and Häbler (1999)

[a] Not all neurons have spontaneous activity

For details about rates of ongoing activity in pre- and postganglionic neurons and reflexes to various afferent stimuli see:

[b] Nisida and Okada (1960), Melnitchenko and Skok (1970), Inoue (1980), Johnson and Purves (1983)

[c] Sillito and Zbrozyna (1970a, b), Gamlin and Clarke (1995), Gamlin (2000)

[d] Gamlin et al. (1994), Gamlin (2000), Kozicz et al. (2011)

[e] Jewett (1964), Katona et al. (1970), Kunze (1972), McAllen and Spyer (1978a), Jänig (2016)

[f] Tomori and Widdicombe (1969), Widdicombe (1966), McAllen and Spyer (1978a), Mitchell et al. (1987), Undem and Potenzieri (2012)

[g] Grundy et al. (1981), Roman and Gonella (1994), see Subchapter 10.7

[h] de Groat et al. (1982, 2015), see Subchapter 9.3

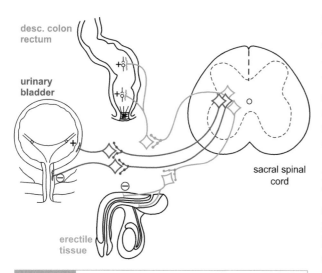

Figure 4.21 Parasympathetic pathways from the sacral spinal cord to the pelvic organs. In the rat the parasympathetic preganglionic neurons are also located in the lumbar segment L6. Excitatory pathway to the body of the urinary bladder (detrusor vesicae), inhibitory pathway to the urethra (transmitters nitric oxide [NO] and vasoactive intestinal peptide [VIP]), inhibitory pathway to the erectile tissue (transmitters NO and VIP) and excitatory pathway to the distal colon/rectum (this pathway possibly consists of three neurons, i.e., the postganglionic neurons from synapses with enteric neurons [myenteric and serosal plexus]).

evacuation (defecation) and continence (the latter together with the upper lumbar sympathetic supply; see Subchapter 9.3). The sacral parasympathetic neurons to the hindgut are excited by stimulation of sacral afferents from the hindgut (most of them being unmyelinated) generated by distension or contraction, and possibly inhibited by stimulation of afferents from the lower urinary tract (urinary bladder and urethra) (see Subchapter 9.3 and Figure 9.10). Stimulation of afferents from the anal canal (which constitute a distinct population of visceral afferents [Bahns et al. 1987; Jänig and Koltzenburg 1991a]) probably inhibits the sacral efferent neurons innervating the hindgut.

Lower Urinary Tract
The lower urinary tract (urinary bladder and urethra) is supplied by at least two sacral parasympathetic pathways. One pathway innervates the bladder body (detrusor vesicae). Its activation leads to contraction of the urinary bladder. Neurons of this pathway are activated by stimulation of sacral bladder afferents and probably inhibited by stimulation of sacral

afferents from the colon or from the anal canal. The other sacral parasympathetic pathway innervates the urethra. Its activation (e.g. by stimulation of sacral vesical afferents during micturition) relaxes the urethra, probably by release of NO and VIP. This parasympathetic pathway to the lower urinary tract is anatomically and functionally less well characterized than the pathway to the bladder body (Jänig 1996b; de Groat 2013; de Groat et al. 2015; see Subchapter 9.3).

Reproductive Organs
The sacral spinal autonomic pathways to the reproductive organs have a complex organization, which is related to the target cells and to the integration of lumbar (sympathetic) spinal systems and sacral (parasympathetic) spinal autonomic systems at the level of the target cells and of the splanchnic pelvic ganglia (McKenna 1999, 2000, 2001, 2013; see Jänig and McLachlan [1987], Jänig [1996c]; see Subchapter 9.3).

The spinal parasympathetic innervation of the reproductive organs consists of at least one pathway innervating the erectile tissues (sinusoids and trabecular tissues of the corpus cavernosum and corpus spongiosum of the penis and the helicine arteries that feed the erectile tissues in males). In males, the postganglionic neurons innervating the erectile tissues project through the cavernous nerve. These neurons are cholinergic and use NO and VIP as transmitters (Jänig 1996c; de Groat 2013; see Figure 9.12). It is unclear whether postganglionic neurons projecting through the cavernous nerve also receive convergent synaptic input from lumbar sympathetic preganglionic neurons or whether the sympathetic pathway responsible for penile erection (e.g., in patients or animals with destroyed sacral spinal cord) is separate from the parasympathetic pathway (see Figure 9.12 and Subchapter 9.3). Neurophysiological studies in vitro support the idea that the two pathways to the erectile tissue are largely separate (Jobling et al. 2003, 2004). Neurons of the parasympathetic pathways of the erectile tissue are reflexly activated by stimulation of pudendal afferents from the penis and surrounding tissue (Figure 9.11). Further characterization of these neurons has not been done. Parasympathetic spinal neurons may also be involved in activation of glands of the reproductive organs.

The role of spinal parasympathetic pathways in the regulation of female external and internal reproductive organs (during sexual arousal) has been little explored. However, it is generally believed that the spinal parasympathetic pathway(s) and the underlying mechanism involved are similar to those in the male. Thus, the erectile tissue of females is innervated by a parasympathetic cholinergic vasodilator pathway, as in the male. Furthermore, engorgement of the vaginal wall with blood and transudation of mucoid fluid through the epithelium of the vagina seems to be generated by reflex activation of spinal parasympathetic neurons, which generate vasodilation and increase of permeability of the capillaries (McKenna 2000, 2002; Giuliano et al. 2001).

4.8.2 Parasympathetic Pathways From the Brain Stem

Heart

The heart is innervated by at least two parasympathetic pathways. One pathway is involved in the regulation of frequency of heart beat, by acting on the pacemaker cells of the sinoatrial node and on the atrioventricular node, and in the regulation of force of contraction of the atria. The axons of most preganglionic neurons of this pathway are myelinated (in the cat, rat and human). The cell bodies of the preganglionic neurons are situated in the external formation of the nucleus ambiguus and the cell bodies of the postganglionic neurons are in the parasympathetic cardiac ganglia associated with the right atrium. Some neurons in this cardiomotor pathway exhibit spontaneous activity. The neurons are excited by stimulation of arterial baroreceptors and exhibit cardiac rhythmicity in their activity (Figure 4.22c). The activity in most cardiomotor neurons of this pathway exhibits respiratory rhythmicity (Figure 4.22b): (in the cat) the neurons are inhibited during inspiration and activated in expiration (mostly postinspiration). This coupling to the central respiratory network is the basis of respiratory sinus arrhythmia of the heartbeat. Stimulation of arterial chemoreceptors, nasopharyngeal receptors or other receptors excites these cardiomotor neurons, leading to bradycardia (McAllen and Spyer 1978a, b; Izzo and Spyer 1997; Cheng and Powley 2000). Chemical stimulation of the cell bodies of the cardiomotor neurons in the nucleus ambiguus leads to decrease in heart rate. In fact excitation of a single parasympathetic preganglionic cardiomotor neuron already slows heart frequency, showing how powerful this parasympathetic pathway is to generate bradycardia (Figure 4.22d; McAllen and Spyer 1978a).

A second parasympathetic cardiomotor pathway, which is entirely separate from the first one, originates in the lateral part of the dorsal motor nucleus of the vagus [DMNX] (Figure 4.22a). Preganglionic neurons of this pathway have unmyelinated axons (in the rat and probably in the cat). Some of these cardiomotor neurons exhibit spontaneous activity. This spontaneous activity is neither modulated by activity in arterial baroreceptors nor by the central respiratory drive. The function of this cardiomotor pathway is unknown. Its activation generates weak bradycardia (Izzo and Spyer 1997; Feigl 1998; Jones et al. 1998; Cheng et al. 1999). Experiments on rats suggest that these preganglionic cardiomotor neurons are involved in regulation of ventricular excitability (Machhada et al. 2015; Gourine et al. 2016; Jänig 2016).

Airways

Tracheobronchial airways of the respiratory tract seem to be innervated by three parasympathetic pathways, two pathways supplying the airway smooth muscle (parasympathetic bronchomotor neurons) and one pathway innervating the glands of the airways (bronchosecretomotor neurons; Canning and Undem 1993; Canning and Mazzone 2005; Undem and Potanzieri 2012). One bronchomotor pathway contracts the airway smooth muscle cells by release of acetylcholine. Neurons of this pathway are activated by stimulation of airway nociceptors, arterial chemoreceptors, upper airway mechanoreceptors or esophageal afferents. The second parasympathetic bronchomotor pathway relaxes the airway smooth musculature by release of nitric oxide (NO) and possibly a peptide (e.g., vasoactive intestinal peptide). This pathway may also be activated by noxious airway stimulation or stimulation of rapidly adapting stretch afferents of the lung. Bronchosecretomotor neurons may be reflex activated by firing of airway nociceptors or by lung stretch receptors.

Most neurons of these bronchomotor pathways seem to be spontaneously active. One type of bronchomotor pathway is active during inspiration and postinspiration and not under control of arterial baroreceptors. It is inhibited by hyperinflation of the lung (generated by increase in transpulmonary pressure [Figure 4.23a]) and excited by stimulation of arterial chemoreceptors and other stimuli that lead to reflex bronchoconstriction. The postganglionic neurons of

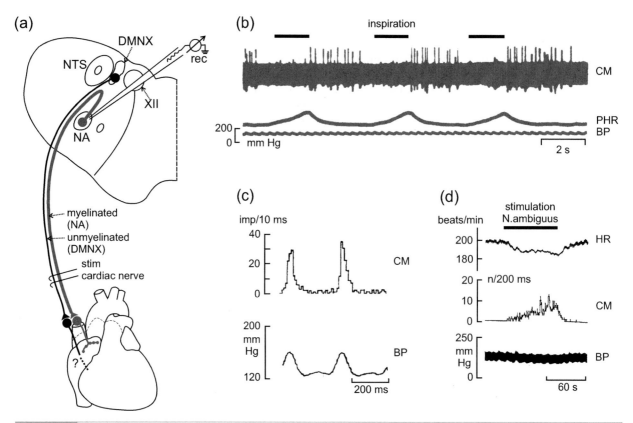

Figure 4.22 Discharge pattern of parasympathetic cardiomotor neurons (CM) in the cat. (a) Experimental setup: recording from the cell bodies with a microelectrode. The cell bodies of the neurons are located in the external formation of the nucleus ambiguus (NA). The neurons project through the vagus nerves to the heart. The neurons were identified by electrical stimulation of their axons in the cardiac branch of the vagus nerve (stim cardiac nerve). Cardiomotor neurons in the NA have myelinated axons. Cardiomotor neurons in the lateral part of the dorsal motor nucleus of the vagus (DMNX) have unmyelinated axons. Their function is unknown (see text). NTS, nucleus tractus solitarii; XII, hypoglossus nucleus. (b) Respiratory modulation of the activity. The CM neuron was active in expiration (mostly postinspiration) and inhibited during inspiration. BP, blood pressure; PHR, integrated phrenic nerve activity. (c) Cardiac rhythmicity of the activity in a cardiomotor neuron in the NA. Blood pressure pulse-triggered histogram of the activity in the neuron. Activity in 256 cardiac double cycles superimposed. Lower record: averaged pulse wave of the arterial blood pressure recorded in the femoral artery. (d) Stimulation of cell bodies of the CM neurons in the NA by ionophoretic application of an excitatory amino acid through a microelectrode decreased heart rate (HR) and BP. In this experiment only a few (possibly only one!) CM neurons were stimulated. Modified from McAllen and Spyer (1978a) with permission.

this bronchomotor pathway may innervate the bronchial smooth muscle cells. The second functional type of bronchomotor neuron is active during expiration and excited by lung hyperinflation (Figure 4.23b). These bronchomotor neurons may innervate secretory glands of the airways, and thus are probably bronchosecretomotor neurons (Mitchell et al. 1987; see Jordan [1997]). The discharge pattern of the type of parasympathetic postganglionic bronchomotor neuron that relaxes the airway smooth muscle cells is unknown; however, these neurons may exhibit spontaneous activity too (Kesler et al. 2002). The cell bodies of the preganglionic neurons of the first type of bronchomotor

neuron are located in the external formation of the nucleus ambiguus, mostly rostral to the cell bodies of the preganglionic cardiomotor neurons with myelinated fibers (McAllen and Spyer 1978a). The location of the preganglionic neurons of the second type of bronchomotor neuron and of the bronchosecretomotor neurons is unknown, but probably also in the external formation of the nucleus ambiguus.

Gastrointestinal Tract

Cranial parasympathetic pathways to the gastrointestinal tract are complex. The preganglionic neurons are located in the dorsal motor nucleus of

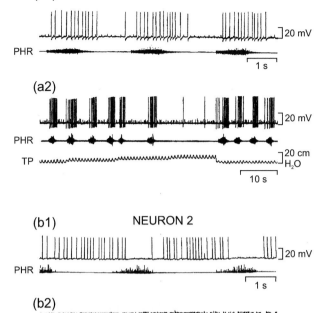

(a1) NEURON 1

20 mV

PHR

1 s

(a2)

20 mV

PHR

TP

20 cm H₂O

10 s

(b1) NEURON 2

20 mV

PHR

1 s

(b2)

20 mV

PHR

TP

20 cm H₂O

10 s

Figure 4.23 Reflex discharge pattern of postganglionic bronchomotor neurons. Intracellular recordings from the cell bodies of neurons in tracheal ganglia in anesthetized cats (upper records). Lower or middle records, activity in the phrenic nerve (PHR). (a) Neuron 1 active in inspiration and postinspiration. The activity of this neuron was depressed by increase of transpulmonary pressure (TP). This type of neuron may innervate the smooth musculature of airways. (b) Neuron 2 largely active during expiration. This neuron was activated by increase of TP. It may innervate tracheobronchial glands. Modified from Mitchell et al. (1987) with permission.

the vagus (DMNX); the postganglionic neurons are neurons of the enteric nervous system. Experimental studies of preganglionic neurons clearly show that these neurons are functionally differentiated with respect to regulation of various gastrointestinal functions (motility, secretion of exocrine glands, secretion of endocrine glands) (details in Subchapters 5.7 and 10.7; see Subchapter 10.7 for recording from preganglionic neurons in the DMNX). For some functions related to regulation of motility, the reflex pathways have

been worked out. For neurons of parasympathetic pathways to exocrine glands or endocrine cells (e.g., G-cells secreting gastrin or the insular cells of the pancreas secreting insulin or glucagon) the reflex patterns and pathways are unknown.

Salivary Glands

Preganglionic neurons projecting to parasympathetic ganglia innervating salivary glands (and possibly nasopharyngeal glands) are located in the superior salivary nucleus (for the submandibular and sublingual salivary glands; for the nasopharyngeal glands) and in the inferior salivary nucleus (for the parotid gland and the lingual glands) (see Figure 1.4). Studies of the biophysical properties and the reflex patterns show that these neurons may consist functionally of two types, secretomotor neurons and vasodilator neurons. The main physiological stimuli activating these neurons are taste stimuli and mechanical stimuli in the naso-oro-pharyngeal cavity (Matsuo and Yamamoto 1989; Matsuo and Kang 1998; Matsuo et al. 1998; Kim et al. 2004; Fukami and Bradley 2005).

Eye

Preganglionic neurons of the pupillomotor pathway (pupilloconstriction) are activated (some inhibited) by light. Preganglionic neurons of the accommodation pathway (contraction of ciliary body) are specifically activated during target tracking. Preganglionic neurons of the vasodilator pathway (vasodilation of the chorioid blood vessels) are activated by light. In *birds* and *monkeys* the preganglionic neurons are organized topically according to their function in the Edinger–Westphal nucleus; the preganglionic pupilloconstrictor neurons are located in the caudal part of the lateral Edinger–Westphal nucleus (only about 3% of the preganglionic neurons in this lateral part are involved in pupilloconstriction). Most neurons in the lateral Edinger–Westphal nucleus are involved in accommodation. Neurons in the medial Edinger–Westphal nucleus are involved in vasodilation of chorioid blood vessels. Each parasympathetic pathway in the nucleus Edinger–Westphal seems to be connected to a distinct set of central pathways, including the pretectal olivary nucleus (pupillary light reflex), the suprachiasmatic nucleus (chorioid vasodilation reflex), the cerebellum and their nuclei (fastigial and interpositus nucleus; accommodation reflex), which determine the distinct discharge patterns (see Reiner et al.

[1983], Gamlin [2000] and McDougal and Gamlin [2015] for review and references).

4.9 | Genetic-Molecular Aspects of Functional Differentiation of Autonomic Neurons: A Summary

The functional organization of the peripheral autonomic nervous system into target-defined channels as worked out in vivo is supported by molecular biological investigations of postganglionic sympathetic neurons in the stellate ganglion and in the upper thoracic ganglia of the mouse 27–33 days postnatally. RNA (ribonucleic acid)-sequencing and quantitative gene expression analysis in individual neurons were performed to work out parts of the transcriptome (sets of RNA) of the sympathetic postganglionic neurons which determine their physiological properties (Figure 4.24). The results describe seven distinct neuron types on the basis of their genetic-molecular characteristics. Five neuron groups are noradrenergic (i.e., express primarily tyrosine hydroxylase [TH], dopamine-β-hydroxylase [DBH], dihydroxyphenylalanine [DOPA] decarboxylase and vesicular monoamine transporter 2). Two neuron groups are cholinergic (i.e., express primarily choline acetyltransferase [ChAT], vesicular acetylcholine transporter [VAChT], often with somatostatin and/or vasoactive intestinal peptide). Two of the noradrenergic neuron types are nipple- or piloerection neurons, both being target-dependent in their final differentiation (* in Figure 4.24). The cholinergic neurons innervate sweat glands or periosteum, the differentiation of sudomotor neurons also being dependent on their target. The targets of the remaining three molecularly distinct types of noradrenergic neurons are unknown and have to be worked out. But there are more than three distinct target tissues for these sympathetic neurons such as blood vessels of skeletal muscle, cutaneous blood vessels, heart, secretory epithelia and smooth musculature of the gastrointestinal tract and possibly others (Rohrer 2011; Furlan et al. 2016; Ernsberger and Rohrer 2018).

Reproduction of this elegant molecular genetic work, as well as its extension to other populations of postganglionic neurons and to preganglionic neurons, will put the organization of the peripheral autonomic nervous system on a sound molecular basis. However, this will not show how these differentiated peripheral autonomic systems function in vivo in the transmission of the centrally generated activity to the target tissues and through the ganglia.

Conclusions

1. The peripheral autonomic nervous system supplies each group of target tissues by one (sometimes two) pathway(s) each consisting of sets of pre- and postganglionic neurons with distinct patterns of reflex activity. This has been established for the lumbar sympathetic outflow to skin, skeletal muscle and viscera, for the thoracic sympathetic outflow to the head and neck, and for some parasympathetic pathways.

2. The principle of organization into functionally discrete pathways is the same in both the sympathetic and the parasympathetic nervous systems, the only difference being that some functional targets of the sympathetic system are widely distributed throughout the body (e.g., muscle blood vessels, skin blood vessels, sweat glands, erector pili muscles, fat tissue) and are substantially more extensive. However, other target tissues are spatially restricted in both sympathetic and parasympathetic systems.

3. Experimental investigations of sympathetic systems innervating skin or skeletal muscle in humans, using microneurography, fully support the idea of functionally discrete sympathetic pathways developed in animal studies.

4. Figure 4.25 shows the peripheral sympathetic pathways to somatic tissues (skin and skeletal muscle of hindlimb and tail) and to pelvic organs (including the distal colon), which have their origin in the upper lumbar spinal cord and which have been studied extensively in the anesthetized cat, many of them at both preganglionic and postganglionic level:

    a. The reflex patterns observed in each group of autonomic neurons are the result of integrative processes in the spinal cord, brain stem and hypothalamus (all of them probably under the control of the forebrain).

    b. The neurons in many of these pathways have ongoing activity, but neurons in some pathways

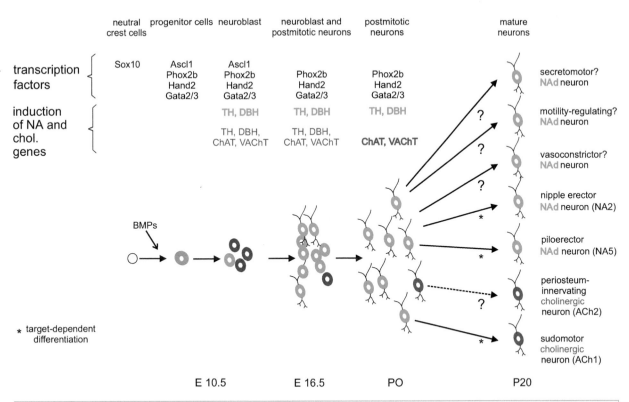

Figure 4.24 Schematic illustration of the sympathetic postganglionic neuron subtype differentiation in the mouse. Signaling by bone morphogenetic protein (BMP) at the dorsal aorta elicits the expression of a group of transcription factors, including Phox2b, Hand2 and Gata3, that induce noradrenergic genes (tyrosine hydroxylase [TH], dopamine-β-hydroxylase [DBH]) and cholinergic genes (choline acetyltransferase [ChAT], vesicular acetylcholine transporter [VAChT]), resulting in a high proportion of cells with a mixed noradrenergic/cholinergic phenotype at the embryonic stages E10.5–E16.5. At birth (P0), the vast majority of postmitotic sympathetic neurons display noradrenergic properties; cholinergic properties are only observed in about 5% of sympathetic neurons. Single-cell RNA-sequencing of mature sympathetic neurons from postnatal day 20 (P20) allowed two subtypes of cholinergic sympathetic neurons (ACh1- and ACh2-neurons labeled by red cell bodies) and five subtypes of noradrenergic sympathetic neurons (NAd1 to NAd5; labeled by blue cell bodies on the right) to be defined. ACh1 and ACh2 correspond to sudomotor neurons and neurons innervating the periosteum. NAd2 and NAd5 neurons have been identified as nipple-erector and piloerector sympathetic neurons. Sudomotor, NAd2 and NAd5 subtype neurons differentiate during postnatal development from noradrenergic neurons under the influence of target-derived differentiation signals (*). Vasoconstrictor (muscle, skin, viscera), visceral secretomotor, motility-regulating sympathetic, sympathetic cardiomotor and other subtypes of sympathetic postganglionic neurons are not yet characterized with respect to their gene expression signature and whether their differentiation is also controlled by target-derived signals. Modified from Ernsberger and Rohrer (2018). Data based on Furlan et al. (2016). For literature, see these publications.

are silent and are activated only under special behavioral conditions.

c. Functionally similar preganglionic and post-ganglionic neurons are synaptically connected in the autonomic ganglia, with little or *no* "cross-talk" between different peripheral functional pathways (see Chapter 6).

d. Vasoconstrictor neurons consist of several subtypes and have a wide spatial distribution. Cutaneous vasoconstrictor neurons are functionally subdifferentiated with respect to

different sections of the vascular tree and different types of skin (hairy, hairless; distal, proximal).

e. The description of motility-regulating neurons that control the pelvic organs is certainly not complete as there probably exist other types of motility-regulating neurons. These neurons innervate spatially restricted groups of target cells in the viscera (e.g., erectile tissue, urinary bladder, hindgut).

FINAL AUTONOMIC PATHWAYS
(lumbar sympathetic system)

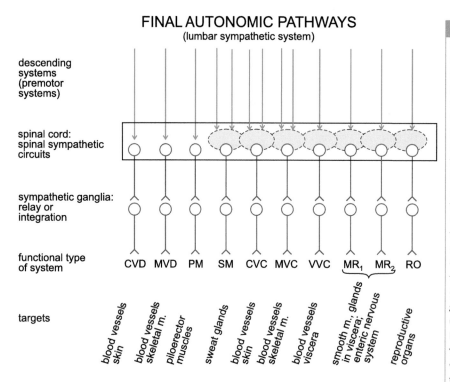

descending systems (premotor systems)

spinal cord: spinal sympathetic circuits

sympathetic ganglia: relay or integration

functional type of system

CVD MVD PM SM CVC MVC VVC MR₁ MR₂ RO

targets

blood vessels skin | blood vessels skeletal m. | piloerector muscles | sweat glands | blood vessels skin | blood vessels skeletal m. | blood vessels viscera | smooth m., glands in viscera; enteric nervous system | reproductive organs

Figure 4.25 Lumbar sympathetic systems supplying skeletal muscle and skin of the hindlimb or pelvic organs (including distal colon) in the cat. The preganglionic neurons of these systems are largely located in the lumbar segments L1 to L5 (see Figure 8.8) and project in the lumbar sympathetic trunk distal to paravertebral ganglion L5 or in the lumbar splanchnic nerves and the hypogastric nerves. The first group projects (with a few exceptions related to pelvic organs) to postganglionic neurons innervating somatic tissues and the second group to postganglionic neurons innervating pelvic organs or colon. The second group includes more than two pathways as shown here (related to smooth musculature or glands in the hindgut, urinary bladder, urethra, erectile tissue, vas deferens). Preganglionic neurons are associated with spinal circuits (yellow areas, see Chapter 9 [only indicated for systems that have been investigated]) and are under multiple supraspinal control via descending systems (descending systems in green, see Chapters 10 to 11). CVC, cutaneous vasoconstrictor; CVD, cutaneous vasodilator; m., muscle; MR, motility-regulating; MVC, muscle vasoconstrictor; MVD, muscle vasodilator; PM, pilomotor; RO, reproductive organs; SM, sudomotor; VVC, visceral vasoconstrictor. Modified from Jänig (1986).

---

f. Release of adrenaline by the adrenal medulla is mediated by a distinct sympathetic pathway. Adrenaline is primarily a metabolic hormone, but also has some other functions.

g. Based on the functional specificity of the reflex patterns and the centrally evoked discharges in the sympathetic neurons, it is postulated that each group of preganglionic neuron receives connections from specific spinal reflex pathways and specific groups of sympathetic premotor neurons that are located in the brain stem and hypothalamus (Chapters 8 to 10).

5. Pre- or postganglionic neurons of only a few parasympathetic pathways have been studied systematically for their reflex pattern. However, where studied (e.g., those to the urinary bladder, gastroduodenal region, heart, airways) the parasympathetic neurons exhibit discharge patterns as predicted from their target cell responses. Neurons of parasympathetic pathways to blood vessels (pelvic erectile tissue, cranial blood vessels) and to glands of the head (salivary, lacrimal, nasopharyngeal) and of pelvic organs have not been studied systematically using neurophysiological methods.

6. These peripheral autonomic pathways are the building blocks for the neural regulation of body functions during internal and external challenges.

They are also the basis for the adaptive responses of the body during different types of behavior, including basic emotions and an important basis for all protective reactions of the body.

7 The concept that the sympathetic nervous system operates in an "all-or-none" fashion, without distinction between different effector organs, is not valid. The same applies to the idea of a simple functional antagonism between the sympathetic and parasympathetic nervous systems. This is corroborated by the finding that circulating noradrenaline has no detectable function under physiological conditions. Circulating adrenaline, the release of which from the adrenal medulla is regulated by a distinct sympathetic pathway, is a metabolic hormone and does not otherwise elicit autonomic effector responses under physiological conditions. The idea of a generally functioning sympatho-adrenal system is refuted by these findings. Under extreme stress, a specific pattern of sympathetic outflow elicited from particular regions of the hypothalamus can appear, which resembles the widely understood "fight or flight" response.

8 The functional organization of the peripheral sympathetic nervous system is supported by molecular-genetic studies of the postganglionic neurons.

Suggested Reading

Furlan, A., La Manno, G., Lubke, M., et al. (2016) Visceral motor neuron diversity delineates a cellular basis for nipple- and pilo-erection muscle control. *Nat Neurosci* **19**, 1331–1340.

Häbler, H. J., Jänig, W. and Michaelis, M. (1994b) Respiratory modulation of activity in sympathetic neurones. *Prog Neurobiol* **43**, 567–606.

Jänig, W. (1985) Organization of the lumbar sympathetic outflow to skeletal muscle and skin of the cat hindlimb and tail. *Rev Physiol Biochem Pharmacol* **102**, 119–213.

Jänig, W. (2016) Neurocardiology: a neurobiologist's perspective. *J Physiol* **594**, 3955–3962.

Jänig, W. (2020) Sympathetic nervous system and pain. In *The Senses: A Comprehensive Reference, Vol 5 – Pain, 2nd edn* (Pogatzki-Zahn, E. and Schaible, H.-G., eds.) pp. 193–226, Elsevier, Amsterdam.

Jänig, W. and McLachlan, E. M. (1987) Organization of lumbar spinal outflow to distal colon and pelvic organs. *Physiol Rev* **67**, 1332–1404.

Jänig, W. and McLachlan, E. M. (1992a) Characteristics of function-specific pathways in the sympathetic nervous system. *Trends Neurosci* **15**, 475–481.

Kirillova-Woytke, I., Baron, R. and Jänig, W. (2014) Reflex inhibition of cutaneous and muscle vasoconstrictor neurons during stimulation of cutaneous and muscle nociceptors. *J Neurophysiol* **111**, 1833–1845.

McAllen, R. M., Salo, L. M., Paton, J. F. and Pickering, A. E. (2011) Processing of central and reflex vagal drives by rat cardiac ganglion neurones: an intracellular analysis. *J Physiol* **589**, 5801–5818.

Morrison, S. F. (2018) Efferent neural pathways for the control of brown adipose tissue thermogenesis and shivering. *Handb Clin Neurol* **156**, 281–303.

All references cited in the text are available online at www.cambridge.org/janig.

Notes

1. Plethysmography: measurement of the change of volume of an organ (here a finger) generated by change in blood flow. Vasoconstriction is indicated by a decrease in volume recorded plethysmographically and a decrease of pulsatile changes.

2. This study was conducted on subjects with the skin temperature of the big toe adjusted to 20 to 22 °C by mild whole-body cooling. Thus, the subjects were in a thermoregulatory state in which the activity in the cutaneous vasoconstrictor neurons was present.

3. Responses of blood flow through glabrous skin in humans (monitored by laser Doppler flowmetry or photoelectrical pulse plethysmography) to arousal, mental stress or deep breath very much depend on the thermoregulatory state of the subjects (generated experimentally by whole-body cooling or warming). At skin temperatures of $\geq$30 °C (when activity in cutaneous vasoconstrictor neurons innervating distal skin of the extremities is low or absent), these stimuli generate vasoconstriction in skin. At skin temperatures of $\leq$25 °C (when activity in cutaneous vasoconstrictor neurons is high), these stimuli generate vasodilation in skin. The vasodilation is generated by decreased activity in cutaneous vasoconstrictor neurons, the vasoconstriction in the warm state by activation of cutaneous vasoconstrictor neurons (Oberle et al. 1988; Wallin et al. 1998).

4. In the cat, the potential recorded from the surface of the hairless skin via a fluid bridge (0.9% NaCl) as shown in Figure 4.11a using non-polarizable silver–silver chloride electrodes (surface versus subcutaneous [extraglandular] electrode) consists of three

components: (1) A direct current (DC) potential, which is negative on the surface of the skin when the sweat glands are *not* activated by sudomotor neurons. (2) This DC potential decreases during activation of sweat glands by the sudomotor neurons. Reflex activation of the sudomotor neurons leads to a slow shift of the skin potential in the positive direction (see Figures 4.12a and b). (3) Activity in the sudomotor neurons generates fast transient negative changes in the skin potential that are preceded by impulses in the postganglionic sudomotor neurons (Figures 4.11b,c, 4.12a; Jänig and Kümmel, unpublished observations).

5. Glabrous skin is the palmar and plantar skin of primates, which is different in its organization from hairless skin of non-primate mammals.

6. It has also been observed that sudomotor neurons supplying glabrous skin of the hands of hyperhydrotic patients (who suffer from bouts of profuse sweating) can be activated by stimulation of low-threshold mechanoreceptors (Pacinian corpuscles and other low-threshold mechanoreceptors of the hand; Marchettini, Torebjörk, Culp and Ochoa, unpublished observation). This reflex appears to be similar to the vibration reflex in cats (Figure 4.12a) and may normally be inhibited by supraspinal centers. It may be activated in healthy human subjects during motor commands which control movements of the hand during manipulation. This parallel activation of sweat glands and skeletal muscles would keep the glabrous skin flexible for optimal somato-sensory discrimination. I hypothesize that the cortically initiated motor commands have access to the neural circuits (e.g., in spinal cord and brain stem) which regulate the activity in the final sudomotor pathway innervating sweat glands in hairless (acral) skin. This regulation of flexibility of hairless skin by the cortex would occur via an inhibitory mechanism. A general decrease of this inhibition would result in hyperhidrosis in the patients.

7. Guanethidine is a compound that is actively taken up by the noradrenergic nerve terminals and concentrated in the neurosecretory vesicles where it displaces noradrenaline. As a consequence of this replacement, the noradrenergic terminals no longer release noradrenaline when excited, which results in a block of noradrenergic transmission.

8. Hexamethonium is a quaternary ammonium agent that blocks cholinergic nicotinic receptors and so blocks transmission in autonomic ganglia (see Chapter 6).

9. It has been proposed that this vasodilation is generated by vasoactive intestinal peptide (VIP), which coexists with acetylcholine in sudomotor neurons, and is released by sudomotor axon terminals when activated (Lundberg 1981). There is evidence against this possibility: (1) Hexamethonium differentially blocks vasodilation and sweat gland activation (i.e., a low concentration of hexamethonium blocks vasodilation in skin but not the activation of sweat glands, whereas a high concentration of hexamethonium blocks both). This can be explained by the size of the excitatory currents produced by the strong synaptic inputs to the postganglionic neurons. (2) Intense activation of sudomotor neurons by vibration does not generate a measurable vasodilation in the skin. (3) Vasodilation induced by released VIP is probably restricted to the tissue around the sweat glands deep below the surface of the skin (see Bell et al. [1985]).

10. Neuropathy generically describes a disease involving peripheral nerves, i.e., primary afferent neurons, autonomic neurons or motoneurons. For example, in severe diabetes mellitus, afferent and autonomic neurons may be affected, thus showing sensory and autonomic neuropathy.

11. Sensations elicited in the skin (e.g. upper arm, back or head) during emotional arousal are most likely due to piloerection produced by activation of pilomotor neurons and subsequent contraction of piloerector muscles. This leads to activation of low-threshold mechanoreceptors innervating the hair follicles and probably also of low threshold, slowly adapting mechanoreceptors that respond to stretch of skin (Grosse and Jänig, unpublished).

12. Muscle spindles and Golgi tendon organs are encapsulated structures in skeletal muscle. Muscle spindles are arranged in parallel with extrafusal muscle fibers and are innervated by fast-conducting (afferent) Ia-fibers (in addition to afferent group II fibers and efferent γ-fibers), which measure the length of the muscle and its derivatives. Golgi tendon organs are located at the junction between extrafusal muscle fibers and the tendon. They are innervated by fast-conducting Ib-fibers, which measure force and its derivatives in extrafusal muscle fibers.

13. The distinct reflexes in these sympathetic neurons are mediated by sacral visceral afferents and not lumbar visceral afferents because they are unchanged after interruption of the lumbar visceral afferents.

14. In the cat, vascular dilation in skeletal muscle is generated by electrical low-frequency (<2 Hz) stimulation of the innervation of the adrenal medulla or by intravenous infusion of adrenaline (<0.5 µg/[kg min]) (Celander 1954). In humans, intra-arterial infusion of 0.05 to 0.1 µg/min adrenaline generates vasodilation in skeletal muscle but vasoconstriction in skin (Golenhofen et al. 1962). This adrenaline-induced vasodilation in skeletal

muscle is most likely not due to the metabolic effect of adrenaline on the skeletal muscle fibers (release of lactic acid) but due to its direct effect on the vascular smooth muscle mediated by β_2-adrenoceptors (Schmidt-Vanderheyden and Koepchen 1967).

15. Some autonomic effector organs, such as smooth muscle, cardiac muscle, exocrine glands and the pineal gland, develop adaptive supersensitivity after denervation and to a certain degree also after decentralization (interruption of the preganglionic axons). This supersensitivity may be interpreted as a compensatory mechanism by which the excitable tissue increases its excitability to extrinsic signals such as neurotransmitters and other compounds. The supersensitivity may be relatively specific (e.g., increased sensitivity of the cardiac muscle to catecholamines) or non-specific. The underlying cellular changes are multiple and include change in postreceptor pathways, membrane potential, electrogenic Na^+–K^+ transport, ion channels, intracellular Ca^{2+} sequestration and other changes. There is no evidence for an increase of density and affinity of receptors for a neurotransmitter in autonomic target cells after denervation. These cellular mechanisms vary between effector tissues and have been poorly investigated (Fleming and Westfall 1988). Denervation in vivo may result in increase of responses of heart, pupil and vasculature to circulating catecholamines. This supersensitivity may even be maintained over a long time when the target tissue is reinnervated (Jobling et al. 1992; Koltzenburg et al. 1995). The change in sensitivity of blood vessels after their denervation and reinnervation and the underlying cellular and subcellular mechanisms have been investigated and discussed by Tripovic et al. (2010, 2011, 2013).

16. *Venular plasma extravasation* is a component of inflammation in all tissues. It is under neural (not in the skin of humans) and neuroendocrine control (see note 2 in Chapter 2). Sensitization of nociceptors for mechanical stimulation leads to *mechanical hyperalgesic behavior*. Both venular plasma extravasation and mechanical hyperalgesic behavior serve to protect body tissue, leading to healing after noxious (tissue-damaging) stimuli. Both are therefore called *protective body reactions*.

Chapter 5

The Enteric Nervous System

In his chapter "The sympathetic and related systems of nerves" in Schäfer's *Textbook of Physiology* (Langley 1900), Langley defined for the first time the idea that the gastrointestinal tract has a nervous system of its own. He called this system the enteric nervous system (Langley 1900). He repeated this idea in his short monograph in 1921 where he clearly described the division of the autonomic nervous system into three parts: sympathetic, parasympathetic and enteric nervous system (ENS). This classification is still used today (Langley 1921). The existence of the neuronal plexuses of Auerbach (plexus myentericus) and Meissner (plexus submucosus) within the wall of the gastrointestinal tract has been known since the second half of the nineteenth century. Langley recognized that this system can act to a large extent independently of the central nervous system. He separated the myenteric and submucosal ganglia from the sympathetic and parasympathetic nervous systems and classified them as a third part of the autonomic nervous system for the following reasons: (1) they have a histology distinct from that of the paravertebral and prevertebral sympathetic ganglia, (2) it was unclear at that time whether they are connected to the central nervous system by sympathetic and/or parasympathetic neurons and (3) the sympathetic postganglionic fibers either send collaterals to or form synapses with the neurons of the enteric nervous system (Langley 1900). Up until about 1970, little or no attention was given to the enteric nervous system; in fact this system was practically ignored. Two further reasons have emerged for considering the ENS as a distinct entity. Comparison of the ENS across the animal kingdom indicates that the ENS developed before the CNS or the sympathetic and parasympathetic divisions of the autonomic nervous system (Furness and Stebbing 2018). In cnidaria (marine invertebrates such as anemones, hydras, jellyfish), there is an ENS but no CNS. Moreover, the ENS contains neurons that project towards sympathetic prevertebral ganglia and even towards the CNS. Thus, the ENS and CNS have reciprocal connections with sympathetic ganglia and with parasympathetic centers in the brainstem and lumbo-sacral spinal cord (Furness et al. 2014; Furness and Stebbing 2018).

Our present knowledge about the neurobiology of the enteric nervous system is chiefly based on systematic experimental studies of this system in the guinea pig and recently in the mouse (including various genetically engineered mice), combining various methods (e.g., neurophysiology, histology, immunohistochemistry, pharmacology and electronmicroscopy, etc.). In the center of these experimental investigations are different types of in vitro preparations of the small intestine and distal colon of the guinea pig, which allow one to study the enteric neurons under visual control and with respect to their function. This type of systematic research has been correlated with research on the intrinsic neural control of the gastrointestinal tract in other species, including the human. Two research groups, represented by John Furness and Marcello Costa, have performed pioneering experimental work in the last 40 years. This work has been extended by their descendants, in particular Simon Brookes and Nick Spencer, to define the afferent and efferent neural pathways controlling the enteric nervous system. Mainly based on this research, I will describe the anatomy, the general concepts and some general functional characteristics of the ENS. For further details, some comprehensive reviews are available (see Furness and Costa [1987]; Kunze and Furness [1999]; Brookes and Costa [2002]; Furness [2006, 2012]; Furness et al. [2014]; Brierley and Costa [2016]).

5.1 Anatomy, Components and Global Functions of the Enteric Nervous System

5.1.1 Anatomy and Global Functions

The gastrointestinal tract serves various global functions: ingestion of energy-rich compounds, water, electrolytes and some other vital substances (e.g., vitamins); transport of its content; enzymatic breakdown of the energy-rich and other vital substances; resorption of the breakdown products, electrolytes, water and vitamins; and evacuation of waste products. To accomplish these functions, the gastrointestinal tract is endowed with a nervous system of its own, the enteric nervous system. Under normal conditions, the central nervous system has delegated many basic functions to the enteric nervous system and does not modify the individual functions of the gastrointestinal tract. It has special commands over the regulation of the intake and the evacuation of the gastrointestinal tract. Furthermore it adapts the way in which the gastrointestinal tract operates during special behaviors of the organism.

Anatomically, the enteric nervous system consists of the myenteric plexus and the submucosal plexus and the axons these supply to various effectors (Figure 5.1). The plexuses contain the neurons of the enteric nervous system. The nerve cell bodies are grouped in small enteric ganglia, which are connected by bundles of nerve cell processes (axons and dendrites). The *myenteric plexus* is located between the circular and longitudinal smooth musculature and the *submucosal plexus* is arranged between the circular musculature and the submucosa. In many species, the submucosal plexus consists of an inner plexus (closer to the mucosa) and an outer plexus (closer to the circular muscle). This plexus is prominent in the small intestines and colon and almost absent in the esophagus and stomach (although there are species differences). The myenteric plexus is present throughout the entire gastrointestinal tract. The enteric nervous system is also found in the gallbladder wall and pancreas, including the bile ducts, all three having developed from the small intestine. Individual ganglia in both plexuses contain up to 200 nerve cell bodies that are arranged in the quasi two-dimensional planes of the plexuses.

The enteric nervous system contains approximately 10^7 to 10^8 neurons (varying according to species and counting procedure; e.g., in humans 2–6×10^8 neurons [Furness 2006]). This number is of the same order of magnitude as the number of neurons in the spinal cord. The myenteric plexus is mainly (but not exclusively) involved in the regulation of different motility patterns, whereas the submucosal plexus is mainly (but not exclusively) involved in the regulation of secretion of water and electrolytes and of local blood flow. The motor neurons of the submucosal plexus project preferentially to target cells in the mucosa, but also to cells of the circular muscles of animals of large body size, but not in rat, mouse and guinea pig. The motor neurons of the myenteric ganglia project preferentially to the smooth musculature, but also to the mucosa and to the submucosal plexus.

The effector cells of the enteric nervous system are smooth muscle cells of the longitudinal and circular musculature, mucosal smooth muscle cells, secretory mucosal cells (which include secretory glands), hormone-secreting cells in the mucosa, mucosal and submucosal arterioles, and intrinsic lymphoid tissues (Chiocchetti et al. 2008). Smooth muscle cells and cells of secretory epithelia are

(a)

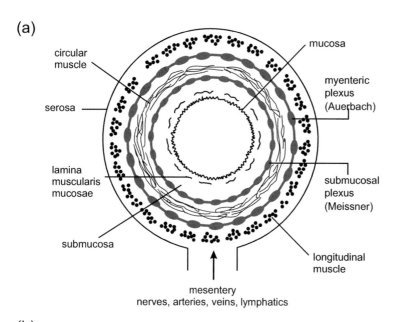

circular muscle

serosa

lamina muscularis mucosae

submucosa

mucosa

myenteric plexus (Auerbach)

submucosal plexus (Meissner)

longitudinal muscle

mesentery
nerves, arteries, veins, lymphatics

Figure 5.1 Transverse section through the small intestine and its mesentery (a) and representation of the enteric plexuses in relation to the layers of the intestine (b). Indicated are smooth muscle layers, neural plexuses (red), submucosa and mucosa viewed macroscopically. Modified from Furness and Costa (1987) with permission.

(b)

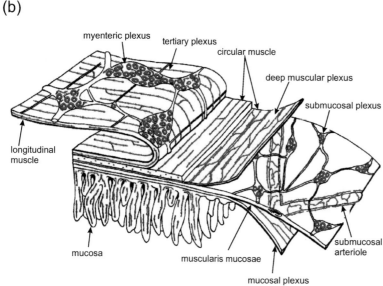

myenteric plexus   tertiary plexus

circular muscle

deep muscular plexus

submucosal plexus

longitudinal muscle

mucosa

muscularis mucosae

mucosal plexus

submucosal arteriole

electrically coupled by gap junctions. Thus, these cells form functional and electrical syncytia that comprise the effector tissues of the enteric nervous system. Interstitial cells of Cajal (ICC), which form several plexuses of electrically coupled cells in the gastrointestinal tract that are arranged in parallel with the smooth muscle cell layers, are also effector cells of the enteric nervous system (see Subchapter 5.4). It is now largely agreed that the ENS innervates the lymphoid follicles (the gut-associated lymphoid tissue [GALT]) (Chiocchetti et al. 2008; Mowat 2003).

5.1.2 Components of the Enteric Nervous System

The enteric nervous system contains three classes of neurons in the myenteric plexus and submucosal plexus: intrinsic primary afferent neurons, motor neurons and interneurons. Each class of neuron consists of several types, which are characterized by their anatomy (location and projection of axons), neurochemical coding (content of neuropeptides, primary transmitters, as well as cotransmitter[s]) (Figure 5.2, Table 5.1) (Note 1).

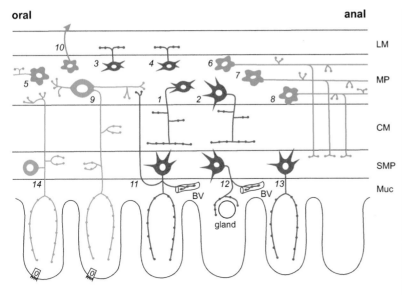

oral   anal

Figure 5.2 Types of neurons of the enteric nervous system in the small intestine of the guinea pig. The neurons have been defined by their functions, cell body morphology, projection to targets, neurochemistry and primary transmitters. Intrinsic primary afferent neurons (IPANs) in blue, motor neurons in red, interneurons in green. Motor neurons innervating the muscularis mucosae or endocrine cells are not shown. The numbers adjacent to the neurons correspond to the numbers in Table 5.1, which lists each of the neuron types by their function, neurochemistry, primary transmitter and percentage of cell bodies in the myenteric or submucosal plexus. BV, blood vessel; CM, circular muscle; LM, longitudinal muscle; MP, myenteric plexus; Muc, mucosa; SMP, submucosal plexus. Modified from Furness et al. (2004) with permission.

Intrinsic Primary Afferent Neurons (IPANs)

About 20% of the enteric neurons in the small intestine are IPANs (Furness et al. 1998, 2004) (Note 2). The cell bodies of these neurons lie in the myenteric and submucosal plexuses. They are activated by various physiological stimuli, such as mechanical stimuli (e.g., shearing and pressure stimuli applied to the mucosa; distension and contraction of the wall of the gut) or intraluminal chemical stimuli (e.g., inorganic acids, bases, short-chain fatty acids or glucose). Excitation of the enteric afferent neurons by chemical or mechanical stimulation of the mucosa is partly mediated by enterochromaffin cells in the mucosa releasing 5-hydroxytryptamine (5-HT), and possibly by other enteric hormone cells in the mucosa (e.g., cells releasing cholecystokinin [CCK] or motilin). Thus, the mechanosensitive enteric afferent neurons would also be, in a strict sense, chemosensitive.

IPANs whose cell bodies are located in the submucosal plexus have their receptive endings in the mucosa. They respond to mechanical distortion of the mucosa (e.g., shearing stimuli exerted by the luminal content) and to intraluminal chemical stimuli. Intrinsic primary afferent neurons located with their cell bodies in the myenteric plexus have their receptive endings in the external muscle layer and/or in the mucosa. They respond to contraction and distension of the enteric musculature and to intraluminal chemical stimuli. In the small

intestine of the guinea pig, most IPANs are polymodal, i.e., they respond to various mechanical as well as chemical stimuli. Some IPANs may have a relative stimulus specificity, i.e., they respond preferentially to one type of adequate stimulus and more weakly to other stimuli. It is unknown whether this relative specificity is functionally important (Furness et al. 2004). In the colon of the guinea pig, the mechanosensitive IPANs consist functionally of two types. One type is stretch-sensitive, but does not respond to contraction. The second type responds preferentially to contraction of the smooth musculature but less to distension of the colonic wall (Spencer et al. 2002, 2003a).

Most IPANs are afterhyperpolarizing (AH) neurons (i.e. they exhibit long-lasting afterhyperpolarization after excitation, which seems to depend on intermediate conductance calcium-activated K^+ channels). These neurons use acetylcholine and tachykinins as transmitters. Enteric afferent neurons connect synaptically to other enteric afferent neurons to form networks of enteric afferent neurons in the myenteric plexus. These networks connect to enteric interneurons and to enteric motor neurons (see Figure 5.6).

IPANs must be distinguished from extrinsic visceral primary afferent neurons which innervate the gastrointestinal tract. These afferent neurons have their cell bodies in the dorsal root ganglia or the

Table 5.1 Types of neurons in the small intestine, some of their defining characteristics and percentage of occurrence found in the enteric nervous system of the guinea pig

Myenteric neurons[a]	Proportion	Chemical coding	Functions/comments
Excitatory circular muscle motor neurons (1)	12%	*Short*: ChAT/TK/ENK/GABA *Long*: ChAT/TK/ENK/NFP	To all regions; PT **ACh**, CT **TK**
Inhibitory circular muscle motor neurons (2)	16%	*Short*: NOS/VIP/PACAP/ENK/ NPY/GABA *Long*: NOS/VIP/PACAP/dynorphin/GRP/NFP	Several CT with varying prominence: NO, ATP, VIP, PACAP
Excitatory longitudinal muscle motor neurons (3)	25%	ChAT/calretinin/TK	PT **ACh**, CT **TK**
Inhibitory longitudinal muscle motor neurons (4)	about 2%	NOS/VIP/GABA	Several CT with varying prominence: NO, ATP, VIP, PACAP
Ascending interneurons (local reflex) (5)	5%	ChAT/calretinin/TK/ENK	PT **ACh**, CT **TK**
Descending interneurons (local reflex) (6)	5%	ChAT/NOS/VIP ± GRP ± NPY	PT **ACh**, CT **ATP**?
Descending interneurons (secretomotor reflex) (7)	2%	ChAT/5-HT	PT **ACh, 5-HT** (at 5-HT_3 receptors)
Descending interneurons (migrating myoelectric complex) (8)	4%	ChAT/SOM	PT **Ach**
Myenteric intrinsic primary afferent (primary sensory) neurons (9)	26%	ChAT/calbindin/TK/NK_3 receptor	PT **TK** and **ACh** (CGRP and ACh in other species)
Intestinofugal neurons (10)	<1%	ChAT/GRP/VIP/NOS/CCK/ ENK	PT **ACh**, mainly from colon
*Motor neurons to gut endocrine cells	N/A	N/A	e.g., myenteric neurons innervating gastrin cells; also in submucosal ganglia
*Secretomotor neurons to gastric glands	N/A	ChAT	Stimulate gastric acid secretion

Submucosal neurons[a,b]	Proportion	Chemical coding	Function(s)/comments
Non-cholinergic secretomotor/vasodilator neurons (11)	45%	VIP/PACAP/GAL	PT **VIP**; a few with cell bodies in myenteric ganglia
Cholinergic secretomotor/vasodilator neurons (12)	15%	ChAT/calretinin/dynorphin	PT **Ach**
Cholinergic secretomotor (non-vasodilator) neurons (13)	29%	ChAT/NPY/CCK/SOM/CGRP/dynorphin	PT **ACh**; a few with cell bodies in myenteric ganglia
Submucosal intrinsic primary afferent (primary sensory) neurons (14)	11%	ChAT/TK/calbindin	PT **ACh** (?TK) (CGRP and ACh in other species)

Table 5.1 (cont.)

Submucosal neurons[a,b]	Proportion	Chemical coding	Function(s)/comments
*Excitatory motor neurons to musculares mucosae	N/A	ChAT/TK	PT **Ach**
*Inhibitory motor neurons to musculares mucosae	N/A	NOS/VIP	PT?, similar to myenteric inhibitory motor neurons

* Types of motor neuron found in other parts of the digestive tract.

Abbreviations: ACh, acetylcholine; ATP, adenosine triphosphate; ChAT, choline acetyltransferase; CCK, cholecystokinin; CGRP, calcitonin gene-related peptide; CT, cotransmitter; ENK, enkephalin; GABA, γ-aminobutyric acid; GAL, galanin; GRP, gastrin-releasing peptide; 5-HT, 5-hydroxytryptamine (serotonin); N/A, not applicable; NFP, neurofilament protein; NK, neurokinin; NO, nitric oxide; NOS, nitric oxide synthase; NPY, neuropeptide Y; PACAP, pituitary adenylyl cyclase activating peptide; PT, primary transmitter; SOM, somatostatin; TK, tachykinin; VIP, vasoactive intestinal peptide. From Furness et al. (2004), with permission, and Brookes (2001).
[a] see Figure 5.2 for numbers.
[b] see also Figure 5.13 for numbers.

vagal ganglia. They are involved in reflex activity via the CNS and in the generation of gut sensations (see Chapter 2).

Motor Neurons

Enteric neurons innervating target cells are called enteric motor neurons. These neurons are specialized with respect to the different groups of target cells they innervate:

- Excitatory muscle motor neurons supplying smooth muscle cells innervate the longitudinal or circular smooth musculature and are involved in descending and ascending reflexes. The cell bodies of these motor neurons are located in the myenteric plexus, representing about 40% of all neurons in this plexus. They are cholinergic and use acetylcholine as the primary transmitter, which acts via cholinergic muscarinic receptors. Tachykinins (substance P, neurokinins A and K) are colocalized with acetylcholine in these neurons and may serve as secondary transmitters. Some excitatory muscle motor neurons also innervate muscle fibers in the lamina muscularis mucosae.
- Motor neurons that induce relaxation of circular smooth muscles are involved in descending inhibitory reflexes and also in accommodation of the stomach. They are located in the myenteric plexus and represent about 16% of all neurons in this plexus. These inhibitory muscle motor neurons use nitric oxide (NO), adenosine triphosphate (ATP) or a related nucleotide, "pituitary adenylyl cyclase

activating peptide" (PACAP) and/or vasoactive intestinal peptide (VIP) as transmitters. In most inhibitory muscle motor neurons, NO may serve as the primary transmitter and the other compounds as secondary transmitter(s). The specific combination of these substances, which potentially serve as inhibitory transmitters, varies between groups of inhibitory motoneurons depending on the section of the gastrointestinal tract and on the species.
- Both excitation and inhibition generated by enteric muscle motor neurons in the smooth muscles are mediated, at least in part, by intramuscular ICC (Burns et al. 1996; Ward et al. 1998; Ward and Sanders 2001; see Subchapter 5.4).
- The lamina muscularis mucosae is also innervated by inhibitory and excitatory motor neurons. The cell bodies of these motor neurons are located in the myenteric plexus.
- Neurons that innervate the mucosal epithelium in the small and large intestines and gallbladder (causing water, electrolyte and bicarbonate secretion) are called secretomotor neurons. Almost all secretomotor neurons are located in the submucosal plexus and represent about 90% of all neurons in this plexus. Neural control of secretion by the enteric nervous system is closely linked to the control of local blood flow by enteric vasodilator neurons. Both effects appear to be exerted by the same populations of secretomotor neurons. Thus, some secretomotor neurons innervate both gland cells and the initial segments of arterioles in the

submucosa and in the outer part of the mucosa. The submucosal blood vessels are the distributing vessels for the blood supply of the mucosa and even in part of the external musculature. About 30% of these secretomotor neurons have only secretory function and the control of mucosal blood vessels by a distinct class of enteric vasodilator neurons cannot be excluded. The secretomotor neurons are either cholinergic and use acetylcholine as the primary transmitter, acting on muscarinic cholinergic receptors, or they are non-cholinergic and use VIP as the primary transmitter. Neurons with dual (vasodilator and secretomotor) function seem to be preferentially non-cholinergic. In the stomach, neural control of parietal cells secreting proton ions is exerted by cholinergic secretomotor neurons. This secretion is accompanied by local vasodilation, which is either also mediated by enteric cholinergic neurons or is reactive consequent to the activation of the parietal cells (reactive or functional hyperemia).

- Several types of enteric endocrine cells are located in the densely innervated mucosa of the gastrointestinal tract. There is evidence that these endocrine cells are innervated too and therefore are under neural control. The best studied example is the control of gastrin release by G-cells in the antral mucosa by enteric motor neurons. It is likely that release of other hormones of the gastrointestinal tract is under neural control as well (e.g., secretin released by S-cells in the duodenal mucosa, hormones [insulin, glucagon, pancreatic polypeptide] released by endocrine cells in the pancreas). The G-cells are innervated by neurons in the myenteric plexus that utilize gastrin-releasing peptide (GRP) as a transmitter. The location and type of motor neurons associated with other enteric endocrine cells are unknown.

Motor neurons of similar types are not synaptically connected with each other and therefore do not form motoneuron networks as do intrinsic primary afferent neurons and interneurons.

Interneurons

The enteric nervous system contains various groups of neurons that have neither afferent nor motor neuron function and that are interposed between these two groups of neuron. So far, in the myenteric plexus of the guinea pig small intestine, three classes of interneuron projecting anally with their axons and one class of interneuron projecting orally with its axons have been identified (Figure 5.2); they form about 16% of all neurons in this plexus. Interneurons seem to be absent in the submucosal plexus of smaller animals but are probably there in larger animals (dogs, humans, pigs). Thus, IPANs are synaptically connected to secretomotor neurons in the submucosal plexus of the smaller animals without intervening interneurons (Figure 5.13).

Probably all interneurons are cholinergic, but synaptic transmission from them to motor neurons and between interneurons is not purely cholinergic. Interneurons of like type are synaptically connected to each other and form chains of like neurons that run either orally or anally (Figure 5.6). The ascending interneurons are involved in regulation of motility and transmit their activity by the nicotinic action of acetylcholine (ACh). The descending interneurons probably use 5-HT (5-hydroxytryptamine = serotonin) (ACh/5-HT descending interneurons that are involved in secretory reflexes) or ATP (ACh/ATP/NOS [nitric oxide synthase] descending interneurons that are involved in inhibitory motor reflexes), in addition to acetylcholine, as a cotransmitter. Whether NO is used as a transmitter by these interneurons is unclear. If it is, its effect is minor. Descending cholinergic interneurons containing somatostatin seem to be involved in the generation of the migrating myoelectrical complex (MMC, see Subchapter 5.4).

The interneurons vary considerably in type between different sections of the gut and are difficult to identify anatomically, histochemically and physiologically. This is not surprising in view of the difficulties in functionally identifying spinal interneurons related to the somatomotor system, to spinal autonomic systems (see Chapter 9) or to sensory systems, or in identifying interneurons in the lower brain stem that are related to the arterial baro- and chemoreceptor reflexes (see Subchapters 10.3 and 10.4).

Finally, intestinofugal neurons (see neuron 10 in Figure 5.2) that project through mesenteric nerves to sympathetic prevertebral ganglia constitute a further type of interneuron. These neurons form cholinergic synapses with noradrenergic neurons projecting to the gastrointestinal tract. Intestinofugal neurons are particularly numerous in the colon and rectum. They are involved in extraspinal intestino-intestinal reflexes that relay signals from more distal to more proximal regions of the gastrointestinal tract and are involved in regulation of motility and possibly also of secretion (see Figures 5.16 and 6.11). Intestinofugal neurons are synaptically activated by IPANs responding to, e.g., distension. Some intestinofugal neurons may be a type of intrinsic primary afferent neuron activated by intestinal distension. Intestinofugal neurons also project to the pancreas, gallbladder, airways, sacral spinal cord and brain stem, but their roles have not been determined (Furness 2012, 2016).

5.1.3 Neurochemical Coding of Enteric Neurons

Enteric neurons contain many (more than 30) substances that could potentially be neurotransmitters. However, only a few substances have been established as neurotransmitters. It is very possible that most substances contained in these neurons are not used as neurotransmitters or neuromodulators. There is consensus that a few substances serve as primary transmitters and that these primary transmitters are more or less uniformly found in the same groups of enteric neurons across species (e.g., acetylcholine, 5-HT, tachykinins [substance P, neurokinin A and K], VIP). Substances that are colocalized with the primary transmitters may serve as secondary or subsidiary transmitters or neuromodulators (see Table 5.1). These vary in distinct groups of enteric neurons and between species. The presence of these different substances, in variable combinations, in enteric neurons is a neurochemical code for these neurons. This code can be used to recognize and identify the neurons and is a valuable tool in the functional experimental studies of enteric neurons (Costa et al. 1996).

5.2 The Enteric Nervous System is an Autonomic System in its Own Right

The global functions of the gastrointestinal tract are intraluminal transport and mixing of its contents, enzymatic and chemical processing of ingested food, absorption of nutrients, water, electrolytes and some other vital substances, evacuation of waste products, vomiting, and protection of the body against poisonous substances and pathogens. These functions are adjusted and coordinated at any moment by the enteric nervous system, in coordination with the brain and in concert with gastrointestinal hormones (e.g., in gastric acid secretion). The enteric nervous system contains a limited repertoire of neural programs to organize these functions according to the state of the gastrointestinal tract (e.g., fasting or digestion). The component parts of the enteric nervous system that are important to accomplish these functions were discussed in Subchapter 5.1. Synaptic connections between intrinsic afferent neurons, interneurons and motor neurons are organized in such a way that excitation of intrinsic primary afferent neurons by physiological stimuli leads to many distinct reflexes mediated by the enteric nervous system; the underlying mechanisms of some of them have been worked out in detail (see Subchapter 5.3). Under physiological conditions, these reflexes are spatially and temporally coordinated and lead to typical behaviors of the gastrointestinal tract. Single reflexes, as they are experimentally analyzed for their underlying mechanisms, are isolated parts of these integrated behaviors and valuable tools in this experimental analysis. This situation is conceptually very similar to that in the experimental analysis of the integrative somatomotor or autonomic processes represented in the spinal cord (see Chapter 9) or in the lower brain stem (e.g., the dorsal vagal complex that consists of the nucleus tractus solitarii, the dorsal motor nucleus of the vagus [DMNX] and the area postrema; see Subchapter 10.7).

The diagram in Figure 5.3 graphically outlines the integrative functioning of the enteric nervous system and its control by the brain. Afferent neurons, interneurons and motor neurons form various reflex circuits, which are defined by the reacting target tissue of the motor neurons and therefore by the function(s) of the motor neurons. Some reflex circuits are monosynaptic between afferent and motor neurons, others are polysynaptic. These reflex circuits include those within the same part as well as those between different parts of the gastrointestinal tract (e.g., gastro-gastric reflexes, duodeno-gastric reflexes [response to glucose], ileo-gastric reflexes [response to lipids], esophageal-gastric reflexes [response to distension], defecation reflexes, etc.). The interneurons, which are defined by their synaptic input, their synaptic output and projection of their axons, probably play an important role in integrating the various reflex circuits. Thus, the population of interneurons is an important component of the various sensorimotor

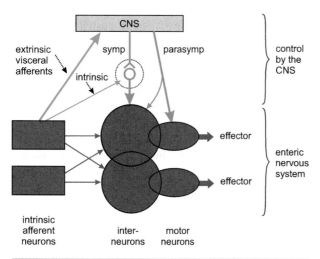

Figure 5.3 Concept of functioning of the enteric nervous system (ENS) and its control by the central nervous system (CNS). The enteric nervous system consists of intrinsic primary afferent neurons, interneurons and motor neurons, which form various reflex circuits. Effector cells can be smooth muscle cells, interstitial cells of Cajal (ICC), secretory epithelia, hormone-secreting cells, blood vessels and possibly immune cells. Each category of neuron is subdivided into several types according to the physiological response properties, morphology (location of cell body, projection of axon and dendrites), immunohistochemistry and transmitter(s) (Table 5.1). The circuits and their reciprocal synaptic connections represent the "sensorimotor programs" of the ENS, which regulate movement patterns and secretory processes. Interneurons are important for the coordination of the different processes. Extrinsic visceral afferent neurons projecting to the spinal cord or to the nucleus tractus solitarii provide detailed information about events in the gastrointestinal tract to the CNS. The CNS acts on the ENS via sympathetic (Sy) and parasympathetic (Parasy) pathways. With some exceptions, it does not regulate single motor functions of the gastrointestinal tract but interferes with the sensorimotor programs of the ENS. For example, activation of sympathetic motility-regulating neurons may interrupt peristalsis by inhibiting enteric circuits and by closing sphincters directly. The CNS has direct control of intake of nutrients, disposal of waste products and vascular diameter/blood flow. Intrinsic neurons (intestinofugal interneurons) project to prevertebral sympathetic ganglia giving afferent feedback to postganglionic secretomotor and motility-regulating neurons. Modified from Wood (1994) with permission.

programs that are represented in the enteric nervous system. This organization is the basis for the autonomous functioning of the enteric nervous system, which has the potential to be independent of the brain. Therefore the enteric nervous system is sometimes also called "brain of the gut." During normal regulation of the gastrointestinal tract, some of these enteric reflex components may not be readily visible (as is the case with the functioning of spinal autonomic circuits; see Chapter 9). However, this does not mean that they are unimportant and secondary.

The central nervous system is continuously informed about the state of the gastrointestinal tract by extrinsic vagal and spinal visceral afferent neurons, by hormones from the gastrointestinal tract and directly as well as indirectly by other non-neural signals:

- The neural afferent feedback signals from the gut are highly differentiated (see Chapter 2; Table 2.1); they include information about the mechanical and chemical states of the gastrointestinal tract, about inflammatory and other noxious processes, and about processes in the immune system of the gut (the GALT) that forms the most powerful defense barrier in the body against the outside world (Mowat 2003). The importance of the afferent feedback signals is reflected in the high number of visceral afferent neurons projecting in the vagus nerves to the lower brain stem (nucleus tractus solitarii; see Chapter 2 and Subchapter 8.3); about 85% of the axons in the subdiaphragmatic vagus nerves are afferent. An important component in the coordination of motility and secretion of different segments of the gut are the sympathetic prevertebral ganglia. Sympathetic secretomotor and/or motility-regulating neurons in these ganglia receive synaptic afferent input via enteric intestinofugal interneurons, probably after activation by intrinsic afferent neurons (Figure 5.3; see Subchapter 6.5). Signals from the central nervous system and the enteric nervous system are thus integrated in prevertebral ganglia (Figure 6.10b; Subchapter 6.5).
- Hormones of the gastrointestinal tract act via the area postrema of the medulla oblongata or the arcuate nucleus of the hypothalamus on central circuits. These hormones consist of gastrin, CCK (cholecystokinin), ghrelin, glucagon-like peptide 1 and peptide YY (see Subchapter 10.7).
- Other non-neural feedback to the central nervous system is humoral (such as glucose and lipid concentration in the blood), from cytokines of the immune system of the gut and from leptin from the white adipose tissue.

The central nervous system influences the functioning of the enteric nervous system via parasympathetic pathways projecting from the dorsal motor nucleus of the vagus (DMNX) through the vagus nerves and from the sacral spinal cord through pelvic splanchnic nerves and via sympathetic systems in the thoracolumbar spinal cord (see Subchapters 4.3 and 4.8). The numbers of preganglionic parasympathetic neurons influencing the gastrointestinal tract are rather small when compared to the total number of neurons in the enteric nervous system (e.g., in the rat approximately 4000–5000 preganglionic parasympathetic neurons project through the vagus nerve to the gut [Prechtl and Powley 1990]). The central nervous system does not interfere directly with most individual effector tissues in the gut, but indirectly by giving commands to the enteric neural circuits. Most noradrenergic non-vasoconstrictor neurons in the prevertebral ganglia innervate enteric circuits presynaptically; the smooth musculature of sphincters is directly innervated by noradrenergic postganglionic neurons. Some sympathetic postganglionic secretomotor neurons may directly innervate the mucosa. Even in the distal colon of rats, most postganglionic parasympathetic neurons of the pelvic splanchnic ganglion that project to the colon innervate the myenteric plexus but not the smooth musculature directly (Luckensmeyer and Keast 1998). Thus, there are also chains of three neurons connected serially between the sacral spinal cord and the effector cells in the distal gastrointestinal tract (Fukai and Fukuda 1985).

At the beginning and the end of the gut, the central nervous system seems to have more or less direct command over some gastrointestinal functions, such as control of some functions of the stomach and regulation of defecation and storage in the colon. This is also reflected in a high innervation density of both parts of the gut by extrinsic afferent neurons that have their cell bodies in the sacral dorsal root ganglia or in the nodose ganglion (ganglion nervi vagi inferius) and is consistent with the idea that these parts of the gut are precisely adapted to the behavior of the organism. The central nervous system also has direct command over the arterial blood flow in the gut exerted via visceral vasoconstrictor neurons. This centrally regulated function is important for the regulation of arterial blood pressure and regional blood flow. The central nervous system regulates fluid balance via control of mucosal and submucosal arterioles and secretomotor neurons.

5.3 Regulation of Motility and Intraluminal Transport in the Small and Large Intestines: The Neural Basis of Peristalsis

5.3.1 Motility Patterns and Slow Waves

The stomach and small and large intestine show two basic patterns of motility in all mammalian species: the interdigestive motility pattern, characterized by the migrating myoelectrical complex (MMC), and the fed pattern of activity.

- The interdigestive motility pattern passes along the intestine at regular intervals (in the human at intervals of 80 to 110 minutes and somewhat more frequently in smaller mammals). It occurs between the feeding and digesting periods. In continuously feeding mammals (e.g., ruminants) it also passes along the intestine during feeding.
- The fed pattern of motility consists of ongoing irregular phasic contractions. Some 30% to 40% of the contractions propagate like peristaltic waves over distances of up to 10 cm towards the anal site. Thus, this pattern includes what is called segmentation, cycling as well as peristaltic movements of the gut.

Figure 5.4 demonstrates electrical activity and mechanical myogenic activity (contractions) of a proximal segment of the mouse small intestine in vitro. Compound electrical activity is recorded extracellularly from the serosal surface of the intestinal segment at three sites with electrodes separated by about 2 cm and pressure is recorded intraluminally at the corresponding sites. At a preset intraluminal pressure gradient of more than about 1 cm water, the electrical activity shows rhythmic waves that are called slow waves. Some groups of slow waves are followed by local rhythmic contractions of the intestinal segment in a 1:1 manner, leading to a rhythmic transient increase in the intraluminal pressure and pulsatile outflow from the intestinal tube. These contractions only occur if the slow waves show action potentials on their plateau phases. Slow waves without action potentials are not followed by contractions. The action potentials (see arrows in Figure 5.4b) are of minimal amplitude in

(a)

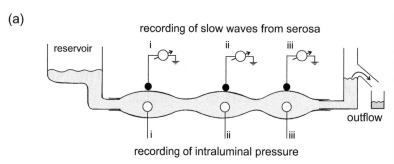

recording of slow waves from serosa

recording of intraluminal pressure

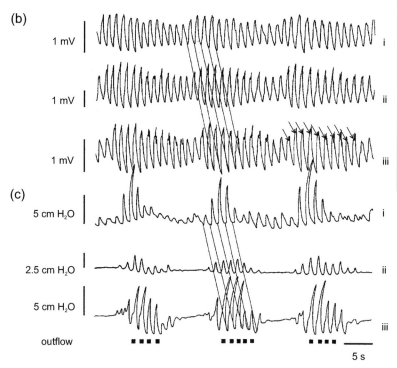

(b)

(c)

5 s

this type of extracellular recording. However, simultaneous recording of potential changes inside the smooth muscle cells and contraction clearly shows that the slow waves without action potentials are not followed by contractions, whereas those with action potentials are (Figure 5.5). Both slow waves and contractile activity occur in the smooth musculature; they are synchronized and propagate in the anal direction at a characteristic velocity, the speed of the latter depending on the section of the gastrointestinal tract and the animal species. The action potentials are generated by inflow of Ca^{2+} through L-type Ca^{2+} channels and the contractions are mediated by an increase in intracellular Ca^{2+} in the cytosol. This coordinated pattern of electrical and contractile activity is the basis of all active motility patterns generated by the gastrointestinal tract (which does not include reactive relaxation and accommodation).

The distinct motility patterns as they occur in vivo under physiological conditions are dependent on the coordinated activity of the following components:

1. myogenic mechanisms;
2. a functioning enteric nervous system;
3. functioning networks of interstitial cells of Cajal (ICCs), which are important in the generation and propagation of slow waves of the gastrointestinal tract and therefore of the MMC and for neuroeffector transmission from enteric muscle motor

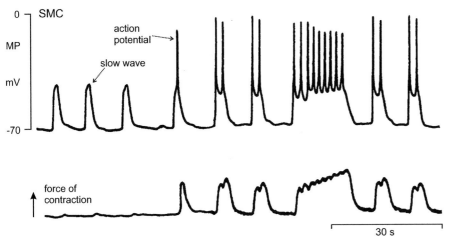

Figure 5.5 Slow waves, action potentials and contractions of smooth musculature. Slow wave potentials recorded intracellularly from a smooth muscle cell (SMC) syncytium with and without action potentials. The action potentials are generated by opening of L-type calcium channels, which trigger intracellularly the excitation–contraction mechanism, leading to contraction of the smooth musculature. Modified from Huizinga et al. (1997).

neurons to the smooth musculature in some parts of the gastrointestinal tract (see Subchapter 5.4).

Extrinsic autonomic (parasympathetic and sympathetic) innervation, including innervation by the prevertebral ganglia, and gastrointestinal hormones are not necessary for the generation of the motility pattern. However, the motility pattern is modulated by these extrinsic neural and hormonal influences.

5.3.2 Peristalsis

The term peristalsis describes the propulsion of intestinal contents from the oral site to the anal site by progressive constriction of the circular intestinal musculature. Bayliss and Starling (1899, 1900) defined peristalsis as contraction of the smooth muscles oral to an intraluminal bolus and the relaxation of the smooth muscles anal to the bolus. Both circular and the longitudinal muscles contract and relax simultaneously, but contraction and relaxation are usually stronger in the circular muscle than in the longitudinal muscle. Bayliss and Starling (1899) called these polarized excitatory and inhibitory reflexes "The law of the intestine." Figure 5.7 illustrates one of the earliest in vivo experiments from Bayliss and Starling (1899) on the dog small intestine, in which they recorded contraction and relaxation of the circular and longitudinal muscles separately. It is interesting to read their own description:

In the experiment from which the curves in Fig. [5.7] were obtained, two enterographs were placed at right angles to one another at a point 130 cm from the pylorus. The position of the levers is shown in Fig. [here 5.7, upper], a and

b being the levers of the longitudinal enterograph (a being the movable lever), c and d the levers of the enterograph recording the contractions of the circular muscle. At the beginning of the observation the intestinal wall was contracting rhythmically, the contractions affecting both coats, and being synchronous in both. At A, a bolus made of cotton-wool coated with vaseline was inserted by an opening into the intestine 4½ inches above the enterographs. It will be seen that the contractions of the circular coat cease instantly, and this inhibition is accompanied by a gradually increasing relaxation. There is some relaxation of the longitudinal coat, but the rhythmic contractions do not altogether cease. On inspection of that intestine it was seen that the introduction of the bolus caused the appearance of a strong constriction above it. This constriction passed downwards, driving the bolus in front of it. The numbers above the tracing of the circular fibers indicate the distance of the bolus in inches from the uppermost enterograph lever. At B the bolus had arrived at the upper longitudinal lever and at C had passed this and was directly under the transverse enterograph, or a little below it. At this point a strong tonic contraction of both coats occurs, expelling the bolus beyond the levers. This strong contraction passes off to be succeeded by another, which like the first is moving down the intestine.

On the basis of their observations, Bayliss and Starling inferred that mechanical stimulation of the mucosa and/or distension of the intestinal wall by a bolus excite(s) mechanoreceptive afferent neurons, which then generate polarized excitatory (oral) and inhibitory (anal) reflexes. Today we know that mechanical as well as intraluminal chemical stimuli in the small intestine elicit peristalsis, both stimuli occurring together under physiological conditions.

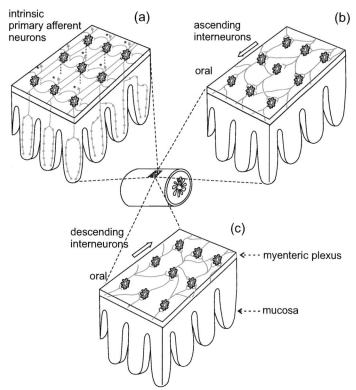

intrinsic
primary afferent
neurons

(a)

ascending
interneurons

(b)

oral

descending
interneurons

oral

(c)

⟵--- myenteric plexus

⟵--- mucosa

Figure 5.6 Assemblies of intrinsic primary afferent neurons (IPANs), ascending interneurons and descending interneurons with cell bodies in the myenteric plexus. These assemblies of neurons are important in the generation of peristalsis (see Figure 5.9). (a) The projections of the IPANs to the mucosa are mechano- and/ or chemosensitive. IPANs are reciprocally connected by slow synaptic excitatory transmission mediated by tachykinins. Their output connects to assemblies of interneurons and to motoneurons. (b, c) The assemblies of interneurons are reciprocally connected by excitatory synapses. They form either ascending (b) or descending chains of neurons (c), which connect synaptically to motor neurons (excitatory or inhibitory; not shown). Modified from Kunze and Furness (1999) with permission.

The underlying neural mechanisms of this propulsive peristalsis can now be almost fully described (Figure 5.9).

The IPANs are mediators of peristalsis. Their cell bodies lie in the myenteric plexus and project to the mucosa. In the small intestine, these neurons are excited by chemical and/or mechanical mucosal stimuli, such as by distension and particularly by contraction of the circular smooth musculature. In the colon, the IPANs involved in peristalsis consist of two separate types, those that are only stretch-sensitive and those that are preferentially contraction-sensitive, similar to the mechanosensitive IPANs in the small intestine. The neurons that are only stretch-sensitive are interneurons in the myenteric plexus of the colon (Spencer and Smith 2004). As mentioned before, IPANs of the same type are synaptically connected to each other and form assemblies of neurons (Figure 5.6a). These assemblies of IPANs are synaptically connected to at least two assemblies of synaptically connected interneurons in the myenteric plexus (Figure 5.6b, c). One assembly of interneurons projects orally and is synaptically connected to

excitatory muscle motor neurons. The other assembly of interneurons projects in the anal direction and is synaptically connected to inhibitory muscle motor neurons. Both groups of muscle motor neurons are not synaptically connected with each other, thus they do not form motor neuron assemblies.

This arrangement of afferent neurons, interneurons and muscle motor neurons, together with the functional properties of the individual classes of involved enteric neurons largely (but not entirely) explains the neural mechanism of oral–anal (aboral) propulsive peristalsis induced by distension (Figure 5.9) with some differences between the small intestine and the colon. These differences are probably related to differences in transport: in the small intestine, the content is transported in a liquid state and, in the distal hindgut, in a more solid state (in guinea pigs as solid fecal pellets).

1. In the small intestine, the polarized reflex organization applies to the circular muscle (CM). Stimulation of IPANs leads to simultaneous

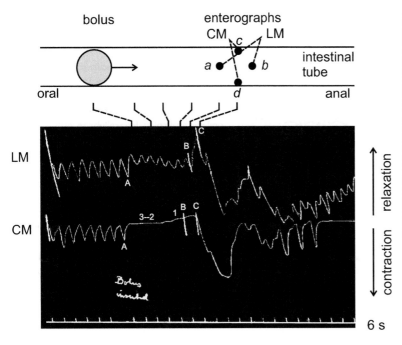

Figure 5.7 Neuronal mechanisms of peristalsis. Contraction and relaxation of the circular (CM) and longitudinal musculature (LM) of the small intestine in a dog in vivo before and during propulsive transport of a bolus from oral to anal. When the bolus was inserted into the intestinal tube about 11 cm (4.5 inch) oral to the recording sites the CM and LM relaxed. When the bolus reached the recording sites both muscles contracted. Contraction and relaxation of the CM and LM were recorded mechanographically across the transverse axis and the longitudinal axis of the intestine, respectively. See text for details. Modified from Bayliss and Starling (1899) with permission.

excitation of the CM orally as well as anally. Simultaneously, but preceding the reflex excitation of the CM, the CM becomes inhibited anally. This inhibition modulates the anal contraction of the CM leading to a decrease of amplitude and rate of rise of its contraction. This inhibition may be responsible for the anal propulsion of the liquid content of the small intestine. The longitudinal muscle (LM) is excited orally and anally to the site of activation of the IPANs (Figure 5.9a). Thus, at least three reflex pathways are involved in peristalsis of the small intestine (Hirst et al. 1975; Spencer et al. 1999).

2. The IPANs involved in the reflexes in the small intestine are polymodal afferent neurons responding to stretch and contraction as well as mucosal chemical stimuli. The neurons are cholinergic and release a tachykinin when excited that generates slow excitatory postsynaptic potentials (slow EPSPs). In this way, the IPANs form a self-reinforcing afferent neuronal network (Figure 5.6a).

3. In the colon, the polarized reflex organization applies to the CM as well as the LM (Figure 5.9b). Thus, both the CM and LM located anally to the stimulation are inhibited and both the CM and LM located orally are excited (Figures 5.8 and 5.9b). However, both the CM and LM located anally to

the stimulation are also excited; this excitation leads to rebound contraction of the colonic musculature following its relaxation (not shown in Figure 5.9b).

4. The IPANs involved in the reflexes in the distal colon consist of two types: (1) Stretch-sensitive IPANs that do not respond to contraction. These IPANs are probably myenteric interneurons. They are cholinergic and do not release a tachykinin during activation. (2) Polymodal IPANs, preferentially responding to contraction, are functionally similar to those in the small intestine.

5. In the colon, a descending assembly of cholinergic interneurons connects synaptically to two populations of inhibitory motor neurons innervating the CM and the LM, respectively (Figure 5.6c). The motor neurons to the CM use NO, ATP and VIP as transmitters (leading to an increase in potassium conductance). The motoneurons to the LM use NO as transmitter. Activation of the inhibitory motor neurons by this assembly of interneurons generates synchronous inhibitory junction potentials (IJPs) in the CM and LM, followed by relaxation of both muscles (Figure 5.8; in this experiment IPANs that are only stretch-sensitive have been activated) (Spencer and Smith 2001; Smith et al. 2003).

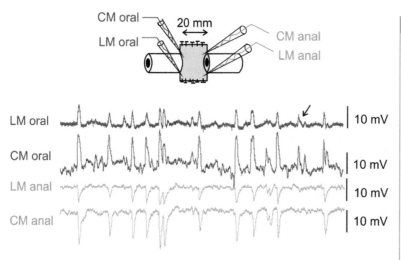

Figure 5.8 Neuronal mechanisms of peristalsis. Simultaneous intracellular recordings from two cells of the circular musculature (CM) and two cells of the longitudinal musculature (LM) in the guinea pig distal colon in vitro. The colon was opened over a length of 20 mm, fixed in a two-dimensional plane and left connected to the intact oral and anal colon. Intracellular records were made from two cells at the oral site of the flattened preparation (LM oral, CM oral) and from two cells at its anal site (LM anal, CM anal) during circumferential stretch of the preparation (stimulating in this way stretch-sensitive intrinsic primary afferent neurons). Excitatory junction potentials (EJPs) in both the CM and LM at the oral end of the colon as well as inhibitory junction potentials (IJPs) in both the CM and the LM at the anal end mostly occur synchronously; a few EJPs are not accompanied by IJPs (arrow). From Spencer et al. (2003a) with permission.

6. An ascending assembly of cholinergic interneurons (Figure 5.6b) connects to two populations of excitatory motor neurons innervating the CM and the LM, respectively. Both groups of motor neurons use acetylcholine as transmitter. Activation of the excitatory motor neurons by this assembly of interneurons generates synchronous excitatory junction potentials (EJPs) in the CM and LM, followed by contraction of both muscles. Excitatory junction potentials in the muscles oral to the stimulation site and IJPs in the muscles anal to the stimulation site are also synchronous (Figure 5.8; Spencer and Smith 2001). The intestinal tube is pulled over its content by the reflex activation of the LM (this is particularly important in the small intestine).

In summary, stimulation of the assembly of IPANs leads to synaptic activation of both assemblies of interneuron (ascending and descending). This synaptic activation triggers the following events (Figure 5.9):

- Reflex contraction of the orally located muscles by activation of excitatory muscle motor neurons.
- Relaxation of the anally located muscles by activation of inhibitory muscle motor neurons and decreased activity in IPANs due to decreased muscle tension.

- Additional activation of orally located IPANs enhances the polarized reflex activity.
- In the colon, a decrease of activity in anally located IPANs, due to relaxation of the circular and longitudinal muscle, probably reduces ascending reflex activation.

5.4 Integration of Enteric Neural, Pacemaker and Myogenic Mechanisms in Generation of Motility Patterns

The enteric reflex pathways and their coordination, as described in the preceding section, do not sufficiently explain the oral–aboral propulsive (and local non-propulsive, pendular or segmental) movement patterns of the gastrointestinal tract as they occur in vivo. These enteric reflex pathways are part of a complex inter-relationship between enteric neurons, smooth muscle cells and a third group of cells that are called interstitial cells of Cajal (ICC). Interaction between these three categories of cells will ultimately explain and clarify the role of the enteric neurons in the generation of the motility patterns of the gastrointestinal tract.

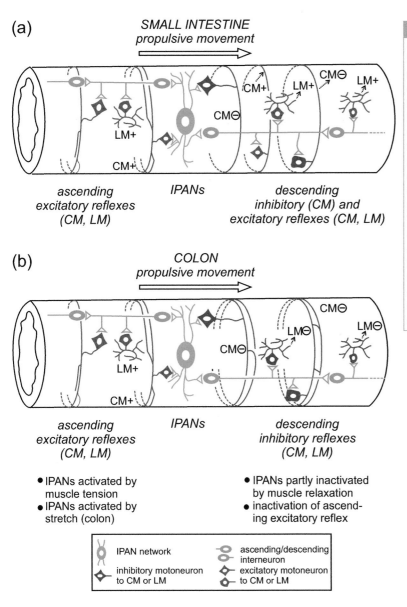

(a)

SMALL INTESTINE
propulsive movement

CM+   LM+   CM⊖   LM+

CM⊖

LM+

CM+

ascending
excitatory reflexes
(CM, LM)

IPANs

descending
inhibitory (CM) and
excitatory reflexes (CM, LM)

(b)

COLON
propulsive movement

CM⊖

LM⊖   LM⊖

CM⊖

LM+

CM+

ascending
excitatory reflexes
(CM, LM)

IPANs

descending
inhibitory reflexes
(CM, LM)

- IPANs activated by
  muscle tension
- IPANs activated by
  stretch (colon)

- IPANs partly inactivated
  by muscle relaxation
- inactivation of ascend-
  ing excitatory reflex

| IPAN network | ascending/descending interneuron |
| inhibitory motoneuron to CM or LM | excitatory motoneuron to CM or LM |

Figure 5.9 Organization of reflex circuits responsible for peristalsis in the small and large intestines. (a) Small intestine: intrinsic primary afferent neurons (IPANs), ascending interneurons and descending interneurons consist of synaptically connected assemblies of neurons (see Figure 5.6). Three reflex circuits to the circular muscles (CM; ascending excitatory, descending inhibitory and descending excitatory) and two reflex circuits to the longitudinal muscles (LM; ascending excitatory and descending excitatory) are indicated. (b) Colon: the ascending reflex pathways are the same as in the small intestine. The two descending reflex circuits are inhibitory both to the CM and to the LM. In (a) and (b), only *one* ascending and descending network of interneurons, respectively, has been indicated. Each may consist of two (ascending) or three (descending) networks. +, excitation; −, inhibition. Modified from Kunze and Furness (1999) and Sanders and Smith (2003) with permission.

5.4.1 The Interstitial Cells of Cajal (ICC) and Slow Waves

Ramón y Cajal (1995) described a group of cells in the wall of the gastrointestinal tract that are distinct in their morphology from smooth muscle cells and from enteric neurons, but closely associated with both of them. He believed that these cells were neurons, being intercalated between the terminals of enteric neurons and smooth muscle cells, and that they were important in generating pacemaker activity in the gut.

Investigation of the development of ICCs shows that they are of mesenchymal origin, as are smooth muscle cells. For their development and differentiation, they need the protooncogene, c-kit, that encodes the receptor tyrosine kinase protein (by which these cells can be recognized histochemically). Loss of c-kit leads to loss of development of ICCs from progenitor cells, which then transform into smooth muscle cells (Sanders et al. 1999). Systematic morphological investigations have shown that ICCs form several

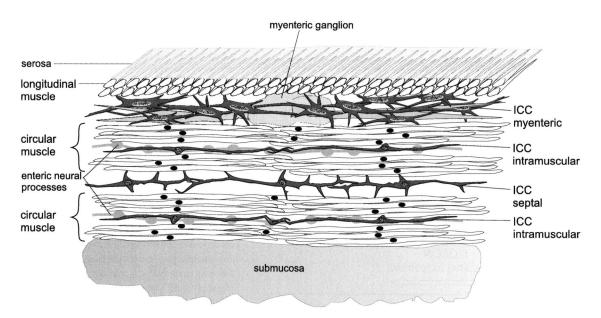

Figure 5.10 Functional organization of the interstitial cells of Cajal (ICC) in the canine gastric antrum. The antral wall contains two layers of smooth muscle cells: the outer longitudinal muscle layer (LM) lacking ICCs and the inner circular muscle layer (CM) in which individual smooth muscle cells are organized into bundles. In this CM layer, intramuscular ICCs (ICC-IM) are distributed through individual CM bundles. A network of ICCs lies between the LM and CM close to the myenteric plexus (ICC-MY). In CM bundles, ICC-IM function both to augment depolarizations reaching them from ICC-MY and as essential intermediaries in the transmission of information from enteric neural processes to nearby smooth muscle cells. Septal ICCs (ICC-SEP) form functional cables that transmit information from pacemaker ICC-MY to deep CM bundles present in the stomach of larger animals. It may well be that ICC-SEP and ICC-MY are directly connected; alternatively ICC-SEP may be electrically excited by activity in CM bundles lying closer to the ICC-MY pacemaker network. From Hirst (2001) with permission.

networks that are oriented along the longitudinal axis of smooth muscle cells or of the enteric nerve plexuses (Figure 5.10):

- A network of ICCs in the same plane as the myenteric plexus between the circular and longitudinal muscle layers (myenteric ICC, ICC-MY) in most regions of the gastrointestinal tract.
- A network of ICCs in the smooth musculature (intramuscular ICC, ICC-IM).
- A network of ICCs at the inner surface of the circular muscular layer of the small intestine (ICC at the deep muscular plexus, ICC-DMP) (not shown in Figure 5.10).
- Groups of ICCs that are located in the connective tissue septa between blocks of circular muscle in the stomach of larger animals (ICC-SEP).

The ICCs of these networks are coupled electrically with each other by close appositions and/or gap junctions forming electrical and functional syncytia. The ICCs also form close appositions or gap junctions with the smooth muscle cells. Finally, ICCs within the smooth muscles of the stomach and possibly elsewhere (but not in the longitudinal muscle of the small intestine and colon) are intercalated between nerve terminals of enteric neurons and smooth muscle cells (Thuneberg 1982; Huizinga et al. 1997; Sanders et al. 1999, 2000) (Note 3).

Functional investigations of various parts of the gastrointestinal tract (antrum, small and large intestines), using intracellular recordings from smooth muscle cells and from ICCs, have shown that the electrical slow waves in the smooth muscle of the gastrointestinal tract are generated by the ICCs (Note 4). Interstitial cells of Cajal of the myenteric plexus normally produce pacemaker potentials. In mutant mice without myenteric ICCs, as studied in the small intestine, pacemaker activity and slow waves are absent. In the stomach, pacemaker potentials generated in myenteric ICCs (ICC-MY) are amplified by ICCs in the musculature (ICC-IM); the

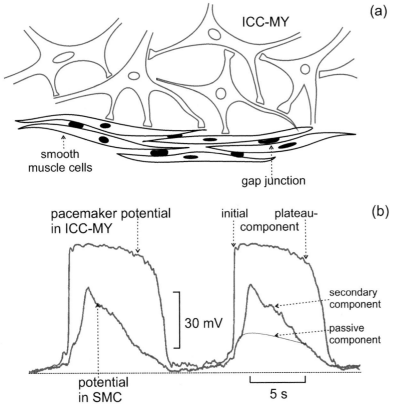

(a)

smooth
muscle cells

gap junction

ICC-MY

pacemaker potential
in ICC-MY

initial   plateau-
component

(b)

secondary
component

30 mV

passive
component

potential
in SMC

5 s

Figure 5.11 Recording from myenteric interstitial cells of Cajal (ICC-MY) and smooth muscle cells (SMC) in the guinea pig stomach. (a) Network of ICC and SMC. The ICCs are coupled electrically by gap junctions with each other and with the SMCs, which are also electrically coupled by gap junctions. Thus, both form electrical and functional syncytia. (b) Simultaneous intracellular recording from ICC-MY and SMC of the circular smooth muscle. The driving potential in the ICC syncytium (pacemaker potential) produces a secondary potential (slow-wave potential) in the SMC syncytium by current flowing through the gap junctions. The driving potential in the ICC has an initial rapid component, which is followed by a long-lasting plateau component. In the SMC, a passive initial component of the slow wave is followed by a secondary component, which is related to the amplifying effects of the intramuscular ICCs. The passive electrotonically transmitted component seen in the SMC in the absence of intramuscular ICCs (i.e., when the amplifying effect of the ICCs is absent) is indicated by the dotted-line curve. In vitro experiment under nifedipine blocking L-type calcium channels in the SMC in order to prevent the generation of action potentials and contractions. Modified from Dickens et al. (1999) with permission.

resultant combined current transmitted to the smooth muscle cells produces slow waves. In the small intestine, the pacemaker currents of myenteric ICCs seem to be sufficiently strong to depolarize the musculature passively, generating slow waves.

Figure 5.11b shows simultaneous recordings from a pacemaker cell of the myenteric plexus (ICC-MY) and from a cell of the circular smooth muscle close-by in the guinea pig stomach in vitro. The (driving) potential generated in the syncytium of myenteric ICC cells is electrically transmitted to the syncytium of smooth muscle cells. The pacemaker potential exhibits an initial fast component and a plateau component. The intracellular record from the circular musculature has two components: a passive component that is transmitted via the gap junctions from the myenteric ICCs to the smooth muscle cells and a secondary regenerative component (Figure 5.11b). In animals with absent intramuscular ICCs, the secondary regenerative

component seen in the smooth muscle cells is absent, but the passive component is present. Thus, the secondary regenerative component is generated by the intramuscular ICCs. This is the way in which transmission of pacemaker potentials from the myenteric ICCs to the smooth muscle cells is augmented (for discussion and literature see Hirst and Ward [2003]). The driving potential is in part generated by opening of Ca^{2+}-dependent chloride channels regulated by regenerative intracellular release of calcium from the sarcoplasmic reticulum (Suzuki and Hirst 1999; van Helden et al. 2000; Hwang et al. 2009) (Note 5).

The induced changes in membrane potential in the smooth muscle cells that follow the pacemaker potential are called slow waves (Figures 5.4 and 5.5). These slow-wave potentials may generate action potentials in smooth muscle cells by opening L-type calcium channels leading to calcium inflow and contraction of the smooth musculature (Figure 5.5). The slow waves in the muscle syncytium propagate from oral to aboral since the frequency of pacemaker activity in the ICCs is higher at the oral site than at the aboral site. The oral–aboral propagation does not occur in the smooth musculature but in the networks of electrically coupled ICCs. Thus, the function of the ICC is not only to generate and augment pacemaker activity, but also to propagate the slow waves (Sanders et al. 2000; Ward and Sanders 2001).

5.4.2 ICC-Myogenic Activity and Enteric Neurons

As mentioned above, intramuscular ICCs in the stomach, which form gap junctions and close appositions with smooth muscle cells, are also closely associated with enteric nerve fibers (Figure 5.10). Morphologically some of these nerve fibers form intimate synaptic contacts with the ICC in the musculature. Excitatory and inhibitory postsynaptic potentials in circular smooth muscle cells generated by electrical stimulation of enteric neurons are absent or reduced in W/W^V mutant mice, which lack ICCs in the musculature (Burns et al. 1996; Ward et al. 2000a; Iino et al. 2004). This shows that the effects of excitatory and inhibitory enteric motor muscle neurons are mediated, at least in part, by the intramuscular ICCs. This is the third main function of the ICCs, in addition to those of generating pacemaker activity and propagating slow waves.

How do the three components, ICCs, smooth muscle cells and enteric neurons, act together to generate the different motility patterns of the gut under normal biological conditions? It has been shown in isolated segments of mouse small intestine that distension-induced peristalsis with pulsatile release of the intraluminal content can be generated experimentally under the following conditions (Huizinga et al. 1998):

- In mutant W/W^V-mice lacking ICCs in the myenteric plexus, which cannot generate pacemaker activity and slow waves, distension-induced peristalsis is present and fully dependent on the enteric neural motor program as described in the preceding section (see Figure 5.5).
- In normal mice that have been treated with tetrodotoxin, blocking active conduction of the enteric neurons, slow waves are present and the distension-induced rhythmic contractions must be initiated by a myogenic mechanism (possibly a stretch-sensitive ionic mechanism in the smooth muscle cells).

- Even in W/W^V mutant mice lacking ICCs in the myenteric plexus, distension-induced peristalsis can be present when action potential conduction in enteric neurons is blocked by tetrodotoxin. In this condition, the distension-induced contraction is fully dependent on myogenic mechanisms.
- However, under these three experimental conditions, in which the myenteric ICCs or enteric neurons, or both, have been eliminated, distension-induced contractions of an isolated intestinal segment are not normal. They lack precise oral–aboral coordination, have a high threshold, lack full pulsatile relaxation (which is generated by the inhibitory muscle motor neurons) or lack the burst-like pattern of contraction. Thus, under biological conditions, cooperation between the motor programs of the enteric nervous system, the slow-wave mechanism linked to the ICCs and the myogenic mechanism is necessary to produce a well-coordinated peristalsis for a proper transit of the intestinal contents.

The way the other local movement patterns (pendular movements, segmentation, cycling) are generated is poorly understood. It is not far-fetched to assume that they require the cooperative action of the mechanisms of the three components too. It has, for example, been shown that local patchy contractions of the small intestine are dependent on slow waves generated by ICCs, which then lead to generation of action potentials in the plateau phase of the slow waves (see Figure 5.5) and local contractions, which may propagate over short but not long distances (Lammers 2000).

The migrating myoelectric complex (MMC) is phase III of the interdigestive movement pattern of the gastrointestinal tract. It is prevented by blockade of cholinergic nicotinic synaptic transmission between neurons with hexamethonium and by blockade of muscarinic synaptic transmission to the smooth musculature with atropine. Thus, the MMC is fully dependent on functioning enteric nerve circuits. However, contrary to expectations, the MMC is still present in the absence of the myenteric ICC network that is responsible for the intrinsic pacemaker activity, as shown in transgenic mice lacking this network (Spencer et al. 2003b). In the MMC, up to 100% of the slow waves are accompanied by action potentials and contractions of the smooth muscle. In the silent phase of the interdigestive movement pattern, slow waves are present but do not generate action potentials and no contractions occur. The

← PROPAGATION OF SLOW WAVES IN ICC NETWORK →

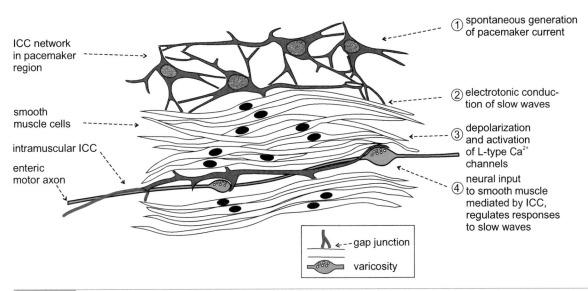

ICC network in pacemaker region

smooth muscle cells

intramuscular ICC

enteric motor axon

① spontaneous generation of pacemaker current

② electrotonic conduction of slow waves

③ depolarization and activation of L-type Ca^{2+} channels

④ neural input to smooth muscle mediated by ICC, regulates responses to slow waves

←-- gap junction

varicosity

Figure 5.12 The rhythmoneuromuscular apparatus to generate gastrointestinal motility. Interstitial cells of Cajal (ICC; specifically of the myenteric plexus of stomach, and small and large intestines) generate the pacemaker potentials. ICCs form electrically coupled networks (syncytia), which in turn are electrically coupled to the smooth muscle syncytium by gap junctions. The pacemaker current flows through the gap junctions and induces in the smooth muscle cells slow-wave potentials, which are amplified by the intramuscular ICCs (see Figures 5.4 and 5.5). The slow-wave potentials lead to activation of voltage-dependent L-type calcium channels with massive inflow of calcium and triggering of smooth muscle contractions. Intramuscular ICCs amplify the pacemaker potentials in the transmission to the smooth muscle cells and mediate inhibitory and excitatory effects of enteric muscle motor neurons. Varicose nerve terminals of these neurons form close (20 nm) specialized junctions with these ICC. Neural influence modulates the slow-wave potentials via the ICC. This in turn modulates the generation of action potentials and therefore contraction of the smooth muscle cells. Modified from Horowitz et al. (1999) with permission.

MMC is not triggered by distension of the gut (the gut is relatively empty!) and is independent of signals in parasympathetic and sympathetic neurons, although it can be suppressed by commands from the brain (e.g., during stress behavior). It is hypothesized that the MMC is linked to an assembly of cholinergic interneurons in the myenteric plexus, which project with their axons aborally and form synapses with inhibitory muscle motor neurons that innervate the circular musculature (see Figures 5.6 and 5.9). In the guinea pig, these interneurons contain somatostatin. This assembly of interneurons receives no or only sparse synaptic input from intrinsic primary afferent neurons, which are important for the initiation of peristaltic reflexes. It is unclear what triggers and maintains the MMC. This triggering may be linked to a local hormone (e.g., motilin).

In summary, ICCs, smooth muscle cells and enteric motoneurons form a "rhythmoneuromuscular apparatus" that generates the pattern of gastrointestinal motility. Figure 5.12 depicts the elements and connections of this elegant model (Horowitz et al. 1999; Sanders et al. 2000; Huizinga et al. 2014):

1. Pacemaker currents are generated in the network of ICCs of both the myenteric plexus (ICC-MY) and the muscular plexus (ICC-IM).
2. These currents are propagated in an oral–aboral direction through the ICC network and are electrotonically transmitted to the smooth muscle cells, thus producing electrical slow-wave potentials.
3. Voltage-dependent L-type calcium channels are opened during the slow-wave depolarization, triggering, in the small intestine, calcium action potentials in the smooth muscle cells when the threshold

is achieved. The inflow of calcium ions triggers contraction of the smooth muscle cells, which manifests as a peristaltic wave of contraction.

4. In some parts of the gastrointestinal tract (e.g., circular muscles of small intestine, colon and stomach), excitatory and inhibitory enteric muscle motor neurons form synaptic contacts with the ICCs within the muscles and in this way (at least in part) influence the smooth muscle cells, increasing or decreasing the effectiveness of slow waves in generating action potentials and contractions.

5.5 | Regulation of Secretion and Transmural Transport

Reflex pathways involved in the regulation of secretory cells and/or local blood vessels (arterioles) have been much less explored than enteric reflex pathways that are involved in regulation of motility. This applies to the organization of the reflex pathways connected to the mucosa and mucosal blood vessels as well as to their coordination with the reflex pathways that are integrated into the regulation of motility. Activation of secretomotor neurons stimulates epithelial cells to secrete chloride ions into the intestinal lumen, taking with them sodium ions and water. The physiological stimuli that induce a reflex activation of the secretomotor neurons are mechanical stimulation of the mucosa (shearing stimuli) and chemical stimuli (e.g., glucose or proton ions). The most important activator of the reflexes is the absorption of water and electrolytes by nutrient transporters. For example, glucose transport involves the Na^+-transporter and each molecule of glucose is accompanied by Na^+, counterions and water. Absorption of 100 grams of glucose is accompanied by 1.8 liters of water (Furness 2006). The purpose of

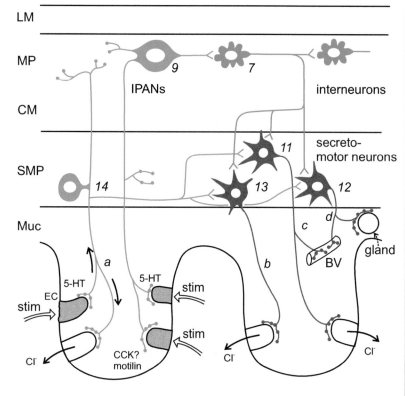

Figure 5.13 Enteric reflex circuits related to secretion and local vasodilation. Intrinsic primary afferent neurons (IPANs) in the submucosal plexus (SMP) or myenteric plexus (MP) are activated by mechanical stimuli (distension, contraction of the musculature; intraluminal shearing) and/or intraluminal chemical stimuli. Intraluminal stimuli may be mediated by enterochromaffin cells (EC) releasing 5-hydroxytryptamine (5-HT) or possibly by other cells releasing, e.g., motilin or CCK. Secretomotor neurons in the SMP are either activated monosynaptically via the SMP or di- or polysynaptically via interneurons in the myenteric plexus. This induces either secretion of chloride ions (reflex b) or secretion of chloride ions as well as dilation of submucosal arterioles (reflex pathways c and d). The first is generated by release of acetylcholine, the second by release of vasoactive intestinal peptide. IPANs themselves may activate mucosal secretory cells (and possibly inhibit arterioles [not shown]) via an axon-reflex-like mechanism (pathway a). BV, blood vessel; CCK, cholecystokinin; CM, circular muscle; LM, longitudinal muscle. The numbers adjacent to the neurons correspond to the numbers in Table 5.1. IPANs, blue; interneurons, green; motor neurons, red. From Cooke (1994, 1998) and Lundgren (1988, 2000). Modified from Furness et al. (2004) with permission.

the secretomotor reflexes in vivo is therefore to preserve whole-body fluid balance. The intraluminal stimuli triggering secretion appear to be the same as those causing enteric motility reflexes in the intestine. The stimuli activate the IPANs via enterochromaffin cells (EC) in the mucosa, which release 5-HT and excite the IPANs, or possibly by other cells releasing CCK or motilin (Figure 5.13). The IPANs excite enteric neurons synaptically by release of acetylcholine and substance P. Intraluminal toxins, such as cholera toxin, lead to pathological activation of secretomotor neurons. This overwhelms the fluid-balance role of the reflexes, causes copious fluid loss and, if unchecked, death, because the fluid ultimately comes from the circulation. Secretomotor reflexes elicited by intraluminal physiological stimuli are always paralleled by enteric vasodilator reflexes mediated via the enteric neurons.

Figure 5.13 illustrates the enteric reflex pathways that lead to activation of the secretomotor neurons resulting in secretion and vasodilation in the mucosa. Based on experimental studies (Lundgren 1988; Cooke 1994, 1998; Cooke and Reddix 1994), there are four configurations by which stimulation of IPANs activates secretory cells of the mucosa via enteric interneurons and motor neurons coordinated with local vasodilation of submucosal arterioles and therefore local increase in blood flow. The dilation of the blood vessels may be generated by the same enteric secretomotor neurons that activate the secretory cells or possibly also by separate ones (not shown in Figure 5.13):

1. Intrinsic primary afferent neurons themselves may directly innervate secretory cells and/or possibly blood vessels, although structural evidence does not support the latter (not shown in Figure 5.13). In this way, both groups of effector cells are influenced by the afferent neurons directly in an axon-reflex-like manner (pathway *a* in Figure 5.13).
2. Reflex secretion triggered by intraluminal chemical or mechanical stimulation is mediated through the submucosal plexus. No interneurons seem to be intercalated between the intrinsic primary afferent neuron and the secretomotor neuron. The secretomotor neurons projecting only to secretory cells use acetylcholine as transmitter (pathway *b* in Figure 5.13).
3. Reflex secretion and vasodilation triggered by intraluminal chemical or mechanical stimulation

are mediated through the submucosal plexus and secretomotor neurons that innervate both secretory cells and blood vessels. These motor neurons use VIP as transmitter (pathways *c* and *d* in Figure 5.13).
4. Reflex secretion generated by cholera toxin is mediated by an interneuron in the myenteric plexus that projects to secretomotor neurons in the submucosal plexus (pathways *c* and *d* in Figure 5.13). It is possible that the reflex pathway via the myenteric plexus also contributes to normal reflexes, e.g., those evoked by mechanoreceptor activation (Reed and Vanner 2003).

5.6 | Defense of the Gastrointestinal Tract and Enteric Nervous System

The gut has developed powerful mechanisms to defend the body against invading antigens derived from food, bacteria and parasites, toxins and other compounds. This includes, as part of the defense, getting rid of toxins through vomiting and diarrhea (Furness et al. 2013). Its epithelial lining constitutes the inner surface of the body that is highly permeable in most parts of the gastrointestinal tract, in particular in the small intestine. The gut contains the largest immune system of the body, collectively called "gut-associated lymphoid tissue" (GALT) that continuously surveys antigens in the lumen of the gut. This immune system of the gut includes the immune cells of Peyer's patches, M-cells of the epithelial lining (modified intestinal epithelial cells [enterocytes]), lymphocytes in the lamina propria, macrophages and mast cells. The GALT is integrated with the enteric nervous system, the gut endocrine system and spinal as well as vagal primary afferent neurons, and constitutes a powerful local defense system that is continuously working and protecting the body. A histological and histochemical expression of the interaction between GALT and the nervous system is the finding that Peyer's patches are innervated by enteric neurons, postganglionic sympathetic neurons and extrinsic primary afferent neurons (Heel et al. 1997; Chiocchetti et al. 2008).

The central nervous system is informed about the actions of this peripheral defense system by activity in vagal and spinal primary afferent neurons, by endocrine signals (hormones in the blood) and by messages from the GALT (cytokines in the blood, such as interleukin-1β [IL-1β], IL-6, tumor necrosis factor α [TNFα]). Activity in both types of extrinsic primary afferent neurons initiates a host of protective reflexes and reactions, which may act back on the local defense mechanisms of the gut via parasympathetic and sympathetic pathways and possibly via circulating hormones. Activity in these afferent neurons triggers discomfort, pain and hyperalgesia of the gut, the latter being elicited by activity in spinal afferents (see Subchapter 2.4). Ideas as to how the enteric nervous system might be involved in this defense system have been discussed in the literature (Downing and Miyan 2000; Furness and Clerc 2000; Holzer 2002a, b; Sharkey and Mawe 2002; Wood 2002; Cervi et al. 2014; Sharkey and Savidge 2014).

The immune system of the intestine is involved in every process of the gastrointestinal tract that potentially leads to its damage (inflammation, infections, injury, erosions by HCl, allergy etc.). This involves M-cells of the intestinal epithelium, which transport antigens across the epithelium to macrophages and dendritic cells. The antigens are processed by these cells and presented to T lymphocytes that stimulate B lymphocytes. The B lymphocytes proliferate in the lamina propria of the mucosa and produce antibodies, preferentially IgA. Some B lymphocytes migrate to mesenteric lymph nodes and continue to mature and to proliferate. They enter the general circulation and localize to the mucosa-associated lymphoid tissue in the intestine and elsewhere.

Signaling molecules of the immune system, such as IL-1β, IL-6 and TNFα, are synthesized and released during injuries by immune cells in the mucosa and muscle layers or by cells associated with the immune system (e.g., enterocytes, monocytes, macrophages, fibroblasts, enteric glia cells). Interleukin-1β and IL-6 increase the excitability of most neurons of the submucosal plexus and of some neurons of the myenteric plexus. This enhances mucosal fluid secretion and motility of the gastrointestinal tract. Cytokines also sensitize and probably activate IPANs of the enteric nervous system and extrinsic spinal and vagal visceral afferent neurons innervating the gastrointestinal tract.

Figure 5.14 summarizes some aspects of the role of the enteric nervous system and other peripheral systems in the protection of the gastrointestinal tract. This diagram demonstrates various hypothetical pathways by which the protective reactions are initiated and maintained, involving enteric neurons, extrinsic afferent neurons, cells associated with the immune system, endocrine cells, enterocytes and cells of blood vessels. Details about the functioning of these pathways and their activation during various harmful or potentially harmful stimuli acting at the epithelial lining have to be worked out. Some of these potentially protective processes are shown in the box on the right side in Figure 5.14:

- Macroscopically, the protective reactions of the gastrointestinal tract consist of the following components: increased mucosal secretion, motility, local blood flow, leukocyte infiltration, sensitivity of enteric neurons and sensitivity of the terminals of extrinsic primary afferent neurons.

- Mast cells can be activated by several agents including antigens (AG), CCK (via the CCK_2 receptor), neurotensin, substance P (SP) and neurokinin A (NKA) released by the terminals of spinal afferent neurons. Activated mast cells can release many signaling molecules, such as leukotrienes, interleukins, prostaglandins, TNFα, tryptase, histamine and 5-HT. They are under the control of enteric neurons of the submucosal plexus, probably influenced by noradrenergic sympathetic postganglionic neurons and possibly under neuroendocrine control. Their activation sensitizes extrinsic afferent nerve fibers, e.g. via release of histamine and other compounds, stimulates enteric neurons, stimulates leukocyte extravasation and generates directly fluid secretion by the mucosa (e.g., by release of platelet-activating factor [PAF] and leukotriene C_4 [LTC_4]). Mast cells are considered to mediate stress-induced barrier defects generated by "psychological" stimuli (Söderholm and Perdue 2001; Yu and Perdue 2001).

- Spinal visceral peptidergic afferent neurons innervating the gut have dual functions: in the periphery they mediate various protective functions; centripetal impulse activity elicits protective reflexes, mediated by spinal cord and brain stem, as well as pain, discomfort and other sensations (see Subchapters 2.2 to 2.4).

- Some vagal visceral afferent neurons innervating the gastrointestinal tract are involved in protective reflexes, central modulation of nociceptive impulse transmission and so-called sickness behavior that may develop during harmful infections of the gastrointestinal tract (Holzer 1998, 2002a, b).

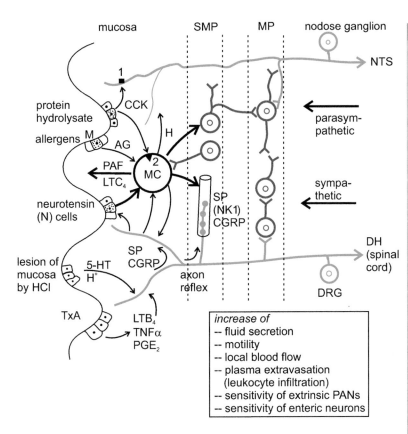

Figure 5.14 Enteric nervous system and protection of the gastrointestinal tract: a summary figure. Emphasized are mast cells (MC), enteric neurons (red) and extrinsic spinal and vagal visceral afferent neurons (blue). Intraluminal processes (related to protein hydrolysates, allergens, toxins [e.g., TxA, toxin A of *Clostridium difficile*], HCl, etc.) that may generate injury activate MC and intrinsic and extrinsic primary afferent neurons (in addition to the activation of the gut-associated lymphoid tissue [GALT]; not shown here). This activation occurs via endocrine cells (cholecystokinin [CCK]; neurotensin [N]), antigens (AG), prostanoids (prostaglandin E_2 [PGE_2]), leukotrienes (e.g., LTB_4), cytokines (e.g., tumor necrosis factor α [$TNF\alpha$], interleukin-1β [IL-1β]), etc. and is in part mediated by substance P (SP) and calcitonin gene-related peptide (CGRP) released by terminals of spinal primary afferent neurons. Mast cells activate enteric neurons, activate and sensitize extrinsic afferent nerve fibers, increase local blood flow, increase plasma extravasation (leading to leukocyte infiltration) and act directly on the enterocytes of the mucosal lining (leading to fluid secretion). These processes are under control of enteric neurons and possibly of extrinsic autonomic neurons. Extrinsic afferent terminals generate neurogenic inflammation (arteriolar vasodilation and venular plasma extravasation) via an "axon reflex" by release of SP and CGRP. They furthermore activate neurons of the myenteric plexus. The global protective effects of these interactions are listed in the lower right. 1, 2: CCK_1 and CCK_2 receptors; NK_1, neurokinin 1 receptor for SP; DH, dorsal horn of the spinal cord; DRG, dorsal root ganglion; MP, myenteric plexus; NTS, nucleus tractus solitarii; PAF, platelet-activating factor; PAN, primary afferent neuron; SMP, submucosal plexus. Modified from Downing and Miyan (2000) and Sharkey and Mawe (2002).

They are not directly involved in the generation of visceral pain (see Subchapters 2.3 and 2.4).

- Lesion of the mucosa by HCl leads to activation of enterocytes as well as acidification of the mucosal interstitial tissue. Peptidergic afferent capsaicin-sensitive fibers are activated. This leads locally (by CGRP and NO, probably released by enteric neurons) to increased blood flow through the mucosa, and secretion of bicarbonate and mucus.

With time, release of substance P and NKA triggers trophic processes (proliferation of endothelial cells, vascular muscle cells and fibroblasts with angiogenesis) and healing (Holzer 2002a, b).

- Toxin A of *Clostridium difficile* activates enterocytes. This leads to release of prostaglandin E_2 (PGE_2), $TNF\alpha$ and leukotriene B_4 (LTB_4) by the enterocytes. These substances activate and sensitize the terminals of spinal afferent neurons that mediate various peripheral effects involving mast cells, enteric neurons and blood vessels.

- Allergens reacting with M-cells in the mucosal lining activate mast cells. This activation is enhanced by cytokines released by cells related to the immune system.
- Protein hydrolysates (and other chemical stimuli) activate enteroendocrine cells in the duodenum, releasing cholecystokinin. CCK activates mast cells (via CCK_2 receptors) and vagal afferents (via CCK_1 receptors). Both together lead to changes in the motility patterns of the small intestine.
- Cholera toxin activates enterochromaffin cells of the mucosa, which release 5-HT and PGE_2. This activates enteric secretory reflex pathways generating active fluid secretion and vasodilation (see reflex pathways c and d in Figure 5.13).

5.7 Control of the Enteric Nervous System by Sympathetic and Parasympathetic Pathways

As mentioned before, the parasympathetic systems have their dominant effects and overall access to target cells at the oral and anal sites of the gastrointestinal tract. Otherwise they do not interfere with single groups of effector cells in the gastrointestinal tract, but influence enteric sensorimotor programs. The sympathetic non-vasoconstrictor systems act throughout the gastrointestinal tract and also largely do not interfere directly with single groups of effector cells, but modulate the enteric sensorimotor programs too. The visceral vasoconstrictor pathways influence visceral blood vessels directly. The numbers of preganglionic parasympathetic and sympathetic neurons involved in gastrointestinal functions are low in comparison to the numbers of enteric neurons, being in the range ≤1%!

5.7.1 Parasympathetic (Vagal) Pathways

Rather little is known about parasympathetic preganglionic neurons in the dorsal motor nucleus of the vagus that project to the gastrointestinal tract. These neurons, also called by John Furness pre-enteric neurons, are probably highly specialized with respect to various motility, secretomotor and enteric endocrine functions. They innervate motor neurons and

interneurons of the enteric nervous system (see Subchapter 4.8 and Table 4.6). Some functional properties of parasympathetic preganglionic neurons that are involved in regulation of gastrointestinal functions will be described in Subchapter 10.7. Figure 5.15 summarizes the way in which parasympathetic preganglionic neurons in the DMNX (see Figures 8.10 and 10.25) may be involved in the regulation of different motility patterns of the proximal gastrointestinal tract. This scheme is hypothetical in several aspects. However, it shows that the brain does interfere, via the preganglionic parasympathetic neurons, with several different functions in which the enteric nervous system is involved. Figure 5.15 may aid in understanding of the complex peripheral mechanisms that are activated by the different classes of preganglionic parasympathetic neurons.

Parasympathetic preganglionic neurons in the DMNX may influence the motility of the gastrointestinal tract (above all stomach, duodenum and ileum) via

- enteric neurons that excite the smooth muscle directly,
- enteric neurons that excite the smooth muscle via ICC,
- enteric neurons that inhibit smooth muscle cells and
- enteric neurons that activate endocrine cells (ENDC) releasing a hormone (e.g., gastrin), which in turn influences smooth muscle cells and enteric neurons that are involved in regulation of motility.

In addition to vagal preganglionic neurons involved in regulation of motility, there exist other types of parasympathetic preganglionic neurons that innervate enteric secretomotor neurons in the submucosal plexus and enteric neurons supplying endocrine cells that are not involved in direct regulation of motility (e.g., G-cells releasing gastrin, S-cells releasing secretin, β-cells of the endocrine pancreas releasing insulin, etc.). The cell bodies of these preganglionic neurons are possibly also located in the DMNX.

To reiterate, first, the number of preganglionic parasympathetic neurons is very small when compared to the number of enteric neurons and, second, the small number of preganglionic neurons is subdifferentiated into several functional types. The sacral parasympathetic pathways to the hindgut has been reviewed by Callaghan et al. (2018).

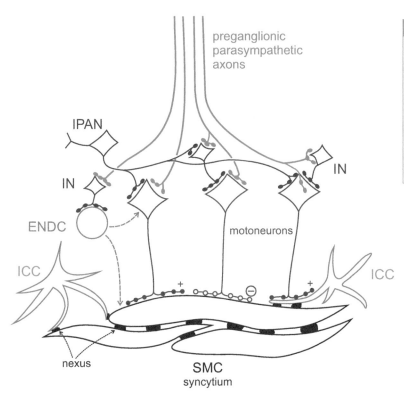

preganglionic
parasympathetic
axons

IPAN

IN

ENDC

ICC

IN

motoneurons

ICC

nexus

SMC
syncytium

Figure 5.15 Schema showing relation between vagal parasympathetic preganglionic neurons (cell bodies in the dorsal vagus motor nucleus) and neurons of the enteric nervous system in regulation of motility. Various peripheral pathways are involved in regulation of the motility of the smooth muscle syncytia. For details see text. ENDC, endocrine cell; ICC, interstitial cell of Cajal; IN, interneuron; IPAN, intrinsic primary afferent neuron; SMC, smooth muscle cell. +, excitation; –, inhibition.

5.7.2 Sympathetic Pathways

The sympathetic innervation of the gastrointestinal tract has been explored for motility control, secretomotor reflex control and vasomotor control, although direct recordings from these neurons in vivo are still scarce. The postganglionic neurons of these sympathetic pathways are located in the prevertebral and some in the paravertebral ganglia.

Most postganglionic visceral vasoconstrictor neurons innervating the vasculature (mainly arterioles) of the gastrointestinal tract seem to be located in the paravertebral ganglia or in the prevertebral ganglia (see Subchapter 6.4). They receive synaptic input from preganglionic neurons in the thoracolumbar spinal cord, but not from peripheral intestinofugal neurons. Furthermore, the postganglionic visceral vasoconstrictor neurons do not receive synaptic input from collaterals of spinal peptidergic primary afferent fibers (Messenger et al. 1999; Gibbins et al. 2003; see Subchapter 2.2).

The population of sympathetic non-vasoconstrictor neurons consists of motility-regulating neurons and secretomotor neurons (Figure 5.16)

and almost certainly neurons innervating the gut-associated lymphoid tissue (GALT; not shown in Figure 5.16 [Lomax et al. 2010]). These groups of neurons are most likely further subdifferentiated with respect to various functions of the gastrointestinal tract. They innervate neurons of the myenteric and submucosal plexus, respectively. Activation of these sympathetic neurons inhibits activity in enteric neurons; this inhibition occurs largely presynaptically by decreased release of excitatory transmitter. A few postganglionic sympathetic secretomotor neurons innervate the mucosa directly and a few sympathetic motility-regulating neurons innervate the non-sphincteric smooth muscles, leading in both cases to inhibition when activated. Sphincter muscles are directly innervated by sympathetic postganglionic fibers and contract when these fibers are excited. Non-vasoconstrictor neurons receive synaptic input from enteric intestinofugal neurons and form extraspinal reflex circuits (see Subchapter 6.5). These intestinofugal neurons are cholinergic and many contain VIP. In the guinea pig, collaterals of spinal peptidergic afferents containing substance P

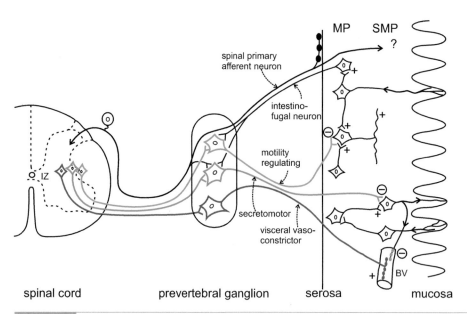

Figure 5.16 Sympathetic outflow to the small intestine. Most sympathetic postganglionic neurons projecting to the intestine are situated in the prevertebral ganglia. These neurons consist of three classes: (1) Vasoconstrictor neurons innervating blood vessels (BV, red). These neurons do not get synaptic input from collaterals of spinal primary afferent neurons (peptidergic) or from enteric intestinofugal neurons (cholinergic). The cell bodies of many visceral vasoconstrictor neurons are located in paravertebral ganglia. (2) Secretomotor neurons innervating neurons of the submucosal plexus (SMP, green). (3) Motility-regulating neurons innervating neurons of the myenteric plexus (MP, blue). Both secretomotor and motility-regulating neurons exert (pre- and postsynaptically) inhibitory effects on enteric neurons; they receive synaptic input from intestinofugal neurons (cholinergic nicotinic) and show integration of preganglionic and peripheral synaptic inputs (but see Subchapter 6.5). Secretomotor neurons additionally receive peptidergic synaptic input from spinal visceral afferent neurons (transmitter Substance P). IZ, intermediate zone; +, excitation; –, inhibition.

appear to influence only postganglionic neurons in prevertebral ganglia that express somatostatin (in addition to noradrenaline). Only these postganglionic neurons that have secretomotor function express the tachykinin NK_1 receptor for substance P, but not the other postganglionic neurons (Messenger et al. 1999; see Subchapter 6.5).

Activity of sympathetic secretomotor neurons is related to the balance of fluid volume and electrolytes in the body. Decrease of both fluid volume and electrolyte concentrations leads to activation of these neurons and consequently to inhibition of chloride and bicarbonate secretion. This results in decreased transport of sodium and water into the intestinal lumen and conservation of body water. The central circuits of this regulation are little known, but their afferent inputs are known, such as baroreceptors, osmoreceptors and atrial stretch receptors. It is unlikely that these circuits are identical to those linked to the visceral vasoconstrictor pathway.

However, it may be speculated that the central pathways linked to sympathetic secretomotor neurons innervating the gastrointestinal tract receive input from vagal atrial stretch receptors and osmoreceptors and that these pathways are connected to the preganglionic neurons or associated interneurons in the thoracolumbar spinal cord. The central circuits linked to the sympathetic motility-regulating and secretomotor neurons are largely unknown (see Subchapter 4.3).

Conclusions

The enteric nervous system is an autonomic nervous system in its own right and can function in many aspects independently of the central nervous system. It contains about as many neurons as the spinal cord and is metaphorically called the "brain of the gut."

1. The enteric nervous system has neurons with cell bodies in the myenteric or submucosal plexus of ganglia and consists of intrinsic primary afferent neurons, interneurons and motor neurons innervating various effectors. Each group of neurons is subdifferentiated according to the physiological stimuli that activate the afferent neurons, the target cells of the motor neurons, their synaptic connections with other neurons, their primary and secondary transmitters, the projection of dendrites and axons and other criteria.

2. Intrinsic primary afferent neurons of functionally similar types are reciprocally synaptically connected with each other and in this way form afferent networks. Interneurons of functionally similar types are also synaptically connected to each other and form several cell assemblies. Motor neurons are not synaptically connected to each other.

3. The primary transmitter in most excitatory enteric neurons is acetylcholine (muscarinic action on effector cells; nicotinic action on neurons). Intrinsic primary afferent neurons use tachykinins as additional transmitters. Inhibitory motor neurons use several cotransmitters (NO, VIP, PACAP, ATP) to varying degrees and at different sites. Some secretomotor neurons use VIP as a transmitter. Enteric neurons can be neurochemically characterized by their colocalization of various neuropeptides. The functions of most of these colocalized neuropeptides are unknown.

4. Afferent neurons, interneurons and motor neurons form reflex circuits. Different reflex circuits related to regulation of motility or secretion are coordinated and represent the sensorimotor programs of the enteric nervous system. These programs underlie the neural regulation of motility, secretion, local blood flow and probably other functions involving gastrointestinal hormones and gut immune function.

5. The regulation of motility patterns is mainly directed by the myenteric plexus. The neural basis of peristalsis, which has been most extensively studied, consists of the coordinated activation of ascending and descending reflex pathways. In the small intestine, the circular and longitudinal muscle layers are influenced by ascending and descending excitatory reflex pathways. The circular muscles are additionally influenced by a descending inhibitory reflex pathway that modulates the contraction of the anally located circular muscle and leads in this way to anal propulsion of the intestinal contents. In the colon, the circular and longitudinal muscle layers are powerfully inhibited by descending inhibitory reflex pathways and excited by an ascending reflex pathway, supporting expulsion of its contents.

6. Inhibitory and excitatory reflex circuits are organized by and coordinated with pacemaker activity of the interstitial cells of Cajal (ICC) and myogenic activity to generate the different movement patterns. The ICCs are electrically coupled and form several networks. These networks are electrically coupled to the smooth musculature. The networks of ICCs generate the pacemaker activity responsible for slow waves, are responsible for oral–aboral contraction and mediate the excitatory and inhibitory synaptic activity of enteric neurons on the circular smooth musculature.

7. Neural regulation of fluid and electrolyte transport, which is less well explored, is largely controlled through the submucosal plexus. Reflex activation of secretomotor neurons is always paralleled by local reflex vasodilation in the mucosa. Secretion and vasodilation may be generated by the same type of secretomotor neuron. Several distinct reflex pathways can be described. The coordination and integration of these reflex pathways with the enteric neural motor programs regulating motility are relatively unexplored.

8. The enteric nervous system is involved, by interaction with the GALT and the gut endocrine system, in protective reactions of the gastrointestinal tract. Intraluminal antigenic and toxic stimuli are sensed by cells of the endothelial lining and lead to concerted actions of these systems resulting in an increase in secretion, motility and mucosal blood flow. Local protective processes are referred by endocrine, immune and extrinsic afferent neural signals to the brain. They are under the neural and hormonal control of the brain.

9. The brain modulates the functions of the enteric nervous system via the parasympathetic and sympathetic nervous system. It receives detailed information from the gastrointestinal tract by impulse activity in visceral vagal and spinal afferent neurons, as well as by gastrointestinal hormones. In this way, functions of the enteric

nervous system are adapted to the behavior of the organism.

10. The efferent extrinsic autonomic (parasympathetic and sympathetic) systems are differentiated with respect to various functions of the enteric nervous system. Except for direct control of the oral and anal sites of the gastrointestinal tract and of blood vessels, the pathways of the two extrinsic autonomic nervous systems do not interfere directly with the final effectors of the enteric nervous system. They give command signals to enteric neural circuits or modulate the activity of these circuits and in this way influence the enteric reflex programs and their coordination.

Suggested Reading

Brierley, S. and Costa, M. (eds.) (2016) *The Enteric Nervous System. Advances in Experimental Medicine and Biology, Vol 891*, Springer Verlag, Berlin, Heidelberg.

Brookes, S. and Costa, M. (2002) *Innervation of the Gastrointestinal Tract, Vol 14 of The Autonomic Nervous System* (Burnstock, G., ed.), Francis and Taylor, London, New York.

Furness, J. B. (2006) *The Enteric Nervous System*. Blackwell Science Ltd, Oxford.

Furness, J. B. (2012) The enteric nervous system and neurogastroenterology. *Nature Rev Gastroenterol Hepatol* **9**, 286–294.

Furness, J. B. (2016) Integrated neural and endocrine control of gastrointestinal function. *Adv Exp Med Biol* **891**, 159–173.

All references cited in the text are available online at www.cambridge.org/janig.

Notes

1. The enteric neurons were originally divided into two electrophysiological classes: S neurons and AH neurons (Hirst et al. 1974; Furness and Costa 1987). (1) S neurons receive fast excitatory synaptic inputs (therefore S, synaptic). They have a distinct morphology and are uniaxonal, most of them being Dogiel type I neurons. The S neurons are interneurons and motoneurons. (2) AH neurons exhibit prolonged afterhyperpolarization following an action potential (therefore AH). They receive no fast excitatory synaptic inputs. They have relatively large cell bodies and multipolar processes (Dogiel type II neurons). These neurons are enteric afferent neurons (intrinsic primary afferent neurons [IPANS]).

Some enteric interneurons can have afferent function (e.g., in the myenteric plexus of the guinea pig colon [Spencer and Smith 2004]). Thus, the term intrinsic primary afferent neuron (IPAN) is functionally defined and does not only include AH neurons but also some S neurons.

2. The percentages given are for the guinea pig small intestine.

3. Cajal stained the cells that later became known as the interstitial cells of Cajal (ICC) using methylene blue and Golgi impregnation. To him, these cells were similar in shape to intraganglionic neurons and resembled an end formation of the sympathetic nervous system. Therefore he originally called these cells sympathetic interstitial neurons. He believed that these interstitial cells form networks or accessory plexuses that are closely associated with intrinsic nerves and target cells, that mediate neural signals to the autonomic target cells (smooth muscle cells, epithelial cells) and are important in the regulation of autonomic effector cells (Cajal 1911/1995). Research starting in the 1980s and intensifying after 2000 clearly shows that these cells are of mesenchymal origin and that they are not restricted to the gastrointestinal tract but are also present in other extradigestive cavity organs of various species (such as corpus spongiosum, prostate, urethra, urinary bladder, uterus, fallopian tube, vas deferens, mesenteric lymphatic vessels, mesenteric artery, portal vein) and even in the pancreas (as already described by Cajal). As in the gastrointestinal tract, they may be involved in pacemaker activity, peristalsis, regulation of neurotransmission and secretion. But this has yet to be shown. The modern criteria to identify ICCs are immunohistochemical staining for the c-kit protein; formation of networks of c-kit positive cells with ≥2 processes that are connected to target cells (smooth muscle cells, epithelial cells) and intrinsic nerve fibers; gap junctions between ICC cells (thereby forming a functional syncytium) and between ICCs and smooth muscle cells; close contacts to intrinsic nerve fibers without interposition of basal lamina (position of ICC between nerve fibers and effector cells) (Thuneberg 1999; Harhun et al. 2005; Huizinga and Faussone-Pellegrini 2005; Popescu et al. 2005a, b).

4. Originally it was thought that pacemaker activity and slow waves of depolarization leading to rhythmic contractions of different sections of the gastrointestinal tract were initiated by the smooth musculature. Thus, it was believed that certain regions of the smooth muscular syncytium had pacemaker properties and that the regenerative process, generated by opening of calcium channels, was

propagated aborally through the smooth musculature, the frequency of the pacemaker potentials being highest in the oral regions of the different sections of the gastrointestinal tract. However, smooth muscle cells isolated from the gastrointestinal tract do not show pacemaker activity and do not generate electrical slow waves.

5. The cellular basis for generation of pacemaker potentials in ICCs and resultant slow waves in smooth muscle is complex and not entirely understood.

1. *Rhythmic electrical (pacemaker) activity of ICCs.* ICC-MY has dual pacemaker mechanisms, one generated by channels with properties similar to T-Type Ca^{2+} channels in the cell membrane and a second caused by rhythmical Ca^{2+} release from intracellular sarcoplasmic reticulum (SR) Ca^{2+} stores that activate chloride channels in the cell membrane. In contrast, ICC-IM has only one of these pacemaker mechanisms, namely the Ca^{2+} store-based pacemaker. This latter pacemaker depends on the following cellular processes: (i) Rhythmic release of Ca^{2+} into the cytoplasm from inositol 1,4,5-triphosphate (IP$_3$)-receptor-operated intracellular Ca^{2+} stores that are located near the cell (plasma) membrane. This is regenerative and is due to the released Ca^{2+} triggering further release of Ca^{2+} from IP$_3$ receptor-operated Ca^{2+} release channels within the same store and in adjacent stores. Resultant emptying of the stores then causes these channels to close. (ii) The consequent increase in Ca^{2+} concentration opens Ca^{2+}-activated chloride-selective channels in the ICC cell membrane. (iii) Intracellular Ca^{2+} stores are then refilled by a Ca^{2+} ATPase pump, which when filled to threshold level triggers re-opening of the IP$_3$ receptor-operated Ca^{2+} release channels

and so the cycle repeats (see Ward et al. [2000b]; Kito et al. [2002]; Hirst and Ward [2003]; van Helden et al. [2010] for discussion and literature).

2. *Generation and propagation of slow waves.* Electrical slow waves in gastrointestinal smooth muscle are generated by current flow from pacemaker potentials generated in ICC-MY and ICC-IM and transmitted through gap junctions to the smooth muscle. Slow waves, when of sufficient amplitude, open voltage-dependent L-Type Ca^{2+} channels, causing contraction of the smooth muscle. The oral–aboral propagation depends entirely on the *propagation of the pacemaker potentials* in the network of electrically coupled ICCs and not on propagation between smooth muscle cells. This propagation depends on the Ca^{2+} store-based pacemaker mechanism in ICCs, namely the oscillatory regenerative release–refill cycle of Ca^{2+} stores and on the resultant oscillatory pacemaker depolarization. It is hypothesized that this activity propagates by a coupled oscillator-based mechanism across the ICC cell networks, which because of strong coupling leads to near synchronous generation of slow waves and resultant contractions in the circumferential direction. However, as the coupling is weaker transversely along the gastrointestinal tract, phase delays arise leading to wave-like propagation (i.e. peristalsis) (see Koh et al. [2003]; van Helden and Imtiaz [2003]; van Helden et al. [2010]) for discussion and literature).

Part III

Transmission of Signals in the Peripheral Autonomic Nervous System

Chapters 3 and 4 introduced the idea of functionally organized "final autonomic pathways" that transmit the central information to peripheral targets. This idea provides the context for the ensuing discussion of transmission of impulses along the final autonomic pathways (i.e., in the autonomic ganglia and to the target cells) as it occurs in vivo. In this part, I focus upon transmission of centrally generated activity through synapses in autonomic ganglia and upon subsequent transmission at the neuroeffector junctions. I will describe the principles of this signal transmission and how it can be modulated by peripheral reflexes and humoral mechanisms. I will not, however, extensively discuss the details of synaptic transmission in autonomic pathways, including the different types of receptors for the neurotransmitters, their pharmacology and postreceptor pathways, and chemical neuroanatomy (see articles in Skok [1973, 1980, 2002]; Burnstock and Hoyle [1992]; Elfvin et al. [1993]; McLachlan [1995]; Gibbins and Morris, [2000, 2006]; Gibbins et al. [2000, 2003a]; Young et al. [2011]; Undem and Potenzieri [2012]).

Chapter 6

Impulse Transmission Through Autonomic Ganglia[1]

Postganglionic neurons are the final autonomic motoneurons. Their cell bodies are aggregated in peripheral autonomic ganglia. As already mentioned in Chapter 1, most sympathetic ganglia are located at some distance from their target cells, whereas parasympathetic ganglia are located close to their targets.

Sympathetic ganglia have fascinated investigators since ancient times. It was believed that these structures are "little brains" which integrate, carry and distribute the "animal spirits" from the brain to the periphery leading to coordinated actions of the peripheral target organs (the "sympathies") in association with the activity of the brain (see Subchapter 1.6).

It is important to note that the great majority of studies of autonomic ganglia have used the superior cervical ganglion, particularly of small laboratory animals, to examine the properties of the neurons and their connections. Many of these sympathetic neurons have vasoconstrictor functions, but the proportions with other targets vary between species, e.g. the specialized innervation of the salivary glands of rodents

and the ear vasculature of rabbits. There have been a number of studies of other paravertebral ganglia leading to similar conclusions about their cellular properties, but relatively few studies of either prevertebral sympathetic ganglia or parasympathetic ganglia. These differ in many respects from those of the paravertebral chain; notably, paravertebral neurons receive only preganglionic synaptic inputs, whereas prevertebral neurons and at least some parasympathetic neurons also receive synaptic inputs from peripheral neurons of the enteric nervous system and, in some cases, collaterals of spinal afferent fibers that innervate peripheral visceral organs.

Modern investigations have led to the conclusion that the core function of most peripheral sympathetic pathways is very basic. They distribute messages to the periphery from relatively small pools of preganglionic neurons to larger pools of postganglionic neurons. Counts of ganglionic neurons and retrogradely labeled preganglionic neurons indicate that the amount of divergence is at least an order of magnitude and that

---

[1] This chapter is dedicated to my friend Elspeth McLachlan. Elspeth introduced me into the scientific problems related to the peripheral autonomic nervous system, in particular the functioning of autonomic ganglia. She introduced me into the Neuroscience Society in Australia and is responsible for my becoming scientifically half Australian. She kept me scientifically on track starting in 1980.

it increases with body size (up to 10- to 20-fold in humans) (Purves et al. 1986; Wang et al. 1995). This particularly applies to the neural regulation of systemic blood pressure, body temperature, gastrointestinal function, evacuative functions (micturition, defecation), sexual functions (e.g. erection), salivation, pupil diameter. Each function is controlled by specific groups of postganglionic neurons. For example, different vascular beds are innervated by functionally different vasoconstrictor neurons and even within vasoconstrictor pathways, identifiable subgroups of neurons terminate on different levels of the arterial tree (Gibbins et al., 2003a). The basic principles of synaptic transmission from preganglionic axons to postganglionic neurons are described in Box 6.1.

Experimental work that began with the application of intracellular glass microelectrodes to ganglia has shown that autonomic ganglia have surprisingly complex neurophysiological, morphological, neurochemical and pharmacological organization (see Karczmar et al. [1986]; McLachlan [1995]; Skok and Ivanov [1987]; Morris and Gibbins [2006]). Since the 1960s, key experiments using intracellular microelectrodes to record from neurons in intact autonomic ganglia have revealed the basic properties of synaptic transmission and its modification under controlled conditions in vitro. Beginning in the 1980s, the advent of tissue culture methods, patch clamp recording and molecular biology techniques accelerated our understanding of receptor structure

---

Box 6.1 Synaptic Transmission in Autonomic Ganglia: A Brief Overview

All preganglionic neurons release acetylcholine (ACh) as their primary neurotransmitter at synapses in ganglia. The rapid excitatory effects of ACh are mediated by neuronal nicotinic acetylcholine receptors (nAChRs), which can be blocked by drugs like hexamethonium or curare. In rodents, subunits of nAChRs present at postsynaptic specializations are $\alpha3\beta4$ with or without $\alpha5$ or $\beta2$ (Del Signore et al. 2004; David et al. 2010). However, deletion of the a3 subunit completely blocks transmission in autonomic ganglia (Rassadi et al. 2005). $\alpha7$-Subunits are also present, but postsynaptic electrical responses are not affected by selective blockade or deletion of $\alpha7$ subunits (Ciuraszkiewicz et al. 2013).

Activation of the preganglionic axon evokes an excitatory postsynaptic current (EPSC), the amplitude of which is determined by the number of postsynaptic neuronal nicotinic receptors (nAChRs) that are opened. The time course of the EPSC reflects the average duration of bursts of opening of the postsynaptic nAChRs and the membrane becomes depolarized (the excitatory postsynaptic potential, EPSP), lasting up to 150 ms, depending on the resting conductance of the neuronal membrane. Temporal summation occurs if the instantaneous frequency is high (>~10 Hz), and spatial summation occurs if EPSPs arise from several preganglionic axons (convergence); when the transmembrane voltage reaches threshold, an action potential is initiated in the postganglionic neuron.

In most paravertebral and some prevertebral sympathetic neurons and most parasympathetic neurons, the amplitude of EPSPs arising from activation of one (or each of a few) of the converging preganglionic axon(s) is large enough to initiate an action potential on every occasion that it discharges. Such a preganglionic axon has been called a "strong" or "dominant" input, whereas the other preganglionic axons that produce only subthreshold EPSPs are called "weak" or "secondary" inputs. Thus, the synapses formed by strong inputs resemble the neuromuscular junctions on somatic muscle fibers. This will be discussed in detail in Subchapter 6.2.

Under some experimental and possibly physiological conditions, repetitive activation of preganglionic axons to some neurons can release enough ACh to activate extrasynaptic muscarinic receptors and/or may release peptidergic cotransmitters. Responses to these interventions are typically depolarizations of a much slower time course than EPSPs. These generally involve a decrease in K^+ conductance (Brown 2010, 2018), which, in addition to moving the membrane towards threshold, amplifies the subthreshold EPSPs and so increases the likelihood of discharge.

and function, and postreceptor molecular signaling pathways. One might assume that the complexities worked out in these in vitro experiments on isolated neurons have implications for impulse transmission through autonomic ganglia during the autonomic regulation of organ function. However, this assumption may not be true at all since dissociating neurons during isolation removes dendrites and destroys ganglionic synapses and limits information concerning synaptic integration.

One of the great challenges in autonomic neuroscience is to understand the functional relevance of the many complex synaptic signaling mechanisms revealed by cellular and molecular studies. How do synaptic divergence and convergence, strong (dominant) and weak synaptic events, fast and slow synaptic transmission, and the phenotypic specialization of ganglionic neurons that innervate different peripheral targets interact in the living animal? These questions are currently best addressed by electrophysiological recordings, not only from the cell bodies of functionally connected ganglion neurons but also using extracellular recordings from single pre- and postganglionic axons in known pathways during reflex activation. Only when this regulation is studied in vivo can the extent to which the in vitro work is applicable to normal function be clarified. Intracellular recording from autonomic neurons in living animals is very difficult and has only been achieved in a small number of laboratories, principally by Skok, Ivanov, Purves, McLachlan, McAllen and their coworkers (Johnson and Purves 1983; Skok and Ivanov 1983, 1987; Ivanov and Purves 1989; Ivanoff and Smith 1995; McLachlan et al. 1997, 1998; Bratton et al. 2010; McAllen et al. 2011).

The main question addressed in this chapter is: How is the centrally generated impulse activity of preganglionic neurons transmitted across autonomic ganglia to postganglionic neurons under physiological conditions? For this purpose, the term "autonomic ganglia" includes sympathetic, para- and prevertebral, and parasympathetic ganglia. It does not include the enteric nervous system (Chapter 5). The transmission of impulses is mainly dealt with here in terms of the division of sympathetic and parasympathetic nervous systems into functional subunits, as defined by their target organs (see Chapter 4).

6.1 | Morphology, Divergence and Convergence in Autonomic Ganglia

6.1.1 Morphology of Postganglionic Neurons and Their Synaptic Inputs

Parasympathetic postganglionic neurons are morphologically comparatively simple, having either no or only a few dendrites, whereas sympathetic postganglionic neurons usually have a number of dendrites. The size of the cell body and the number of dendrites of the sympathetic neurons is dependent on the size of the target tissue innervated by the neurons and the function of those neurons. In the guinea pig (and probably other mammalian species), vasoconstrictor neurons are smaller than all other functional types of sympathetic neurons; pilomotor neurons are smaller than secretomotor neurons (innervation of sweat gland or salivary glands). Their size may correspond to the conduction velocity of the postganglionic axons of these neurons.

Synapses are characterized by close contact between boutons and the postganglionic membrane, by electron-dense membrane specializations at the point of contact and by clustering of vesicles at the presynaptic specialization. Only 1 to 2% of the surface of postganglionic neurons is occupied by synapses, most of the neuron surface being covered by Schwann cells (Figure 6.1). This contrasts with somatic motoneurons in which about 50% of the surface of soma and proximal dendrites is covered by synapses. Less than 50% of the boutons formed by preganglionic axons or (in prevertebral ganglia) by axons of intestinofugal neurons of the enteric nervous system form synapses with the postganglionic neurons. Furthermore, some synapses apparently lack most of the proteins normally required for fast transmitter release and probably do not take part in conventional ganglionic transmission (Gibbins and Morris 2006). Boutons not forming synapses are entirely ensheathed by Schwann cells. It is likely, although not proven, that only boutons forming synapses release ACh on excitation. However, colocalized peptides (e.g., vasoactive intestinal peptide [VIP] in intestinofugal axons; substance P or calcitonin gene-related peptide [CGRP] in some groups of preganglionic axons) may also be released, even by boutons not forming synapses (Note 1).

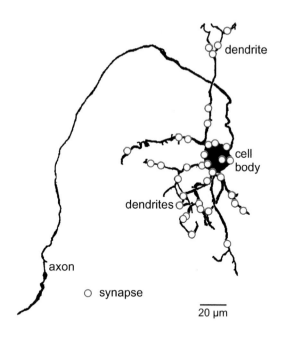

labels: dendrite, cell body, dendrites, axon, synapse, 20 μm

Figure 6.1 Location of synaptic contacts on a sympathetic postganglionic neuron in a thoracic paravertebral ganglion of the mouse. The neuron has been filled with an intracellular injection of neurobiotin and reconstructed from a stack of confocal sections. Note the dendrites and the long axon. Hypothetical distributions of synapses formed by boutons of preganglionic axons are indicated by the circles. Based on systematic investigations using electron microscopy in the guinea pig (Gibbins et al. 1998), this distribution of synapses is random. Approximately 1 to 2% of the surface of the postganglionic neurons is covered by synapses. The density and distribution of synapses are probably similar across species. With permission from Gibbins et al. (2000).

The number of preganglionic fibers innervating one postganglionic neuron, and therefore also the total number of boutons forming synapses, is related to the total surface of soma and dendrites of the postganglionic neuron. For example, in the guinea pig, the postganglionic neurons in the lateral coeliac ganglion, most of which are vasoconstrictor in function, have a small dendritic surface area of about 1300 μm^2. Each neuron receives about 80 synaptic boutons formed by 2 to 10 preganglionic axons. The postganglionic neurons in the medial celiac ganglion, most of which regulate motility or secretion in the intestine, have a large surface area of about 3500 μm^2. They receive about 300 to 400 synaptic boutons formed by both preganglionic axons and axons of intestinofugal neurons (Boyd et al., 1996; Gibbins

et al. 2003c; Gibbins and Morris 2006). However, only about half of these boutons form synapses on the postganglionic neuron (Gibbins et al. 1998). The effectiveness of these dendritic synapses will principally depend on their location with respect to the soma and the site of action potential initiation (on or close to the axon), neither of which is known, although the electrotonic length of the dendrites of guinea-pig sympathetic postganglionic neurons is rather short (Jamieson et al. 2003). What is also not known is how many synapses are made by each preganglionic axon, and specifically by strong and weak ones, and their locations over the soma and dendrites.

6.1.2 Divergence and Convergence

Pre- and postganglionic neurons are synaptically connected in the ganglia by divergence and convergence of preganglionic axons (Figure 6.2). Divergence occurs when a relatively small number of preganglionic neurons connects with a much larger number of postganglionic neurons. Thus, the functional role of divergence is to amplify and distribute the central signal with minimal central representation. Divergence is much larger in larger animals, where the size of the peripheral target is greater. Convergence occurs when several preganglionic neurons form synapses with a single postganglionic neuron. In the CNS, the functional role of convergence is generally thought to be to integrate information from different sources by temporal and spatial summation, but in autonomic ganglia it remains unclear. Since postganglionic neurons receive one (or rarely a few) strong (suprathreshold) preganglionic inputs (see above and Subchapter 6.2), and the other inputs generate quite small EPSPs, the possibility of integration by summation is not great. Is convergence therefore vestigial or is it "designed" by nature for some special functional purpose? The degree of divergence and convergence of preganglionic axons with postganglionic neurons in autonomic ganglia varies between ganglia, between species and, within the same ganglion, between populations of neurons with different functions (i.e. in different final autonomic pathways) (Wang et al. 1995). The selective reinnervation by strong inputs after loss of the original innervation (Ireland, 1999) suggests that their role is to provide the primary drive for the postganglionic neuron. Weak inputs might then be a relic of the developmental process, which also occurs at, e.g., neuromuscular junctions and

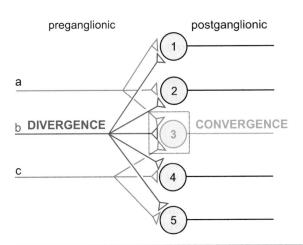

preganglionic   postganglionic

a

b **DIVERGENCE**   CONVERGENCE

c

Figure 6.2 Principles of convergence and divergence in autonomic ganglia as worked out in the sympathetic paravertebral ganglia. The degree of divergence of individual preganglionic neurons on postganglionic neurons is probably a function of the size of target tissue (and therefore body size) and of the type of autonomic final pathway (e.g., low divergence in the pupillomotor pathway and high degree of divergence in vasoconstrictor pathways). The degree of convergence varies between different autonomic pathways. Here preganglionic axon b (red) diverges to contact all postganglionic neurons and postganglionic neuron 3 receives convergent input from preganglionic axons a to c (boxed).

central synapses, when an excess of inputs is formed, many of which are subsequently retracted (Lichtman 1977; Lichtman and Purves 1980). Perhaps this correction is not so well coordinated in the autonomic system. It should be noted that weak inputs have the potential to sprout and become more effective (strong) after partial denervation if the original input does not regenerate.

Studies of the superior cervical ganglion in mammals have shown that the number of preganglionic and postganglionic neurons increases with body size, i.e., with increasing target organ size. The rate of increase in preganglionic cell number is smaller than the rate of increase in postganglionic cell number and both are much smaller than the rate of increase in target numbers (Ebbeson 1968a, b; Purves et al. 1986). For example, the relative body weights of mouse, guinea pig, cat and human (30 g, 300 g, 3 kg and 60 kg) are about 1:10:100:2000, yet the relative numbers of preganglionic neurons (700, 2800, 6000 and 10 000 neurons) projecting to the superior cervical ganglion are about 1:4:9:14 and the relative numbers of postganglionic neurons in the superior cervical ganglion (10 000, 35 000, 100 000 and 1 000 000 neurons) are about

1:3.5:10:100 (Ebbeson 1968a, b; Wesselmann and McLachlan 1984; Purves et al. 1986; see Gabella [1976]). This means that the average ratio between numbers of pre- and postganglionic neurons increases by a factor of approximately 7 (from 14:1 in small animals to 100:1 in humans), whereas the ratio between the size of the target tissue and the number of postganglionic neurons increases by a factor of 20 from mouse to humans with increasing body size. Furthermore, with increasing target size, the mean number of preganglionic neurons converging on each postganglionic neuron in the superior cervical ganglion increases, the numbers in mouse, guinea pig and rabbit being about 5, 12 and 16 preganglionic neurons (Purves et al. 1986; Ivanov and Purves 1989) and possibly higher in larger animals.

Thus, the degree of convergence of sympathetic preganglionic neurons on postganglionic neurons is related to the total surface of the postganglionic neurons and the total surface is related to the size of the target tissue innervated by the postganglionic neurons (Voyvodic 1989). This is an approximation and future investigations will probably show that there are differences between functionally different types of sympathetic pathways (e.g., vasoconstrictor, vasodilator, sudomotor, glandomotor to salivary glands).

Originally it was assumed that the number of converging preganglionic axons matches the number of dendrites of a postganglionic neuron and that each preganglionic axon innervates one dendrite of a postganglionic neuron ("domain theory"; Purves and Hume 1981; Forehand and Purves 1984; Purves and Lichtman 1985; Purves et al. 1988). However, this view is too simplistic since one dendrite may be innervated by more than one preganglionic axon (Forehand 1987; Murphy et al. 1998). On the other hand, in neurons with two strong inputs, the voltage-dependent Ca^{2+} channels associated with the action potential (see Subchapter 6.2) lie in two regions which must be on separate dendrites (Hirst and McLachlan 1986). This is consistent with most of the synapses of a strong input being localized to a single dendrite, but this matter remains to be demonstrated more directly.

The detailed mechanisms involved in this matching between pre- and postganglionic neurons are unknown, although it is believed that retrograde transport of trophic signals from the target tissue to the postganglionic neurons (e.g., nerve growth factor for sympathetic neurons, neurturin for parasympathetic neurons; Heuckenroth et al. 1999) and from the postganglionic neurons to the preganglionic neurons (brain-derived neurotrophic factor, BDNF; Causing et al. 1997) is involved (Purves and Lichtman 1978; Purves 1988).

Thus, the degree of convergence and divergence of preganglionic axons in autonomic ganglia is dependent on the size and type of target organ. This principle is probably universally valid for autonomic ganglia, i.e., there are no major differences between parasympathetic and sympathetic ganglia (Wang et al. 1995).

Increasing the degree of convergence and divergence in autonomic ganglia with body size may be the best strategy to cope with a larger amount of target tissue. This would avoid increasing the number of neurons in order to meet the distribution function of autonomic ganglia under various functional conditions (Purves 1988). Convergence and divergence probably vary between functionally different autonomic pathways. It is possible, although unproven, that convergence and divergence from preganglionic axons to postganglionic neurons are restricted to the same functional autonomic pathway, i.e., within muscle vasoconstrictor, cutaneous vasoconstrictor, pilomotor pathways, etc., but not between functionally different pathways. Alternatively, perhaps only the strong (suprathreshold) synaptic inputs are specific for functional pathways, but not the weak (subthreshold) synaptic inputs (see Subchapter 6.2). Presumably, like in somatic motor units, this is related to the precision of functional control and target size.

6.1.3 Segmental Origin of Converging Sympathetic Preganglionic Neurons

Preganglionic sympathetic axons converging on one postganglionic neuron originate from several contiguous spinal segments. In the guinea pig, postganglionic neurons in paravertebral ganglia are innervated by preganglionic neurons from 4–5 (range 1–7) contiguous spinal segments (Nja and Purves 1977a, b; Lichtman et al. 1979, 1980). The general principle of this organization is that the synaptic input to the postganglionic neurons is dominated by one spinal segment that contributes the highest number of preganglionic axons per segment and elicits, on average, larger excitatory postsynaptic potentials per preganglionic axon. This spinal segment possibly supplies the preganglionic axon forming the strong (suprathreshold) input

to the postganglionic neurons (see Subchapter 6.2). This principle of segmental organization most likely also applies to the thoracic sympathetic outflow of other species such as the rat, cat, rabbit and hamster (Langley 1892, 1894, 1903a, b) and to the lumbar sympathetic outflow to viscera (Krier et al. 1982), as shown by functional responses to stimulation of white rami.

Different functional pathways are represented in different groups of contiguous spinal segments in relation to the position of target organs in the body: some are distributed over the entire thoracolumbar preganglionic cell column (e.g., cutaneous, muscle or visceral vasoconstrictor and pilomotor neurons); others are restricted to groups of contiguous thoracic or lumbar segments (e.g., in the cat, sympathetic pupillomotor [T1–2], sudomotor [T2–3, L1–2], motility-regulating neurons [pelvic organs, L3–4]; parasympathetic preganglionic neurons to pelvic organs [S2–4]). This was quite obvious from experimental studies of the reaction of target organs (vasoconstriction in skin, piloerection, dilation of pupil and palpebral retraction) to electrical stimulation of the segmental preganglionic outflow (Langley 1892, 1894, 1895, 1897; Nja and Purves 1977a, b; Figure 8.8). It is also evident from neurophysiological experiments in which the segmental origin of functionally identified sympathetic lumbar preganglionic neurons projecting to the inferior mesenteric ganglion of the cat (Figure 8.8; Bahr et al. 1986b) and of functionally identified sympathetic thoracic preganglionic neurons projecting to the superior cervical ganglion (Boczek-Funcke et al. 1993) were studied. Finally, it is evident from morphological experiments in which populations of preganglionic neurons have been labeled using tracers that are injected into distinct target tissues and transported retrogradely trans-synaptically by the postganglionic neurons and preganglionic axons to the preganglionic cell bodies (Strack et al. 1988; Pyner and Coote 1994; see Chapter 8 and Table 8.2).

6.2 Strong and Weak Synaptic Inputs From Preganglionic Neurons

The original idea that autonomic ganglia work to integrate convergent synaptic input from several sources by summating a number of subthreshold (weak) EPSPs to initiate an action potential remains attractive and certainly seems to be the case in sympathetic prevertebral ganglia and possibly some parasympathetic ganglia. In the latter examples, cholinergic synaptic inputs from peripheral intestinofugal neurons (see Figures 5.2 and 5.15) in the gastrointestinal tract or possibly from local ganglionic interneurons summate with preganglionic inputs that are not strong. This has been shown to be functionally important for intestino-intestinal reflexes (Kuntz 1940; Crowcroft et al. 1971; Julé and Szurszewski 1983; Julé et al. 1983). However, experimental evidence has accumulated that indicates that, in several functional pathways in sympathetic paravertebral ganglia, in vasoconstrictor neurons in prevertebral ganglia (coeliac ganglion, McLachlan and Meckler 1989; Gibbins et al. 2003c) and in most parasympathetic ganglia (e.g. pelvic ganglion, Keast 1999, 2006; Jobling et al. 2003; submandibular ganglion, Callister and Walmsley 1996; otic ganglion, Callister et al. 1997), many if not all postganglionic neurons receive at least one strong synaptic input that always leads to their discharge. Thus, the pathway is direct and transmits the central signal without modification, as occurs at the peripheral pathway to skeletal muscle fibers, where the neuromuscular junction receives a single suprathreshold input that does not fail. Weak inputs or peptidergic signals arising in the periphery might, however, generate additional signals under particular circumstances.

Investigations in vitro on sympathetic paravertebral ganglia of cat, rabbit, guinea pig, rat and mouse (Hirst and McLachlan 1984, 1986; Cassell and McLachlan 1986; Jobling et al. 2004) and parasympathetic ganglia (cardiac ganglia: Edwards et al. 1995; McAllen et al. 2011) have shown that most postganglionic neurons are normally innervated by one (sometimes two, rarely three) preganglionic axon(s) that, when stimulated, always evoke(s) a suprathreshold EPSP in the postganglionic neuron. Preganglionic axons that always elicit suprathreshold EPSPs in an all-or-none manner are called "strong" inputs. The underlying EPSP elicited by these axons can be up to 100 mV in size, which is seen if the postganglionic neuron is hyperpolarized to prevent generation of action potentials (Figure 6.5c). Action potentials elicited by these large EPSPs have no inflection on their rising phase; the fast Na^+ current is activated before the Ca^{2+} current (see Box 6.2). Other preganglionic axons (up to 15

depending on the functional type of sympathetic neuron, the ganglion and the species; Purves et al. 1986; Ivanov and Purves 1989), when stimulated, evoke subthreshold EPSPs (Figure 6.3). These preganglionic axons eliciting subthreshold EPSPs are called "weak" inputs. The number of quanta released is much smaller than for strong inputs. The synaptic contacts of strong inputs may be located on the neuron's surface in association with the voltage-sensitive Ca^{2+} channels that are exclusive to neurons with strong inputs (see Callister et al. [1997]), but this would have to be tested in postganglionic neurons with dendrites.

In Box 6.2 the essential differences between strong and weak synaptic inputs in autonomic ganglia are described, the key message being that both synaptic inputs are mechanistically two different categories of synaptic input and not the extremes of one category.

From the studies of Hirst and McLachlan (1986), it is an open question whether "one particular preganglionic axon is predetermined to make synaptic contacts on the dendrites that bear a high density of calcium channels or whether the formation of calcium channels in these [postganglionic] neurons is induced by synaptic contacts of particular preganglionic axons." It seems likely that strong inputs have specificity related to the function and, therefore, the target cells of the postganglionic neurons. In the rat lumbar chain ganglia, such contacts develop 7 to 14 days postnatally and at 21 days after birth the majority of the postganglionic neurons in the lumbar paravertebral ganglia receive one or two strong synaptic inputs typical of the adult animal (Hirst and McLachlan 1984, 1986).

In the rat, all postganglionic sympathetic neurons in paravertebral ganglia, some 25% of sympathetic neurons in prevertebral ganglia and probably all parasympathetic postganglionic neurons receive at least one strong synaptic input from preganglionic neurons. Activity in these postganglionic neurons is probably entirely dependent on activity in these preganglionic neurons, which is generated within the central nervous system.

Some sympathetic postganglionic neurons in prevertebral ganglia projecting to the gastrointestinal tract receive mainly weak or just suprathreshold synaptic inputs from preganglionic neurons (Figure 6.4). These neurons receive abundant synaptic inputs from peripheral afferent neurons (intestinofugal enteric neurons, see Subchapter 6.5). Almost all of these latter are subthreshold (weak). These prevertebral neurons

Box 6.2 Synaptic Transmission in Parasympathetic and Sympathetic Paravertebral Ganglia

Differences Between Strong and Weak Excitatory Synaptic Potentials (EPSPs)

When stimulated, preganglionic axons converging on a postganglionic neuron elicit excitatory postsynaptic potentials (EPSPs) of different sizes. The size and shape of each EPSP depends on the size of the underlying postganglionic excitatory postsynaptic current (EPSC) and several other factors (see Jänig and McLachlan [1987]) and can also vary between different functional pathways. The differences between synaptic inputs to postganglionic neurons in paravertebral and prevertebral sympathetic ganglia (Hirst and McLachlan 1984; McLachlan and Meckler 1989; Jobling and Gibbins 1999) and parasympathetic ganglia (Callister et al. 1997; McAllen et al. 2011) have been described.

Most of the features of synaptic transmission resemble those at the neuromuscular junction, except that the majority of the EPSPs in sympathetic neurons are subthreshold and rarely contribute to ganglionic transmission. The behavior of these "weak" synapses resembles that of endplate potentials recorded in low Ca^{2+}/high Mg^{2+} solutions, i.e., the probability of release of quanta is low and facilitation at the beginning of trains of stimuli is marked. At weak ganglionic synapses, both the probability of release and the number of available quanta are low and release can be described by binomial statistics (McLachlan 1975).

As well as several weak EPSPs, most paravertebral neurons in vasoconstrictor pathways receive one or a few suprathreshold "strong" preganglionic inputs that never fail to initiate a discharge. The EPSCs that underlie strong inputs are much larger than those of weak inputs, suggesting that, despite similar synaptic mechanisms, some factor controls whether or not the input is always suprathreshold.

The size of the EPSCs is directly related to the number of quanta of acetylcholine (ACh) released from the preganglionic varicosities and depends on: (1) the number of contacts made between the pre- and postganglionic components of the synapse and (2) their average probability of release (see McLachlan 1995). As the neurons are electrically compact (Jamieson et al. 2003), the location of synapses over the soma and dendrites is unlikely to be a determinant of EPSC amplitude. There may also be differences in the number and/or subtypes of nicotinic acetylcholine receptors (nAChRs) in the subsynaptic membrane (del Signore et al. 2004) at strong and weak synapses, but this has yet to be investigated.

The properties of strong inputs are quite distinct from those of weak inputs, in the following ways:

1. Amplitude histograms of EPSCs evoked from single preganglionic axons in paravertebral neurons show that strong inputs produce >1 nA of inward current and may be as large as 10–15 nA (Callister and Walmsley 1996; McLachlan 2003). Weak EPSCs have a peak at much lower amplitudes (mostly <~ 0.5 nA).
2. Strong EPSCs are relatively invariant in amplitude, implying that the probability of release of quanta is high (close to 1.0) from a large number of release sites. Weak EPSCs are quite variable and steps in amplitude equivalent to those of spontaneous "miniature" EPSCs can often be seen.
3. Consistent with other synapses, the amplitude of weak EPSPs facilitates at the beginning of a train of stimuli at low probability synapses (McLachlan 1978). In contrast, the EPSPs arising from strong inputs usually show depression, as at the neuromuscular junction in normal Ca^{2+} solutions.
4. The majority of the Ca^{2+} channels that determine the release of ACh from strong preganglionic terminals in guinea pig lumbar paravertebral ganglia are of the R-type, with few P/Q-type, whereas at weak terminals P/Q-type rather than R-type are important (Ireland et al. 1999). About 35% of release involves N-type channels at both types of synapse. Differences in presynaptic Ca^{2+} channels have been found at other synapses.

5. The EPSP resulting from the EPSC at strong synapses is amplified by Ca^{2+} influx through voltage-dependent channels that are located near the synapse (Hirst and McLachlan 1986). Neurons receiving one strong synaptic input develop only one discrete Ca^{2+} current on depolarization; neurons receiving two strong preganglionic synaptic inputs develop two distinct Ca^{2+} currents upon depolarization. Hirst and McLachlan (1986) interpreted this to mean that the synaptic contacts of one strong preganglionic axon are associated with a single dendrite (Note 2).

6. The EPSP resulting from the EPSC may also be amplified by Ca^{2+} influx through nAChRs, as the Ca-dependent afterhyperpolarization generated by a strong synaptic input is more prolonged than that triggered by direct stimulation (Callister et al. 1997).

7. Following partial denervation of a paravertebral sympathetic ganglion, sprouting of surviving preganglionic axons within the ganglion resulted in the preferential formation of strong synapses with the same characteristics as those in normal ganglia (Ireland 1999). The single strong input was restored despite a reduced number of inputs, implying that some postganglionic factor is involved in the establishment of strong connections.

These phenotypical differences imply that strong and weak inputs are specialized and not simply due to the number of synaptic contacts, but also that strong inputs ensure an effective transfer of information in particular functional pathways.

Arguments Against the Concept of Strong and Weak EPSPs

There has been some resistance to abandoning the concept of integration in ganglia. The question has been raised that the use of sharp intracellular microelectrodes to record from intact preparations produces a shunt resistance which, by reducing input resistance, reduces the amplitude of the smaller potentials so that they fail to reach threshold (Bratton et al. 2010; Springer et al. 2015; McKinnon et al. 2019). The strongest argument against this is that the rate of discharge in vivo in postganglionic neurons is very similar to that of the preganglionic neurons in the same sympathetic pathways (see Table 6.2).

In a small proportion of neurons recorded with intracellular electrodes, some inputs have been observed to produce EPSPs that sometimes cross the action potential threshold and these have been called "accessory" (Skok and Ivanov 1983) or "secondary" (Bratton et al. 2010) inputs. In larger and/or older animals, these may become additional strong inputs. It has been suggested that such inputs would readily become suprathreshold if membrane conductance decreased (Rimmer and Horn 2010; Springer et al. 2015). Thus a decrease in resting conductance produced by the action of, e.g., a peptide transmitter or a circulating hormone would amplify the EPSPs and recruit such inputs to become effective in initiating action potentials or facilitate summation. Under these conditions, the postganglionic firing frequency would become much higher than that of the individual preganglionic axons.

A number of reports (e.g., Gola and Niel 1993) including a recent one (McKinnon et al. 2019) have shown, using patch clamp recording, that a subset of postganglionic neurons was highly excitable and fired spontaneously at high rates unless hyperpolarized. Surprisingly the rates of activity observed were much higher than has been recorded extracellularly from postganglionic axons in vivo (Table 6.2). Under these conditions, the recorded input resistances are usually much higher than reported with intracellular microelectrodes and it is argued that the EPSPs would therefore really be larger than observed. Neuronal models of sympathetic paravertebral neurons confirm the effects of a shunt resistance in reducing the amplitude of weak inputs (Springer et al. 2015). It is notable, however, that the differences in passive properties are not so great if the intracellular measurements are made only during periods when the membrane resistance has settled to a high and constant level (presumably after the microelectrode has sealed into the cell).

Under these circumstances, application of drugs that block resting potassium conductance can lead to input resistances of >1 GΩ, which implies that the shunt/leak conductance can be very small. Comparison with properties of dissociated neurons can be misleading because of the effects of: (1) removing the dendrites in the preparation process, (2) age and developmental stage, (3) recording temperature, (4) ionic concentrations in the bathing solution, etc. Comparison of recordings made with patch clamp and intracellular electrodes from ganglia of mature animals in vitro at ~35 °C leads to remarkably similar data.

In conclusion, most in vivo data indicates that the majority of vasoconstrictor neurons generate ongoing activity via one or a few single, unitary inputs with a high likelihood of discharging the cell. The configuration of the evoked action potentials is characteristic for different inputs. Temporal summation of subthreshold inputs occurs, but is rare because of the low rate of discharge of individual preganglionic axons. The key questions relate to the connectivity of the strong inputs, i.e., where they originate and the extent of divergence, and whether two strong inputs to the same neuron arise in the same or different functional pathways. In addition, the origin of weak inputs (often from another segment, Lichtman et al. 1979), will impact on their functional importance. The extent and mechanism of modulation of weak EPSPs by slow conductance changes of physiological origin also needs to be investigated.

Elspeth M. McLachlan

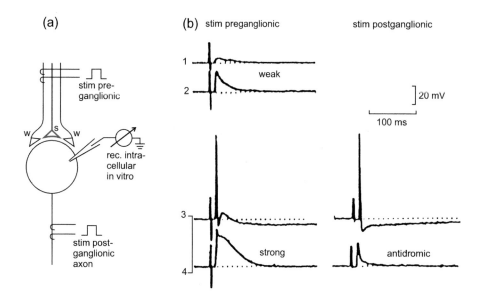

Figure 6.3 Relay function of synaptic transmission in sympathetic (mostly paravertebral) and parasympathetic ganglia. Intracellular recording from a sympathetic postganglionic neuron in a paravertebral ganglion. In vitro experiment. (a) Experimental setup. (b) Electrical stimulation of converging preganglionic axons with single pulses (the stimulus strength increased from 1 to 3) generates several small subthreshold (weak, w) postsynaptic potentials (see 1 and 2) and one large suprathreshold (strong, s) postsynaptic potential resulting in an action potential (see 3 left). Strong synaptic responses can be identified by their "all-or-none" onset and the characteristic form of the postsynaptic potential when the action potential is blocked by hyperpolarization (see record 4 left: brief peak and humped decay phase). Electrical stimulation of the peripheral nerve elicits an antidromically generated action potential. After hyperpolarization, the antidromic response is characterized by its brief decay time course relative to the postsynaptic potential. The relay function, in which only discharge of strong inputs is transmitted across the ganglion, occurs in practically all paravertebral sympathetic neurons, in many prevertebral sympathetic neurons and in parasympathetic neurons. Modified from Jänig and McLachlan (1992) with permission.

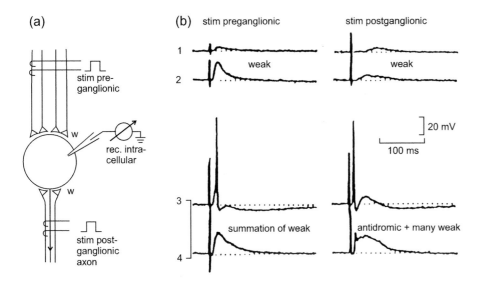

Figure 6.4 Integrative function of synaptic transmission in sympathetic prevertebral ganglia. Intracellular recording from a postganglionic neuron in vitro. (a) Experimental setup. (b) Graded electrical stimulation of the converging preganglionic axons elicits several small (weak) excitatory synaptic potentials with similar latencies. These summate at resting membrane potential to initiate an action potential (see 1 to 3 left). Graded electrical stimulation of a mesenteric (peripheral) nerve containing the postganglionic axon also produces many weak excitatory synaptic potentials with varying latencies and an antidromic action potential (see records 1 to 3 right), which can be identified as occurring earlier than the summed synaptic potentials when the membrane is hyperpolarized (record 4 right). This integration by summation of multiple subthreshold (weak) inputs occurs in sympathetic prevertebral motility-regulating neurons and possibly secretomotor neurons. Modified from Jänig and McLachlan (1992) with permission.

are non-vasoconstrictor in function and involved in regulation of motility and possibly in secretion/absorption of fluid across the gut mucosa (motility-regulating neurons, secretomotor neurons [see Subchapters 4.3 and 5.5]). Some prevertebral postganglionic neurons also receive peptidergic inputs from collateral branches of spinal primary afferent neurons (Figure 6.10b; not shown in Figure 6.4; see also Subchapters 2.2 and 5.7). These postganglionic neurons function by integrating the many synaptic inputs and are therefore activated mainly by summation of weak EPSPs (for correlation between types of synapses in sympathetic ganglia, biophysical membrane properties, "neurochemical coding" and function see Subchapter 6.4).

These findings are conceptually very important. They show that EPSPs elicited by "strong" preganglionic axons represent a class of EPSP that is distinct from EPSPs elicited by excitation of "weak" preganglionic axons (see Box 6.2). Though not yet explicitly investigated, it is likely that the principle of direct transmission via strong inputs generally applies to all

sympathetic pathways through the paravertebral ganglia that innervate targets in somatic tissues, to some sympathetic pathways projecting to the viscera (e.g., the visceral vasoconstrictor pathway) and to many parasympathetic pathways, although these pathways have not been systematically investigated in this respect.

Intracellular in vivo recordings show that most neurons in the ciliary ganglion (Melnitchenko and Skok 1970; Johnson and Purves 1983), most postganglionic neurons of the superior cervical ganglion of the rabbit and rat (Skok and Ivanov 1983, 1987; Tatarchenko et al. 1990; McLachlan et al. 1997) and possibly most postganglionic vasoconstrictor neurons in lumbar ganglia (Bratton et al. 2010) exhibit synaptically evoked action potentials with no inflection on their rising phase. Recordings in autonomic neurons in vitro under voltage clamp (e.g. sympathetic paravertebral neurons [Ireland et al., 1999] and submandibular neurons [Callister and Walmsley, 1996]) have confirmed that single strong preganglionic inputs have very large underlying unitary excitatory currents. Intracellular

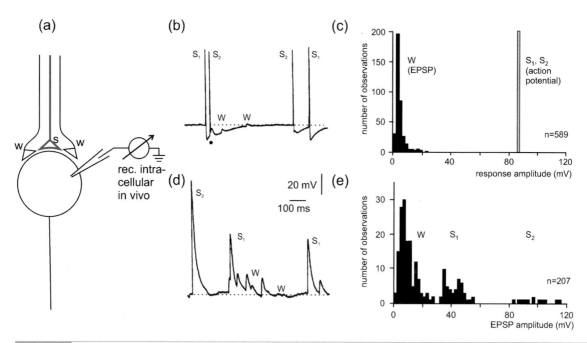

Figure 6.5 Ongoing postsynaptic activity recorded intracellularly in a postganglionic neuron of the rat superior cervical ganglion in vivo. Intracellular recordings were made from a postganglionic neuron of the superior cervical ganglion with its preganglionic innervation intact in a pentobarbital-anesthetized rat. Recordings were made at −50 mV (b, c) and with the neuron hyperpolarized to −130 mV (d, e) to block action potential generation. (a) Experimental setup. (b) Inputs generating EPSPs with amplitudes >20 mV at resting membrane potential triggered action potentials of two configurations (S_1, S_2). S_1 had a larger afterhyperpolarization than S_2, whereas S_2 had a depolarization following the spike, more readily seen during the afterhyperpolarization (dot). (d) At the hyperpolarized membrane potential, all EPSPs were increased in amplitude due to the greater driving potential, but the largest EPSPs (underlying S_1 and S_2) had distinct amplitudes of ~40 mV and ~100 mV, respectively. (c, e) Distribution of peak amplitudes of the responses (n = 589 responses and n = 207 responses in (c) and (e), respectively). Note the difference in amplitude between weak (W) and strong (S) responses. From McLachlan et al. (1997) with permission.

recording of spontaneous activity and reflex activity from postganglionic sympathetic neurons in the superior cervical ganglion in vivo show that spontaneously active neurons (McLachlan et al. 1997, 1998; Figure 6.5):

1. receive one, two or rarely three preganglionic synaptic inputs that are always suprathreshold (strong);
2. also receive several subthreshold (weak) preganglionic synaptic inputs; and
3. are not normally activated physiologically by summation of subthreshold preganglionic synaptic inputs because the firing rates of individual convergent inputs are too low.

In conclusion, the output of paravertebral sympathetic, many prevertebral sympathetic and possibly parasympathetic neurons that is "seen" by the target tissues is only generated by suprathreshold (strong) preganglionic synaptic inputs and not by summation of converging subthreshold (weak) synaptic inputs. It

is unlikely that these observations only apply to synaptic transmission in isolated ganglia or in laboratory rodents in vivo. Extracellular recordings of activity made from axons in sympathetic pathways in anesthetized cats support the concept of single or a few strong inputs. The following observations can only be interpreted this way (Figure 6.6):

1. Electrical stimulation of the preganglionic axons in the lumbar sympathetic trunk of the cat with single pulses at graded stimulus strengths evokes discharges in postganglionic neurons to skin or skeletal muscle (e.g., vasoconstrictor, sudomotor and pilomotor neurons) at constant latencies with a small scatter of mostly less than 1 ms and at well-defined electrical threshold.
2. The scatter of the latency (upper recordings in Figure 6.6b,c) does not change when the strength of the electrical stimulus applied to the preganglionic

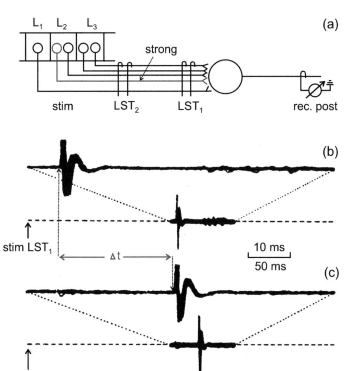

Figure 6.6 Electrical stimulation of preganglionic axons in the sympathetic chain elicits action potentials at distinct latencies and thresholds in postganglionic neurons. Recording from a vasoconstrictor axon innervating the cat hindlimb and electrical stimulation of the lumbar sympathetic trunk (LST) at two sites that were about 60 mm apart (pulse duration 0.2 ms; stimulus strength 2.3 and 5 volt, respectively). (a) Experimental setup. Indicated are one strong preganglionic input (axon in red) and several weak ones (thin axons). L1 to L3, lumbar segments 1 to 3. (b) LST1, stimulation at the distal site. (c) LST$_2$, stimulation at the proximal site. Recordings 10 to 20 times superimposed. Upper traces represent an expanded time scale of the intensified part of the lower traces. Note that the variability of the latency of evoked responses was small and the same for both responses. This and the distinct threshold voltages at which both responses had been elicited argue that *one* strong preganglionic axon was stimulated at both sites of the LST and that it generated a large suprathreshold excitatory postsynaptic potential. Δt (= 27 ms) is the latency difference between the two responses; thus the conduction velocity of the strong preganglionic axon was 2.2 m/s (60 mm/27 ms). Time base: 10 ms applies to the upper records and 50 ms to the lower ones. Modified from Jänig and Szulczyk (1980, 1981) with permission.

axons is raised (recruiting in this way more, mostly weak preganglionic axons), nor is there a difference in scatter of latency in most postganglionic neurons whether the preganglionic axons are stimulated close to the ganglion cell body (Figure 6.6b) or some 30 to 60 mm proximally (Figure 6.6c), which would have been expected to disperse the EPSPs due to the difference in conduction velocity of the stimulated preganglionic axons (Grosse and Jänig 1976; Jänig and Szulczyk 1980, 1981).

These results can only be explained in the following way: the discharges evoked in postganglionic neurons are generated by activation of *one* of the converging preganglionic axons which forms a strong synapse with the postganglionic neuron and generates a large suprathreshold postsynaptic potential. The results are fully consistent with the concept that individual postganglionic vasoconstrictor, sudomotor and pilomotor neurons supplying the skin or skeletal muscle of the cat are innervated by one or a few "strong" preganglionic axons and that summation of postsynaptic potentials generated by activation of weak preganglionic axons

normally does not initiate action potentials in the postganglionic neurons.

6.3 The Autonomic Neural Unit: Structural and Functional Aspects

The "motor unit" of the final common motor pathway of the skeletomotor system consists of the motoneuron and the muscle cells innervated by it. The size of the motor unit varies from a few muscle cells to several hundred muscle cells depending on the function of the skeletal muscle. By analogy, Purves defined the "neural unit" of the final autonomic pathways (Johnson and Purves 1981; Purves and Wigston 1983; Purves et al. 1986). It consists of the number of postganglionic neurons innervated anatomically by one preganglionic neuron. Its mean size for a given autonomic pathway is determined by the ratio of the number of postganglionic to preganglionic neurons and by the mean degree of convergence of preganglionic axons on a postganglionic neuron. The size of an autonomic neural unit is therefore the number of postganglionic

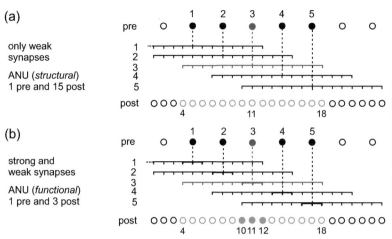

(a)

only weak
synapses

ANU (*structural*)
1 pre and 15 post

(b)

strong and
weak synapses

ANU (*functional*)
1 pre and 3 post

Figure 6.7 The autonomic neural unit (ANU). Schematic representation for a convergence of five preganglionic neurons on one postganglionic neuron. The ratio between post- and preganglionic neurons is assumed to be 3:1. (a) The *structural autonomic neural unit* ("neural unit" of Purves [see Johnson and Purves 1981; Purves and Wigston 1983; Purves et al. 1986]) consists of one preganglionic neuron and 15 postganglionic neurons (which are innervated by each preganglionic neuron). The ANUs exhibit considerable overlap (see units 1–5, brackets). Only postganglionic neurons 10, 11 and 12 receive convergent inputs from these five preganglionic neurons. The postganglionic neurons would discharge only with closely coincident firing of several converging preganglionic neurons if all synaptic connections were subthreshold (weak). (b) Examples of *functional autonomic neural units* which consist of one preganglionic neuron and three postganglionic neurons when each postganglionic neuron receives only one strong (suprathreshold) synaptic input (in addition to weak [subthreshold] synaptic inputs). Now the postganglionic neuron would discharge when the preganglionic neuron forming a strong synapse with it discharges. Functional autonomic units do not overlap when each postganglionic neuron receives one strong synaptic input only. Modified from Jänig (1995).

neurons divided by the number of preganglionic neurons multiplied by the degree of convergence. For example in Figure 6.7a, five preganglionic neurons converge on one postganglionic neuron and the ratio between post- and preganglionic neurons is 24/8 neurons; the autonomic neural unit consists therefore of one preganglionic neuron and 15 postganglionic neurons. The size of the autonomic neural unit varies with the size of the animal, the size of the target organ and the function of the postganglionic neuron (i.e., the type of autonomic final pathway). For the superior cervical ganglion, the mean size of the autonomic neural unit increases from 60 postganglionic neurons in the mouse to 420 postganglionic neurons in the rabbit (Purves and Wigston 1983; Purves et al. 1986; Ivanov and Purves 1989).

The size of the autonomic neural unit is structurally defined in this way. For autonomic systems in which each postganglionic neuron is innervated by only one preganglionic axon (for example, neurons in the submandibular ganglion of the rat and rabbit

[Lichtman 1977] or in some ganglia of lower vertebrates [Blackman et al. 1963]), the synaptic input from that preganglionic axon is generally suprathreshold (i.e., strong) and it is relatively easy to understand how the pattern of discharge is transmitted in these autonomic systems from the CNS to the target tissue. The size of the autonomic neural unit in these systems is therefore structurally and functionally identical. For this case the analogy between skeletomotor and peripheral autonomic pathways is obvious. The main difference from the motor unit of the skeletomotor system is that a structurally defined autonomic neural unit shares the same target cells with other autonomic neural units of the same type. The latter is an assumption, since it is unknown whether all target cells of a structurally defined autonomic neural unit are functionally of the same type. As in the skeletomotor unit, the response of the autonomic target organ or tissue to neural stimulation would depend on the mean rate of activity of the preganglionic neurons and the successive recruitment of different autonomic neural units.

In sympathetic paravertebral and some prevertebral final pathways in which there is considerable convergence of preganglionic axons onto postganglionic neurons, the analogy between the "motor unit" of the final common skeletomotor pathway and the functional autonomic neural unit is less easy to define because several autonomic neural units share subpopulations of postganglionic neurons (Figure 6.7). The size of the autonomic neural unit is usually smaller functionally than structurally because most preganglionic synaptic inputs are subthreshold and only a few are suprathreshold (strong; bold in Figure 6.7b) (see Subchapter 6.2). This applies to most paravertebral and parasympathetic ganglia in mammals. The size of the functional autonomic neural unit probably varies depending on the functional type of final common autonomic pathway. However, the overlap between functional autonomic neural units is relatively small. This follows from the finding that most postganglionic neurons of sympathetic final pathways to somatic tissues, postganglionic neurons of some sympathetic pathways to viscera and postganglionic neurons of parasympathetic pathways receive only one (and rarely two or three) strong synaptic preganglionic input(s) and their output depends only on this and not on the summation of weak synaptic inputs. These systems therefore behave relatively simply as relay stations in the pathway to the target (see Box 6.2). The situation differs for some sympathetic motility-regulating and possibly secretomotor pathways innervating the gastrointestinal tract that receive many peripheral synaptic intestinofugal inputs and weak preganglionic synaptic inputs, but few strong preganglionic synaptic inputs. These postganglionic neurons are activated by summation of synaptic potentials (see Subchapter 6.5).

In conclusion, the autonomic neural unit was originally structurally defined by the number of postganglionic neurons innervated by one preganglionic neuron. Its size increases with increasing degrees of divergence of preganglionic axons. The functional autonomic neural unit is for paravertebral and some prevertebral sympathetic systems much smaller because most synaptic inputs from preganglionic neurons are subthreshold and do not elicit discharges in the postganglionic neurons.

6.4 Electrophysiological Classification, Ion Channels and Relation to Functions of Sympathetic Postganglionic Neurons

General electrophysiological properties of postganglionic neurons, as well as mechanisms underlying fast and slow synaptic potentials, have been extensively reviewed in the literature and will not be discussed here (Adams and Harper 1995; Tokimasa and Akasu 1995). Experimental investigations in vitro of postganglionic neurons in paravertebral and prevertebral ganglia of the guinea pig show that these sympathetic neurons can be classified by way of their responses to suprathreshold depolarizing current pulses passed through an intracellular microelectrode into three types (Figure 6.8): phasic neurons (rapidly adapting), tonic neurons (slowly adapting) and neurons with a prolonged long afterhyperpolarization following the action potential (LAH neurons). Phasic neurons respond with a burst of action potentials at the beginning of the suprathreshold current pulse. Tonic neurons discharge rhythmically throughout the current pulse. LAH neurons discharge only one action potential at the beginning of the current pulse (Note 3).

These three classes of electrophysiologically classified sympathetic postganglionic neurons exhibit differential distributions in different sympathetic ganglia (Figure 6.9) and have the following phenomenological characteristics (Figures 6.8, 6.9; Table 6.1):

1. Almost all postganglionic neurons in the paravertebral ganglia and some 15 to 25% of the postganglionic neurons in the prevertebral ganglia are phasic neurons. Most of these neurons in paravertebral ganglia contain, in addition to noradrenaline, neuropeptide Y (NPY). They receive one or two strong and several weak preganglionic synaptic inputs and very rarely peripheral synaptic input. In prevertebral ganglia, their cell bodies are the smallest of the three classes of neurons and their total dendritic length lies between that of the tonic and the LAH neurons. Phasic neurons in the paravertebral ganglia are involved in regulation of target organs in skin and deep somatic tissues (blood vessels, arrector pili muscles, sweat glands).

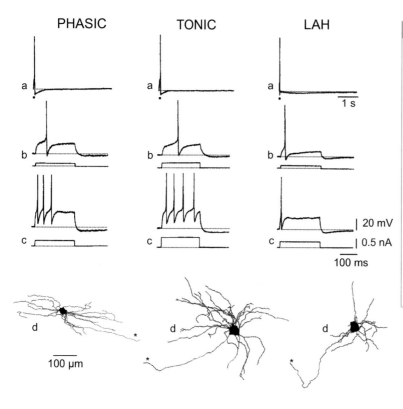

Figure 6.8 Three major classes of sympathetic postganglionic neuron in the guinea pig celiac ganglion defined by discharge characteristics and morphology. Individual neurons are characterized neurophysiologically: (a) Action potentials elicited by 50 ms current steps (dots) showing relative duration of afterhyperpolarization in each class of neuron. (b,c) Voltage responses to long intracellular depolarizing current pulses (lower traces: in b just threshold; in c approximately twice threshold). (d) Neurophysiologically characterized neurons were filled with biocytin. The cell bodies, dendrites and axons (indicated by *) of the biocytin-filled neurons were reconstructed and analyzed quantitatively. Modified from McLachlan and Meckler (1989) (neurophysiology) and Boyd et al. (1996) (morphology).

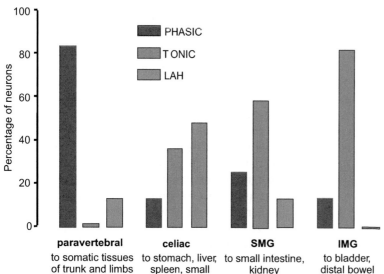

Figure 6.9 Proportions of neurons of different classes in various sympathetic ganglia of the guinea pig. The target tissues of the neurons are indicated at the bottom. Data for celiac ganglia (N = 175), superior mesenteric ganglia (SMG, N = 80) and inferior mesenteric ganglia (IMG, N = 156) from Keast et al. (1993). Data for paravertebral ganglia in the lumbar sympathetic chain (N = 100) from Ireland (unpublished), Davies (unpublished), Christian and Weinreich (1988) and Hamblin et al. (1995). Same data as under "Anatomical distribution" in Table 6.1.

Some of the phasic neurons in the prevertebral ganglia are probably involved in regulation of vascular resistance in, e.g., spleen (Jobling 1994). Phasic neurons located in the inferior mesenteric ganglion are probably involved in the regulation of the vas deferens and other functions related to the pelvic organs. All of these neurons are fully under the control of the central nervous system.

2. Tonic postganglionic neurons are numerous in prevertebral ganglia and are almost absent from paravertebral ganglia. In guinea pigs, they contain, in

Table 6.1 Biophysical properties of sympathetic postganglionic neurons of guinea pigs and their correlation with the content of peptides and function.

	Phasic	Tonic	LAH
Discharge during just suprathreshold depolarization	Transient burst	Rhythmic	Single
Morphology			
Relative soma size	0.75	1.25	1.0
No of primary dendrites	16	20	13
Total dendritic length (μm)	2336	3574	1325
Anatomical distribution			
SCG	85%	<1%	15%
LSC	95%	<1%	<5%
CG	15%	35%	50%
IMG	18%	18%	2%
Resting membrane potential	−55 mV	−61 mV	−55 mV
Specific membrane resistivity	27 KΩ cm²	40 KΩ cm²	15 KΩ cm²
Action potential repolarization			
charybdotoxin-sensitive	BK channels	few or no BK channels	few BK channels
source of Ca^{2+}	L- and N-type	not L-type	not L-type
Afterhyperpolarization (gKCa1)			
apamin-sensitive	SK channels	SK channels	SK and some BK channels
source of Ca^{2+}	L-type and N-type	partly L-type	L-type and N-type
Long afterhyperpolarization (gKCa2)	5%	absent	100%
kinetically slow			BK, SK and resistant K^+ channel
source of Ca^{2+}			CICR triggered by L-, N- and P-type
Prominent K^+ channel			
M	many	a few	some
A (half-inactivation)	−84 mV	−71 mV	not tested
D (decay constant)	rare	415 ms	not tested
Synaptic input			
from CNS (preganglionic)	1–2 strong several weak	several weak some small strong	1 strong several weak
from periphery (visceral afferent)	very rare weak	numerous weak	rare weak
Peptide content	most neuropeptide Y	many somatostatin	many neuropeptide Y

The three classes of neuron are distributed between paravertebral (mainly phasic) and prevertebral ganglia. Ganglia: CG, celiac ganglion; IMG, inferior mesenteric ganglion; LSC, lumbar sympathetic chain; SCG, superior cervical ganglion. Potassium channels (see Alexander et al. 2011; Adams and Harper 1995): *A channel*: voltage-sensitive, Ca^{2+}-independent rapid activation and inactivation; *BK (big potassium) channel*: large-conductance Ca^{2+}-activated; *D (dendritic) channel*: voltage-sensitive slowly activating and inactivating; *M channel*: muscarine-sensitive, voltage-sensitive (slowly activating, non-inactivating); *SK channel*: small-conductance Ca^{2+}-activated; *"resistant-K^+" channel*: Ca^{2+}-activated, resistant to known blockers. Voltage-sensitive Ca^{2+} channels: L-type (nifedipine-sensitive); N-type (omega-conotoxin GVIA-sensitive); P-type (agatoxin IVA-sensitive). CICR: Ca^{2+} induced Ca^{2+}-release from intracellular stores (ryanodine-sensitive). Modified from Jänig and McLachlan (1992) by Elspeth McLachlan. Electrophysiological data from neurons studied in vitro using high-resistance intracellular microelectrodes with single electrode voltage clamp. Published in Boyd et al. (1996), Cassell et al. (1986), Cassell and McLachlan (1987), Ireland et al. (1999), Jamieson et al. (2003), Jobling et al. (1993), Keast et al. (1993), Davies et al. (1996, 1999), McLachlan and Meckler (1989), Martinez-Pinna et al. (2000). Immunohistochemical data also from Macrae et al. (1986), Parr and Sharkey (1996).

addition to noradrenaline, either no known peptide or somatostatin. They receive weak preganglionic inputs and in most cases a strong one that is not as large as those in the paravertebral ganglia. Many other weak inputs originate from peripheral neurons (e.g., from intestinofugal neurons of the enteric nervous system, see Chapter 5). This also applies to tonic neurons in the inferior mesenteric ganglion that project through the hypogastric nerve and innervate pelvic organs (Crowcroft et al. 1971; Cassell et al. 1986). Tonic neurons have large cell bodies and many dendrites, giving a large total dendritic length. In the gastrointestinal tract, tonic neurons containing somatostatin largely innervate the myenteric plexus and are involved in regulation of secretion and/or motility in the gastrointestinal tract. Tonic neurons containing no known peptide project to the submucous plexus and are probably involved mainly in the regulation of secretion (see Subchapter 5.7 and Figure 5.15; see Furness and Costa [1987]). Tonic postganglionic neurons appear to be normally under peripheral control and the centrally generated signals in preganglionic neurons may facilitate synaptic input from peripheral neurons in order to be effective (see Subchapter 6.5).

3. Most LAH neurons are also found in prevertebral ganglia and are almost exclusively located in the celiac ganglion and superior mesenteric ganglion; a few are located in the paravertebral ganglia, in particular the superior cervical ganglion. Many of them contain, in addition to noradrenaline, neuropeptide Y. They receive one strong and several weak preganglionic inputs and very rarely receive synaptic inputs from peripheral neurons. They have medium-sized cell bodies and a small dendritic arbor. In the gastrointestinal tract, they may innervate the submucosal plexus and mucosal cells involved in secretion and absorption important for regulation of fluid balance (see Sjövall et al. [1987]; Lundgren [1988]). These neurons are under the primary control of the central nervous system. LAH neurons in the celiac ganglion also project to the spleen. Their function may be vasoconstrictor or they may modulate immune cells (Jobling, unpublished observations).

This description shows, with the exception of vasoconstrictor neurons, that there are no straightforward correlations between the functions of these postganglionic neurons, as defined by their target cells, and their neurophysiological properties. Indeed this description probably covers the most well-characterized group of neurons. Furthermore, the peptide content of these neurons can only be used as a functional label to a limited degree. There are variations between species in the peptide content of different neurophysiologically characterized postganglionic neurons.

The mechanisms underlying the neurophysiological characteristics of the postganglionic neurons (action potential, afterhyperpolarization, responses to depolarizing current pulses) have been extensively studied, mainly in the guinea pig and rat. The details differ between species. These characteristics depend on the presence (or absence) of different voltage- and calcium-dependent potassium channels, which are differentially expressed in the membranes of these neurons. The main potassium channels that are involved are listed in Table 6.1. For example:

- The phasic responses of sympathetic neurons to current steps (Figure 6.8) depend on the presence of the M-type potassium channel (muscarine-sensitive K^+ channel). Opening of this channel by depolarization increases the K^+ current and limits the discharge of phasic neurons. After blockade of this channel, by a muscarinic agonist, phasic neurons exhibit a tonic response to suprathreshold depolarizing current pulses.
- The rhythmic firing of tonic neurons is determined mainly by A-type and also by D-type K^+ channels with distinct voltage characteristics that make it dominate membrane behavior in the subthreshold voltage range.
- The long-lasting afterhyperpolarization in LAH neurons is generated by various calcium-dependent K^+ channels (BK, SK and other K^+ channels; see Table 6.1).

6.5 Different Types of Autonomic Ganglia and Their Functions In Vivo

6.5.1 Paravertebral Sympathetic Ganglia

The function of sympathetic paravertebral ganglia is to transmit discharges from preganglionic neurons to postganglionic neurons innervating somatic tissues without integrating additional synaptic inputs, either from other preganglionic neurons or from the periphery. Experimental investigations of sympathetic neurons in vivo in the cat and rat show that the rate of ongoing discharge is remarkably similar in pre- and postganglionic neurons of the same functional type under the same experimental conditions (Table 6.2) (Note 4). Thus, convergence of many preganglionic axons on one postganglionic neuron, which appears to occur in all paravertebral sympathetic systems, rarely leads to a higher suprathreshold activity in the postganglionic neurons. The simplest explanation for this finding is that each postganglionic neuron receives strong synaptic inputs from one preganglionic axon (Figure 6.10a). Occasionally the firing rate is higher because ~25% of neurons receive two preganglionic inputs. Evidence for this has been presented for paravertebral ganglia in the rat, guinea pig and rabbit as described in Subchapter 6.2 (see Box 6.2; Skok and Ivanov 1983; Cassell et al. 1986; Hirst and McLachlan 1986; McLachlan et al. 1997).

What is the function of the subthreshold EPSPs, generated by weak converging preganglionic axons, that do not summate to suprathreshold events but whose collective rate is higher than the rate of action potentials in most postganglionic neurons? Is the existence of these subthreshold potentials left over from the development of the connectivity between preganglionic axons and postganglionic neurons (Hirst and McLachlan 1984), i.e., do they have any function relevant to the ongoing regulation of the target organs?

The following questions remain to be addressed:

1. Are all synaptic events in individual postganglionic neurons of the same functional type, i.e., do all converging preganglionic neurons have the same functional properties (e.g., are they muscle vasoconstrictor, cutaneous vasoconstrictor, sudomotor, etc. neurons)? Evidence so far available suggests that this is the case in some neurons (Skok and Ivanov 1987; McLachlan et al. 1997; Bratton et al. 2010).
2. What is the degree of convergence of preganglionic neurons in different types of final autonomic pathways? For example, it is known that, in vasoconstrictor neurons, the degree of convergence is high and in secretomotor neurons to salivary glands it is low.
3. How many of the preganglionic neurons converging on postganglionic neurons with spontaneous activity are silent, at least under anesthesia? This question is relevant in view of the fact that 40 to 70% of sympathetic preganglionic neurons are silent and exhibit no reflex activity under experimental conditions (Table 4.5).
4. Do central synchronizing mechanisms contribute to spatial and temporal summation of subthreshold EPSPs and in this way to synaptic activation of postganglionic neurons that receive a strong (suprathreshold) input (Skok and Ivanoff 1987)? This idea is not supported by experiments so far conducted (McLachlan et al. 1997, 1998), but is often included in models of ganglionic transmission (Karila and Horn 2000; Springer et al. 2015).
5. How do strong suprathreshold synaptic inputs to sympathetic postganglionic neurons develop postnatally with respect to the target cells? Strong synaptic inputs form at about the same time as the connections of postganglionic axons with peripheral targets (Hirst and McLachlan 1984). There must exist functional matching between preganglionic neurons and postganglionic neurons, otherwise it would be impossible to get correct restoration of function after denervation following complete or partial lesion of preganglionic axons (Langley 1895; Murray and Thompson 1957; Guth and Bernstein 1961; Nja and Purves 1977a).

6.5.2 Prevertebral Sympathetic Ganglia

The sympathetic prevertebral ganglia have a number of different functions during ongoing regulation of the abdominal organs, pelvic organs and blood vessels. They contain different types of neurons, as judged by morphological, electrophysiological, neurochemical and other criteria (Table 6.1). Many neurons in these ganglia receive multiple synaptic inputs from the spinal cord, from the periphery and from collaterals of visceral primary afferent axons (Figure 6.10b; see Note 5). In this context it is worth noting that many postganglionic vasoconstrictor neurons projecting to abdominal and pelvic organs are situated in the paravertebral ganglia (Costa and Furness 1973; Kuo et al. 1984; Hill et al. 1987; see Jänig and McLachlan [1987]).

Mediation of Peripheral Reflexes

Peripheral extraspinal reflexes have been well established for the gastrointestinal tract in the guinea pig;

Table 6.2 Discharge rates of single sympathetic axons in vivo in the cat and rat

| Neuron type | Resting activity | | Maximal activity | | Refs |
	Preganglionic imp/s	Postganglionic imp/s	Preganglionic imp/s	Postganglionic imp/s	
MVC_L	1.8 ± 1.3 (26)		approx. 12	approx. 10	8,9
	(0.1–4.6)	(0.5–3)			
		1.4 ± 0.5 (44)			*6*
		(0.3–2.4)			
MVC_C	1.1 ± 0.8 (54)				
	1.1 ± 0.8 (36) [a]	*0.7 ± 0.4 (21)* [b]			6,3,4
	(0.2–3.5)	*(0.2–1.5)*			
VVC_L	1.6 ± 0.9 (46)	1.1 ± 1.1 (14)	<5		2,9
	(0.3–4)	(0.2–2.5)			
CVC_L	0.9 ± 0.6 (47)	1.2 ± 0.7 (44)			8,9
	(0.1–3.4)	(0.4–4)			
		1.2 ± 0.6 (65) [c]			*6,7*
		(0.3–2.4)			
CVC_C	1.5 ± 1.1 (30)				5
SM_L	Low	0.2 ± 0.1 (15)		approx. 5	8,9
MR_L	0.8 ± 0.7 (91)	0.7 ± 0.5 (67)	5.3 ± 1.5 (54)	2.7 ± 1.5 (22)	1,2,10
	(0.1–3.8)	(0.1–2.6)	(max 8)	(max 5)	
INS_C	1.4 ± 1.4 (24)				5

The measurements were taken under chloralose anesthesia in artificially ventilated cats or in pentobarbital-anesthetized and artificially ventilated rats (rat data in italics). Resting activity was recorded extracellularly from the axons of the neurons at mean arterial blood pressure of ≥100 mmHg and end-tidal CO_2 of 4%. Rates of maximal activity were estimated from reflex responses to systemic hypoxia (MVC_L, SM_L, VVC_L), to mechanical shearing stimuli applied to the mucosa of the anal canal (MR_L) and to mechanical stimulation of the nasopharyngeal mucosa (MVC_C, INS_C). C, thoracic sympathetic outflow to the superior cervical ganglion; CVC, cutaneous vasoconstrictor; INS, inspiratory type; L, lumbar sympathetic outflow to skin, skeletal muscle or pelvic organs; MR, motility-regulating; MVC, muscle vasoconstrictor; SM, sudomotor; VVC, visceral vasoconstrictor; means ± SD (n), range of activity in parentheses.

[a] Cervical sympathetic trunk in rat: most neurons behave like MVC neurons
[b] Postganglionic neurons to submandibular gland in rat with spontaneous activity and high cardiac rhythmicity
[c] Rat tail data for CVC 1.1 ± 0.7 imp/s (51), range 0.2–2.6 imp/s (Häbler et al. 1999)

References: 1. Bahr et al. (1986a); 2. Bahr et al. (1986b); 3. Bartsch et al. (1996); 4. Bartsch et al. (2000); 5. Boczek-Funcke et al. (1993); 6. Häbler et al. (1994); 7. Häbler et al. (1999); 8. Jänig (1985); 9. Jänig (1988); 10. Jänig et al. (1991). From Jänig (1995).

distension of one part of this tract leads to inhibition of the motility of other parts (e.g., colocolonic, gastro-colic reflexes) mediated via the inferior mesenteric ganglion and the celiac plexus (Kreulen and Szurszewski 1979a, b; see Szurszewski and King [1989]). These reflexes also exist in other mammals, such as the cat and dog, and probably in humans. They were first described by Kuntz in the dog (inset (a) in Figure 6.11; Kuntz 1940; Kuntz and Saccomanno 1944). The neurons involved have their cell bodies in the plexus myentericus of the wall of the gut (intestinofugal neurons) and can be synaptically activated by intrinsic primary afferent neurons (IPANs; see Subchapter 5.1) in the enteric nervous system (Crowcroft et al. 1971). Synaptic

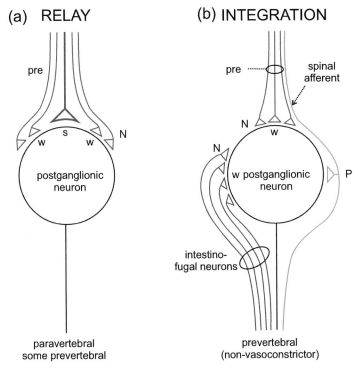

(a) RELAY

(b) INTEGRATION

Figure 6.10 Relay and integrative functions of autonomic ganglion cells. (a) Postganglionic neuron with one (and sometimes two or three) strong (s; suprathreshold) preganglionic synaptic input(s) and several weak (w; subthreshold) synaptic inputs. This connectivity occurs in most paravertebral sympathetic neurons, some prevertebral sympathetic neurons and parasympathetic neurons. These connections mainly function to transmit the activity from specific preganglionic neurons to postganglionic neurons. (b) Postganglionic sympathetic neuron with synaptic inputs from both preganglionic neurons and intestinofugal neurons of the enteric nervous system and also from collaterals of spinal visceral afferents. The first two are cholinergic and nicotinic (N) but subthreshold (weak, w); the intestinofugal afferents may also contain neuropeptides, which may function as transmitters (e.g., vasoactive intestinal peptide in guinea pig). The collaterals of spinal visceral afferent neurons release substance P (P), which produces a slow depolarization of the postganglionic neuron (calcitonin gene-related peptide that is colocalized with substance P in the afferent neuron is probably also released but has no known function). These postganglionic neurons innervate neurons of the enteric nervous system and other target tissues in the viscera. They fire only after integration of several subthreshold inputs with or without the peptide-induced slow depolarization.

transmission to the postganglionic neurons is nicotinic cholinergic, but may also be non-cholinergic (i.e., peptidergic) (Figure 6.11).

These peripheral reflex pathways may also exist for other target tissues of the sympathetic prevertebral neurons in the gastrointestinal tract and its appendages (such as the submucosal tissue, pancreas, gallbladder), of sympathetic neurons in the stellate and possibly middle cervical ganglion projecting to the heart, and of parasympathetic neurons in cardiac ganglia (see Subchapter 6.5.4 "Intrinsic Cardiac Nervous System"). These peripheral autonomic neural circuits may be of considerable importance for the understanding of neural regulation of the internal organs in health and disease, yet we need more rigorously controlled physiological experiments to demonstrate their recruitment and relative importance in organ regulation.

Integration of Impulse Activity From Spinal Cord and Periphery in Prevertebral Ganglia

Most peripheral synaptic and central synaptic inputs to tonic prevertebral sympathetic postganglionic neurons that innervate non-vascular target tissues, in particular

in the gastrointestinal tract, are subthreshold (see Szurszewski [1981]; Jänig and McLachlan [1987]):

- Spatial summation of synaptic inputs is necessary in order to excite the neurons. By lowering or increasing synaptic afferent activity from the periphery, the state of the peripheral tissues determines the conditions under which the central messages reach the target organs.
- Alternatively, one could argue that the impulse activity in the preganglionic neurons sets the firing threshold of the prevertebral postganglionic neurons for the peripheral afferent synaptic input (Figure 6.11).
- Peripheral integration of this type is probably important for pathways to some non-vascular target cells of the gastrointestinal tract, unimportant for regulation of vascular resistance and probably unimportant for regulation of motility and secretion of pelvic organs. However, experimental data showing that the prevertebral abdominal ganglia function in vivo in this integrative mode are lacking.

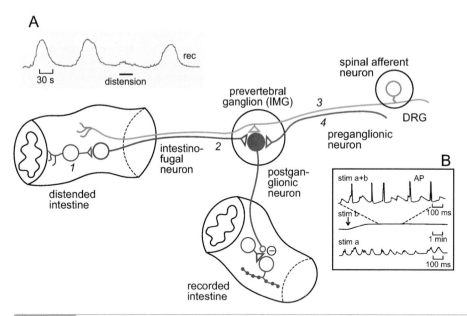

Figure 6.11 Peripheral reflexes involving the enteric nervous system and sympathetic prevertebral ganglia. Distension of the bowel activates afferent terminals of local enteric neurons (neuron 1) are linked to intestinofugal neurons (neuron 2). It also activates visceral primary afferent neurons (neuron 3) with cell bodies in the dorsal root ganglia (DRG). The intestinofugal neurons project to prevertebral ganglia, where they excite postganglionic neurons projecting to another, mostly more proximal, part of the bowel. This leads to inhibition (−) of enteric excitatory muscle motor neurons and to relaxation. Collateral branches of primary afferent neurons (neuron 3) release substance P around the same postganglionic neurons, depolarizing them and summing with EPSPs generated by inputs from intestinofugal and preganglionic neurons (neurons 2 and 4). Inset A: Recording of the intraluminal pressure in an isolated proximal segment of the colon in the cat during distension of the rectum. The inferior mesenteric ganglion (IMG) was decentralized by section of the preganglionic axons in the lumbar splanchnic nerves. The regular contraction waves of the proximal colon were inhibited during distension of the rectum. This inhibition was mediated by the IMG. From Kuntz (1940). Inset B: lower trace, ongoing subthreshold cholinergic postsynaptic potentials elicited in a prevertebral postganglionic neuron during activity in intestinofugal (neuron 2) and preganglionic neurons (neuron 4); middle trace, long-lasting postsynaptic potential generated by activity in peptidergic spinal visceral afferent neurons (via decrease in K^+ conductance); upper trace, enhancement of nicotinic postsynaptic potentials when peptidergic synapses are activated, leading to an increase in size and duration of postsynaptic potentials with generation of action potentials (AP). Idealized in vivo behavior derived from in vitro experiments. Modified from Jänig and McLachlan (2013).

- As already discussed in Chapter 5, sympathetic pathways to the gastrointestinal tract by which the central nervous system directly controls target tissue have strong preganglionic synapses and are not controlled by peripheral reflexes. This applies to the neural control of vascular resistance and in part to the neural control of the oral and anal parts of the gastrointestinal tract.

- The sympathetic pathways involved in regulation of motility are not normally under dominant control by the central nervous system and are modifiable by peripheral reflexes.

- The sympathetic pathways regulating secretion and absorption may be under both dominant central control and peripheral control.

In vivo experiments on animal models need to be done to test the idea that there is reciprocal integration of central and peripheral cholinergic synaptic input in prevertebral postganglionic neurons. The main question to be tested is: can central reflex activation of the postganglionic neurons be gated by the peripheral input from the gastrointestinal tract and vice versa?

Putative Function of Peptidergic Synapses Made by Visceral Afferents

Postganglionic neurons in the prevertebral abdominal ganglia may receive synaptic input from collaterals of spinal visceral afferent neurons that have their cell bodies in the thoracolumbar dorsal root ganglia. These afferents may form synaptic connections with postganglionic neurons in the inferior mesenteric ganglion (Dalsgaard et al. 1982; Matthews and Cuello 1984; Matthews et al. 1987). These collaterals form boutons associated with non-vascular postganglionic neurons. The peptides present in these collaterals are substance P and calcitonin gene-related peptide (CGRP) (for review see Elfvin et al. [1993]).

In the guinea pig, repetitive electrical stimulation of the visceral afferents in the upper lumbar dorsal roots, which have been sectioned between the spinal cord and the stimulation electrodes (so as to prevent spinal reflex activation of preganglionic neurons), elicits long-lasting postsynaptic potentials in some postganglionic neurons of the prevertebral ganglia (produced by an increase of membrane resistance, probably due to closure of potassium channels). Electrical stimulation of the mesenteric nerves elicits slow EPSPs in tonic postganglionic neurons and prolonged inhibition of the long afterhyperpolarization in postganglionic LAH neurons (Zhao et al. 1996). Both of these changes increase excitability of the prevertebral neurons. The changes in the postganglionic neurons are generated by impulses in unmyelinated visceral afferents. The transmitter involved in this is probably substance P (SP) acting via NK_1 (neurokinin 1) receptors on the postganglionic neurons. However, there is no match between SP-immunoreactive baskets around sympathetic prevertebral neurons and the distribution of NK1 receptors. So the peptide must diffuse some unknown distance to reach the receptors (Messenger and Gibbins 1998). Calcitonin gene-related peptide, which is probably also released by the afferent fibers, has no known function on the postganglionic neurons. The anatomical data argue that substance P acts by volume conduction on the postganglionic neurons in the prevertebral ganglia and not by direct synaptic action (for the biophysical and pharmacological properties of this effect of substance P released by afferent axons see Tsunoo et al. [1982]; Dun [1983]; Katayama and Nishi [1986]; Tokimasa and Akasu [1995]).

What is the function of this peptidergic transmission from collaterals of spinal visceral afferents to prevertebral sympathetic neurons? These visceral afferents respond to various mechanical and chemical stimuli, most being polymodal and many having low mechanical thresholds. They are involved in spinal and supraspinal reflex discharges mediated by sympathetic and skeletomotor systems and in various forms of visceral sensations, the most important being visceral pain and discomfort (see Chapter 2). Reflexes and sensations elicited by stimulation of these afferents are integrative components of a protective behavior, which is elicited when, for example, the gastrointestinal tract or other visceral organs are abnormally affected (e.g., by inflammation of the organs, by overdistension, by obstruction). Activation of the spinal visceral afferents would induce slow non-cholinergic depolarizations of the prevertebral neurons, which would enable the preganglionic and peripheral afferent cholinergic synaptic potentials to reach threshold (see Figure 6.11, inset [B]). This peripheral mechanism would enhance inhibitory intestino-intestinal reflexes mediated by sympathetic prevertebral ganglia to the gastrointestinal tract, decreasing contractions and contributing to the protection of the organ. Evidence for this hypothesis comes from experiments conducted on postganglionic neurons in the guinea pig inferior mesenteric ganglion with an attached segment of the colon in vitro: distension of the colon elicits non-cholinergic depolarizations in many neurons, leading to increased excitability (Crowcroft et al. 1971; Kreulen and Peters 1986; see also Krier and Szurszewski [1982]). Similar slow depolarizations can be elicited in neurons of the inferior mesenteric ganglion by distension of a mesenteric vein attached to the ganglion (Keef and Kreulen 1986) and by distension of the ureter (Amann et al. 1988).

6.5.3 Parasympathetic Ganglia

Parasympathetic ganglia differ from sympathetic ones in some anatomical and functional ways. As already discussed in Chapter 1, the postganglionic neurons are mostly located in small ganglia close to their targets. Most parasympathetic postganglionic neurons are structurally relatively homogeneous, having few or no dendrites, but this varies between species. They typically receive a small number of preganglionic synaptic inputs, often one or more of them being strong. Parasympathetic ganglia are commonly considered to have only relay function. This may not be true for all pathways and may also be related to the fact that parasympathetic postganglionic neurons have not been studied as extensively as sympathetic ones (Akasu and Nishimura 1995). No evidence for interneurons or peripheral synaptic inputs has been detected in cranial parasympathetic ganglia (e.g., the ciliary, otic, submandibular and pterygopalatine ganglia) and ganglia of the intrathoracic airways (Undem and Potenzieri 2012).

Ganglia in pancreas or gallbladder, both having the same embryological origin as the enteric neurons, are similar to enteric ganglia, but are also typical of parasympathetic ganglia. The neurons in these ganglia are involved in regulation of exocrine and endocrine functions of the pancreas or of motility and secretion of the gallbladder. They receive synaptic input from enteric neurons as well as from preganglionic parasympathetic neurons and probably have integrative function. These ganglia are considered to be accessory enteric ganglia (Mawe 1995, 1998).

Intracardiac parasympathetic ganglia have been studied in more detail using neurophysiological methods (Edwards et al. 1995; McAllen et al. 2011). In these ganglia only a proportion of the ganglion cells receive input from preganglionic axons and project to cardiac muscle. A subpopulation of neurons that cannot be activated synaptically may be afferent neurons (P neurons in Figure 6.12). These cells have intrinsic activity, which might be responsible for ongoing synaptic activity recorded in other neurons within the ganglia. A third group of smaller neurons receives local synaptic inputs and may also terminate on cardiac muscle (S neurons in Figure 6.12). Both the location of the endings of the putative afferent neurons and the adequate stimuli that excite them remain unclear. However, these peripheral connections are obviously a feature of parasympathetic cardiac ganglia.

Pelvic ganglia contain postganglionic neurons supplying pelvic viscera and are often considered to be parasympathetic. However, this is misleading. Most cholinergic neurons receive synaptic input from preganglionic neurons in the sacral spinal cord (and in rodents the sixth lumbar spinal segment) projecting through the pelvic nerve. Some postganglionic neurons in pelvic ganglia are noradrenergic and receive synaptic input from preganglionic neurons in the upper lumbar spinal cord projecting through the hypogastric nerves (see Note 3). A few postganglionic neurons in the pelvic ganglia receive convergent synaptic input from both the sacral spinal cord and the upper lumbar spinal cord. Interneurons are absent or rare in the pelvic ganglia. Most cholinergic vasodilator neurons in pelvic ganglia of guinea

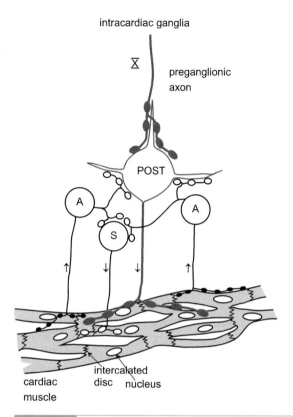

Figure 6.12 Integration in parasympathetic cardiac ganglia. Diagram of the component neurons of intracardiac ganglia of the guinea pig. Only one neuron type (POST, postganglionic) receives preganglionic synaptic inputs via the vagus nerve (X). The postganglionic cells and another neuron type (S, synaptic) receive synaptic input arising from the third neuron type, which is spontaneously active (A, afferent). The A cells may be sensory neurons with afferent terminals within the heart. The physiological stimuli to activate them are unknown. Modified from Edwards et al. (1995) and Jänig and McLachlan (2013).

pigs that project to, e.g., uterine vasculature are activated either by sacral or by upper lumbar preganglionic neurons, very few by both (Jobling et al. 2003, 2004). Pelvic neurons supplying distal colon and rectum (and innervating myenteric plexus or circular musculature) may receive additional synaptic input from intestinofugal neurons located in the myenteric plexus or the serosal ganglia (Félix et al. 1998). Overall there are considerable species differences in organization of the pelvic ganglia but the properties of the postganglionic neurons of these have been less well studied than those of other ganglia (Jänig and McLachlan 1987; Keast 1995, 1999).

6.5.4 The Intrinsic Cardiac Nervous System

Armour and Ardell have developed an interesting idea about the autonomic regulation of the heart (Armour 2008; Ardell et al. 2016; Ardell and Armour 2016). They propagate the concept that the heart is associated with an "intrinsic cardiac nervous system" (ICNS) which is sometimes called metaphorically "the little brain of the heart." This ICNS consists essentially of four groups of neurons: parasympathetic postganglionic cardiomotor neurons, sympathetic postganglionic cardiomotor neurons (located in the stellate ganglion), local afferent neurons and interneurons called "local circuit neurons" (LCN) (Figure 6.13): (1) Postganglionic cardiomotor neurons are the output neurons of the ICNS. They are under neural control of the preganglionic cardiomotor neurons located in the spinal cord or lower brain stem and of the LCNs. (2) Local afferent neurons are mechanosensitive and/or chemosensitive. These local neurons project within the cardiac ganglia forming excitatory synapses to the LCNs. (3) LCNs are functionally specific interneurons that subserve integrative control of cardiac functions. They are the centerpiece of the ICNS and mediate intrinsic cardiac reflexes to the postganglionic parasympathetic and sympathetic cardiomotor neurons. They do not project outside of the ganglion in which their cell body is located. They are synaptically activated by preganglionic neurons and by local afferent neurons and form excitatory synapses with postganglionic cardiomotor neurons.

As interesting as the idea from Armour and Ardell may be, the ICNS is certainly not comparable with the enteric nervous system (see Chapter 5). The way the ICNS works under physiological conditions, employing excitatory as well as inhibitory synapses, is entirely unclear. Several open questions to be answered require in vivo experimentation in which the activity of the neurons of the ICNS has to be measured intracellularly:

- The synaptic transmission from preganglionic to postganglionic CM neurons is mediated by strong synapses in parasympathetic cardiac ganglia (McAllen et al. 2011). In the stellate ganglion, the activity in postganglionic CM neurons is dominated by one or a few strong preganglionic synaptic inputs and the presence of peripheral inputs has not been shown. Cardiac and non-cardiac neurons in this ganglion are not different in morphology and electrophysiological properties (Selyanko and Skok 1992; Mo et al. 1994; Wallis et al. 1996). How can this strong synaptic transmission be modulated by local circuits of the ICNS?
- What are the functional characteristics of local cardiac afferent neurons? Do these afferent neurons project to remote cardiac ganglia (Bosnjak and Kampine 1982, 1984, 1985)? Are these the same as A neurons in cardiac parasympathetic ganglia (Figure 6.12)?
- How do the LCNs in the ICNS integrate activity in local afferent neurons and in preganglionic CM neurons?
- It is claimed the LCNs project to the stellate ganglion; but what is the evidence for this?

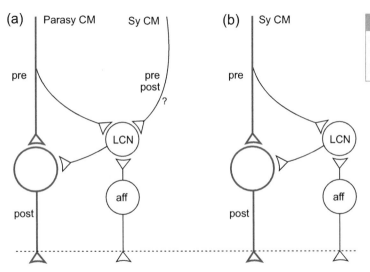

Figure 6.13 Neurons of the intrinsic cardiac nervous system. Aff., local afferent neuron; CM, cardiomotor; LCN, local circuit neuron; parasy, parasympathetic; post, postganglionic; pre, preganglionic; Sy, sympathetic.

- How do LCNs integrate activity in both parasympathetic and sympathetic preganglionic CM neurons?

6.6 Non-Nicotinic Transmission and Potentiation Resulting From Preganglionic Stimulation in Sympathetic Ganglia

Studies of sympathetic ganglia of amphibians and some mammals have shown that electrical stimulation of sympathetic preganglionic axons elicits not only fast nicotinic EPSPs, but also slow muscarinic and slow noncholinergic EPSPs (see Elfvin [1983]; Karczmar et al. [1986]; North [1986]). In most cases, the slow electrical events require repetitive stimulation at nonphysiological frequencies to be detected. The presence of these events has led to the speculation that fast nicotinic synaptic transmission in autonomic ganglia is modulated by long-lasting (muscarinic and noncholinergic) conductance changes and that peptides may be acting as transmitters (Akasu and Koketsu 1986; Katayama and Nishi 1986). In fact the only neuropeptide in autonomic ganglia that has been thoroughly studied so far and shown to have postsynaptic effects as a putative transmitter is a luteinizing hormone-releasing hormone (LHRH)-like peptide in the bullfrog. This peptide coexists with acetylcholine in sympathetic preganglionic neurons with unmyelinated axons that project to vasoconstrictor neurons in paravertebral ganglia (C neurons) regulating blood vessels. It is absent in sympathetic preganglionic neurons that synapse with postganglionic secretomotor neurons (B neurons) in the same paravertebral ganglia that regulate cutaneous glands. The peptide is released when the preganglionic neurons innervating the C neurons are excited repetitively and leads to long-lasting postsynaptic potentials in the B neurons (after diffusing to them). Furthermore, acetylcholine, which is released after repetitive stimulation of the preganglionic axons, generates slow EPSPs by muscarinic action. Both conductance changes are generated by the closing of potassium channels of the M-type (see Table 6.1) (Jan et al. 1979, 1980a, b; Jan and Jan 1982). It has not been shown up to now, even in this well-established example, whether non-nicotinic transmission is relevant in vivo during neural regulation of skin glands and blood vessels in the bullfrog (but see Jobling and Horn [1996]).

There are some reports in the literature indicating that in mammals postganglionic sympathetic neurons projecting to the heart (cardiomotor neurons) and postganglionic muscle vasoconstrictor neurons can be activated in vivo from the central nervous system or through a central reflex pathway via non-nicotinic synaptic mechanisms, i.e., when nicotinic transmission in autonomic ganglia is blocked (Brown 1967, 1969; Henderson and Ungar 1978). Furthermore, blood pressure responses in humans during asphyxia (Freyburger et al. 1950a, b) or during tilting (Fielden et al. 1980) are not completely abolished by blockade of nicotinic transmission in autonomic ganglia.

Questions to be addressed are:

1. Can postganglionic neurons supplying skeletal muscle or skin be activated via non-nicotinic mechanisms in paravertebral ganglia during electrical stimulation of the preganglionic axons?
2. Can the postganglionic neurons be activated or their physiological discharges be modulated by non-nicotinic mechanisms in vivo?

To answer these questions, activity was recorded from postganglionic axons isolated from skin and muscle nerves of the hindlimb and tail of the anesthetized cat. The preganglionic neurons innervating the postganglionic neurons were stimulated electrically or physiologically (by a reflex) (Figure 6.15a). The postganglionic neurons were identified to be vasoconstrictor (skin, skeletal muscle), sudomotor or pilomotor in function.

6.6.1 Responses to Electrical Stimulation of Preganglionic Axons

Decentralized Preparations

In decentralized preparations (preganglionic axons cut, see Figure 6.15a), repetitive supramaximal electrical stimulation of preganglionic axons in the lumbar sympathetic trunk with short trains of impulses (50 stimuli at 25 Hz) elicits (early) high-frequency responses during the train in all postganglionic neurons projecting to the hindlimb and (late) low-frequency responses after the train in many postganglionic neurons. The early high-frequency response is generated by nicotinic action of acetylcholine (i.e., it is blocked by an antagonist of nicotinic receptors such as hexamethonium). The late response is resistant to blockade of nicotinic transmission and is therefore non-nicotinic. These

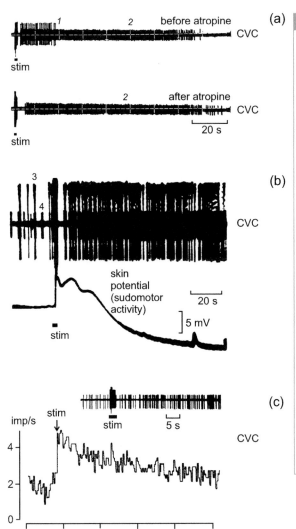

(a)

(b)

(c)

non-nicotinic responses have the following characteristics (Hoffmeister et al. 1978; Jänig et al. 1982, 1983, 1984; Figure 6.14a):

1. They start at a latency of 2 to 10 seconds following the burst of fast (nicotinic) responses and last up to 2 minutes.
2. Sometimes the early component of the slow response can be blocked by atropine (which blocks muscarinic cholinergic receptors), but the late part cannot, even at high concentrations of atropine.
3. The responses in the postganglionic neurons are elicited with trains of 50 stimuli applied to the preganglionic axons at a minimum of 3 to 4 Hz or by 3 to 10 stimuli at 25 Hz.

4. The responses can only be elicited when slowly conducting, mostly unmyelinated, preganglionic axons are stimulated repetitively, i.e., repetitive electrical stimulation of myelinated preganglionic axons only at 25 to 50 Hz for 2 to 5 seconds does not elicit the late responses. Nicotinic responses in the same postganglionic neurons are also elicited when low-threshold faster conducting preganglionic axons are stimulated. Preganglionic neurons with unmyelinated axons that have functional properties of muscle or cutaneous vasoconstrictor neurons have been identified in the lumbar sympathetic outflow and in the sympathetic outflow to the head and neck (Jänig and Szulczyk 1980, 1981; Boczek-Funcke et al.

1993). The physiological firing frequencies of these preganglionic neurons may reach 10 Hz, e.g., by chemoreceptor stimulation during hypoxia (see Table 6.2).

5. The slow non-nicotinic responses occur in most postganglionic neurons supplying skeletal muscle and in about 30% of the postganglionic neurons supplying hairy skin of the cat hindlimb, both being most likely vasoconstrictor in function.

6. Postganglionic pilomotor neurons supplying the tail skin and sudomotor neurons supplying sweat glands in the paw pads do not exhibit late, long-lasting discharges following repetitive electrical stimulation of the preganglionic axons (Figure 6.14b).

These results obtained in vivo in cats clearly demonstrate that impulses can be elicited in sympathetic postganglionic neurons in vivo via non-nicotinic transmission from the preganglionic site in the same way as in vitro, that this synaptic transmission appears to be specific for vasoconstrictor neurons in muscle and skin nerves and that preganglionic neurons with slowly conducting, unmyelinated axons have to be recruited to activate the postganglionic neurons via muscarinic and/or non-cholinergic synaptic mechanisms. This effect probably involves a maintained depolarization (with decreased conductance) of the postganglionic neuron.

Intact Preparations

Can the rate of ongoing discharge present in postganglionic vasoconstrictor neurons in vivo (when the preganglionic axons are not interrupted) be enhanced by non-nicotinic mechanisms following repetitive electrical stimulation of the preganglionic axons? To answer this question, the same experimental design was used as for the experiments on the decentralized preparation, but the preganglionic axons were left intact and spontaneous activity (which is fully dependent on the synaptic input from preganglionic axons) was recorded from the postganglionic neurons (Blumberg and Jänig 1983a; Figure 6.14b, c):

1. Ongoing discharge in most preparations with cutaneous and muscle vasoconstrictor neurons was enhanced for 4 to 40 minutes or longer following repetitive electrical stimulation of preganglionic axons for 2 seconds at 25 Hz. This was not the case for sudomotor neurons (Figure 6.14b).

2. One to two minutes after the train the enhancement reached peak values of 120 to 600% of the control rate of ongoing discharge before the train.

3. The enhancement could only be elicited by stimulus strengths at which the nicotinic response was maximal, i.e., when slowly conducting largely unmyelinated preganglionic axons in the sympathetic trunk were activated.

4. The enhancement could be elicited heterosynaptically. Repetitive electrical stimulation of preganglionic axons in a cut white ramus could enhance ongoing activity in postganglionic neurons generated by intact preganglionic axons converging on the postganglionic neurons.

5. The enhancement was abolished or partially abolished by blockade of muscarinic transmission (by atropine) in some preparations but not in others.

6. The enhancement of activity in cutaneous vasoconstrictor neurons was associated with a long-lasting reduction of blood flow through the skin (Jänig and Koltzenburg 1991).

These results warrant speculation that the enhancement of ongoing discharge occurs in postganglionic vasoconstrictor neurons that receive many weak convergent preganglionic axons or that receive just subthreshold preganglionic synaptic input called "accessory" or "secondary" (Skok and Ivanov 1983; Bratton et al. 2010). After repetitive activation of the small-diameter preganglionic axons, some of these small ineffective synaptic events could be enhanced by an increase in membrane resistance generated by closure of potassium channels (e.g., of the M-type).

These slow responses generated in vivo in sympathetic postganglionic by repetitive electrical stimulation of preganglionic axons could never be reproduced in vitro in the guinea pig, rat or rabbit (McLachlan, unpublished observations).

6.6.2 Reflexes in Vasoconstrictor Neurons Mediated by Non-Nicotinic Mechanisms

Stimulation of arterial chemoreceptors (e.g., by systemic hypoxia: ventilation of the animal with a gas mixture of 8% O_2 in N_2) elicits reflex activation of muscle vasoconstrictor neurons and reflex inhibition of cutaneous vasoconstrictor neurons, both being among the strongest reflex responses known in these neurons. This reflex is mediated by neuronal circuits in the medulla oblongata for the muscle vasoconstrictor neurons and probably also through the hypothalamus for the cutaneous vasoconstrictor neurons (Jänig 1975; Gregor and Jänig, 1977; see Subchapter 10.4) (Figure 6.15b, left). After blockade of nicotinic transmission (with hexamethonium) in sympathetic ganglia, which leads to the disappearance of the centrally generated spontaneous activity in the vasoconstrictor neurons and to disappearance of fast nicotinic responses generated by electrical single-pulse stimulation of preganglionic axons, muscle vasoconstrictor neurons can still be activated reflexly, as in the control (before blockade of nicotinic transmission). This response is accompanied by an increased blood pressure and is either partially or completely blocked by atropine or not affected (Figure 6.15b, c, left side). Corresponding to the reflex activation of the muscle vasoconstrictor neurons via a non-nicotinic mechanism, the postganglionic neurons exhibited afterdischarges to repetitive

electrical stimulation of the preganglionic axons (Figure 6.15b, c right side). Cutaneous vasoconstrictor neurons that were normally reflexly inhibited during arterial chemoreceptor stimulation were not activated after blockade of nicotinic transmission and after additional blockade of muscarinic transmission. However, they showed late discharges in response to repetitive electrical stimulation of the preganglionic axons (not shown in Figure 6.15).

These results clearly show that:

1. postganglionic vasoconstrictor neurons can be physiologically activated after complete blockade of nicotinic transmission or, in some cases, blockade of both nicotinic and muscarinic transmission in the paravertebral ganglia, and
2. the artificially elicited synchronous discharges in the preganglionic neurons, as they occur during electrical stimulation of the preganglionic axons, are not necessary for driving the postganglionic

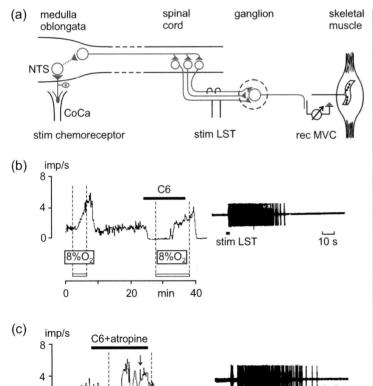

Figure 6.15 Reflex activation of a postganglionic muscle vasoconstrictor (MVC) neuron projecting to the cat hindlimb via non-nicotinic transmission in a paravertebral ganglion. Activity was recorded in a single MVC neuron. (a) Experimental setup. CoCa, common carotid artery; LST, lumbar sympathetic trunk; NTS, nucleus tractus solitarii. (b,c) Stimulation of arterial chemoreceptors (ventilation of the animal with a gas mixture of 8% O_2 in N_2 [lower open bars]) activated the MVC neuron (b) before and after intra-arterial (i.a.) injection of hexamethonium (C6, 12.1 mg/kg infused over 13 min) and (c) after i.a. injection of C6 (26 mg/kg infused over 19 min) in the presence of atropine (1 mg/kg i.a.). Drugs were injected retrogradely into the internal iliac artery close to the caudal lumbar paravertebral ganglia. At 276 min in (c) an additional dose of 0.4 mg atropine was injected i.a. (arrow). The records on the right show the responses of the MVC neuron to repetitive electrical stimulation of the preganglionic axons in the LST (stim. LST; 50 stimuli at 25 Hz, 8 V/0.2 ms) during block of nicotinic transmission by C6 before (b) and after (c) atropine. Note that the early part of the long-lasting response in the MVC neuron was blocked by atropine. Nicotinic blockade generated by C6 was regularly confirmed by the absence of responses of the postganglionic neurons to single-pulse stimuli applied to the preganglionic axons in the LST at 1 per 5 s. Time scale in (b) and (c) (left) indicates time after start of the experiment. Modified from Jänig et al. (1983).

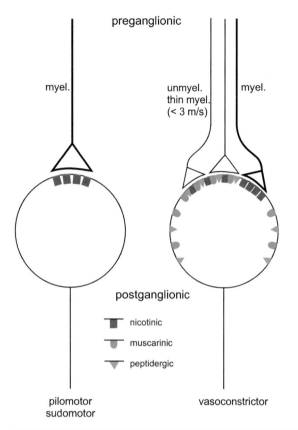

pilomotor
sudomotor

vasoconstrictor

Figure 6.16 Transmission of impulses from pre- to postganglionic vasoconstrictor neurons in paravertebral ganglia in the cat via a non-nicotinic mechanism. Stimulation of myelinated preganglionic fibers (conduction velocity >3 m/s) with single pulses or repetitively (at 25 to 50 Hz for 2 to 5 s) excites the postganglionic neurons only via nicotinic synaptic transmission. Stimulation of unmyelinated and some small-diameter myelinated preganglionic axons (conduction velocity <3 m/s) may excite the postganglionic neurons via nicotinic and muscarinic mechanisms and via a non-cholinergic (possibly peptidergic) mechanism. The receptors for the muscarinic and non-cholinergic mechanisms may be located subsynaptically and extrasynaptically. Postganglionic sudomotor and pilomotor neurons cannot be excited via these non-nicotinic mechanisms.

neurons via non-nicotinic mechanisms in the paravertebral ganglia.

In conclusion (Figure 6.16), nicotinic transmission in postganglionic vasoconstrictor neurons can undergo a long-lasting enhancement when preganglionic neurons with slowly conducting axons are activated. This enhancement can also be elicited heterosynaptically (e.g., enhancing ongoing activity by stimulation of a cut white ramus), and involves muscarinic and non-cholinergic mechanisms. It is specific for vasoconstrictor pathways. The membrane events that mediate long-term synaptic processes and the transmitter(s) (peptides?) that mediate(s) the non-cholinergic discharges in the vasoconstrictor neurons are unknown.

In view of the unphysiologically high-frequency stimulation of the preganglionic axons that has to be used, it is assumed that the cholinergic muscarinic and putative peptidergic synaptic transmission is mediated by both subsynaptic and extrasynaptic receptors in the postganglionic cell membrane involving volume transmission. However, three experimental findings argue that the long-lasting non-nicotinic discharges are preferentially mediated subsynaptically: (1) High-frequency electrical stimulation of myelinated preganglionic axons conducting at ≥ 3 m/s did not elicit long-lasting discharges in the postganglionic neurons (Jänig et al. 1984); thus, the non-nicotinic responses can only be generated by stimulation of preganglionic axons conducting at ≤ 3 m/s. (2) The non-nicotinic responses can only be generated in postganglionic vasoconstrictor neurons, but not in pilomotor or sudomotor neurons (Figure 6.14). (3) Massive reflex activation of muscle vasoconstrictor neurons by strong stimulation of arterial chemoreceptors did not activate cutaneous vasoconstrictor neurons (Jänig et al. 1983).

Finally, I hypothesize that the central nervous system could use this mechanism of long-lasting enhancement of synaptic transmission in sympathetic ganglia to regulate the level of ongoing activity in postganglionic vasoconstrictor neurons by means of short bursts of activity of at least 3–4 Hz intraburst frequency and at long intervals between the bursts, being in the range of several minutes in preganglionic neurons with slowly conducting largely unmyelinated axons.

6.6.3 Non-Cholinergic Ganglionic Transmission to Postganglionic Vasodilator Neurons Supplying the Uterine Artery

Arteries of the female internal sexual organs of guinea pigs are innervated by vasodilator neurons located in the paracervical ganglia that receive synaptic input from sympathetic preganglionic neurons projecting through the lumbar splanchnic and hypogastric nerves. Each postganglionic vasodilator neuron receives synaptic input from about two preganglionic axons, one being strong (Jobling et al. 2003). Activation of the preganglionic neurons in vitro generates vasodilation by release of nitric oxide (NO) and VIP from the postganglionic vasodilator fibers. Repetitive electrical stimulation of the sympathetic preganglionic axons at 10 Hz generates repetitive discharge of the postganglionic vasodilator neurons, produced by a slow excitatory postsynaptic potential, and a vasodilation, both outlasting the train of stimulation for a considerable period. Continuous activation of postganglionic neurons and vasodilation are only slightly reduced by blockade of nicotinic transmission in the paracervical ganglia. The ganglionic transmitter involved is unknown, but unlikely to be substance P, adenosine triphosphate, 5-hydroxytryptamine, glutamate or acetylcholine (muscarinic action) (Morris et al. 2005). The continuous discharge of the postganglionic neurons cannot be a long-term potentiation of cholinergic transmission since it also occurs after complete block of cholinergic transmission and since synaptic transmission normally occurs via a strong cholinergic synapse.

This mechanism to generate and maintain activity in pelvic vasodilator neurons (and possibly secretomotor neurons) ties up with observations, made in the cat, that preganglionic non-vasoconstrictor neurons (here collectively called motility-regulating neurons) projecting in the lumbar splanchnic nerves can be activated reflexly for up to 12 minutes by short-lasting mechanical stimulation of sacral afferents (e.g., from the anal canal) as described in Subchapter 4.3 (see Figure 4.15; Bahr et al. 1986a). The mechanism underlying this long-lasting reflex activation lies in the sacro-lumbar spinal pathways. Thus, a centrally potentiated spinal reflex in preganglionic neurons would be further amplified by non-cholinergic synaptic transmission in the paracervical ganglia. This sequential cascade of amplification of a central signal could be important in the neural regulation of reproductive organs.

Conclusions

1. Synaptic transmission from preganglionic to postganglionic neurons in autonomic ganglia is cholinergic nicotinic. Most autonomic ganglia transmit the central message with high accuracy to the postganglionic neurons. This concurs with the idea that the target tissues innervated by the neurons in these ganglia are predominantly under control of the central nervous system.

2. A relatively small number of sympathetic preganglionic neurons connect with a large number of postganglionic neurons by divergence of the preganglionic axons. The number of postganglionic neurons is lower in parasympathetic pathways. This divergence has primarily a distribution function. In addition, postganglionic neurons receive convergent synaptic input from several preganglionic neurons. The degree of divergence and convergence varies between different final autonomic pathways and between species.

3. Almost all neurons in sympathetic paravertebral and parasympathetic ganglia and some neurons in sympathetic prevertebral ganglia with convergent synaptic input generally receive one (sometimes two or rarely three) strong (suprathreshold) preganglionic synaptic inputs, the other synaptic inputs being weak (subthreshold). Discharges in these postganglionic neurons are generated by these strong synaptic inputs, but usually not by summation of several weak synaptic inputs.

4. Based on neurophysiological properties and mainly the presence of voltage- and calcium-dependent potassium channels, sympathetic postganglionic neurons in guinea pigs and rodents consist electrophysiologically of three broad classes:

   a. Phasic neurons respond with a burst of action potentials at the beginning of suprathreshold current steps. Almost all paravertebral and 15% to 25% of the prevertebral neurons are phasic. These neurons receive one or two strong synaptic inputs from preganglionic axons and are fully under the control of the central nervous system. They rarely receive peripheral synaptic input.

   b. Tonic neurons discharge rhythmically throughout a current step. These neurons are numerous in prevertebral ganglia and practically absent in paravertebral ganglia. They receive weak preganglionic synaptic inputs and many receive weak synaptic inputs from the periphery (mainly from intestinofugal neurons of the gastrointestinal tract). They have an integrative function. They are non-vasoconstrictor, being mainly involved in regulation of motility and secretion in the gastrointestinal tract.

c. Neurons with long afterhyperpolarization following an action potential (LAH neurons) discharge one action potential at the beginning of a current step. Most LAH neurons are located in the celiac ganglion and a few in paravertebral ganglia. They receive one strong synaptic input and rarely peripheral synaptic inputs. They are fully under the control of the central nervous system and have relay function. They are non-vasoconstrictor and are mainly involved in secretion and absorption and/or motility.

5. The number of postganglionic neurons innervated by one preganglionic neuron is called the autonomic neural unit (ANU). Functionally defined ANUs are smaller than anatomically defined ANUs, since only postganglionic neurons that receive a strong synaptic input from a preganglionic neuron are activated. The size of ANUs varies according to function; e.g., ANUs of a vasoconstrictor pathway are larger than ANUs of the pupillomotor pathway.

6. Some neurons in sympathetic prevertebral ganglia receive, in addition to several preganglionic inputs and cholinergic synaptic inputs from peripheral intestinofugal neurons, peptidergic synaptic inputs from collaterals of spinal visceral afferents. These postganglionic neurons are involved in the regulation of non-vascular functions.

7. In many sympathetic neurons of the prevertebral ganglia, and in some parasympathetic ganglia, the central synaptic input is weak or even may play a subordinate role. The way in which central synaptic input and peripheral synaptic inputs are integrated in vivo by these prevertebral postganglionic neurons is unclear. In cardiac parasympathetic ganglia, postganglionic neurons may receive, in addition to strong preganglionic inputs, usually small peripheral afferent synaptic inputs and probably inputs from interneurons. Their function is not known.

8. Nicotinic synaptic transmission in sympathetic ganglia can be enhanced by muscarinic and non-cholinergic (peptidergic) mechanisms. For vasoconstrictor systems, it has been shown in vivo that ongoing activity can be enhanced for up to tens of minutes by these non-nicotinic mechanisms following short bursts of activation from a subgroup of preganglionic neurons.

9. Reflex activity can be transmitted to postganglionic vasoconstrictor neurons by non-nicotinic mechanisms. This leads to amplification of the efferent signal in the time domain in vivo.

Suggested Reading

Gibbins, I. L., Jobling, P., Messenger, J. P., Teo, E. H. and Morris, J. L. (2000) Neuronal morphology and the synaptic organisation of sympathetic ganglia. *J Auton Nerv Syst* **81**, 104–109.

Gibbins, I. L., Jobling, P., Teo, E. H., Matthew, S. E. and Morris, J. L. (2003a) Heterogeneous expression of SNAP-25 and synaptic vesicle proteins by central and peripheral inputs to sympathetic neurons. *J Comp Neurol* **459**, 25–43.

Gibbins, I. L. and Morris, J. L. (2006) Structure of peripheral synapses: autonomic ganglia. *Cell Tissue Res* **326**, 205–220.

Keast, J. R. (2006) Plasticity of pelvic autonomic ganglia and urogenital innervation. *Int Rev Cytol* **248**, 141–208.

McLachlan, E. M., Davies, P. J., Häbler, H. J. and Jamieson, J. (1997) On-going and reflex synaptic events in rat superior cervical ganglion cells. *J Physiol (Lond)* **501**, 165–181.

McLachlan, E. M., Häbler, H. J., Jamieson, J. and Davies, P. J. (1998) Analysis of the periodicity of synaptic events in neurones in the superior cervical ganglion of anaesthetized rats. *J Physiol* **511**, 461–478.

Morris, J. L. and Gibbins, I. L. (2006) Structure of peripheral synapses: autonomic ganglia. *Cell Tissue Res* **326**, 205–220.

Skok, V. I. (2002) Nicotinic acetylcholine receptors in autonomic ganglia. *Auton Neurosci* **97**, 1–11.

Young, H. M., Cane, K. N. and Anderson, S. R. (2011) Development of the autonomic nervous system: a comparative view. *Auton Neurosci* **165**, 10–27.

All references cited in the text are available online at www.cambridge.org/janig.

Notes

1. Release of acetylcholine requires the presence of SNARE (soluble NSF [N-ethylmaleimide-sensitive factor] attachment protein receptors) proteins in the presynaptic boutons, which are necessary for the fusion of the synaptic vesicle membrane with the presynaptic plasma membrane. Release of peptides does not seem to require SNARE proteins and is therefore insensitive to botulinum toxin. SNARE proteins are present in presynaptic specializations, but absent or reduced in boutons not forming synapses (Gibbins et al. 2003b). Furthermore, there may be differences between synapses formed by

peripheral afferent neurons and those formed by preganglionic fibers.

2. Voltage clamp recordings from sympathetic neurons in the presence of tetrodotoxin (TTX, to block the primary Na^+ component of the action potential) revealed that, in neurons with only one strong preganglionic input, a single high-threshold Ca^{2+} "spike" was initiated by depolarization of the soma, presumably because voltage control of the site of initiation of this action potential was incomplete. This suggests that the voltage-dependent Ca^{2+} channels that were activated by the EPSP lay somewhere (electrically distant) on the dendritic tree. In neurons with two strong inputs, two unclamped Ca^{2+} spikes with distinct depolarization thresholds and different configurations were recorded (Hirst and McLachlan 1986). This raises the possibility that each strong input is associated with a cluster of voltage-dependent Ca^{2+} channels and that, if there is more than one, they are isolated from each other by the somatic voltage clamp, i.e., they lie on separate dendrites.

3. Similarly, phasic and tonic neurons have been identified in rat, mouse, rabbit and cat autonomic ganglia; subtypes with slightly different characteristics have sometimes been defined (e.g., rat superior cervical ganglion, Wang and McKinnon [1995]; guinea pig inferior mesenteric ganglion, Weems and Szurszewski [1978], King and Szurszewski [1988]; rat intracardiac ganglia, Rimmer and Harper [2006]), generally by using suprathreshold depolarization.

4. The ongoing discharge in sympathetic paravertebral postganglionic neurons projecting to the hindlimb in cats or rats is physiologically entirely of central origin. Decentralization of paravertebral ganglia (transection of the preganglionic axons innervating the postganglionic neurons) in cats or rats always abolishes the ongoing activity in the postganglionic neurons supplying skin or skeletal muscle (Häbler and Jänig, unpublished observation). Furthermore, ≥99% of the ongoing activity in

postganglionic neurons in the inferior mesenteric ganglion of the cat that project through the hypogastric nerve to the pelvic organs are of central origin (Jänig et al. 1991). The neurons have vasoconstrictor and non-vasoconstrictor functions. These data seem at variance with data obtained on isolated ganglia in vitro showing that a subpopulation of prevertebral postganglionic neurons may generate spontaneous activity without synaptic input from preganglionic neurons and from peripheral neurons (celiac ganglion [Gola and Niel 1993]; ganglia on the serosal surface of the cat colon [Krier and Hartman 1984]; intracardiac ganglia [Xi et al. 1991; Selyanko 1992]); inferior mesenteric ganglion [Cassell and McLachlan, 1986; Julé and Szurszewski 1993a]; vesical pelvic ganglia [Griffith et al. 1980]). These ganglia are associated with visceral organs. It was postulated that the ganglia contain pacemaker cells which may synaptically transmit their activity to other ganglion cells (Gola and Niel 1993; Julé and Szurszewski 1993a, b). However, McLachlan and Meckler (1989) found spontaneous activity in a small number of postganglionic neurons of the inferior mesenteric ganglion and no pacemaker activity in postganglionic sympathetic neurons of the celiac ganglion in vitro. The recording conditions (intracellular vs. patch electrodes), ionic concentrations, etc., may be responsible.

5. In the cat, about 90% of the efferent axons in the hypogastric nerve are postganglionic and 10% preganglionic (Baron et al. 1985b). In the male rat less than 30% of the efferent axons in the hypogastric nerve are postganglionic and 70% preganglionic (Baron and Jänig 1991). The same applies to the hypogastric nerve of the male guinea pig; in the female guinea pig about 50% of the efferent axons are preganglionic (McLachlan 1985). These histological data imply that many sympathetic postganglionic neurons innervating pelvic organs are located in the caudal part of the inferior mesenteric ganglion in cats and in the pelvic ganglia of rats and guinea pigs.

Chapter 7

Mechanisms of Neuroeffector Transmission

Impulse activity in the preganglionic neurons is the result of integrative processes in the spinal cord and brain stem (see Chapters 9 and 10). Such top-down signaling (i.e., the central message) is not generally distorted in the ganglia of the final autonomic pathways. It is modified by synaptic input from peripheral neurons in a few autonomic pathways to the viscera (see Subchapters 5.7 and 6.5). The central message is distributed to a large population of postganglionic neurons, but confined to the respective autonomic pathways. Thus, transmission of impulses from preganglionic neurons to postganglionic neurons occurs within the same final autonomic pathway, but not between autonomic pathways. In this chapter I will discuss some mechanisms by which centrally generated messages are transmitted from postganglionic neurons to the target cells (effectors).

The mechanism of neuroeffector transmission varies considerably between target tissues. This is a consequence of there being many different functional types of cells innervated by postganglionic neurons (see Table 1.2). However, autonomic neuroeffector transmission has been studied in only a few cases. These studies clearly demonstrate that the impulse activity in postganglionic neurons is transmitted to the effector cells in a rather specific way and this may apply to *all* autonomically innervated

effector cells. This view does not preclude the idea that the activity in some autonomic effector cells is also modified by multiple non-neural influences and that these non-neural components may operate during ongoing regulation of the target tissues. However, in the context of this book, the important points in the neural regulation of autonomic effector cells are: (1) that the central message reaches the target tissue via differentiated structures and (2) that specific mechanisms occurring at neuroeffector junctions are an important basis for the precise regulation of autonomic target organs and tissues by the brain.

In the last part of this chapter I will: (1) summarize the interaction of the centrally generated neural signal with other neural and non-neural signals in the regulation of target cells and (2) describe some unconventional functions of sympathetic postganglionic axons that are not dependent on the generation of action potentials or on the release of noradrenaline.

7.1   Transmitter Substances in Postganglionic Neurons

The principles of chemical transmission were originally defined in the peripheral autonomic nervous system based on the release of the "conventional" neurotransmitters, acetylcholine and noradrenaline. However, it is now clear that, in addition to acetylcholine and noradrenaline, other putative neurotransmitters are contained within individual autonomic neurons. These may have multiple actions on effector tissues (Furness et al. 1989; Morris and Gibbins 1992; Hoyle et al. 2002):

- Most sympathetic postganglionic axons release noradrenaline, but sympathetic sudomotor and, in some species, muscle vasodilator axons are cholinergic. Whether these cholinergic vasodilator axons exist in human beings remains controversial (see Subchapter 4.2). Significantly, not all effects generated by stimulation of postganglionic sympathetic nerve axons can be abolished by antagonists of either adrenoceptors or muscarinic receptors.
- All parasympathetic postganglionic neurons are cholinergic, defined by the presence of choline acetyltransferase (ChAT) in these neurons (Keast 1995; Keast et al. 1995; McLachlan 1995). However, not all effects of stimulating parasympathetic nerve axons are blocked by muscarinic antagonists; these must therefore be mediated by another transmitter or transmitters. Nicotinic cholinergic receptors are absent from effector cells supplied by parasympathetic postganglionic neurons.
- Postganglionic autonomic neurons, the excitatory effects of which are not in any way modified by antagonists to the conventional transmitters acetylcholine or noradrenaline, have been called non-adrenergic non-cholinergic (NANC) neurons and by analogy the transmission is referred to as NANC transmission.
- NANC transmission has been studied extensively in the enteric nervous system, where this transmission is thought to mediate inhibition of gastrointestinal smooth muscle by enteric neurons. The compounds that may be involved in NANC transmission are nitric oxide (NO), adenosine triphosphate (ATP) or a neuropeptide (e.g., vasoactive intestinal peptide [VIP], neuropeptide Y [NPY], galanin [GAL], etc.). "Nitrergic" nerves (containing the enzyme neuronal nitric oxide synthase [NOS]) are vasodilator or relaxant in several tissues. Neuropeptides (tachykinins, calcitonin generelated peptide [CGRP], etc.) released from sensory

nerve endings, when activated, also take part in NANC transmission (see Subchapter 6.5).

Responses of tissues (contraction, secretion, etc.) to nerve-released noradrenaline or acetylcholine mostly only occur following repetitive activation of many axons. In addition, high-frequency stimuli, particularly in bursts, may be required to recruit effector responses due to the concomitant release of a neuropeptide.

Immunohistochemistry has revealed the presence of many peptides in the postganglionic neurons (cell bodies and nerve terminals). This has led to the concept of "neurochemical coding" of autonomic neurons (Subchapter 1.4). However, there are quite some differences between species and only a few of these peptides have been demonstrated to modify effector function after release from nerve terminals in vivo and the functional role of these peptides during ongoing regulation of the target cells still awaits clarification. Some known examples follow:

- Neuropeptide Y in sympathetic vasoconstrictor axons evokes vasoconstriction in some arteries, whereas in others it potentiates the effects of noradrenaline on the contractile apparatus (Lundberg 1996). In the heart, NPY released by sympathetic cardiomotor neurons acts prejunctionally to attenuate the decrease of heart frequency produced by activation of parasympathetic cardiomotor neurons (Potter 1987).
- Vasoactive intestinal peptide is thought to be the primary *vasodilator* transmitter released from cholinergic vasodilator, sudomotor and secretomotor axons (Gibbins 1994; Lundberg 1996).

Vasoconstriction in some vascular beds, such as those in the skin and mesentery, is in part regulated by interactions between sympathetic axons and the terminals of primary afferent nociceptive neurons that express substance P and CGRP. However, it is a matter of debate whether this interaction only occurs postjunctionally at the level of the vascular smooth muscle or also involves prejunctional interactions between the two types of neuronal terminals (Häbler et al. 1997b). CGRP released by axon reflex activation (Note 1) of afferent terminals during inflammation is a potent vasodilator (Holzer 1992, 2002a, b). Substance P released by axon reflex activation also contributes to precapillary vasodilation, but mainly to venular plasma extravasation (Häbler et al. 1997b, 1999).

Table 7.1 lists transmitter substances (primary transmitters) or putative transmitter substances in autonomic postganglionic neurons. In most neurons, the primary transmitter is either acetylcholie or noradrenaline; in a few neurons, another compound has been established as a transmitter. In most postganglionic neurons with colocalized neurotransmitter, the functions of the peptides are entirely unclear. The presence of a neuropeptide in an autonomic neuron, the release of that neuropeptide during nerve stimulation and the presence of the receptors for the same neuropeptide on the target cells (neurons or effector cells) do not reveal whether the neuropeptide is normally, or under pathophysiological conditions, used during neural regulation of that target tissue. For example, no entirely convincing experiment has been performed that illustrates a functional context for neurally released NPY on autonomically innervated target tissues, although it has been shown that this peptide is released into the blood during activity of muscle vasoconstrictor neurons and that its concentration increases during exercise (Morris et al. 1986; Pernow 1988). The same is true for VIP, which is colocalized with acetylcholine in sympathetic postganglionic neurons innervating sweat glands (Lundberg 1981) and in parasympathetic postganglionic neurons innervating the erectile tissue of sexual organs (de Groat and Booth 1993; de Groat 2013).

7.2 Principles of Neuroeffector Transmission in the Autonomic Nervous System

The membranes of the autonomic effector cells contain a large number of receptors that are activated by signaling molecules to which the cells are potentially exposed, leading to modulation of cellular effectors (ionic channels, contractile proteins, transcription, metabolic processes, secretion). Three functional types of membrane receptors regulate cellular effectors: ligand-gated receptors, G-protein-coupled receptors and catalytic receptors. The high number and differential expression of membrane receptors, the multiple intracellular pathways that potentially regulate cellular effectors, as well as the interactions between these intracellular pathways lead to an enormous variety of responses of autonomic effector organs. However, where the postjunctional actions of postganglionic autonomic neurons have been studied under physiological conditions, only a limited

Table 7.1 | Transmitter substances in autonomic neurons

System	Neuron	Transmitter	Cotransmitters
Parasympathetic	Preganglionic	ACh	
	Postganglionic	ACh	VIP and/or NO
Sympathetic	Preganglionic	ACh	
	Postganglionic	NAd	ATP and/or NPY
Enteric	[Vagal and pelvic inputs ACh]		
	[Sympathetic inputs NAd]		
	Intrinsic afferent neurons	Substance P (tachykinins)	
	Interneurons	ACh	Some ATP
	Motor neurons excitatory	ACh	Substance P (tachykinins)
	Motor neurons inhibitory	NO/VIP/PACAP/?ATP	
	Secretomotor	ACh	VIP

ACh, acetylcholine; ATP, adenosine triphosphate; NAd, noradrenaline; NO, nitric oxide; NPY, neuropeptide Y; PACAP, pituitary adenylate cyclase activating peptide; VIP, vasoactive intestinal polypeptide

For further data about cotransmitters and neuropeptides in enteric neurons see Table 5.1.
Modified from Jänig and McLachlan (2013).

population of membrane receptors are activated by the released transmitter(s) and these act on tissue-specific cellular pathways to generate the cellular effector responses. However, the conditions in in vivo experiments are very variable and can explain the diversity of responses. This is the basis for the diversity of the autonomic effector responses generated by neural signals (see Table 7.1).

In peripheral tissues, the effects of activity in autonomic nerve terminals can be due to the release of several different compounds. However, failure to block effector responses by either adrenoceptor or muscarinic receptor antagonists at concentrations that entirely abolish the response to exogenously applied transmitter is not proof for the existence of NANC transmitters. This is because exogenous transmitter predominately acts on extrajunctional receptors (i.e., located at sites outside the neuroeffector junctions), whereas neuronally released transmitter primarily acts on junctional receptors (i.e. selectively located at the neuroeffector junctions) and these may be different. Furthermore, reuptake mechanisms in prejunctional terminals and tissue acetylcholine esterase can markedly reduce the concentration of exogenously applied transmitter that reaches the junctional receptors. It is also possible that the extrajunctional and junctional receptors are similar, but they mediate their effects by differing intracellular mechanisms. The effects of exogenously applied transmitter substances on cellular functions are known for many tissues, but the mechanisms of activation of these tissues by neurally released transmitters (see Table 7.1) have been under-investigated. This latter type of activation is biologically the most important, as it transmits the centrally generated neural signal from the postganglionic neurons to the target cells. Where these studies have been performed, the mechanisms of neuroeffector transmission have been found to be diverse. The important concept that has emerged from these studies is that the mechanism utilized by endogenously released transmitter is often not the same as that activated by exogenous transmitter substances or their analogs (Hirst et al. 1992, 1996).

Excitation or inhibition may involve a range of cellular events (Note 2):

- Brief openings of ligand-gated channels (as at many neuronal synapses) or slower conductance changes mediated by second-messenger systems.

- An ensuing membrane voltage change may open or close voltage-dependent channels. For example, depolarization may open voltage-dependent calcium channels leading to Ca^{2+} influx.
- Receptor activation may cause G-protein activation and release of Ca^{2+} from intracellular Ca^{2+} stores or modulation of the Ca^{2+} sensitivity of the contractile/secretory mechanism.
- Receptor activation (e.g., β-adrenoceptors) may be linked to adenylate cyclase and modify cell function by changing intracellular levels of cyclic adenosine monophosphate (cAMP).
- Inhibition (relaxation) often involves the activation of cyclic guanosine monophosphate (cGMP)-dependent protein kinases.

7.2.1 The Autonomic Effector Cells and Their Innervation

The autonomic effector cells are very diverse, the most common types being smooth muscle cells, cardiac muscle cells and secretory epithelia (Table 1.2). The cytoplasm of the adjacent cells, when of the same type, in these autonomic effector tissues is usually connected by gap-junction channels that allow electrical and chemical signals to pass directly between neighboring cells. Thus, the cells in these tissues form *functional syncytia*, with neurally evoked signals spreading directly from cell to cell. This means that not all effector cells need to be directly innervated. In smooth muscle innervated by sympathetic nerves (e.g., vas deferens and arterial vessels), the current injected by the action of transmitter released spontaneously onto individual cells flows rapidly through low-resistance gap-junction channels into neighboring cells and as a consequence potential change at the point source is brief. When nerves are stimulated, the transmitter is released at many points (i.e., from many varicosities) throughout a smooth muscle, and the current spreading through the gap-junction channels from each point source uniformly changes the membrane potential of the whole tissue. In this case, where the tissue is uniformly polarized, the time course of the potential change will be determined by a relatively slow process of charge dissipation across the cell membrane; i.e., the membrane time constant of decay is dependent on the resistance and capacitance of the cell membranes. This behavior of the electrically coupled cells makes the study of synaptic transmission from postganglionic autonomic axons to the effector cells technically difficult and difficult to interpret (Note 3). The responses of the syncytia are generally mediated by intracellular signaling (Ca^{2+} etc.) in and between the postjunctional cells and may not involve membrane potential changes.

The axons of a postganglionic autonomic neuron branch extensively within the tissues they innervate and form many varicosities along the nerve terminal axons. These varicosities are about 1 μm or less in diameter with the intervaricosity axon being 0.1–0.2 μm in diameter. The varicosities contain numerous vesicles (up to ~1000) that store transmitter substances and contain the biochemical machinery for synthesis, release, reuptake and metabolization of the transmitter substances. Each postganglionic axon forms hundreds to thousands of varicosities in their terminal branches, the number of which depends on the size of the target tissue and its function. Axons of sympathetic postganglionic vasoconstrictor neurons have up to 10 000 varicosities, while parasympathetic postganglionic axons projecting to the eye or axons of enteric motoneurons acting locally on circular or longitudinal smooth muscles have several hundred varicosities.

At the skeletal neuromuscular endplate, acetylcholine is released in quanta from the stores of vesicles in the nerve terminals into the synaptic cleft at the neuromuscular endplate. After release, the transmitter reaches a high concentration in the synaptic cleft for a short time and reacts with acetylcholine receptors in the postsynaptic membrane close to the site of release. This causes transient opening of specific non-selective cation channels via nicotinic acetylcholine (ACh) receptors, resulting in a brief excitatory synaptic current and a consequent endplate potential. The enzyme acetylcholinesterase, present in the synaptic cleft, breaks down acetylcholine to form choline and acetic acid in about 0.1 ms and thereby limits the action of acetylcholine and prevents diffusion of acetylcholine out of the synaptic cleft. This process of chemical transmission of an electrical signal from the terminal of motor axons to the skeletal muscle fibers is restricted to the neuromuscular endplate and shows a high safety factor for transmission (i.e., a single action potential in the motor nerve always evokes a single muscle action potential and muscle twitch because the endplate potential is much larger than the threshold).

Chemical transmission at autonomic neuroeffector junctions is also often spatially restricted but does not exhibit the high safety factor.

A widely held misconception that arose from early electron microscopic studies is that tissues innervated by postganglionic autonomic neurons do not have a specialized neuroeffector apparatus. Rather, varicosities were found to be located at variable distances from the effector cells with few varicosities in close apposition to the effector cells. The consequences of this arrangement would be that the transmitter is released at variable distances with neurotransmitters acting like a local hormone to activate widely distributed receptors on the effector cells. This type of neuroeffector communication has been assumed to be the *status quo*, particularly for the sympathetic postganglionic axons. It has fostered the belief that the effect of postganglionic noradrenergic neurons on the effector cells can be equated with the effect of noradrenaline or a cotransmitter that is superfused over the preparation, i.e., that endogenous and exogenous neurotransmitters act in the same way. However, experimental, morphological and functional studies in tissues from experimental animals that have investigated the process of neuroeffector transmission radically contradict this conventional concept:

1. In many autonomically innervated target tissues so far investigated, quantitative structural analysis of the neuroeffector apparatus at the electron microscopic level clearly shows that many varicosities located within 1–2 μm of the tissue form close contacts with effector cells and make structurally specialized neuroeffector contacts (Table 7.2).
2. Transmitter released from these varicosities often produces responses that are quite different from those of the same transmitter applied exogenously to the preparation. Neurally released transmitter interacts with specialized junctional receptors, which can have different properties from extrajunctional receptors activated by the same transmitter when exogenously applied (Hirst et al. 1992, 1996).

There is no doubt that, in some tissues where close neuroeffector junctions have not been identified, nerve-released transmitter may stimulate receptors over the surface of the effector cells and, during continuous nerve activation, transmitter concentration can build up in the "biophase." Whether or not this situation actually occurs in vivo is not clear.

7.2.2 Morphology of the Neuroeffector Junction

Precise transmission of the signals in postganglionic neurons to the effector cells requires a spatially close association between the varicosities and the effector cells. However, random histological thin sections give the false impression that most varicosities do not make close contact with the effector cells, that the gaps between varicosities and effector cells are very variable and that close contacts with the innervated tissue are rare. This is also true of skeletal muscle, unless the sections are sampled from the middle of the muscle in the vicinity of the endplates, particularly when ultrathin sections are taken for electron microscopy. The shortcoming of such sampling is that the relationship between a varicosity and the target tissue is assumed to be retained throughout the entire surface of the varicosity. This turns out *not* to be the case when electron microscopy is used to investigate serial sections of varicosities and the relationships between pre- and postjunctional membranes are revealed in three-dimensional reconstructions. Such an approach has been used for various autonomically innervated tissues (for references see Table 7.2) and the following parameters were assessed quantitatively: percentage of varicosities forming junctions, size of the area on the effector cell surface occupied by the junction and volume of the varicosity (for detailed data and references see Table 7.2).

The sympathetic and parasympathetic neuroeffector junctions investigated so far have the following characteristics (Figure 7.1, Table 7.2):

- Most varicosities that lose part of their Schwann cell sheath form organized neuroeffector junctions with nearby target cells. These junctions cover from 0.1% to 1% of the effector cell surface.
- At the junction, the basal laminae covering the effector cell and the varicosity fuse.
- The neuroeffector gap is >50 nm wide.
- In the varicosities forming neuroeffector contacts, the small vesicles that contain the transmitter(s) accumulate at the membrane facing the junctional cleft. In contrast, large vesicles that contain neuropeptides, in addition to a classical transmitter, do not have a preferential location within

varicosities. In varicosities, which are exposed through a gap in the Schwann cell covering but do not form neuroeffector contacts (no fused basal laminae), both small and large synaptic vesicles are homogeneously distributed.

- Prejunctional membrane specialization (i.e., thickening with vesicles accumulating to the point of contact) has been reported for some varicosities but no postjunctional membrane specializations have been detected.

These morphological characteristics of the neuroeffector junctions clearly indicate that chemical transmission may occur at these sites. The physiological function of non-contacting varicosities remains unclear. There appears to be a difference in the proportion of varicosities forming neuroeffector junctions between arterioles and muscular arteries. In the guinea-pig submucosal arteriole, 80–90% of varicosities form close neuroeffector contacts, whereas ≤50% of the varicosities form close neuroeffector junctions in the rat tail artery, about 15% in the rat mesenteric artery (Luff et al. 1987, 1995, 2000; Luff, personal communication) and about 70% in iris arterioles (Sandow et al. 1998).

7.2.3 Electrophysiology of the Neuroeffector Transmission

Experimental investigations of a few effector tissues show that the mechanism of neuroeffector transmission is tissue specific. There is now full agreement that the transmitter or combination of a "classical" (primary) transmitter and one (or more) peptide transmitter(s) are localized in the synaptic vesicles. Importantly, as for other synapses, release of transmitter at these junctions occurs in quanta with a low probability of release from individual varicosities. Despite strong evidence supporting the quantal (vesicular) release of neurotransmitter from postganglionic sympathetic neurons, it was long held in contention whether the release of transmitter from individual varicosities of autonomic nerve axons occurs through emptying of the entire content of a synaptic vesicle or through fractional release of a vesicle's content (Folkow and Nilsson 1997; Folkow 2000).

Evidence for quantal release was first gleaned from electrophysiological experiments in which the following conditions were fulfilled (Hirst et al. 1996):

1. The transmitter released must act at *ligand-gated* ion channels. This leads to a *rapid* opening of the

Table 7.2 | Properties of neuroeffector junctions on autonomic effector cells determined by successive sections of tissues using the electron microscope

Tissue	Percentage of varicosities forming junctions	Area of target tissue occupied by junctions (μm^2) mean ± SEM	Varicosity volume (μm^3) mean ± SEM	Ref.
(a) Sympathetic neuroeffector junctions in blood vessels				
Rabbit juxtaglomerular arterioles:				
Afferent	70	0.48 ± 0.32 (n = 4)	0.52 ± 0.25 (n = 8)	1
Efferent	69	0.38 ± 0.05 (n = 6)	0.36 ± 0.13 (n = 8)	1
Guinea pig submucosal arterioles*	90	1.26 ± 0.29 (n = 11)	1.2 ± 0.25 (n = 11)	2
Guinea pig mesenteric veins*	98	0.64 ± 0.08 (n = 47)	0.81 ± 0.15 (n = 17)	4
(b) Sympathetic neuroeffector junctions on cardiac muscle and in structures associated with the rat iris dilator muscle				
Toad sinus venosus*	88	0.44 ± 0.07 (n = 25)	0.68 ± 0.39 (n = 4)	3
Guinea pig sinoatrial node*	90	0.15 ± 0.03 (n = 9)	0.31 ± 0.06 (n = 9)	5
Rat iris dilator myoepithelium*	26	0.23 ± 0.07 (n = 6)	0.21 ± 0.07 (n = 4)	6
Rat iris dilator melanophores	35	0.21 ± 0.05 (n = 8)		6
(c) Parasympathetic neuroeffector junctions on cardiac muscle and in structures associated with the rat iris dilator muscle				
Toad sinus venosus*	96	0.45 ± 0.06 (n = 28)	0.60 ± 0.16 (n = 9)	3
Guinea pig sinoatrial node*	85	0.21 ± 0.04 (n = 13)	0.48 ± 0.07 (n = 13)	5
Rat iris dilator myoepithelium*	36	0.50 ± 0.12 (n = 14)	0.36 ± 0.09 (n = 14)	6
Rat iris dilator melanophores	71	0.44 ± 0.08 (n = 27)		6

*Autonomic effector structures in which neuroeffector transmission has been studied
References: 1. Luff et al. (1992); 2. Luff et al. (1987); 3. Klemm et al. (1992); 4. Klemm et al. (1993); 5. Choate et al. (1993b); 6. Hill et al. (1993). From Hirst et al. (1996). See also Sandow et al. (1998).

ionic channels and to a postsynaptic potential at *short latency* and with a brief duration. If the transmitter were to act on the ionic channels through a G-protein and second-messenger system, it would be impossible to detect the unitary postsynaptic events upon release of single quanta because the kinetics of the intracellular multi-stage reaction pathways between membrane receptors and ionic channel are too slow.

2. The transmitter must be released at a close neuroeffector junction that leads, upon the release of the content of a vesicle, to a short-lasting high concentration of the transmitter in the cleft. In wide clefts, the transmitter released prejunctionally would be diluted by the second power of the distance between release site and membrane receptor.

3. The recording of the postjunctional potential must be made either from a neuroeffector junction involving a varicosity on a single electrically isolated cell or from a small syncytial conglomerate of electrically coupled cells that behaves

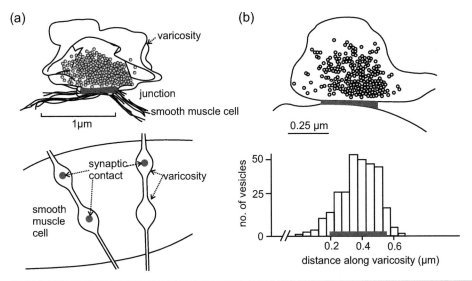

(a)

varicosity

junction

smooth muscle cell

1 µm

synaptic contact

varicosity

smooth muscle cell

(b)

0.25 µm

no. of vesicles

50

25

0

0.2   0.4   0.6

distance along varicosity (µm)

Figure 7.1 Morphology of a neuroeffector synapse to smooth muscle cells. (a) Three-dimensional reconstruction. The varicosity and its postjunctional cell were serially sectioned and reconstructed. The varicosity forms a close contact with a smooth muscle cell (on a small part of its surface). The neuroeffector cleft is >50 nm wide. The varicosity loses part of its Schwann cell sheath and the basal laminae of the varicosity and the smooth muscle fuse. The lower panel shows schematically that some varicosities form a synaptic contact with the effector cell at only a small part of their surface. (b) Outline of a varicosity and the position of individual vesicles (small open circles) close to the neuroeffector cleft (red bar). Lower diagram: distribution of vesicles along the varicosity showing that the highest density of vesicles is located along the neuroeffector cleft. Histological unpublished data supplied by Susan Luff.

approximately like a single, spherical cell. As the former situation has not yet been identified, the latter was obtained by cutting a segment of an arteriole much shorter than its length constant.

With these limitations, it has been shown for several blood vessels that transmitter is released from the varicosities in quanta.

Figure 7.2b shows an intracellular recording from a short segment of an arteriole of about 200 µm length, which is innervated by two to four noradrenergic postganglionic axons with about 200 varicosities, some of which make neuromuscular junctions with the smooth muscle. This short segment of arteriole contains only about 100 to 200 electrically coupled smooth muscle cells and current injected into a single cell uniformly polarizes the whole segment, so it behaves electrically like a single spherical cell. This preparation exhibits postsynaptic electrical events that are similar to those recorded at many synapses of the skeletal neuromuscular junction. *First*, electrical activation of the postganglionic axons by single pulses evokes stimulus-locked excitatory junction potentials (EJPs). *Second*, in the absence

of stimulation, spontaneous excitatory junction potentials (sEJPs) are recorded that are believed to be produced by spontaneous release of the transmitter content of a single vesicle (quantum). These junction potentials are generated by excitatory junction currents (EJCs), which have a rise time of about 10 ms and a decay time of about 100 ms. In the short arteriolar segments, the duration of both the EJPs and sEJPs is about 1 second, because the time course of the preparation is determined by the membrane time constant of decay.

It should be appreciated that intact smooth muscle syncytia do not usually behave in the same way as this preparation. Multiple layers of electrically coupled smooth muscle cells that extend along and around a vessel attenuate the voltage change produced by the currents that originate at varicosities on its external surface. Thus, the time course of the sEJP recorded in surface cells is much briefer than that of the EJP recorded when many axons are activated throughout the syncytium (Jobling and McLachlan 1992). During activation by sympathetic axons in vivo, summation of asynchronous sEJPs from sites around the vessel is likely to produce a general depolarization that leads to

(a)

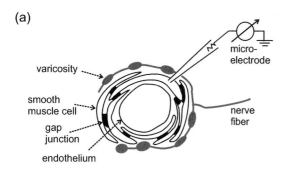

(b)

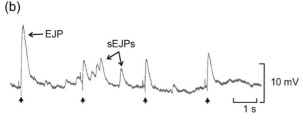

(c)

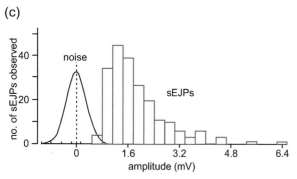

Figure 7.2 Neuroeffector transmission in arterioles.
(a) Experimental setup. Intracellular recording from a 200 μm segment of an arteriole isolated from the guinea pig submucosa. The innervation was electrically stimulated transmurally with single impulses of 0.5 ms duration. (b) Recording of excitatory junction potentials (EJPs) evoked by nerve stimulation (at arrows below trace) and of spontaneous excitatory junction potentials (sEJPs) occurring randomly. Note that the EJPs fluctuate in amplitude and the amplitude of the EJPs in this preparation is close to that of the sEJPs. (c) Comparison of the amplitude frequency histogram of the sEJPs with the normal distribution of the recording noise. Spontaneous EJPs have a separate unimodal amplitude distribution. All responses are the result of transmitter release from sympathetic varicosities. With permission from Hirst and Neild (1980).

Ca^{2+} entry, contributing to activation of vasoconstriction (see Brock et al., 1995).

Because the time course of the sEJP and EJP in these short arteriolar segments is similar, it is possible to determine the relationship between these two events

directly. The amplitude distribution of the sEJPs is unimodal and their amplitudes correspond to the smallest evoked EJPs recorded. The unimodal distribution of sEJP amplitudes indicates that transmission must occur at a population of varicosities that make similar close neuroeffector contacts with the smooth muscle. Assuming that the EJP is composed of quantal units having the same size as the sEJP, the amplitude distribution of EJPs indicates that the majority of EJPs in this preparation had a quantal content of one to four. Furthermore, since all varicosities in this preparation are excited by the electrical stimulation of the postganglionic axons with single pulses it follows that only about 1% of the varicosities release a quantum of transmitter when the innervation is activated by a single electrical stimulus, i.e. the probability of release is low. These findings indicate that transmitter release from an individual varicosity occurs in quanta (i.e., is not fractional).

These results have been fully confirmed by extracellular recording of electrical activity at sympathetic neuromuscular junctions in both vas deferens and muscular arteries by using a suction microelectrode (Figure 7.3a). This technique allows recording of both evoked and spontaneous junction currents (EJCs and sEJCs) from small populations of varicosities and has demonstrated that the two events recorded at the same site have a similar amplitude and time course (Figure 7.3b,c). This finding indicates that both events result from release of a single quantum of transmitter. During trains of low-frequency stimuli, evoked junction currents occur intermittently, consistent with the low probability of quantal release from the individual varicosities. The extracellular recording technique also allows recording of the nerve terminal action potential (NTAP in Figure 7.3b,c) and demonstrates that electrical excitation of the postganglionic axon leads to action potential invasion into *all* the varicosities. Therefore, the probability of releasing single quanta of transmitter from the invaded varicosities is very low (range of probability of 0.01 to 0.1, depending on the frequency of excitation) (Cunnane and Stjärne 1982; Brock and Cunnane 1988, 1992, 1993; Lavidis and Bennett 1992).

In conclusion, quantal release of transmitter from individual varicosities occurs with probabilities ranging between 0.01 and 0.1, with the majority having very low probabilities of release. These individual EJCs recorded in this short length of arteriole, where the varicosities lie close to all the cells recorded from, are identical in shape and duration to the sEJCs generated

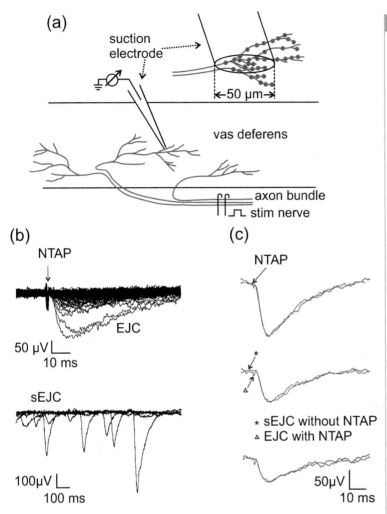

Figure 7.3 Extracellular recordings of nerve terminal action potentials and smooth muscle junction currents generated by transmitter release from varicosities using a suction microelectrode. (a) Experimental setup. The suction microelectrode is attached to the surface of the vas deferens, generating a high resistance between the inside and outside of the microelectrode. The inner diameter of the microelectrode is, at its tip, about 50 μm; a small number of varicosities located on the nerve terminal(s) of a single neuron are within the membrane patch covered by the microelectrode (inset upper right). This arrangement allows extracellular recording of the action currents in the nerve terminal (nerve terminal action potential, NTAP) together with the excitatory junction currents (EJCs) in the smooth muscle cells generated by the release of transmitter from the varicosities. While the extracellular postjunctional signals are recorded as changes in voltage, their time course follows that of the junctional current. (b) Spontaneous excitatory junction currents (sEJCs) and EJCs evoked by nerve stimulation. The sEJCs and evoked EJCs had similar time courses and amplitudes consistent with the quantal release of transmitter. Each stimulus during a train of pulses at 1 Hz leads to an action potential in the nerve terminal but to only intermittent occurrence of evoked EJC. (c) Three pairs of similar sEJC (without NTAP) and evoked EJC (with NTAP) in the same preparation are shown. These three pairs of junction currents were most likely generated by the release of transmitter from three individual varicosities. Modified from Brock and Cunnane (1988) with permission.

by spontaneous release from the varicosities of the same preparation.

In the arterial vessels investigated and the vas deferens, which are both supplied by sympathetic nerves, neither the sEJPs nor the evoked EJPs could be blocked by α- or β-adrenoceptor antagonists. This shows that these junction potentials are not mediated by noradrenaline. The compound that is believed to elicit the junction potentials is ATP acting at P2X1-purinoceptors. This is believed to be colocalized with noradrenaline in the small vesicles and released together with noradrenaline from the varicosity, either spontaneously or when the postganglionic axon is excited. The evidence that the junction

potentials are generated by release of ATP is as follows:

- They are blocked by P2X-purinoceptor antagonists (e.g. suramin).
- They are blocked by α-β-methylene-ATP, a purinoceptor agonist that rapidly desensitizes the purinoceptors.
- They are absent in tissues of transgenic mice in which P2X1-purinoceptors have been knocked out (vas deferens; Mulryan et al. 2000). This is the best evidence for ATP as a transmitter to date.

Ironically, we know more about the molecular mechanisms of ATP release than about those of noradrenaline release (see further discussion below in the context of neurovascular transmission).

7.3 Specific Neuroeffector Transmissions

In the following Subchapter, I will describe neuroeffector transmission for three groups of effector tissues: sinoatrial node in mammalian heart and the sinus venosus of toad heart, smooth muscle in small blood vessels, and the longitudinal muscle of the gastrointestinal tract. In these three cases, stimulation of the autonomic (sympathetic, parasympathetic or enteric) nerves and superfusion of the preparation with the respective transmitter, acetylcholine or noradrenaline, causes the same responses in the effector. However, detailed examination of the changes in membrane potential of the effector cells following the neural release of the transmitter and following exogenous application of the transmitter to the preparation reveals that the mechanisms leading to the effector responses are quite different. This, together with the morphology of the neuroeffector junctions, supports the notion that the transmission of neural signals to the effector cells occurs through these junctions.

7.3.1 Innervation of the Heart

Neuroeffector transmission in the heart has been studied in the toad and in some mammals (in particular the guinea pig). For parasympathetic control, there are parallels between toad and mammals. For sympathetic control, there are some differences. These differences do not change the overall message that the transmission of the neural signals to the heart is mediated through junctionally located receptors.

Parasympathetic Cardiomotor Neurons
Stimulation of the preganglionic cardiomotor axons in the vagus nerve slows action potential firing in atrial pacemaker cells. During nerve stimulation, the rate of the action potentials decreases without any change in their configuration and without membrane hyperpolarization. The pacemaker potential exhibits a slower depolarization and therefore the time to reach threshold for initiation of the action potential is increased. This neurally induced slowing

of the pacemaker depolarization is generated by inhibition of sodium channels (that are distinct from non-selective calcium channels [Edwards et al. 1993]), which is accompanied by an increase in membrane resistance. These sodium channels are normally open, tending to depolarize the pacemaker cells (Figure 7.4b,d). Stronger stimulation of the vagus nerve leads to further inhibition of these sodium channels and complete abolition of pacemaking.

Exogenous acetylcholine superfused over the preparation also slows firing of the pacemaker cells. However, the membrane is hyperpolarized and the amplitude and duration of the action potentials are reduced. Exogenous acetylcholine opens potassium channels causing hyperpolarization (Figure 7.4c,d; Bolter et al. 2001) and the resultant increase in membrane conductance decreases the size and duration of action potentials.

When pacemaking is abolished by blocking the muscle calcium channels (e.g., by nifedipine), the membrane potential of the pacemaker cells settles to values of about −35 to −40 mV because of ongoing activity of the pacemaker-associated sodium channels. Both electrical stimulation of the vagus nerve and the rapid focal application of acetylcholine to the preparation now hyperpolarize the pacemaker cells. However, the onset of hyperpolarization following nerve stimulation is much faster and shorter than that following acetylcholine (Figure 7.5). The mechanism underlying hyperpolarization generated by exogenous acetylcholine and the mechanism underlying hyperpolarization from nerve stimulation are different. The response to exogenous acetylcholine superfusion is prevented by blockade of potassium channels with barium ions (Ba^{2+}) in the arrested preparation and therefore is generated by opening of potassium channels. The hyperpolarization to nerve stimulation is not affected by Ba^{2+}, but is generated by blockade of sodium channels (Figure 7.5b). In relation to both neurally released and exogenously applied acetylcholine, the hyperpolarization in arrested preparations and the effects on the time course and rate of action potentials in beating hearts are blocked by atropine, an antagonist for muscarinic cholinergic receptors. However, as the mechanisms underlying the postreceptor conductance changes clearly differ, the muscarinic receptors activated by acetylcholine released by the vagal axons cannot be

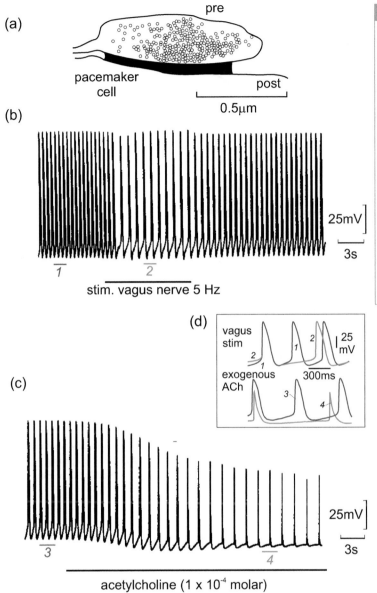

(a) pre
pacemaker cell
post
0.5μm

(b)
stim. vagus nerve 5 Hz

25mV
3s

(d)
vagus stim
exogenous ACh
300ms
25 mV

(c)
acetylcholine (1 x 10⁻⁴ molar)

25mV
3s

Figure 7.4 Effect of vagus nerve stimulation and acetylcholine on cardiac pacemaker cells. (a) Schematic outline of a cholinergic neuromuscular junction on a cell of the guinea pig sinoatrial node. (b, c) Intracellular record from a pacemaker cell in an in vitro preparation with attached vagus nerve. Expanded records of time periods marked with numbers *1* to *4* are shown in the inset (d). The cell shows pacemaker potentials with action potentials. Electrical stimulation of the vagus nerve at 5 Hz (b) shows no change in action potential configuration and no hyperpolarization, but a reduced slope of the pacemaker potential (upper records in inset). Exogenous acetylcholine (ACh) (c) hyperpolarizes the membrane and shunts the action potentials (due to opening of potassium channels and decrease in membrane resistance), reducing their amplitude and duration (lower records in inset). (a) According to Choate et al. (1993a). (b, c) Modified from Campbell et al. (1989) with permission.

the same as those to which exogenous acetylcholine binds (Campbell et al. 1989).

Further investigations have shown that the postreceptor pathways connecting muscarinic receptors to ionic channels are different for the junctional and the extrajunctional acetylcholine receptors. The junctional receptors are connected via a yet to be defined intracellular pathway or even directly to the sodium channels. By contrast, the extrajunctional acetylcholine receptors are connected via a G-protein that increases the activity of adenylate cyclase and the production of cAMP, which in turn regulates the activity of potassium channels and other channels (see Demir et al. [1999]). Since it is unlikely that significant acetylcholine escapes from the neuroeffector junction during neural stimulation (due to acetylcholinesterase near the synaptic cleft), it is likely that the extrajunctional acetylcholine receptors play no role in the control of heart rate under physiological conditions. As mentioned before (see Subchapter 7.2), ≤1% of the

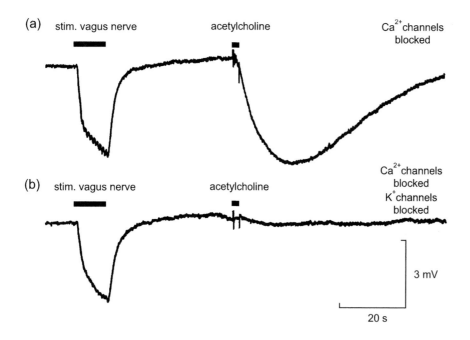

Figure 7.5 Inhibition of pacemaker activity generated by electrical stimulation of the vagal nerve and by applied acetylcholine (ACh) is mediated by different cellular mechanisms. Intracellular recording in the sinus venosus of toad *Bufo marinus* in vitro with attached vagus nerve. The pacemaker cells are arrested by blocking the calcium channels with nicardipine (10 μM). Under this condition the membrane potential settles at about −35 mV because of the high Na+ permeability. (a) Vagal stimulation for 10 s at 1 Hz hyperpolarizes the pacemaker cells. Ionophoretic application of ACh applied through a micropipette for 2 s (10-4 M, 50 nA) also hyperpolarizes the cells. Onset and decay of the hyperpolarization are longer when generated by exogenously applied ACh than during vagus nerve stimulation. (b) Recording from the same cell about 15 min later after adding Ba2+ (1 mM), which blocks potassium channels, to the physiological saline superfusate. Response to vagus nerve stimulation is unaffected but the response to ionophoretically applied ACh is abolished. Acetylcholine released by vagus nerve stimulation leads to closing of sodium channels coupled to junctionally located muscarinic receptors. Superfused ACh leads to opening of potassium channels coupled indirectly via a G-protein and cAMP to extrajunctionally located muscarinic receptors. Modified from Hirst et al. (1991) with permission.

surface of the pacemaker cells is covered by neuro-effector junctions. Thus, the biologically important transmission of neural signals from parasympathetic cardiomotor neurons to these pacemaker cells occurs only at these junctions.

Sympathetic Cardiomotor Neurons

Similar investigations have been conducted on the sympathetic innervation of pacemaker cells, which increase the rate of pacemaking when activated. In *mammals*, both neurally released and exogenous noradrenaline activate β-adrenoceptors. In the *toad*, sympathetic postganglionic cardiomotor neurons use adrenaline as the transmitter. Nerve-released adrenaline activates junctional adrenoceptors that are neither α- nor β-adrenoceptors; applied adrenaline activates β-adrenoceptors (Note 4). Noradrenaline or

adrenaline released from the nerve terminals of the sympathetic cardiomotor neurons modifies the pacemaker current, whereas application of exogenous noradrenaline or adrenaline produces its effect by increasing cAMP in the pacemaker cells, leading to phosphorylation of voltage-dependent ionic channels, which are activated during pacemaker activity (Choate et al. 1993a).

Thus, as for vagal innervation of the heart, it is likely that the signals arising from the sympathetic innervation of the heart are mediated by junctional adrenoceptors. At least in the toad, the intracellular postreceptor pathways to the ionic channels are different for the junctional adrenoceptors and the extrajunctional adrenoceptors: the extrajunctional adrenoceptors act through an increase in cAMP, whereas the intracellular pathway used by junctional adrenoceptors has not been identified, but may involve inositol 1,4,5-trisphosphate, which triggers the release of calcium ions from intracellular stores (Bramich et al. 2001).

The function of the extrajunctional adrenoceptors in neuroeffector transmission in the heart is unknown. However, they may play a role in mediating the effects of circulating adrenaline; whether this is functionally important under physiological conditions remains to be shown (see Subchapter 4.5 and Figure 4.17; see here that circulating noradrenaline, in physiological concentration, increases neither heart rate nor blood pressure). It may become important in the sympathetically denervated heart (e.g., in the transplanted heart or in patients with severe diabetic neuropathy in whom the sympathetic postganglionic neurons to the heart are metabolically destroyed), where the adrenoceptors may have dramatically changed in number, affinity and coupling to the postreceptor pathways.

7.3.2 Sympathetic Innervation of Blood Vessels

Small Arteries and Arterioles

Postganglionic vasoconstrictor neurons have long axons and form many branches in the adventitia of blood vessels with thousands of varicosities (Figure 7.6). Many of the varicosities on small muscular blood vessels with diameters <0.5 mm form close neuromuscular junctions, as described above. The proportion that does not form junctions varies between vessels at different sites throughout the vascular bed (Luff and McLachlan 1989; Luff et al. 1995, 2000; see Table 7.2). The neural signal is transmitted from these varicosities to the vascular smooth muscle cells, which form a functional syncytium. The small vesicles in the varicosities contain noradrenaline and ATP; the large vesicles (which are much less frequent than the small ones) contain noradrenaline, ATP and NPY. In some vascular beds (e.g., of the skin) different vascular sections (e.g., large arteries, small arteries, arterioles, veins) are innervated by vasoconstrictor neurons with neurochemically different phenotypes (see Subchapter 1.4).

Most blood vessels constrict when exogenous noradrenaline is applied to them. This pharmacological action is largely mediated by α_1-adrenoceptors, but also by α_2-adrenoceptors located extrajunctionally (note that only about 1% of the surface of autonomic effector cells [e.g., arterioles, heart] are occupied by

synapses). Most of the Ca^{2+} triggering vasoconstriction to exogenous noradrenaline is released from intracellular stores by second messengers. Nerve stimulation evokes brief depolarizations (EJPs) in the vascular smooth muscle cells (Figure 7.2b), which are followed in some blood vessels by long-lasting depolarizations. The brief depolarizations have durations of about 1 second and a time constant of decay of 200 to 300 ms, and cannot be blocked by adrenoceptor antagonists. As they are blocked by purinoceptor antagonists (e.g., by suramin) or by desensitization of P2X purinoceptors with α-β-methylene-ATP, they are believed to be mediated by ATP. The receptor involved is the P2X1 purinoceptor (Mulryan et al. 2000), which is a ligand-gated cation channel. The excitatory junction potentials evoked by single stimuli usually do not evoke vasoconstriction, but during trains of stimuli at frequencies above 1 Hz they summate to depolarize the membrane potential to the threshold for opening of voltage-sensitive calcium channels. Calcium entering via these channels can cause a transient constriction in some small arterial vessels. The slow depolarization that follows the EJPs reflects the action of noradrenaline on α_2-adrenoceptors, which causes maintained constriction (Jobling et al. 1992; Hirst et al. 1996).

Constriction of some small arteries during sympathetic nerve activity is abolished by α-adrenoceptor antagonists, but is only partly dependent on membrane depolarization (Brock et al. 1997). In contrast, in some small arterioles (e.g., the arterioles of the submucosa of the gastrointestinal tract), vasoconstriction produced by nerve stimulation is unaffected by α-adrenoceptor blockade and is entirely dependent on opening of voltage-dependent calcium channels (Evans and Surprenant 1992). However, in other small arterioles (e.g., those in the rat iris), vasoconstriction produced by nerve stimulation is due solely to release of noradrenaline and activation of α_1-adrenoceptors. Activation of these receptors stimulates the formation of inositol 1,4,5-triphosphate (IP3), which in turn triggers the release of calcium from intracellular stores. Cytosolic calcium activates the contractile apparatus (vasoconstriction) and opening of calcium-activated chloride channels in the cell membrane with the outflow of chloride ions (along their electrochemical gradient) resulting in depolarization (Gould and Hill 1996; see Note 5).

Thus, neural control of constriction in the small arteries and arterioles involves multiple transmitters

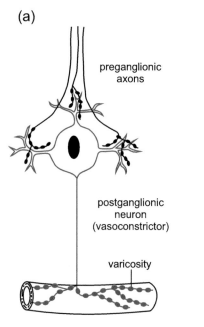

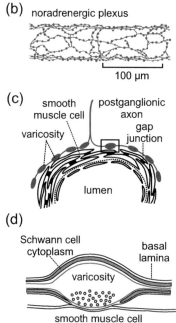

Figure 7.6 Morphology of sympathetic postganglionic vasoconstrictor neurons and the vascular neuroeffector synapse. (a) Schematic representation of the relationship between a sympathetic postganglionic neuron and a blood vessel. The neuron has a long axon and forms a plexus of many thousands of varicosities at the surface of the blood vessel. (b, c) The terminal branches of the postganglionic axon form a plexus of nerve terminal axons at the adventitial medial border. Some varicosities lie close to the smooth muscle cells. Smooth muscle cells are electrically coupled by gap-junction channels, forming a functional syncytium. (d) The neuroeffector synapse formed by a varicosity. The varicosity forms close contact with the smooth muscle cells without intervening Schwann cell cytoplasm. The basal laminae of smooth muscle cell and varicosity fuse. The vesicles are arranged close to the synaptic cleft.

(such as ATP and noradrenaline) and both voltage-dependent and voltage-independent mechanisms in different parts of the arterial vascular tree. In addition, there is evidence that the relative role of the cotransmitters changes, depending on the pattern of nerve stimulation (e.g., Evans and Cunnane 1992). However, the way in which signals generated by the cotransmitters and the membrane receptors that they activate are integrated by the vascular smooth muscle (Figure 7.7), so as to regulate vascular tone and control of blood flow through tissues, remains a puzzle.

This apparent paradox may be resolved in the future if one looks at comparable densely innervated arteries in the same species, such as fine branches of the superior mesenteric artery and the tail artery of the rat. The fine branches of the superior mesenteric artery have about four layers of smooth muscle cells and a lumen diameter of approximately 200 μm. The rat proximal tail artery has several layers of smooth muscle cells (up to 15) and a lumen diameter of 400 to 800 μm:

- In the *rat mesenteric artery*, electrical nerve stimulation at 10 Hz produces ATP-mediated junction potentials, but no α-adrenoceptor-mediated slow depolarizations (Brock and van Helden 1995). However, a part of the contraction produced by

electrical stimulation of the vascular innervation can be prevented by an α-adrenoceptor blocker, another part by blockade of purinergic transmission (Luo et al. 2003). Contraction produced by exogenous noradrenaline is closely correlated with the depolarization produced by this agent (Nilsson et al. 1994). However, unphysiological concentrations greater than 1 μM are required to produce significant depolarization (Mulvany et al. 1982). This shows that exogenously applied noradrenaline does *not* mimic the effect of nerve stimulation, although it may increase the release of both noradrenaline and ATP from varicosities of postganglionic axons involving β-adrenoceptors (Brock et al. 1997). Electrochemical studies show that the concentration of noradrenaline at the adventitia during short trains of electrical nerve stimulation at 10 Hz can reach levels in the *micromolar range* (Dunn et al. 1999). These micromolar concentrations can presumably activate adrenoceptors located at a distance from the release sites (i.e., extrajunctionally). They cannot be produced by circulating noradrenaline under physiological conditions, which is in the picomolar range in the rat (see Subchapter 4.5 and Figure 4.17).

- In the *rat tail artery*, electrical nerve stimulation with trains of impulses at 10 Hz produces ATP-mediated junction potentials and a slow depolarization, mediated by noradrenaline acting at α-adrenoceptors (Jobling and McLachlan 1992). However, nerve-evoked contractions of this artery are primarily generated by released noradrenaline with only a minor role of ATP (depending on the frequency and duration of stimulation) (Bao et al. 1993; Al Dera et al. 2012). In contrast to the mesenteric artery, the electrical and contractile effects of nerve-released noradrenaline in the tail artery are mimicked by exogenously applied α-adrenoceptor agonists (Brock et al. 1997). Thus, the nerve-induced constrictions of the rat tail artery are mediated by noradrenaline acting at both junctional and possibly extrajunctional α-adrenoceptors that are activated by concentrations of noradrenaline in the micromolar range.

These examples, and the example of the submucosal arterioles where neurally evoked contraction is fully dependent on a purinergic mechanism, demonstrate that the mechanisms of nerve-induced constriction can differ greatly in different arterial vessels. Neuropeptide Y can play a neuromodulatory role by potentiating the contractile response to nerve stimulation in some blood vessels (Macarthur et al. 2011). However, as high bursts of activity are necessary to elicit NPY release and such activity is normally absent in postganglionic vasoconstrictor neurons it remains unclear as to the importance of this mechanism.

Veins and the Pulmonary Artery

Veins (portal, mesenteric) and the pulmonary artery contain sympathetic neuroeffector junctions. Rapid focal application of noradrenaline to mesenteric veins mimics the effect of noradrenaline released by the sympathetic nerve axons, both causing a fast excitatory junction potential, and a slow depolarization and constriction. These effects are abolished by α-adrenoceptor blockers. It is likely that the adrenoceptors in the venous smooth muscle cells are linked to an intracellular pathway that involves inositol 1,4,5-trisphosphate. This triggers the release of calcium from intracellular stores that produces contraction and the opening of calcium-activated chloride channels, which are responsible for the fast EJPs (Note 5). The mechanism underlying the noradrenaline-induced slow depolarization has not been resolved. Purinoceptor-mediated mechanisms

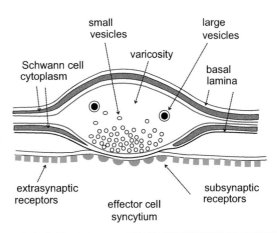

Figure 7.7 Simplified scheme of neuroeffector transmission to autonomic target cells (arterioles, heart). Subsynaptic receptors mediate the effect of transmitter released by the nerve terminals during excitation under physiological conditions. The cell surface at which this nerve–effector communication occurs is ≤1% of the total effector cell surface. These subsynaptic receptors are ligand gated or second-messenger-coupled to cellular effectors (e.g., ionic channels). Extrasynaptic receptors for the transmitter are either different from the subsynaptic ones and/or are coupled by different intracellular second-messenger pathways to the cellular effectors. The functions of the extrajunctionally located receptors are unclear for most innervated effector organs. Nerve-induced constriction of small arteries is entirely or partially mediated by noradrenaline acting on junctionally and possibly extrajunctionally located adrenoceptors. Small vesicles containing the transmitter are located close to the synaptic cleft. Large vesicles are also present in many varicosities. In these large vesicles, neuropeptides are colocalized with "classical" transmitters. Large vesicles are not located close to the synaptic cleft. The physiological role of the neuropeptides is, in most cases, unclear.

do not seem to play a role in sympathetic neuron-induced constriction of rat mesenteric veins although these vessels are very reactive to exogenously applied ATP (van Helden 1988a, b, 1991; Hirst et al. 1996).

7.3.3 Transmission to Smooth Muscle of the Ileum

The longitudinal muscle of the ileum is innervated by cholinergic neurons of the myenteric plexus. The varicose terminals of these neurons form close junctions with the smooth muscle cells, which are the sites of signal transmission between enteric neurons and effector cells (Klemm 1995). Nerve-evoked contractions and contractions induced by exogenous acetylcholine are both mediated by muscarinic receptors and therefore abolished by atropine. Both elicit membrane potential changes (depolarizations) at relatively long latencies of 500 to 600 ms, Ca^{2+} action potentials and muscle contractions. The long latency of the depolarizations shows that both activate complex intracellular pathways and are not generated by activation of ligand-gated ionic channels. However, the mechanisms underlying both are entirely different (for details see Cousins et al. [1993, 1995]; Hirst et al. [1996]; Figure 7.8):

- Nerve-released ACh generates EJPs that trigger Ca^{2+} muscle action potentials and muscle contraction. However, when the action potentials are prevented (by calcium channel blockers), EJPs still evoke contractions. Excitatory junction potentials probably open channels with high Ca^{2+} selectivity. This is supported by the observation that EJPs and the transient increase of intracellular Ca^{2+} in the smooth muscle cells occur simultaneously.

- Ionophoretically applied ACh opens non-selective cation channels (for Na^+, Ca^{2+} and K^+), yet the Ca^{2+} entering the muscle cells is negligible. The depolarization following opening of these channels opens voltage-dependent calcium channels, generating action potentials and contraction (through inflow of Ca^{2+}). Additionally, ionophoretically applied ACh causes increase of intracellular Ca^{2+} from an intracellular store. This release of Ca^{2+} is pulsatile and involves the inositol IP3 pathway (Note 6).

These results suggest that increase in intracellular Ca^{2+}, and subsequent contraction, caused by neurally released ACh or by ionophoretically applied ACh, involves different intracellular pathways, the latter involving IP_3 and pulsatile release of Ca^{2+} from an intracellular store, and the former not. This difference is supported by different sensitivities to organic Ca^{2+} antagonists of the responses to nerve-released ACh and to applied ACh.

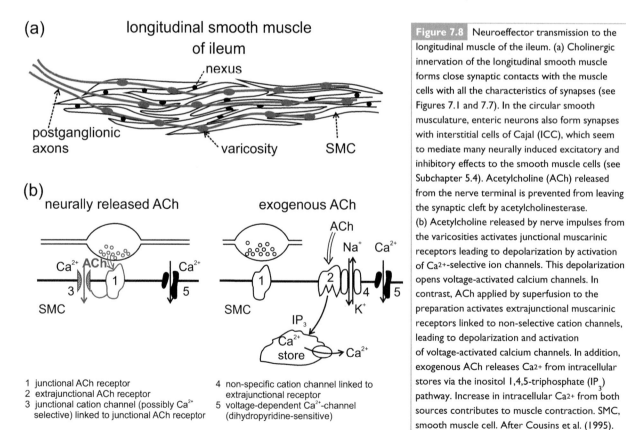

(a) longitudinal smooth muscle of ileum

nexus

postganglionic axons

varicosity   SMC

(b)

neurally released ACh

Ca^{2+} ACh Ca^{2+}
3   1   5
SMC

exogenous ACh

ACh
Na^+ Ca^{2+}
1   2   4   5
SMC
K^+
IP_3
Ca^{2+} store → Ca^{2+}

1 junctional ACh receptor
2 extrajunctional ACh receptor
3 junctional cation channel (possibly Ca^{2+} selective) linked to junctional ACh receptor
4 non-specific cation channel linked to extrajunctional receptor
5 voltage-dependent Ca^{2+}-channel (dihydropyridine-sensitive)

Figure 7.8 Neuroeffector transmission to the longitudinal muscle of the ileum. (a) Cholinergic innervation of the longitudinal smooth muscle forms close synaptic contacts with the muscle cells with all the characteristics of synapses (see Figures 7.1 and 7.7). In the circular smooth musculature, enteric neurons also form synapses with interstitial cells of Cajal (ICC), which seem to mediate many neurally induced excitatory and inhibitory effects to the smooth muscle cells (see Subchapter 5.4). Acetylcholine (ACh) released from the nerve terminal is prevented from leaving the synaptic cleft by acetylcholinesterase.

(b) Acetylcholine released by nerve impulses from the varicosities activates junctional muscarinic receptors leading to depolarization by activation of Ca^{2+}-selective ion channels. This depolarization opens voltage-activated calcium channels. In contrast, ACh applied by superfusion to the preparation activates extrajunctional muscarinic receptors linked to non-selective cation channels, leading to depolarization and activation of voltage-activated calcium channels. In addition, exogenous ACh releases Ca^{2+} from intracellular stores via the inositol 1,4,5-triphosphate (IP_3) pathway. Increase in intracellular Ca^{2+} from both sources contributes to muscle contraction. SMC, smooth muscle cell. After Cousins et al. (1995).

These findings suggest that muscarinic receptors involved in transmission from cholinergic nerves to the longitudinal smooth muscle of the ileum are restricted to the junctional membrane and differ from those activated by exogenous acetylcholine. The findings also suggest that the intracellular pathways leading to contraction differ (Cousins et al. 1993, 1995). Thus, neural transmission in this smooth muscle occurs at organized neuroeffector junctions. The function of the extrajunctionally located ACh receptors is unknown. Acetylcholinesterase in or near the junctional cleft prevents ACh from leaking out of the cleft and hence ACh is unlikely to activate extrajunctionally located ACh receptors.

Interstitial cells of Cajal (ICC) in the smooth musculature of the gastrointestinal tract mediate, at least in part, the excitatory and inhibitory effects of enteric motor neurons to circular smooth muscle cells (see Subchapter 5.4; Burns et al. [1996]; Ward et al. [2000]) and possibly also to longitudinal muscle cells (Tanahashi et al. 2014). It appears that the nerve terminals of the motor neurons also form synapses with the ICC (see Burns et al. [1996]; Ward et al. [2000]; Iino et al. [2004]; Subchapter 5.4).

7.4 | Integration of Neural and Non-Neural Signals Influencing Blood Vessels

The reactions of many autonomic effector cells depend not only on impulses in the autonomic postganglionic neurons. They also depend on impulse activity in peptidergic afferent neurons, on circulating compounds (hormones), on intrinsic properties of the effector cells, on locally released compounds and directly on physical stimuli (mechanical, thermal). These remote and local neural and non-neural influences vary between effector cells and in different functional conditions of the micromilieu of the effector cells. For example, contraction of the smooth muscles in the iris of the eye is only dependent on impulses in the postganglionic neurons innervating it. In contrast, contraction and relaxation of arterioles and small arteries in viscera, skeletal muscle, skin, etc., while *dependent on their innervation by vasoconstrictor neurons*, are also dependent on several other factors. There are differences between different types of blood vessels with

regard to these neural and non-neural influences. Potential long-range and local influences acting on blood vessels are exemplified in Figure 7.9:

- Some vascular beds are innervated by sympathetic or parasympathetic vasodilator neurons. For example, small arteries in skeletal muscle are innervated by sympathetic cholinergic vasodilator neurons in some species (see Subchapter 4.2). Sinusoids and helical arteries of the erectile tissue of sexual organs are innervated by sacral parasympathetic vasodilator neurons, whereas cerebral arteries are innervated by cranial parasympathetic cholinergic vasodilator neurons (see Subchapter 4.8).

- Remote non-neural influences on blood vessels are blood borne (e.g., circulating catecholamines, angiotensin, vasopressin). These blood-borne substances act on vascular muscle cells or on the varicosities of the postganglionic axons, modulating transmitter release. It is unclear how important many of these long-range influences are in generating or attenuating vasoconstriction under physiological conditions. For example, it is unlikely that circulating noradrenaline is important in the regulation of innervated blood vessels. Circulating adrenaline may generate β_2-adrenoceptor-mediated vasodilation in skeletal muscle (see Subchapter 4.5). However, the endothelium is relatively impermeable to these catecholamines at physiological concentrations (Lew et al. 1989), limiting their access to the smooth muscle.

- Many blood vessels are innervated by peptidergic afferent nerve axons (e.g., superficial cutaneous, visceral, deep somatic and intracranial blood vessels). These nerve axons have nociceptive function. Their excitation elicits arteriolar vasodilation and venular plasma extravasation, both responses being peripheral protective reactions that do not require the spinal cord. Vasodilation is mediated by CGRP and to a lesser extent by substance P; plasma extravasation is mediated by substance P (Holzer 1992; Häbler et al. 1999). It is likely that subpopulations of peptidergic afferents are specialized with respect to these functions (see Subchapter 2.2, Note 2). Vasodilation due to impulses in the peptidergic afferents at frequencies of ≤1 Hz (or higher) overrides the constriction generated by impulse

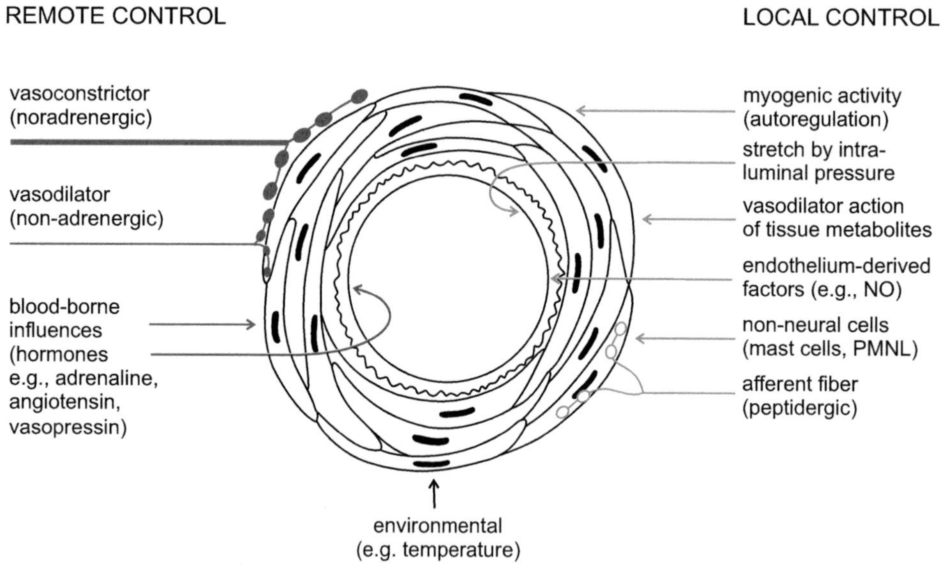

REMOTE CONTROL   LOCAL CONTROL

vasoconstrictor
(noradrenergic)

vasodilator
(non-adrenergic)

blood-borne
influences
(hormones
e.g., adrenaline,
angiotensin,
vasopressin)

myogenic activity
(autoregulation)

stretch by intra-
luminal pressure

vasodilator action
of tissue metabolites

endothelium-derived
factors (e.g., NO)

non-neural cells
(mast cells, PMNL)

afferent fiber
(peptidergic)

environmental
(e.g. temperature)

Figure 7.9 Blood vessels are under multiple remote and local controls. *Left side:* Remote controls. Vasoconstrictor neurons (ongoing activity). Vasodilator neurons (normally silent; only in some blood vessels). Blood-borne influences: vasopressin (e.g., during water deprivation or severe blood loss); angiotensin (e.g., during severe blood loss); adrenaline (vasodilation; only blood vessels in skeletal muscle and during special behavioral conditions; see Subchapter 4.5). *Right side:* Local control. Spontaneous myogenic activity. Stretch-evoked contractions. Endothelium-induced vasodilation (e.g., by nitric oxide [NO] released by the endothelial cells by shearing forces exerted by blood flow changes). Vasodilation generated by tissue metabolites (e.g., in skeletal muscle during exercise; in brain vessels by increase in P_{CO2}; in coronary arteries by decrease in P_{O2}). Vasodilation during inflammation involving mast cells, polymorphonuclear leukocytes (PMNL) and other cells. Vasodilation by peptides (calcitonin gene-related peptide, substance P) released by unmyelinated and small-diameter myelinated afferent axons. Environmental temperature (e.g., enhancement of neuroeffector transmission from vasoconstrictor nerve terminals to skin blood vessels during cold). Modified from Folkow and Neil (1971).

activity in vasoconstrictor neurons in the physiological range (≤ 5 Hz) (Häbler et al. 1997b, 1999).

- Some blood vessels (e.g., in skeletal muscle and kidney) generate spontaneous myogenic activity and react to stretch (increase in transmural pressure). These properties are the basis for autoregulation of vascular beds. The mechanisms underlying spontaneous myogenic activity, myogenic responses to distension of the blood vessels and interaction between myogenic activity and nerve-induced vasoconstriction (e.g., in resistance vessels), however, remain unclear (see Note 3 in Chapter 5). Rhythmic spontaneous contractions of blood vessels that are independent of their innervation may involve cyclic Ca^{2+} release from intracellular stores without contribution of voltage-dependent calcium channels in the cell

membranes. This rhythmic intracellular release of Ca^{2+} is entrained between different muscle cells of the syncytium by the oscillating membrane potential via gap-junction channels (Hill et al. 1999; Peng et al. 2001). Stretch-activated myogenic responses involve mechanosensitive ionic channels and complex intracellular pathways leading to intracellular increase of Ca^{2+} and contractions (for review see Davis and Hill [1999]; Hill et al. [2001]; Tykocki et al. [2017]).

- Mechanical shearing forces exerted by pulsating blood flow at the luminal endothelial surface trigger synthesis and release of nitric oxide (NO) by endothelial cells. NO leads to relaxation of the vascular smooth muscle cells and to vasodilation. This local mechanism seems to operate continuously in various arterioles and small arteries. It is unclear whether this endothelium-derived production of

NO and therefore the vasodilation are also under some neural control (see Häbler et al. 1997a), and whether there are differences between the endothelia of different vascular beds with regard to this mechanism of vasodilation. Furthermore, there are several other ways in which the endothelium can influence vascular smooth muscle. The physiological relevance of most of these paracrine activators and neural influences on these agents or their actions is unclear (Vanhoutte et al. 2016).

- Skeletal muscles undergo dramatic changes during exercise, resulting in the accumulation of several metabolites (e.g., lactate, phosphate), decrease in pH and P_{O2}, increase in P_{CO2}, increase in osmolality, increase in adenosine, etc. It is believed that during exercise these changes directly influence the vascular muscle to generate a vasodilation that attenuates neurally evoked vasoconstriction. However, the mechanisms of local vasodilation are still poorly understood and no single factor that dilates blood vessels under physiological conditions has so far been identified. Furthermore, the neural vasoconstrictor influence on blood vessels in skeletal muscle during exercise does not seem to be diminished by the metabolic changes (for discussion see Rowell [1993]; Marshall [2015]).
- Local mechanisms related to inflammation influence blood vessels, generating precapillary vasodilation and postcapillary plasma extravasation. These changes are brought about by compounds released by inflammatory cells (e.g., mast cells, leukocytes), which either act directly on the muscle cells, via the endothelium or via peptidergic afferents.
- Environmental temperature changes may influence cutaneous blood vessels directly or indirectly by changing neurovascular transmission from vasoconstrictor nerve terminals. Warming dilates these vessels and attenuates neurovascular transmission; cooling constricts these blood vessels and enhances neurovascular transmission (Cassell et al. 1988; Johnson and Kellogg 2010; Johnson et al. 2014; Smith and Johnson 2016; Flavahan and Flavahan 2020).

This summary of the different components that may influence the reactivity of the vascular smooth musculature shows that this autonomic effector tissue is potentially under multiple local and remote controls. These interact with impulses from vasoconstrictor neurons. Local and remote non-neural influences may also influence other autonomic effector tissues (e.g., sweat glands [Smith and Johnson 2016]) and interact with their innervation. However, here I want to emphasize that: (1) for most of these processes the mechanisms of interaction with the neural influence are not very well explored, and (2) the neural signal in the vasoconstrictor neurons seems to have preference over most other signals under several physiological conditions.

7.5 Unconventional Functions of Sympathetic Noradrenergic Neurons

New emerging ideas are whether noradrenergic sympathetic terminals have functions that are not dependent on centrally generated impulse activity, not on their excitability and even not on release of noradrenaline. Arguments will be given showing that sympathetic terminals may be involved in bradykinin-induced plasma extravasation and as a mediator element in the sensitization of nociceptors by the inflammatory mediator bradykinin (and possibly by other inflammatory mediators). Thus, terminals of sympathetic noradrenergic neurons may have functions that are entirely different from their conventional function of transmitting centrally generated impulses to peripheral target tissues.

7.5.1 Involvement of the Sympathetic Postganglionic Axons in Neurogenic Inflammation

The synovium of joints continuously secretes fluid into the joint cavity. This secretion occurs on the venular side of the synovial vascular bed; it is essential for adequate functioning of joints and is finely adjusted to joint activity. Decreased secretion of synovial fluid leads to joint damage and finally to arthrosis; increased synovial secretion occurs during synovial inflammation and also leads to a restriction of joint function. Here I describe experiments demonstrating that synovial secretion is dependent on the sympathetic innervation of the synovia and that the role of the sympathetic postganglionic axons is, first, to control blood flow (as expected) and, second, to serve as a mediator element in the control of venular plasma extravasation (Jänig and Green 2014).

Bradykinin (Note 7) is a potent inflammatory mediator and generates plasma extravasation by increasing the permeability of the postcapillary venules. Perfusion of the knee joint cavity of the rat hindlimb with bradykinin solution at a concentration of 160 ng/mL (1.5×10^{-7}M) increases the synovial plasma extravasation about fivefold (open circles in Figure 7.10d):

- Resting and bradykinin-evoked plasma extravasation are not dependent on the innervation of the joint capsule by unmyelinated afferent axons (Coderre et al. 1989), but are to some extent dependent on the innervation of the synovia by sympathetic postganglionic nerve axons. Both are significantly reduced 7 to 14 days after surgical sympathectomy (Figures 7.10d and 7.11; Miao et al. 1996b).

- Cutting the preganglionic axons to chronically decentralize the lumbar sympathetic ganglia that contain the postganglionic neurons to the rat hindlimb does not significantly change the bradykinin-induced plasma extravasation in the knee joint capsule (Figure 7.10d). Similarly, acute interruption of the lumbar sympathetic chains during ongoing bradykinin-induced plasma extravasation does not reduce this plasma extravasation (Miao et al. 1996b). Finally, perfusion of the joint cavity with the sodium channel blocker tetrodotoxin, in addition to bradykinin, does not significantly change bradykinin-induced plasma extravasation. These interventions leave the postganglionic axons intact and argue that bradykinin-induced plasma extravasation is not dependent on their excitation/electrical activity.

- However, as might be expected, activation of the sympathetic postganglionic neurons by electrical stimulation of the sympathetic chain reduces both resting and bradykinin-evoked plasma extravasation because of a reduction in blood flow through the synovia.

- Quantitative analysis of the synovial plasma extravasation generated by different concentrations of bradykinin in the perfusate shows that the sympathetically mediated component is particularly large at bradykinin concentrations that have been measured in inflamed tissues (between 10^{-8} and 10^{-7} M; Hargreaves et al. 1993; Swift et al. 1993) and almost undetectable at higher (pharmacological) concentrations, probably because bradykinin also acts directly on the endothelial cells and because this direct

endothelial effect is maximal at pharmacological bradykinin concentrations (Figure 7.11; Miao et al. 1996a).

These experiments suggest that bradykinin-induced plasma extravasation is dependent on the presence of the terminals of the sympathetic postganglionic axons in the synovia but not on action potentials in these axons.

These types of experiments suggest that sympathetic postganglionic neurons innervating the joint capsule and its synovium have two functions (Figure 7.12), to regulate blood flow (vasoconstrictor function) and to mediate vascular permeability. The latter function is a newly described component of neurogenic inflammation. The first occurs at the precapillary resistance vessels by vesicular release of transmitter(s), which induces vasoconstriction and which is regulated by action potentials in the sympathetic vasoconstrictor neurons. The second function occurs at the postcapillary venules by non-vesicular release of a chemical substance(s) (possibly prostaglandin E_2 and/or related substances) (Sherbourne et al. 1992), which is independent of the electrical activity in the sympathetic neurons. Whether this substance is released by the sympathetic terminals or by other cells in association with these terminals is unknown. This sympathetically mediated component of neurogenic inflammation is an entirely peripheral function of the sympathetic terminals. Whether the two functions of the sympathetic postganglionic neurons are represented in the same class of neuron or in distinct ones remains to be studied. This study should include the role of mast cells and of cells related to the immune system, such as polymorphonuclear leukocytes (Figure 7.12).

The results obtained from experiments investigating bradykinin-induced plasma extravasation in the rat knee joint raise questions as to whether:

- the noradrenergic sympathetic neurons are involved in the maintenance of inflammatory processes that normally occur in various compartments of the body (e.g., the skin, the viscera, the deep somatic tissues);

- inflammatory mediators other than bradykinin generate increases in permeability of postcapillary venules via the sympathetic noradrenergic varicose terminals (Pierce et al. 1995); and

- an interaction between sympathetically mediated neurogenic inflammation and afferent-mediated

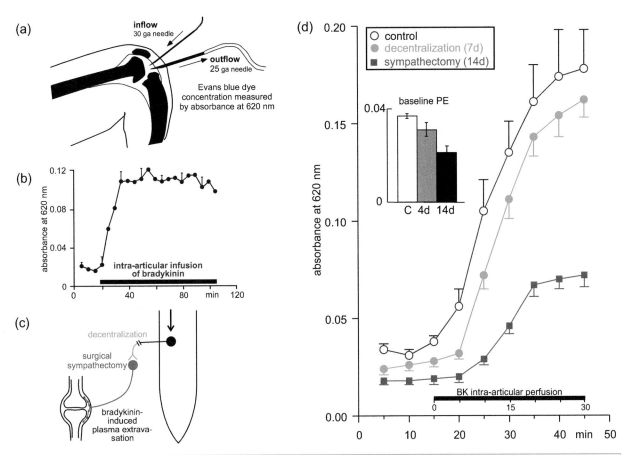

Figure 7.10 Bradykinin-induced plasma extravasation in the synovia of the knee joint is largely dependent on the sympathetic innervation but not on activity in the sympathetic neurons. (a) The rat knee joint was perfused with saline at a constant rate of 250 μL/min in the anesthetized rat. Rats were pretreated with Evan's blue dye given i.v. (Evan's blue binds to albumin and does not normally leave the vascular space). Plasma extravasation of the synovia into the knee joint cavity was determined by measuring Evan's blue dye extravasation into the perfusate in 5 min samples. The concentration of Evan's blue, determined spectrophotometrically at a wave length of 620 nm, is proportional to the degree of extravasation (ordinate scale in [b,d]). Bradykinin (BK, 160 ng/mL, 1.5×10^{-7} M), an inflammatory mediator, was added to the perfusate 15 min after the beginning of the perfusion and the perfusion lasted for at least 30 min. (c) Three preparations were used: intact lumbar sympathetic system; decentralized lumbar sympathetic system (preganglionic axons interrupted 7 days before the experiment by sectioning the white rami); surgical sympathectomy 14 days before the experiment (removal of the paravertebral ganglia [see Baron et al. [1988]). (d) Increased plasma extravasation induced by BK in control rats (open circles, n = 12 knees). This increase was significantly smaller 14 days after sympathectomy (closed red squares, n = 12 knees) but was not significantly different from control after decentralization (closed green circles, n = 12 knees). Inset: baseline plasma extravasation (PE) over 15 min preceding infusion of BK was also lower in animals 4 days and 14 days after sympathectomy than in control (C) animals. (d) Modified from Miao et al. (1996b) with permission; from Jänig and Green (2014).

neurogenic inflammation occurs and what the nature of this interaction is (see Note 2 in Subchapter 2.2).

Bradykinin-induced plasma extravasation in the synovia can be modulated by the hypothalamus–pituitary–adrenal axis and by the sympatho-adrenal axis. Activation of both neuroendocrine axes (e.g., by noxious cutaneous or visceral stimulation) depresses this experimental inflammation. This depression is mediated by corticosterone and adrenaline, which are released by the adrenal cortex and the adrenal medulla, respectively. The effects of activation of the hypothalamus–pituitary–adrenal axis and of intravenously administered corticosterone on the

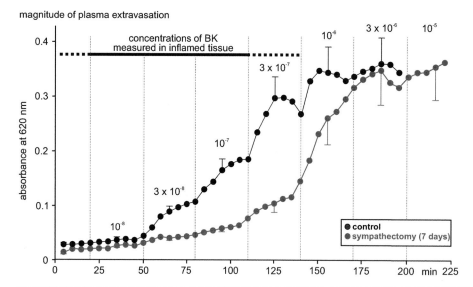

Figure 7.11 Concentration-dependent bradykinin-induced plasma extravasation in control rats and in sympathectomized rats (see Figure 7.10c). For experimental procedure, see legend to Figure 7.10. Bradykinin was added cumulatively from 10^{-8} to 10^{-5} M to the perfusate. The measured bradykinin concentrations in inflamed tissues (Hargreaves et al. 1993; Swift et al. 1993) are indicated. In sympathectomized rats, the extravasation is significantly reduced between 3×10^{-8} and 3×10^{-7} M bradykinin. At higher (pharmacological) concentrations ($> 10^{-6}$M), sympathectomy has no effect because the effect of bradykinin is generated via pathways other than the sympathetically mediated one. Modified from Miao et al. (1996a) with permission.

bradykinin-induced plasma extravasation in the synovia are dependent on the presence of the sympathetic terminals in the synovia. This shows that the sympathetic axons are in a strategic, yet unexpected, position in the control of synovial plasma extravasation by the brain (Green et al. 1995, 1997). The depression of bradykinin-induced plasma extravasation in the synovia by adrenaline released by the adrenal medulla is not mediated by vasoconstriction in the synovia; its mechanism is unknown (Jänig et al. 2000; Miao et al. 2000, 2001).

7.5.2 Involvement of the Sympathetic Postganglionic Axons in Sensitization of Nociceptors and Mechanical Hyperalgesia

Sensitization of nociceptors during peripheral inflammation leading to hyperalgesia (increased sensitivity to painful stimuli) may depend on the sympathetic innervation of the inflamed tissue (Note 8). An animal model of hyperalgesic behavior in which the sympathetic postganglionic nerve axons are supposed to be involved has been proposed.

Cutaneous Mechanical Hyperalgesia Elicited by the Inflammatory Mediator Bradykinin

The paw-withdrawal threshold to mechanical stimulation is a behavioral measure of pain elicited by this stimulus. This, as studied in rats, is dose-dependently decreased by intracutaneous injection of bradykinin at the site of stimulation. Following a single intracutaneous injection into the dorsal skin of the hindpaw, the decrease in threshold to mechanical stimulation lasts for more than 1 hour (Taiwo and Levine 1988). This mechanical hyperalgesic behavior is mediated by the B_2 bradykinin-receptor (Khasar et al. 1995, 1998) and does not develop when bradykinin is injected subcutaneously, i.e., into the subcutaneous fat of the dorsal hindpaw away from the superficially located cutaneous nociceptors (Khasar et al. 1993). The decrease in paw-withdrawal threshold to mechanical stimulation generated by bradykinin is caused by prostaglandin (prostaglandin E_2), which is an arachidonic acid metabolite and sensitizes cutaneous nociceptors. Blockade of arachidonic acid metabolism by indomethacin (injected intraperitoneally 30 minutes before the measurements and injected together with bradykinin intracutaneously),

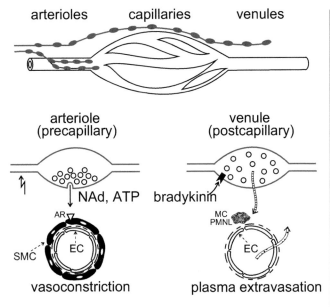

arterioles   capillaries   venules

arteriole
(precapillary)

venule
(postcapillary)

NAd, ATP   bradykinin

AR

SMC   EC

MC
PMNL

EC

vasoconstriction   plasma extravasation

Figure 7.12 Schematic diagram illustrating that sympathetic axons innervating the synovia have two functions. *Left side:* varicosities of vasoconstrictor axons form close synaptic contacts with the smooth muscle cells of the precapillary resistance vessels (arterioles). Impulse activity in these postganglionic neurons leads to vesicular release of transmitter(s) (NAd, ATP) and to constriction of the resistance vessels. *Right side:* reaction of bradykinin with bradykinin receptors in the varicosities leads to activation of the cyclooxygenase pathway of arachidonic acid metabolism and to synthesis and release of a prostaglandin (probably prostaglandin E). This release occurs by *de novo* synthesis and not by vesicular release, and leads to opening of the endothelial gaps of venules and subsequent increase in plasma extravasation. This process is independent of activity in the sympathetic neurons. It is unknown whether synthesis and release of prostaglandin occurs from the varicosities or from other cells in association with the varicosities. It is furthermore unknown whether vasoconstriction and plasma extravasation are generated by the *same* group of sympathetic postganglionic neurons or by *different* groups of sympathetic postganglionic neurons. AR, adrenoreceptor; ATP, adenosine triphosphate; EC, endothelial cell; NAd, noradrenaline; MC, mast cells; PMNL, polymorphonuclear leukocytes; SMC, smooth muscle cells. Modified from Miao et al. (1996b) with permission.

prevents the release of prostaglandin and therefore also the mechanical hyperalgesia.

The cutaneous mechanical hyperalgesic behavior can no longer be generated by intracutaneous injection of bradykinin after *surgical sympathectomy* of the rat hindlimb (removal of the sympathetic paravertebral ganglia; performed ≥8 days before the behavioral measurements). However, *decentralization* of the lumbar sympathetic trunk (cutting the preganglionic axons and leaving the postganglionic neurons in the paravertebral ganglia intact) does not change the mechanical hyperalgesic effect of bradykinin. It is hypothesized that sensitization of the cutaneous nociceptors to mechanical stimulation by a prostaglandin is dependent on the sympathetic terminals but not on activity in the sympathetic neurons. The release of prostaglandin, either from the sympathetic terminals or from cells in association with the sympathetic innervation of the skin, is triggered by bradykinin via B_2-receptors, presumably in the sympathetic terminals.

This role of sympathetic postganglionic axons as mediators in the sensitization of cutaneous nociceptors, independently of nerve firing, is an interesting idea, which assigns to the sympathetic nerves a function that is entirely different from its usual one. However, this interpretation based on the evidence of behavioral studies raises several open and critical questions (see Jänig and Häbler 2000). The mechanisms of bradykinin-induced sensitization of cutaneous nociceptors for mechanical stimulation and of sympathetic axons in facilitating this effect are rather unclear and have to be more closely investigated. It is necessary to perform neurophysiological experiments on cutaneous nociceptive afferents in vivo and/or in vitro in order to directly demonstrate that the nociceptors or a subpopulation of them are sensitized by bradykinin for mechanical stimulation and that this effect is dependent on the presence of the sympathetic terminals.

Conclusions

Axons of postganglionic neurons branch many times close to their effector cells and have hundreds to thousands of varicosities, which contain transmitter(s) packed in vesicles. Excitation of the postganglionic neurons spreads over all its branches and normally invades all varicosities.

1. Signal transmission from postganglionic neurons to most effector cells occurs through neuroeffector synapses, which are characterized by a close junction between varicosities and membranes of the effector cells, by fusion of the basal laminae and by accumulation of synaptic vesicles close to the synaptic junction.

2. Release of transmitter during excitation of the postganglionic neuron occurs in quanta (i.e. release of the entire contents of a vesicle). Individual varicosities have a low probability (about 0.01) of releasing the transmitter when the discharge rate is low. This probability of transmitter release may increase up to 10 times with increasing discharge rate of the postganglionic neurons.

3. The release of the content of a vesicle from a varicosity leads to a short-lasting increase in the concentration of the transmitter in the junctional cleft, which may reach into the millimolar range, and the subsequent interaction of the transmitter with junctional receptors in the effector cells.

4. In the heart, acetylcholine released by varicosities of parasympathetic cardiomotor axons reacts only with junctional muscarinic receptors that are coupled via a distinct intracellular second-messenger pathway to the cellular effectors (e.g., ionic channels). Extrajunctional cholinergic muscarinic receptors are not activated by neuronally released acetylcholine. The extrajunctional muscarinic receptors are coupled by another intercellular second-messenger pathway to the cellular effectors. Their function during neural organ regulation is unclear.

5. In the heart, noradrenaline released by the varicosities of the sympathetic cardiomotor axons reacts with junctional β_1-adrenoceptors, which are coupled via a yet unknown intracellular pathway to ionic channels modifying the pacemaker current. It is unclear whether an extrajunctional pathway operating via cAMP is also used during ongoing regulation of the heart by the sympathetic neurons.

6. Arterioles and small arteries are influenced by neural release of noradrenaline and ATP from the varicosities of the vasoconstrictor axons. The ATP reacts with junctional purinoceptors and opens ligand-gated cation channels, which depolarize the membrane, causing activation of voltage-sensitive calcium channels and resultant action potentials. Noradrenaline released from the postganglionic vasoconstrictor terminals reacts with junctionally and possibly extrajunctionally located α-adrenoceptors leading to slow depolarization in some blood vessels.

- Nerve-induced constriction of small arterioles in the submucosa of the gut is only mediated by ATP and purinoceptors, but in other arterioles it is mediated by noradrenaline and α_1-adrenoceptors.
- Nerve-induced constriction of some larger arteries (e.g., the rat tail artery) is mediated by noradrenaline and α-adrenoceptors.
- Nerve-induced constriction in some arteries is mediated by both the purinergic and adrenergic mechanisms. The integration between these cellular processes during ongoing regulation of small arteries and arterioles is unclear.
- Circulating catecholamines are unlikely to be involved in direct regulation of these innervated blood vessels in the concentrations that occur in vivo.

7. Contractility of veins and the pulmonary artery is likely regulated by neuronal release of noradrenaline via adrenoceptors coupled to an intracellular pathway involving inositol 1,4,5-triphosphate (IP3).

8. Cholinergic neurons of the enteric nervous system that innervate the longitudinal musculature of the ileum activate the smooth muscle cells via junctional muscarinic receptors. This activation leads, via an intracellular second-messenger pathway, to opening of *calcium channels* and subsequently to contraction. The cellular mechanisms mediating contraction evoked by activation of junctional and extrajunctional muscarinic receptors are different.

9. The functions of neuropeptides in neuroeffector transmission have been little explored and are, in most cases, unknown.

10. The influence exerted by autonomic neurons on their effector tissues may be modulated by local and remote non-neural signals. The influence of

the local signals varies between different effector tissues.

11. Experimental bradykinin-induced inflammation of the knee joint synovia and experimental bradykinin-induced mechanical hyperalgesic behavior in rats indicate that sympathetic post-ganglionic nerve axons may have entirely unexpected functions that are independent of their function to evoke neurotransmitter release onto effector cells. These functions include the mediation of venular plasma extravasation and the sensitization of nociceptors generated during inflammation.

12. The mechanisms of neuroeffector transmission in different targets of the autonomic nervous system are diverse. Nerve-generated signals are transmitted to the autonomic effector cells by distinct cellular pathways linked to the neuroeffector junctions. The traditional ideas about the ability of conventional transmitters to mimic effects of nerve activity are being reconsidered.

13. As no exceptions have yet been found, it is not far-fetched to assume that neuroeffector transmission is specific for all target cells innervated by postganglionic neurons. To best understand nerve-mediated effects in vivo, it is more useful to determine which specific antagonists reduce or abolish the effects of nerve activity than to know which receptor subtypes are present in the tissue.

14. In conclusion, activity in postganglionic sympathetic and parasympathetic neurons is generated by the integrative action of central autonomic circuits. This activity is reliably transmitted by various neuroeffector mechanisms to the target cells, leading to the precise regulation of autonomic effector organs.

Suggested Reading

Brock, J. A. and Cunnane, T. C. (1988) Electrical activity at the sympathetic neuroeffector junction in the guinea-pig vas deferens. *J Physiol* **399**, 607–632.

Campbell, G. D., Edwards, F. R., Hirst, G. D. S., and O'Shea, J. E. (1989) Effects of vagal stimulation and applied acetylcholine on pacemaker potentials in the guinea-pig heart. *J Physiol* **415**, 57–68.

Green, P. G., Jänig, W., and Levine, J. D. (1997) Negative feedback neuroendocrine control of inflammatory response in the rat is dependent on the sympathetic post-ganglionic neuron. *J Neurosci* **17**, 3234–3238.

Hirst, G. D. and Edwards, F. R. (1989) Sympathetic neuroeffector transmission in arteries and arterioles. *Physiol Rev* **69**, 546–604.

Jänig, W. and Green, P. G. (2014) Acute inflammation in the joint: its control by the sympathetic nervous system and by neuroendocrine systems. *Auton Neurosci* **182**, 42–54.

Jänig, W. and McLachlan, E. M. (2013) Neurobiology of the autonomic nervous system. In *Autonomic Failure*, 5th edn (Mathias, C. J. and Bannister, R., eds) pp. 21–34, Oxford University Press, New York, Oxford.

Miao, F. J.-P., Jänig, W. and Levine, J. D. (1996b) Role of sympathetic postganglionic neurons in synovial plasma extravasation induced by bradykinin. *J Neurophysiol* **75**, 715–724.

All references cited in the text are available online at www.cambridge.org/janig.

Notes

1. See Note 2 on the axon reflex concept in Chapter 2.
2. For intracellular signaling involving receptor-activated G-proteins and second-messenger systems see Schulman (2013).
3. The passive electrical properties of functional syncytia of electrically coupled smooth muscle cells can be treated as one-, two- or three-dimensional systems, depending on the type of syncytium. In small arterioles, current spreads approximately in one dimension; in thick-walled arteries or gastrointestinal smooth muscles (e.g., of the stomach or the colon), current spreads in three dimensions. This electrical geometry influences the time course of potential changes and the distance of electrotonic spread of a potential generated by current injection in the syncytia. For resting arterioles that can be treated approximately as one-dimensional cables, the time constant is in the range of 300 to 700 ms (time of the potential to decrease to $1/e$ [37%]; product of specific membrane resistance and capacitance) and the length constant in the range of 1.5 mm (distance taken for electrotonic potentials to decrease to $1/e$ [37%]; square root of ratio of membrane resistance to axial resistance). The electrical behavior of the syncytia of electrically coupled cells is described in the literature (Jack et al. 1975; Tomita 1975; Hirst and Edwards 1989).
4. The argument that nerve-released adrenaline in the toad activates adrenoceptors that are neither α nor β is based on pharmacological experiments. These show that the

postsynaptic effects (generation of junction potentials) following nerve stimulation: (1) are not abolished by α- or β-adrenoceptor blockers, (2) are abolished after depletion of adrenaline from the postganglionic terminals by bretylium and (3) are blocked by dihydroergotamine (that blocks the effect of applied adrenaline, but not of applied ATP, by acting on non-α, non-β adrenoceptors). Furthermore, the experiments show that the actions of applied adrenaline on the sinus venosus are blocked by a β2-adrenoceptor antagonist, arguing that applied adrenaline reacts with extrajunctionally located β2-adrenoceptors (Morris et al. 1981; Bramich et al. 1990, 1993).

5. Venular smooth muscle cells have a high intracellular chloride concentration due to transport of chloride from extracellular to intracellular. This results in a chloride equilibrium potential that is more positive than the membrane resting potential (in the range of 30 mV). Opening of the chloride channels by elevated intracellular calcium generates an outflow of chloride along its electrochemical gradient, producing a depolarization (i.e. excitatory junction potentials; van Helden 1988a, b). This mechanism applies to arterioles in the rat iris too (Gould and Hill 1996).

6. The pulsatile Ca^{2+} release from the intracellular store not only activates the contractile machinery but also potassium channels in the muscle cell membrane. This leads to transient membrane hyperpolarizations superimposed on the membrane depolarizations generated by the opening of non-specific cation channels.

7. Bradykinin is a peptide and is released in inflamed tissues. It mediates multiple functions, one of them being the generation of plasma extravasation through post-capillary venules.

8. With the exception of the parenchyma of the liver and brain, all tissues are innervated by primary afferent neurons that are activated by tissue-damaging stimuli or by stimuli indicating impending damage (thermal, mechanical, chemical stimuli). These afferent neurons are called nociceptive neurons. They have unmyelinated or small-diameter myelinated axons. *Sensitization of nociceptors* occurs during inflammation; it is characterized: (1) by a decrease in threshold to heat and mechanical stimulation, (2) by the development of spontaneous activity, (3) by increased responses to noxious stimuli and (4) by the recruitment of nociceptive primary afferent neurons that cannot normally be activated (or have extremely high threshold for activation) (see Subchapter 2.4). *Hyperalgesia* denotes increased pain generated by a stimulus that is normally painful and excites nociceptors. The mechanisms of hyperalgesia are peripheral (sensitization of nociceptors) and central (sensitization of central neurons, e.g., in the dorsal horn of the spinal cord). *Animal models of hyperalgesic behavior* are used to investigate the peripheral and central mechanisms of hyperalgesia. Standardized reactions of the animals to mechanical or thermal stimuli are measured and quantified (e.g., paw-withdrawal threshold to mechanical stimulation of the hindpaw; latency of paw withdrawal to a heat stimulus applied to the hindpaw; latency of tail flick to heat stimulation, etc.) (Belmonte and Cervero 1996; Ringkamp et al. 2013).

Part IV

Representation of the Autonomic Nervous System in the Spinal Cord and Lower Brain Stem

In the preceding chapters I have described how sympathetic and parasympathetic systems consist of many functionally *separate* pathways that supply the peripheral target organs. The neurons in these pathways have characteristic reflex discharge patterns, which are centrally generated. The final central output neurons are the preganglionic neurons in the spinal cord and the brain stem. Integrative processes in general do not seem to occur *between* functionally distinct autonomic pathways, but only *within* some non-vasoconstrictor pathways to viscera (see Chapter 4). The discharge patterns measured in postganglionic neurons are unlikely to be generated by qualitatively different discharge patterns in subpopulations of preganglionic neurons converging on the same postganglionic neuron, although we have no direct experimental proof for this. This does not clash with the finding that neurochemically different preganglionic neurons may converge on the same postganglionic neuron (Murphy et al. 1998). Thus, in the autonomic ganglia, the discharge patterns are not changed qualitatively, but may be modified quantitatively, e.g., enhanced by the converging synaptic input. At the neuroeffector junctions, temporal and spatial aspects of the neural signals transmitted to the effector cells contribute to transmission; furthermore, various non-neural signals may modulate neuroeffector transmission pre- and postjunctionally

(see Subchapter 7.4). The final response of the effector tissue is determined by its own functional properties.

This part will focus on some principles of the organization of central regulation of peripheral autonomic pathways integrated into the spinal cord, brain stem and hypothalamus. I will not describe the central regulation of specific autonomic functions that are related to the regulation of the cardiovascular system, pelvic organs, gastrointestinal tract, body core temperature, metabolism, etc. in detail (see Loewy and Spyer [1990]; Blessing [1997]; Appenzeller [1999]; Robertson et al. [2012]; Bujis and Swaab [2013]; Mathias and Bannister [2013]; Romanovsky [2018]), only use some of these data to exemplify what is known about the organization of autonomic systems in the spinal cord and lower brain stem.

The reference point for this description is the *functional specificity* of the peripheral autonomic pathways with respect to the target organs derived from the measurements of the reflexes in post- and preganglionic neurons (see Chapter 4). It should be kept in mind that these reflexes are mostly isolated fragments of neural regulating systems; they are, as such, experimental artifacts (such as the monosynaptic stretch reflex as used in research on somato-motor physiology). Some reflexes may easily be interpreted as functionally meaningful, such as baro- and chemoreceptor reflexes in vasoconstrictor neurons (to regulate cardiovascular function; see Chapter 10); locally restricted inhibitory nociceptive reflexes in cutaneous or muscle vasoconstrictor neurons (to increase blood flow through damaged tissue; see Subchapter 4.1); thermoregulatory spinal and supraspinal reflexes in cutaneous vasoconstrictor neurons; vibration reflexes generated by stimulation of Pacinian corpuscles in sudomotor neurons [to keep the stratum corneum flexible during sensory manipulation; see Subchapter 4.2); excitatory and inhibitory sacro-lumbar reflexes in sympathetic motility-regulating neurons innervating pelvic organs (to regulate continence; see Subchapter 4.3). The application of the reflex concept provides an insight into the neuronal structure underlying regulation of autonomic target organs. The advantage of this approach is obvious, as it was in the analysis of the somatomotor system (Granit 1981):

1. the types of efferent neurons being controlled are known;
2. the afferent neurons stimulated are known;
3. the experimental conditions are defined;
4. the reflexes can be studied in various types of preparation (e.g., in vivo brain-intact, decerebrate or spinal animals; in vitro whole-heart-brain-stem preparation with attached heart in which the afferent and efferent pathways are intact; Paton 1996a, b);
5. the mechanisms of synaptic transmission in these well-defined reflex pathways can be studied;
6. once the reflexes, their pathways (including interneurons) and the underlying mechanisms are well defined, how these pathways function and interact during ongoing regulation of the autonomic target organs can be elucidated.

The central representations of the autonomic systems are organized caudorostrally in spinal cord, brain stem, hypothalamus and telencephalon. This organization exhibits some hierarchy in the degree of functional complexity, simple functions being represented at the level of the spinal cord and most complex autonomic functions at the forebrain level (hypothalamus and telencephalon). The description of the central representations of autonomic functions will therefore follow this general idea:

1. The first level of integration occurs in the spinal cord for sympathetic systems and sacral parasympathetic systems and is represented in the various autonomic reflex pathways and their mutual synaptic connections via interneurons (see Subchapter 8.3). Here I will use the term *spinal autonomic systems* (Nilsson 1983). An analogous situation exists for the parasympathetic systems in the brain stem (see Subchapter 10.7).

2. Integration is more complex in the lower brain stem (medulla oblongata and pons). It mainly involves: (a) regulation of arterial blood pressure to maintain perfusion of the body's tissues with blood, (b) regulation of the transport of oxygen and carbon dioxide (regulation of respiration) and (c) regulation of gastrointestinal function (ingestion, digestion, and absorption of nutrients and fluid). These three global *homeostatic regulations* (Figure 10.1) are closely integrated. Included in them are the spinal autonomic systems and equivalent parasympathetic systems in the brain stem. Additionally, the lower brain stem represents regulation of evacuative functions (urinary bladder, hindgut) and reproductive organs. The underlying supraspinal mechanisms of these regulations are largely unknown and will not be further discussed here (see Jänig [1996a, b]; de Groat [2013]; McKenna [2000, 2001, 2013]).

3. Integration in the hypothalamus and mesencephalon is related to thermoregulation, regulation of energy balance and metabolism, regulation of body protection (including the immune system [Jänig 2014]), etc. These regulations include autonomic, somatomotor and neuroendocrine systems. Integrated in these regulations are the homeostatic regulations represented in the lower brain stem and the spinal autonomic systems.

4. The most rostral level of autonomic integration occurs in the telencephalon. The homeostatic autonomic regulations are adapted to the needs of the organism according to environmental challenges (e.g., when the organism is physically threatened, is potentially in a state of starvation, etc.) (Note 1).

The concept of hierarchical organization of central autonomic systems is not absolute and must not be taken too literally. It is not new, as can be seen from previous discussions of control of the cardiovascular system by the brain (see Rushmer and Smith [1959]; Bard [1960]). However, it helps to understand the structural and physiological basis of the regulation of peripheral autonomic pathways by the brain. Here

I would like to put a word of caution: in the last 30 to 40 years we have made considerable progress in research on the central autonomic nervous pathways; however, we are far from understanding how the multiple homeostatic regulations are generated, integrated with each other and integrated with the behavior of the organism.

In Chapters 9 to 11, spinal cord, brain stem and hypothalamus are separated. This separation is helpful because it reflects to a certain degree the functional hierarchy in the organization of the central autonomic regulations mentioned above. Chapter 11 describes some overall aspects of homeostatic regulation of autonomic functions that are represented in the upper brain stem, and hypothalamus and associated structures, without going into detail in describing autonomic hypothalamic and telencephalic functions.

This part will be introduced by Chapter 8 on the anatomy of the central autonomic systems, which concentrates mainly on the preganglionic neurons, the sympathetic and spinal parasympathetic premotor neurons and the neurons that are antecedent to the autonomic premotor neurons. Further aspects of the anatomy of central autonomic systems are described in Chapter 10, in relation to the description of the physiology of central autonomic systems in the lower brain stem.

Notes

1. The adaptation of homeostatic regulations represented in brain stem and hypothalamus in response to internal and environmental challenges (during exercise, temperature load, lack of fluid, lack of nutrients, physical threat, mental stress) is sometimes called *allostasis* (Sterling and Eyer 1988; McEwen 2001; Schulkin and Sterling 2019). This concept will be discussed in Chapter 11.

Chapter 8

Anatomy of Central Autonomic Systems

8.1 Tools to Investigate the Anatomy of the Central Autonomic Systems

The functional specificity of the autonomic regulation of target organs and the neurophysiological recordings from peripheral autonomic neurons (see Chapter 4) argue that central autonomic systems must be differentiated. It seems likely then that the central organization is reflected in the micro- and macroanatomy of the central autonomic systems. Originally, central stimulation and lesion studies, involving recordings from autonomic nerves or autonomic effector responses (e.g., blood pressure, heart rate, gastrointestinal motility), gave clues about the location of the autonomic centers in the neuraxis. However, the results from these studies were imprecise so that it was not possible to identify anatomically distinct populations of central neurons as being associated with distinct autonomic output systems. Furthermore, focal electrolytic lesioning and focal electrical stimulation did not discriminate between destruction or excitation of cell bodies and passing axons. With the introduction of chemical stimulation of cell bodies (by microiontophoretic application of excitatory amino acids, such as glutamate, aspartate or DL-homocystic acid, or of inhibitory amino acids,

such as γ-aminobutyric acid [GABA] or glycine) it was possible to topically excite or inhibit small populations of central neurons selectively. This technique turned out to be a valuable tool in physiological experimentation.

The breakthrough in unraveling aspects of the microanatomy of the central organization of autonomic systems came: (1) with the introduction of axon tracer methods in the 1970s and (2) with the introduction of retrograde transneuronal labeling of neuron populations using neurotropic viruses at the end of the 1980s by Arthur Loewy's group (Strack et al. 1989a, b):

- The first method allows the localization of the cell bodies of autonomic pre- and postganglionic neurons, as well as of central autonomic neurons (e.g., sympathetic and parasympathetic premotor neurons) with substances that were applied to their cut axons or axon terminals, taken up by the axons and transported retrogradely by axoplasmic flow to their cell bodies (e.g., horseradish peroxidase [HRP], wheat-germ agglutinin horseradish peroxidase, cholera toxin subunit B [CTb], C-fragment of tetanus toxin, Fluoro-Gold [FG], Fast Blue [FB]; Figure 8.1, right side). Other markers applied close to the cell bodies are taken up and transported orthodromically to the axon terminals (e.g., the lectin *Phaseolus vulgaris* leuko-agglutinin [PHA-L]; Gerfen and Sawchenko 1984) or tracers are transported bidirectionally (e.g., bio-tinylated dextran amines). The markers can be histochemically visualized, allowing quantitative analyses of location, number and structure of the labeled cells or terminals.

- The second method principally allows the local-ization of whole networks of neurons that are connected with a specific autonomic output sys-tem (Loewy 1998). A suspension of a live neuro-tropic virus is injected into a peripheral tissue (e.g., heart, a gland, urinary bladder wall, etc.) or autonomic ganglion (e.g., stellate ganglion, celiac ganglion, pterygopalatine ganglion, etc.). The virus is taken up by nerve terminals and trans-ported to the cell bodies. Within the cell bodies, the virus undergoes replication in the nucleus. The virions exit the nucleus and acquire an enve-lope derived from the nuclear membrane. The newly formed viruses are transported intracellu-larly by the endoplasmic reticulum and Golgi apparatus. In order to trace functionally related neurons of a neuronal network it is critical to use viruses that are transported by *trans-synaptic mech-anisms* and not by unspecific release through the cell membranes of the neurons, which would infect neighboring neurons via the extracellular space, glial cells or other cells in an unspecific way (Figure 8.1, left side). This has been achieved using weak suspensions of herpes viruses and the Bartha strain of the pseudorabies virus (PRV), which turned out to be particularly useful as a highly specific retrograde transneuronal synap-tic marker in the autonomic nervous system (Card et al. 1990; Strack and Loewy 1990; Jansen et al. 1993; Enquist and Card 2003; for references see Tables 8.2 and 8.3). With this strain of PRV (or genetically engineered substrains) and careful monitoring, transneuronal synaptic transport of the virus and labeling of first-, second-, third- or fourth-order neurons depend on time after virus application. Taking these aspects and some other limiting factors into account, only neurons that are synaptically connected to the cell bodies of the infected neurons should be labeled (Figure 8.1, left side).

- Combining the retrograde trans-synaptic labeling technique with "classical" tracing methods, or com-bining two different substrains of a neurotropic virus that can be differentiated histochemically are powerful anatomical tools to label central groups of neurons that form direct or indirect con-nections with the preganglionic neurons of the per-ipheral autonomic pathways. Various neuronal networks in spinal cord, brain stem, hypothalamus and cerebral hemispheres involved in the regula-tion of the final autonomic pathways have been described.

- The axonal tracing techniques can be com-bined with other techniques labeling neuro-peptides, enzymes, etc. in the neurons or their axon terminals, using immunohistochem-istry. They can be combined with neurophysio-logical experiments in which reflex activity is recorded from functionally identified neurons. Examples are:
  - Single neurons that are functionally character-ized with neurophysiological techniques can be labeled by tracers injected intracellularly or applied juxtacellularly (Pinault 1996; Pilowsky and Makeham 2001; see Note 3 in Chapter 10; Figures 8.3, 8.9, 10.10).
  - Experiments can be performed on animals in which distinct populations of neurons have been eliminated by a toxin that is conjugated with an agonist for a specific membrane receptor or with a specific enzyme. The toxin–agonist–receptor or toxin–enzyme complex is taken up and internal-ized by the neurons (e.g., by the cell bodies or axon terminals of catecholaminergic neurons or serotonergic neurons projecting to the spinal cord; by neurons expressing specific receptors, e.g. the neurokinin 1 receptor in the respiratory rhythm generator in the medulla oblongata). The internalized toxin then leads to selective suicide of the neurons (see Note 9 in Chapter 10).
  - Expression of *c-fos* messenger RNA (mRNA) and its protein in neurons during their activation can be used as a marker for activa-tion of populations of functionally related neurons during physiological stimuli (e.g., stimulation of arterial baro- or chemorecep-tors) (see Note 1 in Chapter 10 and Schulman [2013]).

Knowledge about the functional anatomy of cen-tral autonomic systems that was obtained with older tracing and degeneration techniques has been con-firmed and considerably extended. In this way the basis for future physiological studies on the central

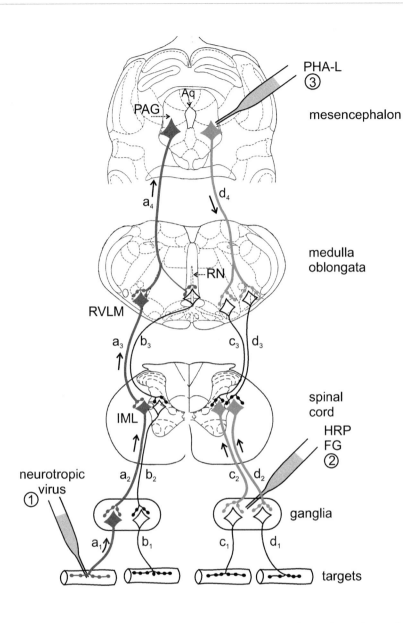

Figure 8.1 Schematic drawings to illustrate the design of experiments in which autonomic neurons are labeled by a neurotropic virus (left side) or by markers not transported trans-synaptically (right side). (1) A neurotropic virus (e.g., Bartha strain of the pseudorabies virus) is injected in the target tissue. The virus is transported retrogradely and replicates in the synaptically connected neurons a_1 to a_4 (red neurons) but not in the neurons b_2 and b_3. (2) A marker that is taken up by the axon terminals and transported to the cell bodies, but not transported trans-synaptically, is injected into an autonomic ganglion or into the target tissue (e.g., horseradish peroxidase, HRP, or Fluoro-Gold, FG). This marker is found in the cell bodies of neurons c_2 and d_2 (green neurons), but not in the cell bodies of the other neurons. (3) A marker that is taken up by the cell bodies and transported orthogradely to the synaptic terminals is applied close to the cell bodies of the neurons d_4 (e.g., *Phaseolus vulgaris* leuko-agglutinin, PHA-L; blue neuron). This marker is found in the synaptic terminals on neurons c_3 and d_3 but not in the other synaptic terminals. These marker techniques can be combined. Aq, cerebral aqueduct; IML, intermediolateral cell column; PAG, periaqueductal gray matter; RN, raphe nuclei; RVLM, rostral ventrolateral medulla.

organization of the different autonomic systems has been laid down.

In this chapter I will summarize the data about the anatomy of central autonomic systems, including the location of preganglionic neurons in the spinal cord and brain stem, and the nucleus tractus solitarii (NTS). The point of reference of all experimental investigations about central autonomic neurons and their functions are the different groups of preganglionic neurons. Details about the anatomy of central autonomic systems (mostly in rats; some in pigeons, pigs and cats) are described and discussed by Cabot (1990), Cechetto and Saper (1990), Loewy (1990a), Loewy and Spyer (1990), Saper (1995) and Blessing (1997). In future the mouse will be used in this anatomical experimental work. This shift will enable the use of genetically engineered animals. Tables 8.2 and 8.3 list the groups of neurons in the different nuclei of the spinal cord, brain stem, hypothalamus and cerebral hemispheres that have been transneuronally labeled from various target tissues using a neurotropic virus (in most cases the Bartha strain of PRV).

8.2 | Morphology and Location of Preganglionic Neurons

8.2.1 Sympathetic Preganglionic Neurons and Interneurons

Preganglionic Neurons

Sympathetic preganglionic neurons lie in the intermediate zone of the thoracolumbar spinal cord, extending from the white matter to the central canal (Figure 1.2). This zone is identical to the dorsal part of lamina VII and lamina X of the spinal gray matter according to Rexed (1952, 1954). The intermediate zone has been subdivided into four subnuclei (Petras and Cummings 1972; Oldfield and McLachlan 1981): the funicular part of the intermediolateral nucleus (ILf) for neurons lying in the white matter, the principal part of the intermediolateral nucleus (ILp) for densely packed neurons lying just medial to the border between white and gray matter, the intercalated spinal nucleus (IC) for neurons lying in bands medial to the ILp across the intermediate zone and the central autonomic nucleus (CA) for neurons lying lateral and dorsal to the central canal, which is located in lamina X of Rexed (Figure 8.2) (Note 1).

Sympathetic preganglionic neurons have cell bodies that are larger than most dorsal horn neurons but significantly smaller than those of motor neurons. They have various groups of dendrites extending mainly rostrocaudally in the lateral intermediate zone and some medially across the intermediate zone or laterally into the white matter. The dendritic field of the preganglionic neurons is almost strictly confined to the intermediate zone. A few dendrites may project ventrally or dorsally along the border between white and gray matter (Figure 8.3). The distances over which the dendrites project along the rostrocaudal axis are considerable, reaching 1.5 to 2.5 mm in the cat (Dembowsky et al. 1985). The surface of the cell bodies is much smaller than the surface of the dendrites, thus most synaptic inputs occur at the dendrites (Cabot et al. 1994; Cabot 1996). The preganglionic neurons project their axons around the lateral edge of the ventral horn and into the ventral root. The majority of preganglionic axons do not have recurrent axon collaterals in the spinal cord (in analogy to the collaterals of the axons of motor neurons that form synapses with Renshaw cells). Some examples have been demonstrated but the function of these collaterals is unknown (see Weaver and Polosa [1997]).

The preganglionic cell bodies are arranged in clusters with intercluster distances varying from 100 to 500 μm (Figure 8.2b C). There is no indication that preganglionic neurons of individual clusters are homogeneous in function; thus, different preganglionic neurons of the same cluster may project into different nerves and to postganglionic neurons with different functions (e.g., to the adrenal medulla or to the superior cervical ganglion or to the stellate ganglion; Jansen et al. 1993). Furthermore, there is no direct evidence that axons of individual preganglionic neurons branch and project into functionally different nerves (e.g., both in lumbar splanchnic nerves and in the lumbar sympathetic trunk distal to the most caudal lumbar splanchnic nerve) or up and down in the sympathetic trunk. This does not preclude that an individual preganglionic axon may form synapses with several postganglionic neurons in adjacent paravertebral ganglia. Finally, sympathetic preganglionic neurons projecting to distinct sympathetic ganglia or the adrenal medulla are segmentally organized. For example, in the cat, preganglionic neurons projecting to the superior cervical ganglion are located in the segments T1 to T7, those projecting in the lumbar sympathetic trunk distal to the paravertebral ganglion L4 in the segments T12 to L5 (Note 2), and those projecting in the lumbar splanchnic nerves in the segments L2 to L5 (Figure 8.8b) (see Jänig [1985]; Jänig and McLachlan [1987]). Similar distinct segmental distributions of different groups of preganglionic neurons have been shown to exist in the rat (Strack et al. 1988). Table 8.2 (column spinal cord) lists the segmental location of sympathetic preganglionic neurons that are associated with different target tissues in the rat, as has been studied using trans-synaptic transport of a neurotropic virus injected into the target tissues. These data correspond to the results of experiments in which autonomic effector responses elicited by electrical stimulation of preganglionic axons in ventral roots were recorded (see Figure 8.8a).

Since Langley, preganglionic sympathetic neurons in the lumbar spinal cord have been most extensively studied, in several species, using morphological, immunohistochemical and neurophysiological methods. These neurons project in the lumbar sympathetic trunk, lumbar splanchnic nerves and

(a)

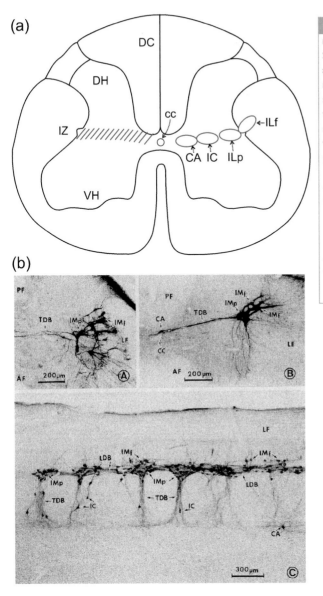

(b)

Figure 8.2 Location and morphology of sympathetic preganglionic neurons in the spinal cord. (a) Diagram of transverse section. Subnuclei in the intermediate zone (IZ) in the cat: ILf, ILp, funicular and principal part of the intermediolateral nucleus; IC, intercalate nucleus; CA, central autonomic nucleus. (b) Photomicrographs showing sympathetic preganglionic neurons labeled with cholera toxin subunit B in transverse sections (A, B) and in a horizontal section (C) of the rat. A. Spinal level C8. Preganglionic neurons are widely distributed in the ILp and ILf. B. Spinal level T2. Labeled preganglionic neurons are located in the IML (here named IMf and IMp) and some in the CA. C. Preganglionic neurons form periodic clusters at intercluster distances of 300 to 600 μm connected by longitudinal dendritic bundles (LDB). Most dendrites are oriented rostrocaudally and some dendrites are oriented mediolaterally in bundles across the intermediate zone. A few dendrites are oriented dorsally or ventrally. AF, LF, PF, anterior, lateral and posterior funiculus; cc, central canal; DC, dorsal columns; DH, dorsal horn; TDB, transversal dendritic bundle and axons of the neurons in the CA; VH, ventral horn. From Hosoya et al. (1991) with permission.

hypogastric nerves; they are involved in various functions (see Tables 4.1 and 4.3) in somatic tissues, pelvic organs and colon (Figure 8.6a). Therefore, I will describe these sympathetic preganglionic neurons in the cat more extensively. The results of these experiments show (Baron et al. 1985a, b, c; Jänig and McLachlan 1986a, b):

- Almost all preganglionic neurons that project in the lumbar sympathetic trunk distal to the most caudal lumbar splanchnic nerve (Figure 8.6a), which are involved in regulating target cells in skin and skeletal muscle, lie in the ILf or ILp (Note

3). Very few neurons are located medial to the ILp (Figure 8.4). Most preganglionic neurons are situated in segments L1 to L4 with a few in segments T12, T13 and L5 (Figure 8.8b). Practically all preganglionic neurons are ipsilateral (Figure 8.4a).

- All preganglionic neurons that project in the lumbar splanchnic nerves lie in the intermediate zone medial to the border between white and gray matter. Many of these neurons are located in the ILp, but lie somewhat medial to those that project caudally in the lumbar sympathetic trunk and innervate postganglionic neurons projecting to

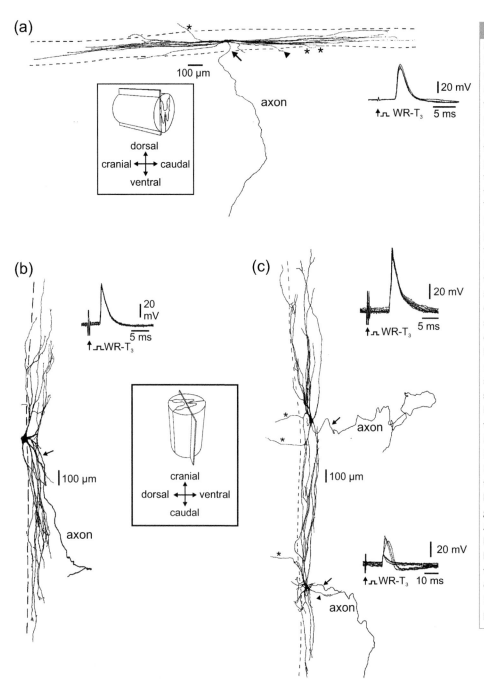

Figure 8.3 Morphology of single preganglionic neurons located in the intermediolateral cell column in the thoracic segment T3 in the cat. Activity was recorded from the preganglionic neurons using an intracellular microelectrode filled with horseradish peroxidase (HRP). The neurons were identified by stimulating their axons in the white ramus T3 (WR-T3) with single pulses (see the superimposed action potentials). After identification, the neurons were filled with HRP. After filling the neurons, the animals were perfused, the spinal cord was removed and cut longitudinally in serial sections (30 to 50 μm thick) either parasagittally or horizontally. The neurons were reconstructed from the serial sections. (a) Neuron in a parasagittal plane. The dashed lines mark the dorsal and the ventral border of the intermediate zone. (b, c) Neurons in a horizontal plane. In (c) two neurons labeled in the same animal. The dashed lines mark the border between gray and white matter. Asterisks, dendrites projecting laterally or dorsally; arrow head, dendrites projecting ventrally; arrows, origin of axon. Modified from Dembowsky et al. (1985) with permission.

somatic tissues. Many preganglionic neurons projecting in the lumbar splanchnic nerves are located medial to the Ilp, extending across to the central canal. These preganglionic neurons are situated in segments L2 to L5, most of them in segments L3 and L4 (Figure 8.8b). Practically all preganglionic neurons are located ipsilaterally (Figure 8.5).

- All preganglionic neurons that project in the hypogastric nerves lie in the intermediate zone medial to the border between white and gray matter. However, most of these neurons are located in the ILp and only very few medial to the ILp. Again these preganglionic neurons are situated medial to those projecting in the lumbar sympathetic trunk.

(a)

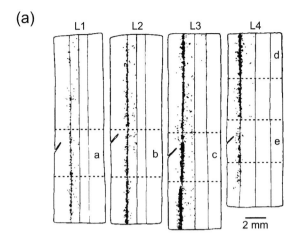

(b)

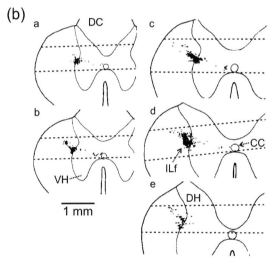

Spatial distribution of preganglionic cell bodies in lumbar segments L1 to L4 innervating postganglionic neurons that project to somatic tissues in the cat. Horseradish peroxidase (HRP) was applied to the cut lumbar sympathetic trunk distal to the most caudal lumbar splanchnic nerve (see Figure 8.6a). The enzyme is transported retrogradely to the preganglionic cell bodies two days after application and the reaction product is demonstrated histochemically in the cell bodies. Horizontal sections of the spinal segments are cut serially and the location of the HRP-labeled preganglionic cell bodies reconstructed by superimposing their position in sections through the entire intermediate region. (a) Rostrocaudal distribution of cells. The labeled cell column stops in the caudal half of segment L4. Note that all labeled preganglionic cell bodies are located ipsilaterally. (b) The lengths of L1 to L4 marked by broken lines in (a) (a–e, each about 4 mm long) have been rotated by 90 degrees and displayed transversely. The broken lines in the transverse sections indicate the limits of the horizontal sections that were included in this analysis. Note that many cell bodies are located in the ILf and very few medial to the ILp (see Figure 8.2). For abbreviations see legend of Figure 8.2. From Jänig and McLachlan 1986a) with permission.

About 20% of these preganglionic neurons are located in the contralateral intermediate zone.

• When subtracting the position of the preganglionic neurons that project through the hypogastric nerves to the pelvic organs from those projecting through the lumbar splanchnic nerves (Figure 8.5) one obtains the position of preganglionic neurons that synapse with postganglionic neurons in the inferior mesenteric ganglion, many of them being associated with target tissues in the hindgut. These preganglionic neurons are also located medial to those projecting in the lumbar sympathetic trunk, many of them lying in the gray matter extending up to the central canal.

• The approximate positions of the three groups of preganglionic neurons (associated with somatic tissues, pelvic organs and colon, respectively) are schematically outlined in Figure 8.6b,c. In the cat, these lumbar preganglionic neurons exhibit some viscerotopic organization:

    ▪ Almost all neurons projecting in the lumbar sympathetic trunk are located in the "classical" intermediolateral cell column and most of them in the white matter (ILf). Most of these neurons are vasoconstrictor in function (1 in Figure 8.6b,c).

    ▪ Almost all neurons projecting in the hypogastric nerves are located medial to those projecting in the lumbar sympathetic trunk, extending in clusters up to the central canal (3 in Figure 8.6b,c).

    ▪ Most preganglionic neurons that synapse in the inferior mesenteric ganglion are also located in the gray matter in the ILp, but medial to those projecting in the lumbar sympathetic trunk and ventral to those projecting in the hypogastric nerves (2 in Figure 8.6b,c). Most of these neurons and those projecting in the hypogastric nerve are probably not vasoconstrictor in function but involved in regulation of visceral organs (Bahr et al. 1986).

Similar results on the location of lumbar sympathetic preganglionic neurons projecting to viscera or somatic target tissues have been obtained in the guinea pig (Dalsgaard and Elfvin 1982; McLachlan 1985) and in the rat (Baron and Jänig 1991; see Tables 8.2 and 8.3 for references). However, in these species, the medially located preganglionic neurons in the central autonomic nucleus that project to the viscera are situated in a continuous closely packed

(a)

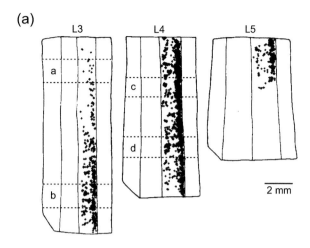

(b)

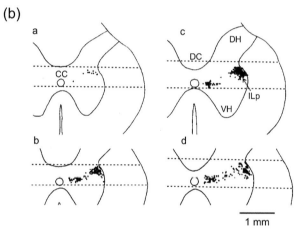

Figure 8.5 Spatial distribution of preganglionic cell bodies in lumbar segments L3 to L5 innervating postganglionic neurons that project to pelvic organs or colon in the cat. Horse radish peroxidase was applied to the cut lumbar splanchnic nerves (see Figure 8.6a). (a) Superimposed horizontal sections showing the rostrocaudal distribution of cells in the intermediate zone. All labeled cell bodies are located ipsilaterally. (b) The length of L3 (1.6 mm) and L4 (1.4 mm) marked by the broken lines in (a) have been rotated by 90 degrees and displayed transversely. Broken lines indicate the limits of the horizontal sections that were included in the analysis. Note that no neurons were located in the ILf and that many neurons were located medial to the ILp. For abbreviations see legend of Figure 8.2. From Baron et al. (1985c) with permission.

column overlying the central canal, the dorsal commissural nucleus (Hancock and Peveto 1979).

This principle of organization also applies to the sympathetic outflow of the thoracic spinal cord in the rat: populations of preganglionic neurons projecting to the superior cervical ganglion, stellate ganglion or

adrenal medulla, respectively, are arranged in horizontal columns in the intermediolateral nucleus (mainly principal part; Figure 8.7) (Pyner and Coote 1994).

Figure 8.8 projects the topographical anatomical situation on the functional situation for the preganglionic neurons of the lumbar sympathetic outflow, which project in the lumbar sympathetic trunk and the lumbar splanchnic nerves of the cat. From one side of the spinal cord about 4500 preganglionic neurons project in the lumbar sympathetic trunk and 2300 neurons in the lumbar splanchnic nerves. Not included in these numbers are preganglionic neurons that innervate only postganglionic neurons in paravertebral ganglia projecting into segmental nerves (ventral and dorsal rami) that supply the skin and deep somatic tissues of the trunk since these preganglionic neurons were not labeled in the tracing experiments (see Figure 8.6a) (see Baron et al. [1995]). These are probably numerically small.

Based on the stimulation studies performed by Langley and coworkers and some other investigators in the cat (see legend of Figure 8.8), most preganglionic neurons involved in regulation of target cells in somatic tissues, pelvic viscera and colon are situated in the segments L1 to L5. This fully corresponds to the neurophysiological studies on pre- and postganglionic neurons of the lumbar sympathetic outflow, as reported in Chapter 4. Segments L3 and L4 contain the highest density of preganglionic neurons; they consist of at least ten functionally different types of preganglionic neurons (see Tables 4.1 and 4.3). There is no indication that the preganglionic neurons are arranged in the different subnuclei of the intermediate zone with respect to their function, although up to now it has not been possible to test this explicitly.

Spinal Interneurons and Propriospinal Neurons Associated With Preganglionic Neurons

Sympathetic preganglionic neurons labeled transsynaptically from the target tissue or postganglionic neurons are commonly associated with labeled neurons in the spinal cord that cannot be labeled retrogradely by tracers that do not cross synapses (e.g., horseradish peroxidase or Fluoro-Gold). Thus, these neurons do not project with their axons through the ventral roots. It is hypothesized that these neurons are interneurons, which form synapses with the preganglionic neurons (Deuchars 2011, 2015; Deuchars and Lall 2015). Three major groups of putative autonomic

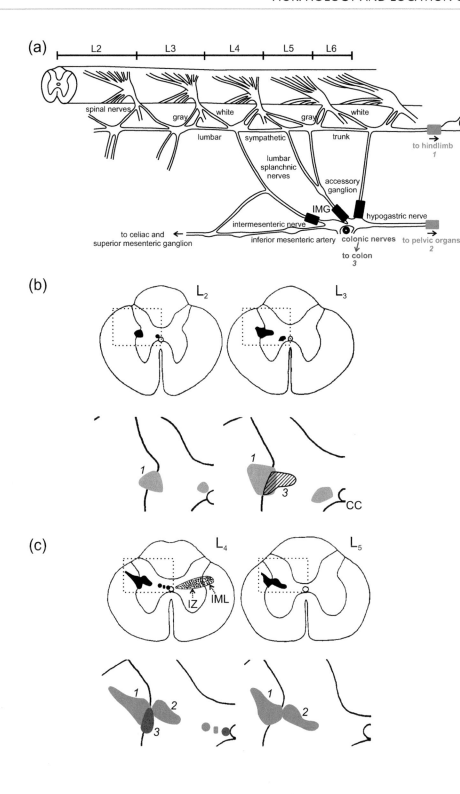

Figure 8.6 Topographic organization of sympathetic preganglionic neurons in the lumbar spinal cord projecting in the different nerve trunks of the cat. (a) Diagram of the anatomy of the lumbar nerve pathways in the cat, indicating various sites at which horseradish peroxidase was applied. (b, c) Transverse sections illustrate the regions containing the highest density of preganglionic neurons in the most rostral 2 mm of each segment L2 to L5. The lower parts in (b) and (c) show enlargements of the intermediate zone (see boxes) of cells labeled from the lumbar sympathetic trunk (blue, *1*) and from the hypogastric nerve (green, *2*), together with those projecting in the lumbar splanchnic, but not hypogastric, nerves (red, *3*). The latter group has been derived from the first two and is likely to be involved with innervation of the colon. IMG, inferior mesenteric ganglion; IML, intermediolateral nucleus; IZ, intermediate zone. From Jänig and McLachlan (1986b) with permission.

interneurons detected after labeling of preganglionic or postganglionic neurons with a trans-synaptically transported virus have been identified in this way:

1. Interneurons that are situated in the same, or neighboring, spinal segments, as the preganglionic neurons. These interneurons are found in

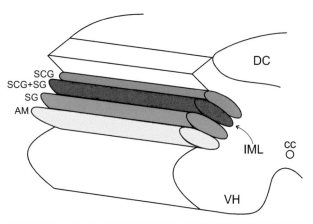

Figure 8.7 Arrangement of functionally distinct sympathetic preganglionic neurons in horizontal columns in the rat thoracic spinal cord. Diagram of the gray matter on the right side of the spinal cord indicating the location in the intermediolateral nucleus of different groups of sympathetic preganglionic neurons in the thoracic segment T5. Note the arrangement of the preganglionic neurons in horizontal rostrocaudal columns. Preganglionic neurons projecting to the superior cervical ganglion (SCG, green) are located dorsally and neurons projecting to the adrenal medulla (AM, yellow) ventrally. Neurons projecting to the stellate ganglion (SG, blue) are located in between and close to the neurons projecting to the AM. SCG + SG (red), region containing both groups of preganglionic neurons. In more rostral thoracic segments there is little AM representation, whereas at more caudal segmental levels (such as T10) there is little representation of SG and no SCG. Sympathetic preganglionic neurons to each of the three targets were simultaneously labeled with fluorescent dyes, either Fluoro-Gold, Fast Blue or Diamidino Yellow. cc, central canal; DC, dorsal column; IML, intermediolateral nucleus; VH, ventral horn. From Pyner and Coote (1994) with permission.

laminae I, II, V, VI, IX and X (close to the central canal) (Note 4) of the gray matter, as well as close to the preganglionic neurons in the intermediate zone (Table 8.2, Figure 8.15). Experimental evidence suggests that all interneurons within the region of the intermediolateral nucleus have activity related to the activity in sympathetic preganglionic neurons, suggesting that these neurons are antecedent to the sympathetic preganglionic neurons. It has been shown in spinal cord slices that interneurons in the intermediolateral region exhibit a fast firing pattern, which is dependent on the presence of specific voltage-gated potassium channels. Interneurons labeled transneurally from the adrenal gland contain the

channel subunit Kv3.1 of these potassium channels (Deuchars et al. 2001; Brooke et al. 2002; Deuchars 2015; Deuchars and Lall 2015). Figure 8.9 illustrates the morphology and electrophysiology of such an interneuron.

2. Propriospinal neurons located in spinal thoracolumbar segments remote from the labeled preganglionic neurons in laminae I, V, VII and X (e.g., in segments C1 to C6; Jansen and Loewy [1997]; Smith et al. [1998]).

3. Propriospinal neurons lying within the white matter of the cervical spinal cord. These spinal interneurons are found in the lateral funiculus and in the lateral spinal nucleus of spinal segments C1 to C4 (Jansen et al. 1995a, b; Jansen and Loewy 1997; see Table 8.2, Figure 8.15).

Although no spinal sympathetic interneuron has been functionally identified and characterized so far, it is not far-fetched to assume that these interneurons are particularly important in the generation of the differentiated reflex patterns in sympathetic pre- and postganglionic neurons that have been worked out in neurophysiological experiments (see Chapters 4 and 9).

8.2.2 Parasympathetic Preganglionic Neurons and Interneurons

Sacral Parasympathetic Systems

The sacral spinal cord contains at least three groups of parasympathetic preganglionic neurons, which are involved in the regulation of lower urinary tract, hindgut and sexual organs. In the cat, some morphological differentiation and viscerotopic organization are present.

- Preganglionic neurons associated with the hindgut are small, lie in the dorsal band of the intermediate zone and have primarily a mediolateral orientation of their dendrites.

- Preganglionic neurons associated with the urogenital tract lie in the lateral band of the intermediate zone. These neurons have a complex dendritic organization, one type projecting its dendrites mainly into the (superficial) lamina I of the dorsal horn and into the ventral funiculus and the second type having its major dendritic projections into the dorsolateral and lateral funiculi of the white matter and medially. These two types of sacral preganglionic neurons may innervate the

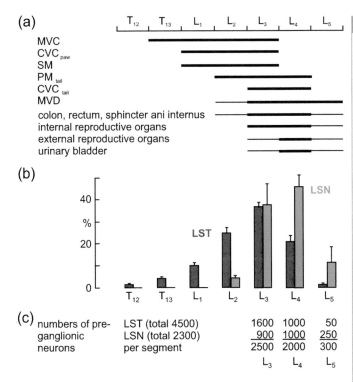

Figure 8.8 The lumbar spinal sympathetic outflow: functional systems, segmental distribution and numbers of preganglionic neurons in the cat. (a) Segmental distribution of sympathetic spinal systems. Autonomic effects generated by electrical stimulation of the ventral roots in the cat. MVC, MVD: muscle vasoconstriction and vasodilation in the hindlimb (Sonnenschein and Weissman, 1978). *CVC:* cutaneous vasoconstriction in paw and tail skin (Langley 1894b). *SM:* sudomotor activity and sweat secretion on foot pads (Langley 1891, 1894b). *PM:* pilomotor activity and piloerection on the tail (Langley and Sherrington 1891; Langley 1894a). *Colon, rectum, sphincter ani internus:* decrease of motility, contraction, pallor (Langley and Anderson 1895a). *Internal reproductive organs: contraction, pallor* (Langley and Anderson 1895d). *External reproductive organs:* pallor, contraction, retractor penis and cutaneous smooth muscles (Langley and Anderson 1895c). *Urinary bladder:* short contraction (Langley and Anderson 1895b). (b) Segmental distribution of preganglionic neurons that project in the lumbar sympathetic trunk (LST) distal to paravertebral ganglion L5 (distal to the most caudal lumbar splanchnic nerve, red columns) and in the lumbar splanchnic nerves (LSN, blue columns) of the cat. These experimental distributions were determined from experiments as described in Figures 8.2, 8.4 and 8.5. Mean + SEM. LST, n = 9 (Jänig and McLachlan 1986a). LSN, n = 4 (Baron et al. 1985c). (c) Numbers of preganglionic neurons. These numbers were derived from the animals with the highest numbers of horseradish peroxidase-labeled cells (LST, n = 6; LSN, n = 3) (Baron et al. 1985c; Jänig and McLachlan 1986a, b). Modified from Jänig (1986) with permission.

urinary tract and reproductive organs, respectively. Axons of the preganglionic neurons in the lateral band exhibit extensive intraspinal collaterals, which project bilaterally to various regions of the ventral and dorsal horn (Morgan et al. 1993; de Groat et al. 1996).

In the rat, the preganglionic neurons projecting to pelvic organs are located in the sacral preganglionic nucleus lying across the intermediate zone in the segments S2, S1 and L6. Several groups of putative interneurons have also been found here that are labeled by a trans-synaptically transported neurotropic virus after application to the sacral parasympathetic preganglionic axons or when injected into the walls of the pelvic organs. These do not project through the ventral roots and are not labeled by a classical (not trans-synaptically transported) tracer applied to the preganglionic axons. These interneurons are located in lamina I of the dorsal horn, in lamina X, in the dorsal commissural nucleus

and in the intermediate zone just dorsal to the preganglionic neurons (see Table 8.3). Some of the interneurons have been characterized using neurophysiological techniques (see Chapter 9 and Figure 9.8).

Cranial Parasympathetic Systems

The location of the preganglionic neurons of the cranial parasympathetic systems have been extensively studied, mainly in the rat, but also in other species, using retrograde labeling and other techniques. Table 8.1 and Figure 1.4 show, for different functional groups, the location of the cranial preganglionic neurons, the cranial nerves through which the preganglionic neurons project and the location of the postganglionic neurons (see also Table 8.3).

- Almost all parasympathetic preganglionic neurons with myelinated axons innervating the heart (cardiomotor neurons) and parasympathetic neurons innervating airways and lung (bronchomotor

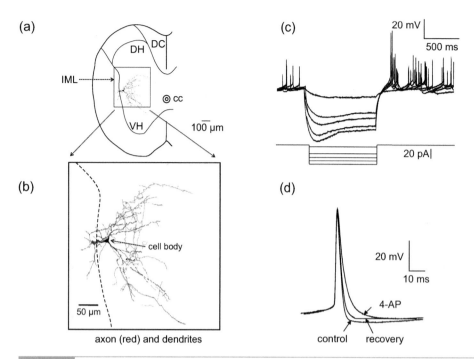

Figure 8.9 Morphology and electrophysiology of an autonomic interneuron in the thoracic segment T9. The neuron was recorded intracellularly in a transverse spinal cord slice (300 μm thick). The neuron showed characteristic high-frequency discharges and short action potentials following hyperpolarizing pulses (c), both being due to a specific type of voltage-gated potassium channel. The neuron was sensitive to the potassium-channel blockers 4-aminopyridine (4-AP; d) and tetraethylammonium, suggestive of the presence of the Kv3 potassium channel. It has been shown that autonomic interneurons labeled transneuronally from the adrenal medulla contain the Kv3.1 subunit of these channels (Deuchars et al. 2001; Brooke et al. 2002). After recording the neuron was filled through the microelectrode with biotinamide. The spinal cord slice was serially sectioned and the neuron was reconstructed (axon arborization, dendrites and cell body). (a) shows the reconstructed neuron in a transverse section. In (b) cell body, dendrites and axon ramifications (red) of the neuron are shown. cc, central canal; DC, dorsal columns; DH, dorsal horn; IML, intermediolateral nucleus; VH, ventral horn. From Deuchars et al. (2001) with permission.

neurons, probably also secretomotor neurons) are located in the external formation of the nucleus ambiguus (NA). A few are located in the intermediate region between the NA and dorsal motor nucleus of the vagus (DMNX). However, this issue is controversial. Those parasympathetic cardiomotor neurons that are located in the DMNX have unmyelinated axons. They are probably located in the most lateral part of the DMNX (lateral to those neurons projecting to the cecum [Figure 8.10]). In this region, there seem to exist some species differences (Bieger and Hopkins 1987; Altschuler et al. 1989, 1992; Izzo et al. 1993; Hopkins et al. 1996). The functions of the cardiomotor neurons in the DMNX are unknown (Jones et al. 1998; see Subchapter 4.8).

• Preganglionic parasympathetic neurons innervating the proximal part of the gastrointestinal tract (stomach, duodenum, small intestine, including pancreas and liver) are located in the DMNX. This nucleus is, in practice, the motor nucleus of the foregut in which the stomach has the highest representation. In the rat it contains about 10 000 neurons (5000 neurons on each side), 7500 neurons being preganglionic and projecting to the gastrointestinal tract, the remaining neurons being interneurons or other types of preganglionic neurons projecting to visceral organs in the thoracic cavity (Fox and Powley 1985, 1992; Powley et al. 1992) (Note 5).

• The preganglionic neurons in the DMNX projecting through the subdiaphragmatic vagus nerves to the gastrointestinal tract are topographically organized. The rat subdiaphragmatic vagus nerves consist of five branches, which innervate different

Table 8.1 Classification of cranial parasympathetic motor neurons

Peripheral target	Brain stem nucleus[a]	Cranial nerve	Final motor neuron
Iris muscle (constriction of pupil)	Edinger–Westphal nucleus, lateral division	III	Ciliary ganglion
Ciliary muscles (accommodation)	Edinger–Westphal nucleus, lateral division	III	Ciliary ganglion
Chorioid blood vessels (vasodilation)	Edinger–Westphal nucleus, medial division	III	Ciliary ganglion, pterygopalatine ganglion[b]
Lacrimal gland	Superior salivary nucleus[c]	VII[d]	Pterygopalatine ganglion
Sublingual and submandibular glands	Inferior salivary nucleus[c]	VII[e]	Submandibular ganglion
Lingual (von Ebner) glands	Inferior salivary nucleus[c]	IX	Intralingual ganglia in posterior tongue
Parotid gland	Inferior salivary nucleus[c]	IX[f]	Otic ganglion
Mucosal glands	Probably salivary nuclei[c]	VII, IX	All cranial ganglia (except ciliary ganglion)
Cranial blood vessels (vasodilation)	Probably with salivary and lacrimal preganglionic cells	VII, IX	All cranial ganglia (except ciliary ganglion)
Airways and lungs	Nucleus ambiguus	X	Ganglia in airways
Heart (pacemaker, atria)	Nucleus ambiguus (external formation)	X	Cardiac ganglia
Stomach and other abdominal organs[g]	Dorsal motor nucleus of the vagus	X	Enteric neurons

III, oculomotor nerve; VII, facial nerve; IX, hypoglossal nerve; X, vagus nerve. Modified from Blessing (1997). For eye see Reiner et al. (1983), Gamlin (2000) and Neuhuber and Schrödl (2011).

[a] Location of cell bodies of preganglionic neurons mostly based on tracing studies in animals.

[b] Synonym sphenopalatine ganglion.

[c] Salivatory nuclei are not very well defined (see Table 1.1). The *superior salivary nucleus* is located in the lateral reticular formation medial to the oral subnucleus of the spinal trigeminal nucleus at the level (dorsolateral) of the rostral part of the facial nucleus. The *inferior salivary nucleus* extends rostrocaudally adjacent to the medial border of the rostral part of the nucleus tractus solitarii (NTS) and somewhat rostrally (Contreras et al. 1980; Matsuo and Kang 1998; Kim et al. 2004; Paxinos and Watson 2014).

[d] Via greater petrosal and zygomaticotemporal nerves.

[e] Via chorda tympany and lingual nerve.

[f] Via tympanic and lesser petrosal nerves.

[g] Various functions related to contraction, relaxation, exocrine secretion, endocrine secretion (see Table 1.2; Chapter 5 and Subchapter 10.7).

parts of the gastrointestinal tract with some overlap (left and right gastric branches, hepatic branch, left accessory celiac branch and right celiac branch [Prechtl and Powley 1985, 1990]). The preganglionic neurons in the DMNX are organized in rostrocaudal cell columns. The neurons projecting in the gastric branches are located medially and the neurons projecting in the celiac branches laterally. Neurons projecting in the hepatic branch are located in a cell column

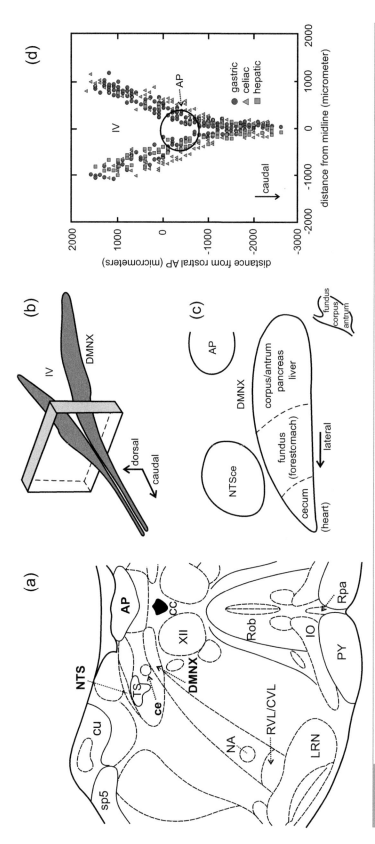

Figure 8.10 Topographic organization of the dorsal motor nucleus of the vagus (DMNX) in the rat. (a) Transverse section through the medulla oblongata at the level of the area postrema (AP) showing the location of the DMNX in relation to other nuclei, in particular the nucleus tractus solitarii (NTS) and the AP. (b) The DMNX viewed from a three-dimensional dorsocaudal perspective. The level of the transverse section in (a) and (c) is indicated. (c) Mediolateral viscerotopic organization of the DMNX at the rostral level of the AP. (d) The distribution of preganglionic neurons projecting through the gastric (circles, red), celiac (triangles, blue) and hepatic (squares, green) branches of the subdiaphragmatic vagus nerves as viewed in the horizontal plane from dorsal. The neurons were labeled with Fast Blue. Fast Blue was injected intraperitoneally in rats four to six days before perfusing the animals. In these experiments, various combinations of abdominal vagal branches (two gastric, two celiac, one hepatic) were transected leaving one or two vagal branches intact. Fast Blue is taken up by the terminals of the intact vagal preganglionic axons and transported to the cell bodies. The DMNX was cut in horizontal 100 μm thick sections. In these sections preganglionic cell bodies are visualized under ultraviolet epifluorescence and intracellularly filled via a glass micropipette with the dye Lucifer yellow. In this way, cell bodies, dendrites and axons of the neurons can be visualized and reconstructed. cc, central canal; ce, central nucleus of the NTS; cu, cuneate nucleus; IO, inferior olive nucleus; LRN, lateral reticular nucleus; NA, nucleus ambiguus; PY, pyramid; Rob, raphe obscurus; Rpa, raphe pallidus; RVL/CVL, rostral ventrolateral medulla/caudal ventrolateral medulla; sp5, spinal trigeminal tract; TS, tractus solitarius; IV, fourth ventricle; XII, hypoglossus; (a) modified from Hopkins et al. (1996) with permission. (b, d) modified from Paxinos and Watson (2014); (b, d) modified from Fox and Powley (1992); (c) modified from Hopkins et al. (1996) with permission.

between the medial (gastric) and the lateral (cecal) cell column of the right DMNX. The dendrites of these preganglionic neurons are almost confined to the cell columns projecting rostrocaudally, but also extend dorsally to the subnuclei of the NTS (Fox and Powley 1992; Powley et al. 1992) (Figure 8.10) (Note 6). Most preganglionic parasympathetic neurons innervating the lower esophageal sphincter are probably also located in a medial rostrocaudal cell column of the DMNX (Rossiter et al. 1990).

- Preganglionic neurons regulating glands of the head (lacrimal, salivary and mucosal) are located dorsal to the rostral portion of the facial nucleus in areas called the superior and inferior salivary nuclei.

- In monkeys and birds, preganglionic parasympathetic neurons regulating the inner muscles of the eye (constrictor pupillae and ciliary muscle [accommodation]) are located in the Edinger–Westphal nucleus of the mesencephalon and project through the oculomotor nerve to the ciliary ganglion. Most neurons in the lateral Edinger–Westphal nucleus are associated with accommodation; neurons in the caudal part of this lateral nucleus are associated with pupilloconstriction) (Note 7). Preganglionic parasympathetic vasodilator neurons innervating cranial blood vessels seem to be located in the same nuclei that contain the parasympathetic secretomotor neurons. This population of vasomotor neurons has not been investigated at all. In birds, preganglionic neurons generating active vasodilation of the chorioid blood vessels of the eye are situated in the medial Edinger–Westphal nucleus (see Reiner et al. [1983]; Gamlin [2000]; McDougal and Gamlin [2015]).

8.3 | Nucleus Tractus Solitarii

The nucleus tractus solitarii (NTS) is located in the dorsomedial part of the medulla oblongata and extends as columns of neurons that are arranged around the tractus solitarius (TS) from rostral to caudal (Figure 8.11). Left and right NTS unite distal to the obex of the medulla oblongata (commissural nucleus); here the NTS is closely associated with the area postrema (AP). The NTS (with the AP) is the important neuronal input structure from gustatory receptors, from vagal afferents innervating the respiratory system (lung, airways), from vagal afferents innervating the cardiovascular system (arterial baro- and chemoreceptors; afferents innervating the heart, the portal vein and caval vein) and from vagal afferents innervating the gastrointestinal tract. The AP is a neurohemal (circumventricular) organ of the NTS, which conveys blood-borne information (and possibly information from the cerebrospinal fluid) to the central nervous system. Thus, the afferent information from the thoracic and abdominal internal organs and from the blood, which is important for regulation of respiration, the cardiovascular system and gastrointestinal functions, is channeled through the NTS to different nuclei in the brain stem and forebrain (Figure 8.13).

The projection of gustatory and vagal visceral afferent neurons to the NTS exhibits some viscerotopic organization with respect to the rostrocaudal and mediolateral axes of the NTS and with respect to several subnuclei of the NTS, which have been defined anatomically by cytological criteria (Figure 8.11). There is controversy about the cytoarchitectonic criteria that divide the NTS into subnuclei, about the number of subnuclei and about their parcellation (see Blessing [1997]). Independent of this, it is intuitively clear that:

1. subdifferentiation of the NTS must exist,
2. this anatomical subdifferentiation must be in some way related to function and
3. different types of afferents from the three visceral organ systems must exhibit distinct projections to the subnuclei of the NTS.

Figure 8.11 shows, schematically for the rat, the subnuclei of the NTS on two transverse sections at the level of the AP (b) and at a level rostral to the AP as described by Loewy and Burton (1978), Altschuler et al. (1989) and Herbert et al. (1990). The gustatory afferents project to the rostral part of the NTS and the other groups of afferents to the caudal half (Figure 8.12). There is some overlap in projection between cardiovascular, respiratory and gastrointestinal afferents:

- Afferents from the subdiaphragmatic *gastrointestinal tract* project preferentially to the gelatinous, medial and commissural nuclei, but not to the central, interstitial, intermedial and ventrolateral nuclei. Afferents from the esophagus project to

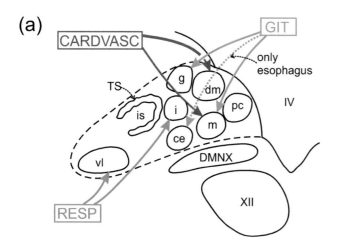

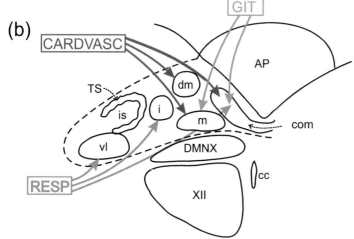

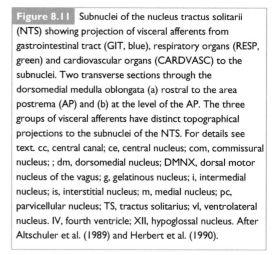

Figure 8.11 Subnuclei of the nucleus tractus solitarii (NTS) showing projection of visceral afferents from gastrointestinal tract (GIT, blue), respiratory organs (RESP, green) and cardiovascular organs (CARDVASC) to the subnuclei. Two transverse sections through the dorsomedial medulla oblongata (a) rostral to the area postrema (AP) and (b) at the level of the AP. The three groups of visceral afferents have distinct topographical projections to the subnuclei of the NTS. For details see text. cc, central canal; ce, central nucleus; com, commissural nucleus; ; dm, dorsomedial nucleus; DMNX, dorsal motor nucleus of the vagus; g, gelatinous nucleus; i, intermedial nucleus; is, interstitial nucleus; m, medial nucleus; pc, parvicellular nucleus; TS, tractus solitarius; vl, ventrolateral nucleus. IV, fourth ventricle; XII, hypoglossal nucleus. After Altschuler et al. (1989) and Herbert et al. (1990).

the central nucleus of the NTS. Figure 8.12d demonstrates the projection of afferents from the soft palate, pharynx, esophagus, stomach and cecum to the NTS. It shows that the afferent neurons from the different sections of the alimentary canal are organized topographically with limited overlap. This organization has three distinct characteristics: (1) Afferents from different organs project to different subnuclei of the NTS (Figure 8.12a–c). (2) The afferent projections have a mediolateral and caudorostral segregation (Figure 8.12d). (3) The organization of afferent projections is related to the mediolateral organization in the underlying DMNX of the preganglionic neurons that project to the gastrointestinal tract (Figure 8.12e). This topographical organization of projecting afferents from and efferent neurons to the alimentary tract is

the anatomical basis of the neural control of the gastrointestinal tract (stomach, duodenum, small intestine; see Subchapter 10.7). The NTS subnuclei related to the gastrointestinal tract, the ventrally located DMNX and the area postrema are also called the *dorsal vagal complex* (DVC; see Subchapter 10.7).
- Afferent neurons innervating the *respiratory system* project to the commissural, intermedial and ventrolateral nuclei (Kalia and Richter 1985a, b, 1988a, b).
- *Cardiovascular afferents* (arterial baro- and chemoreceptor afferents) project to the dorsomedial, medial and commissural nuclei and to the AP (see Ciriello et al. [1994]).

The topography of projection of visceral afferents was obtained on the basis of tracing experiments in which distinct populations of afferent neurons were labeled. Information is not available on the projections

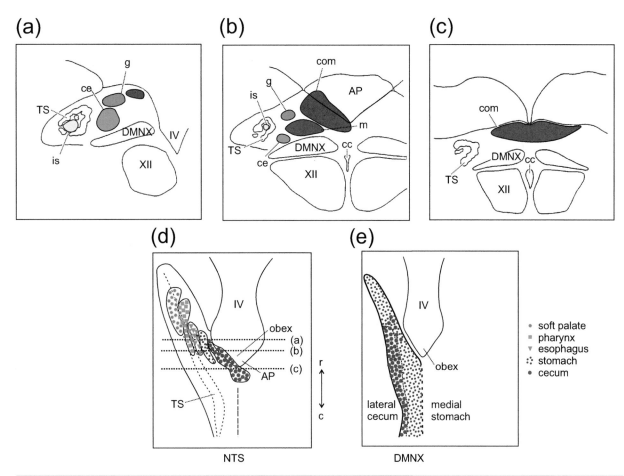

Figure 8.12 Topographic projection of afferents from different sections of the alimentary canal to the nucleus tractus solitarii (NTS). (a–c) Schematic transverse sections through the rat dorsomedial medulla oblongata containing the NTS and dorsal motor nucleus of the vagus (DMNX) just rostral to the area postrema (AP) (a), through the AP (b) and caudal to the AP (c). See location of the transverse sections in (d). IV, fourth ventricle; for abbreviations of subnuclei see Figure 8.11. (d) Horizontal (longitudinal) section through the NTS showing rostrocaudal and mediolateral topography of the projections of the afferents from the oropharynx, esophagus, stomach and cecum. (e) Horizontal (longitudinal) section through the DMNX showing mediolateral topography of the location of preganglionic neurons projecting to the stomach or cecum (see Figure 8.10d). Modified from Altschuler et al. (1991) with permission.

of functionally distinct groups of afferents. For example, arterial baroreceptor afferents and arterial chemoreceptor afferents have widely overlapping projection fields in the NTS (Ciriello et al. 1994). No convincing topographical functional differentiation of the second-order neurons in the NTS with respect to their afferent synaptic inputs from respiratory, cardiovascular and gastrointestinal organs has been found so far, using neurophysiological and other methods. Thus, functionally identified NTS neurons appear to lack viscerotopic organization (Paton 1999; Paton and Kasparov 2000; Paton et al. 2005; for discussion and

references see Blessing [1997]). This is puzzling in view of the many distinct reflex pathways associated with the gastrointestinal tract, the respiratory system and the cardiovascular system.

Neurons in the NTS either project to various regions of the brain stem, hypothalamus and forebrain or are interneurons that are confined in their projection to the NTS. Both types of neuron can be excitatory or inhibitory. Furthermore, anatomical tracing studies (including those with neurotropic viruses) show: (1) that neurons of the NTS are synaptically influenced from many sites in the spinal cord,

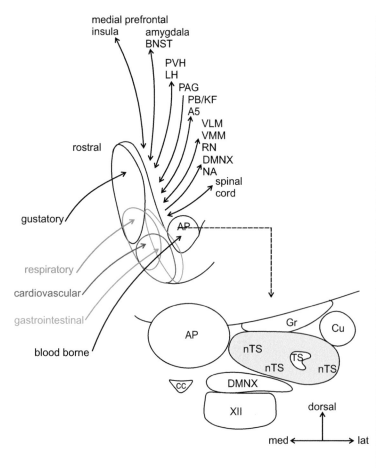

Figure 8.13 Afferent and efferent connections of the nucleus tractus solitarii (NTS) and area postrema (AP). The peripheral synaptic inputs from gustatory afferents, afferents of the respiratory system (including the trachea), cardiovascular afferents (including afferents from arterial chemoreceptors and arterial baroreceptors) and gastrointestinal afferents (including afferents from the oropharyngeal structures) are topographically organized. However, a topographic organization of synaptic inputs to the second-order neurons of the NTS from functionally different types of afferent neurons of a particular type of visceral organ seems to be absent. "Afferent" blood-borne inputs are relayed by neurons in the AP. Neurons in the NTS and AP project to various nuclei in the neuraxis including forebrain; neurons in most of these nuclei project back to the NTS/AP. *Lower right*: transverse section through the dorsomedial part of the medulla oblongata at the level of AP. The subnuclei of the NTS (nNTS), which are arranged around the tractus solitarius (TS), are not shown. A5, pontine A5 nucleus (most of the neurons are noradrenergic); BNST, bed nucleus of the stria terminalis; Cu, Gr, cuneate and gracile nuclei; cc, central canal; DMNX, dorsal motor nucleus of the vagus; LH, lateral hypothalamus; NA, nucleus ambiguus; PAG, periaqueductal gray; PB/KF, parabrachial and Kölliker–Fuse nuclei; PVH, paraventricular nuclei of the hypothalamus; RN, raphe nuclei (raphe magnus, obscurus and pallidus); VLM, ventrolateral medulla; VMM, ventromedial medulla; XII, nucleus of the hypoglossal nerve. Modified from Loewy (1990a), Saper (1995) and Blessing (1997).

lower and upper brain stem, hypothalamus and telencephalon, and (2) that projection neurons in the NTS project to the same brain regions from which the NTS receives its synaptic inputs (Figure 8.13) (Note 8).

The general functions of the NTS are as follows (see numbers in Figure 8.14):

1. The activity in vagal and gustatory afferents is synaptically transmitted to the projection neurons and relayed to various brain centers.
2. The synaptic transmission is locally modulated by inhibitory and excitatory interneurons in the NTS, which also receive synaptic input from primary afferents. This modulation can occur pre- or postsynaptically.
3. The projection neurons and interneurons in the NTS are under inhibitory and excitatory control from various brain centers.

4. The neuronal circuits in the NTS are modulated by blood-borne substances via the AP, such as angiotensin, corticotropin-releasing hormone (CRH), thyrotropin-releasing hormone (TRH), gastrointestinal hormones (see Subchapter 10.7) or signals from the immune system.
5. The synaptic transmission in the NTS is modulated by local signals related to the blood vessels (e.g., nitric oxide [NO]; Paton and Kasparov 2000; Paton et al. 2005).

This shows that the neurons in the NTS do not only transmit activity in a relay-like fashion to other nuclei, but that NTS circuits also have integrative functions and are under powerful control of the brain. The degrees of relay and integrative functions probably vary between different functional systems. Details about the integrative functions of the NTS and their underlying mechanisms with respect to specific

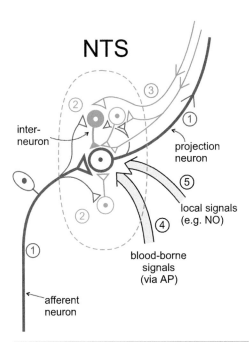

NTS

inter-
neuron

projection
neuron

local signals
(e.g. NO)

blood-borne
signals
(via AP)

afferent
neuron

Figure 8.14 Functions of the nucleus tractus solitarii (NTS). The NTS has relay function transmitting the activity in gustatory and vagal afferents to other brain centers (*function 1, red*). The impulse transmission is modulated by local circuits involving excitatory and inhibitory interneurons (*function 2, blue*), by brain centers in spinal cord, brain stem, hypothalamus and telencephalon that project to the NTS (*function 3, green*), by blood-borne substances via the area postrema (AP; *function 4*) and by local signals (e.g., related to blood vessels, nitric oxide [NO]; *function 5, yellow*).

artificially perfused but attached to the beating heart and the ventilated lung by vagal afferents (Paton 1996a, b).

8.4 | Sympathetic and Parasympathetic Premotor Neurons in the Brain Stem and Hypothalamus

Neurons in the brain stem, hypothalamus and cerebral hemispheres that project to the territory of preganglionic neurons in the spinal cord and brain stem have been called *autonomic premotor neurons*. The autonomic premotor neurons have been localized by retrograde labeling of their cell bodies with tracers. These neurons are sometimes called presympathetic or preparasympathetic neurons, although they may form synapses with interneurons that are situated in close proximity to the preganglionic neurons rather than with the preganglionic neurons directly. Thus, the term premotor neuron does not always mean that these autonomic neurons form direct synaptic contacts with the preganglionic neurons (this also applies to premotor neurons projecting, e.g., through the pyramidal tract, that form synapses with somatomotor neurons in the ventral horn and associated interneurons). Furthermore, these premotor neurons may form synapses with propriospinal neurons (e.g., in the cervical spinal cord) that project to the intermediate zone in the thoracolumbar spinal cord (see Subchapter 8.4.1; Jansen and Loewy 1997).

The cell bodies of the autonomic premotor neurons can be located by tracers applied to the terminal fields of the axons of these neurons (e.g., in the spinal intermediate zone, the external portion of the nucleus ambiguus, the DMNX). Alternatively, a neurotropic virus, which is transported retrogradely and transsynaptically, can be applied to the termination fields of postganglionic axons (e.g., in the kidney, rat tail artery, skin, heart, etc.) or of preganglionic axons (e.g., in the adrenal medulla, stellate ganglion, the pterygopalatine ganglion, etc.; see Tables 8.2 and 8.3). These two techniques may be applied together in the same experiment or combined with histochemical techniques that visualize the putative transmitters in the neurons (Figure 8.1). Furthermore, two different tracers or two different neurotropic viruses may be applied in the same experiment. Taking the limitations of these labeling techniques into account (Jansen et al. 1993,

afferent inputs (e.g., from arterial baro- or chemoreceptors or from specific gastrointestinal afferents), and with respect to specific homeostatic regulation, are virtually unknown (Paton 1999; Paton and Kasparov 2000; Paton et al. 2005; Andresen and Paton 2011; see Subchapter 10.7). The bewildering functional anatomy of the NTS, with its intrinsic integrative processes, its multiple peripheral and central synaptic inputs and its multiple efferent projections, clearly shows that the mechanisms operating in the NTS during regulation of autonomic functions can only be worked out using a multidisciplinary approach, which includes in vivo experimentation on animal models with full experimental control over the autonomic systems under study. One promising preparation to be used in these experiments is the working-heart-brain-stem preparation of the mouse and rat in which the lower brain stem is

1995a) it has been demonstrated that several distinct groups of neurons in the brain stem and hypothalamus project to the preganglionic neurons or the interneurons that are closely associated with them.

With a few exceptions (e.g., Siberian hamster, brown adipose tissue), most transneuronal labeling studies have been performed in the rat. Most functional studies about the central organization of the autonomic nervous system have been performed in this species in the recent past and will probably be performed in future. However, there is a need for more information about mammalian species other than the rat.

8.4.1 Sympathetic Premotor Neurons

Sympathetic premotor neurons that project to the sympathetic preganglionic neurons and/or their interneurons (see Subchapter 8.1) are mainly found in the following nuclei of brain stem and hypothalamus (Figures 8.15 and 8.16; marked by red # in Table 8.2) (see Note 9):

- *Neurons in the ventrolateral medulla (VLM)*: these neurons are located in the rostral ventrolateral medulla (RVLM) and in the lateral paragigantocellular nucleus (LPGi). About half to two-thirds of the neurons in the RVLM projecting to the preganglionic neurons are adrenergic (i.e., contain phenyl-N-methyltransferase, an enzyme that converts noradrenaline into adrenaline) and belong to the C1 cell group (for review see Guyenet et al. [2001]; Subchapter 10.2, Figure 10.3). Some neurons contain peptides (e.g., enkephalin, substance P, TRH or vasoactive intestinal peptide [VIP]). Neurons in the LPGi are serotonergic or non-serotonergic; some are also adrenergic and belong to the C1 cell group.
- *Neurons in the ventromedial medulla (VMM)*: sympathetic premotor neurons are located in the gigantocellular reticular nucleus, alpha and ventral (GiA and GiV), and in the parapyramidal region or nucleus (PPy) (see Note 9). Many of these projecting autonomic premotor neurons are serotonergic (i.e., contain 5-hydroxytryptamine [5-HT] as the putative transmitter). Some neurons contain the neuropeptides enkephalin, VIP and/or substance P.
- *Neurons in the caudal raphe nuclei*: these nuclei consist of the raphe magnus, the raphe pallidus and the raphe obscurus. Many of these are serotonergic. Some neurons contain neuropeptides such as enkephalin, substance P or other peptides.

- *A5 cell group in the caudal ventrolateral pons*: 90% of these neurons are catecholaminergic and use noradrenaline as the putative transmitter.
- *Neurons in the paraventricular nucleus of the hypothalamus (PVH)*: these sympathetic premotor neurons are located in the parvocellular nuclei of the PVH and may contain oxytocin, CRH or vasopressin as the putative transmitter.
- *Neurons in the lateral hypothalamus (LH)*: these neurons may contain the neuropeptide orexin as the putative transmitter (Geerling et al. 2003).
- *Propriospinal neurons* located in the gray matter of the spinal segments C1 to C6 and in the lateral funiculus and lateral spinal nucleus of the segments C1 to C4 (see Subchapter 8.2.1). It is a matter of semantics to call these neurons propriospinal interneurons or sympathetic premotor neurons.

These results clearly illustrate that there are several candidates for sympathetic premotor neurons in the brain stem and hypothalamus, as postulated in neurophysiological studies of sympathetic preganglionic and postganglionic neurons (see Chapters 4 and 9). The types of premotor system are characterized by their supraspinal origin, their histochemistry (types of neuropeptide colocalized in the neurons) and whether the premotor neurons synapse directly with the preganglionic neurons, with the segmental autonomic interneurons or with the propriospinal autonomic neurons (Figure 8.15).

Many sympathetic premotor neurons use glutamate (or perhaps aspartate) as the excitatory transmitter. The role of adrenaline, noradrenaline or 5-HT as transmitter during ongoing regulation of the activity in the sympathetic preganglionic neurons is unclear. Action of these monoamines can be inhibitory. Inhibitory pathways from the brain stem probably use GABA too. Furthermore, it is unclear whether, and in which functional context, the neuropeptides colocalized in the sympathetic premotor neurons are used as neurotransmitters (see Subchapter 9.1.2 for details).

Premotor neurons in the RVLM have been most thoroughly studied. These neurons are largely involved in cardiovascular regulation (see Subchapters 10.2 to 10.4). Sympathetic premotor neurons in the raphe nuclei may be involved in regulation of cutaneous blood flow for thermoregulation and also of brown adipose tissue (see Subchapter 10.5). The functions of

Table 8.2 | Sympathetic nervous system

TARGET	SPINAL CORD Preggl. (IML,IC,CA)	SPINAL CORD INN RN	VMM GiA	VMM GiV	VMM PPN	VLM LPGi	VLM RVLM	RAPHE N. M	RAPHE N. O	RAPHE N. P	PONS A5	PONS PB (KF)	PONS BN	PAG	HYP PVH	HYP LH	HYP DMH (VMH)	HYP OTHER	BNST	MPO	CeAM	Cortex	REFS.
ADRENAL MEDULLA	X T4–T13	I,II,IV,VII C1–C4 LF,LSN	X			X	X	X	X	X	X	X	X	X	X pc			Periformical		X			[1]
CUT. VC (TAIL)	X T11–L2	I,V,VII,IX,X C1–C4	X	X		X	X Adren	X	X	X	X LC,SC	X	X	X dm,dl	X pc	X		Periformical ZI	X	X	X		[2]
SPLEEN	X T3–T12	C1–C4	X Ventromedial medulla			X	X LC,SC	X	X	X	X LC,SC	X	X	X	X pc	X	X						[3]
KIDNEY	X T3–T12	T1–T13	X Ventromedial reticular formation				X Adren	X	X	X	X	X	X	X	X pc	X		Retrochiasmatic	X	X			[4]
HEART	X T1–T7		X Ventromedial medulla				X	X Raphe nuclei						X				Retrochiasmatic Periformical				Insula Infralimbic	[5]
STELLATE GANGLION	X	I,II,IV,VII,X C1–C4 LF,LSN	X	X	X	X	X	X	X	X	X LC,SC	X	X	X vl,EW	X pc	X		Periformical		X	Septum	Insula Frontal Infralimbic	[6]
PINEAL GLAND	X T1–T3	X	X			X	X	X	X	X	X LC	X	X	X	X			SCN		X			[7]
BROWN ADIPOSE TISSUE	X	X	X			X	X	X	X	X	X	X	X	X vl,l	X	X		SCN	X	X	Septum		[8]
WHITE ADIPOSE TISSUE	X	X	X			X	X Adren	X	X	X	X	X	X	X d,v	X	X	X	SCN	X	X	Septum		[9]
	#	#	#	#		#	#	#	#	#		#	#		#								

[1] Strack et al. 1989a,b; Jansen et al. 1995a; Jansen and Loewy 1997; Westerhaus and Loewy 1999, 2001. [2] Smith et al. 1998. [3] Cano et al. 2000, 2001. [4] Schramm et al. 1993; Sly et al 1999; Huang and Weiss 1999; Cano et al. 2000. [5] ter Horst et al. 1996. [6] Jansen et al. 1995a,b; Jansen and Loewy 1995a,b; Jansen and Loewy 1997; Westerhaus and Loewy 1999, 2001. [7] Larsen et al. 1998. [8] Bamshad et al. 1999. [9] Bamshad et al. 1999. Sites of labeled neurons are indicated by **X** or are specified. Location of premotor neurons is indicated by **#** on the lower margin.

Abbreviations:

Spinal cord: IML, intermediolateral nucleus; IC, intercalate nucleus; CA, central autonomic nucleus (dorsal commissural nucleus); INNRN, interneurons; I, II,V,VII,IX,X spinal laminae of the gray matter; LF, lateral funiculus; LSN, lateral spinal nucleus; Pregl, preganglionic; C, cervical; T, thoracic.

Ventromedial medulla (VMM): GiA, GiV, nucleus gigantocellularis reticularis medialis pars alpha and ventralis; PPN, parapyramidal nucleus.

Ventrolateral medulla (VLM): Adren, adrenergic; LPGi, nucleus paragigantocellularis lateralis; RVLM, rostral ventrolateral medulla.

Raphe nuclei: M, magnus; O, obscurus; P, pallidus.

Pons: A5, A5 area (nucleus); BN, Barrington nucleus (pontine micturition center); KF, Kölliker–Fuse nucleus; LC, locus ceruleus; PB, parabrachial nuclei; SC, locus subceruleus.

Periaqueductal gray matter (PAG): EW, Edinger–Westphal nucleus; d, dorsol; dl, dorsolateral; dm, dorsomedial; l, lateral; v, ventral; vl, ventrolateral;.

Hypothalamus: DMH, VMH, dorso- and ventromedial hypothalamus; LH, lateral hypothalamus; PVH, paraventricular hypothalamus (pc, parvocellular); SCN, subchiasmatic nucleus; ZI, zona incerta.

Telencephalon: BNST, bed nucleus of the striae terminalis; CeAM, central nucleus of the amygdala; MPO, medial preoptic nucleus (area).

Preganglionic neurons, interneurons, propriospinal neurons, premotor neurons and neurons antecedent to the premotor neurons of the sympathetic system labeled by a neurotropic virus injected into the target tissue, target organ or a sympathetic ganglion.

the other sympathetic premotor neurons have been very little studied and how the different sympathetic premotor neurons relate to the different sympathetic pathways is practically unknown.

8.4.2 Parasympathetic Premotor Neurons

The parasympathetic premotor neurons have the following distribution (Figure 8.17, Table 8.3):

• Parasympathetic premotor neurons that project to the parasympathetic preganglionic neurons in the *external formation of the nucleus ambiguus, DMNX* or *salivary nuclei* have a similar pattern of distribution as sympathetic premotor neurons. The neurons are located in the ventromedial medulla, in the caudal raphe nuclei, some in the ventrolateral medulla (including adrenergic [C1] and noradrenergic neurons [A1]), in the ventrolateral pontine A5 area, in the paraventricular nucleus of the hypothalamus, in the lateral hypothalamus and in the preoptic area, as well as in the central nucleus of the amygdala.
• Parasympathetic premotor neurons projecting to the *sacral parasympathetic neuronal circuits* (preganglionic neurons and interneurons) are located in the ventromedial medulla (parapyramidal nucleus), the ventrolateral medulla (RVLM, LPGi), the raphe nuclei, the pontine A5 area, Barrington's nucleus, the paraventricular nucleus of the hypothalamus, the lateral hypothalamus and the preoptic area (Table 8.3). In most virus tracing studies of the central autonomic innervation of the pelvic organs, lumbar sympathetic systems were included since the nerves containing sympathetic pre- or postganglionic axons that supply pelvic organs were not cut.

The pattern of labeled sacral premotor neurons is, first, similar for all pelvic organs and, second, similar to the pattern of premotor neurons labeled trans-synaptically via cranial preganglionic parasympathetic neurons (e.g., from heart, pancreas, airways, glands; Table 8.3). Thus, no pattern of trans-synaptically labeled neurons is seen that is characteristic for individual pelvic organs or organs innervated by the vagus nerve. Furthermore, with the exception of the labeling of neurons in the nucleus gigantocellularis medialis from the cranial organs, no pattern has emerged that is distinct for these organ groups.

8.4.3 Autonomic Neurons Antecedent to Sympathetic or Parasympathetic Premotor Neurons

In addition to the autonomic premotor neurons there are other groups of neurons in the brain stem, hypothalamus and telencephalon that have been labeled using a retrogradely trans-synaptically transported virus. Prominent groups of labeled neurons were present in the parabrachial and Kölliker–Fuse nuclei, in the periaqueductal gray matter (PAG; most of them located ventromedial, ventrolateral or dorsolateral), in the preoptic region of the hypothalamus (Westerhaus and Loewy 1999) and in the telencephalon, including cortical structures (e.g., insula, infralimbic cortex, medial prefrontal cortices [Westerhaus and Loewy 2001]). These neurons have been labeled via autonomic premotor neurons. For example, labeled neurons in the PAG are infected via premotor neurons in the ventromedial medulla, ventrolateral medulla, raphe nuclei, the A5 area and the paraventricular nucleus of the hypothalamus (Farkas et al. 1998) (Tables 8.2 and 8.3). Labeled neurons in the septum, amygdaloid complex, insula, infralimbic cortex, anterior cingulate cortex, medial prefrontal cortex, etc., may be infected via premotor neurons in the hypothalamus (Westerhaus and Loewy 1999, 2001).

8.4.4 Patterns of Central Autonomic Neurons Labeled From Distinct Targets: Strengths and Limitations

Unfortunately, the results obtained with the transsynaptic tracing technique give only rather limited information about the *central organization of functionally distinct autonomic systems*. However, the differences between functionally distinct autonomic systems must exist, otherwise it would be impossible to explain: (1) the characteristic reflex discharge patterns in the neurons of the different types of autonomic pathways and (2) the precise neuronal regulation of autonomic target organs. It is perhaps not unexpected that labeled neurons do not exhibit obvious differences in experiments in which the virus has been injected in the stellate ganglion, celiac ganglion or other sympathetic ganglia. In the rat, the stellate ganglion contains cardiomotor, cutaneous vasoconstrictor, muscle vasoconstrictor, sudomotor, pilomotor, lipomotor (innervating brown adipose tissue) neurons and possibly other functional types of neurons (Baron et al. 1995). The celiac ganglion contains various types of postganglionic

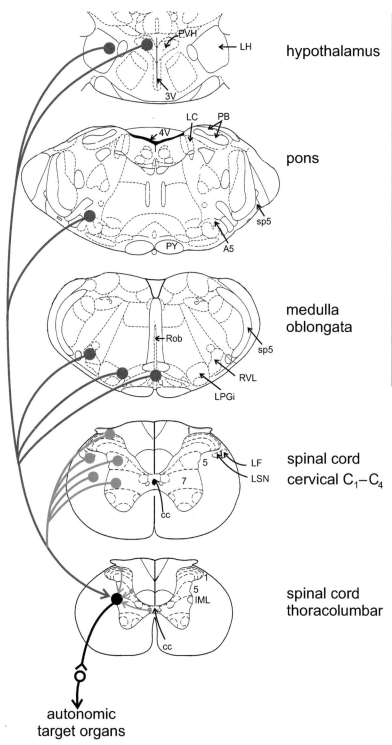

hypothalamus

pons

medulla
oblongata

spinal cord
cervical C$_1$–C$_4$

spinal cord
thoracolumbar

autonomic
target organs

Figure 8.15 Premotor neurons in the brain stem and hypothalamus, spinal segmental interneurons and propriospinal neurons projecting to sympathetic preganglionic neurons. Sympathetic premotor neurons (red) project to preganglionic neurons and to spinal autonomic interneurons (not shown). They are located in the rostral ventrolateral medulla (RVLM), in the caudal raphe nuclei of the medulla oblongata (raphe magnus, pallidus and obscurus [Rob]), in the A5 area of the caudal ventrolateral pons, in the lateral hypothalamus (LH) and in the paraventricular nucleus of the hypothalamus (PVH). Autonomic interneurons are located in laminae 1, 2, 5, 6, 9 and 10 of the spinal cord (blue). Propriospinal neurons are located in laminae 1, 5, 7 and 10 of the cervical spinal segments C1 to C6, in the lateral funiculus (LF) and in the lateral spinal nucleus (LSN) of the cervical segments C1 to C4 (green). cc, central canal; PY, pyramidal tract; sp5, spinal trigeminal tract; 3V, third ventricle; 4V, fourth ventricle. For further abbreviations see Table 8.2. Modified from Jansen et al. (1995b) and Jansen and Loewy (1997) with permission.

neurons innervating the gastrointestinal tract (secreto-motor, motility-regulating, visceral vasoconstrictor neurons; see Subchapters 4.3 and 5.7), spleen (vasoconstrictor neurons, neurons innervating the immune tissue, neurons innervating the capsule), kidney and other targets.

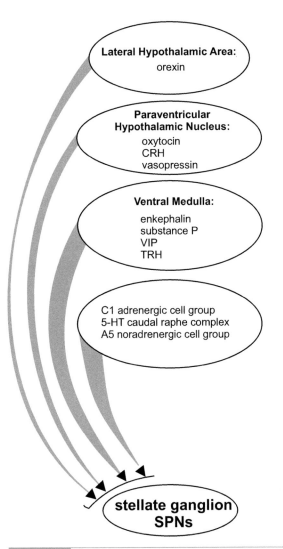

Figure 8.16 Putative transmitters present in sympathetic premotor neurons. In many (all?) sympathetic premotor neurons, glutamate is the fast excitatory transmitter and GABA may be the fast inhibitory transmitter. Data obtained in sympathetic premotor neurons labeled by a neurotropic virus or by a tracer applied to the intermediate zone in the spinal cord. Monoamine synthesizing enzymes (e.g., tyrosine hydroxylase, phenyl-N-methyl transferase) and neuropeptides have been localized immunohistochemically. CRH, corticotropin-releasing hormone; 5-HT, 5-hydroxytryptamine; SPNs, sympathetic preganglionic neurons; TRH, thyrotropin-releasing hormone; VIP, vasoactive intestinal peptide. Modified from Jansen et al. (1995b), Westerhaus and Loewy (1999) and Stornetta et al. (2001) with permission.

However, when considering those experiments in which rather distinct targets have been labeled by the virus, the situation is different. The apparent lack of central differentiation probably results because the differentiation occurs in the central microcircuits, i.e., the excitatory and inhibitory synaptic connections between neurons, the transmitters used, etc. The transported virus does not discriminate between excitatory and inhibitory synapses, nor does it identify their relative effectiveness. The lack of central differentiation is unlikely to result from technical deficits of the transneuronal tracing technique (e.g., by non-specific retrograde transfer of the virus between neurons via the extracellular space or via glia; see Card et al. [1990]; Jansen et al. [1993]; Enquist and Card [2003]). It may partly be related to the projection of vasoconstrictor neurons to most autonomically innervated target tissues. But even this argument is not entirely convincing to explain the relative uniformity of the central labeling with this technique when one compares, e.g., the neuronal networks associated with the adrenal medulla, pineal gland, heart, spleen and urinary bladder, all five having entirely different functions of their non-vasoconstrictor innervation. Furthermore, the innervation of the blood vessels in the heart, spleen or urinary bladder also has different functions. The labeled central neuronal networks associated with these five target tissues are rather similar and resemble the neuronal network labeled from the cutaneous blood vessels of the rat tail, which are involved in thermoregulation (Smith et al. 1998; see Table 8.2).

In summary, trans-synaptic labeling studies have laid down the groundwork for the anatomy of central autonomic circuits and will be one basis for further functional and anatomical studies of these circuits. Unfortunately, few, if any, of these labeling studies conducted so far provide much of a basis for understanding the differential regulation of final autonomic motor pathways.

Conclusions

Neurophysiological investigations of the peripheral sympathetic and parasympathetic neurons strongly support the notion that autonomic systems have a distinct organization in the central nervous system, including the spinal cord and brain stem. Anatomical investigations, using various anterograde, orthograde and trans-synaptic tracing techniques, have provided

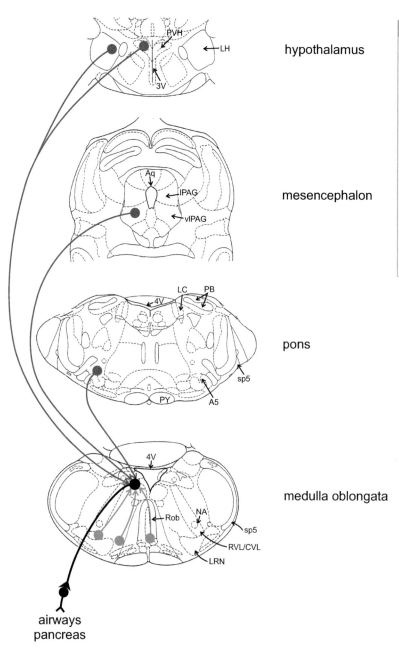

hypothalamus

mesencephalon

pons

medulla oblongata

airways
pancreas

Figure 8.17 Premotor neurons for parasympathetic preganglionic neurons projecting to airways and pancreas. The premotor neurons (red) synapse with parasympathetic preganglionic neurons and/or interneurons (blue) associated with these preganglionic neurons. The premotor neurons have been labeled by a neurotropic virus (Bartha strain of the pseudorabies virus), which was injected into the wall of the airways or the pancreas. Aq, aqueduct; LRN, lateral reticular nucleus; PY, pyramidal tract; sp5, spinal trigeminal tract; 3V, third ventricle; 4V, fourth ventricle. For other abbreviations see Table 8.2. Data from Haxhiu et al. (1993, 1998), Loewy and Haxhiu (1993), Loewy et al. (1994) and Haxhiu and Loewy (1996).

an important basis for this postulated functional organization of central autonomic systems. The structural organization will be the basis for future functional studies of the central autonomic systems.

1. Sympathetic preganglionic neurons are located in the intermediate zone of the thoracic and upper lumbar spinal cord. These neurons exhibit some broad mediolateral topographic organization with

respect to the efferent innervation of the visceral and somatic body domains. Otherwise functionally different groups of preganglionic neurons are intermingled. Most preganglionic neurons supplying somatic tissues are located laterally in the funicular and principal part of the intermediolateral nucleus. Preganglionic neurons supplying viscera have a more medial location.

Table 8.3 | Parasympathetic nervous system

TARGET	SPINAL CORD		DORS. MED. OBL./NA				VMM			VLM		RAPHE N.			PONS			PAG	HYPOTHALAMUS				TELENCEPHALON			REFS.
	IML	INNRN	NTS	AP	NA	DMNX	GiA	GiV	PPN	LPGi	RVLM	M	O	P	A5	PB	BN		PVH	LH	DMH/VMH	Other	BNST	MPO	CeAM	
CRANIAL SYSTEMS																										
HEART	X	SPN, DCN	X	X	X	X									X	X		X	X	X	X	Retro-chiasmatic	X	X	Lateral septum	[1]
PANCREAS		DH (I), X	X	X		X	X	X		X	X	X	X	X	LC,SC		X	X (v,lm)	X	X	X	Perifornical	X		X	[2]
AIRWAYS		SPN, DCN	X	X	X		X	X	X	X	X	X	X	X	SC	X	X	X (vl)	X	X		Dorsal hypothal.	X	X		[3]
GLANDS (SM, PTPG)		SPN, DH (I), X	X			Sup. sal. n.	X	X	X	X	X	X	X	X	LC,SC	X	X	X (vl, ventr. tegm.)	X (pc)			Perifornical / Periventricular	X	X	X	[4]
							#	#	#	#	#	#	#	#	#		#	#	#	#						
SACRAL SYSTEMS																										
(* includes sympathetic systems)																										
URINARY	X	SPN, DCN						X		X		Raphe nuclei			X		X	X	X	X						[5]
BLADDER	SPN	DH (I), X; L5–S1													SC											
URINARY	X	SPN, DCN					X		X	X		X			X (SC)		X	X (vm)	X (pc)	X		Perifornical		X		[6]
BLADDER*, EUS*	SPN	DH (I), X; L1/L2							X						SC		X									
URETHRA*	X	DCN, DH; SPN L6/S1, L1/L2					Gigantocell. ret. n.					X			LC, SC		X	X (vl)	X							[7]
PENIS*,	X	DCN, X; L5–S1							X	X	X	X		X	X		X	X (vl)	X (pc)	X				X		[8]
CLITORIS*, PROSTATE*	L5–S1; T12–L4	dors. IML																								
BULBO/ISCHIO-	X								X	X	X			X	X		X	X (vl)	X (pc)	X				X		[9]
CAVERNOSUS*		L/S, T/L													LC,SC		v,l vm	X	X (pc)	X	X					
UTERUS*	X	DCN, X, DH; intermed. gray	X			X							X		X		v,l vm	X	X	X						[10]
COLON*	X	SPN, IML	X	X	X	X					X	Raphe nuclei			X (LC,SC)		X	X	X (SO)	X		Medial/ frontal lobe				[11]
			#	#	#	#	#	#	#	#	#	#	#	# #	#		#	#	#	#						

[1] ter Horst et al. 1996. [2] Loewy and Haxhiu 1993; Loewy et al. 1994. [3] Haxniu et al 1993, 1998; Haxhiu and Loewy 1996; Hadziefendic and Haxhiu 1999. [4] Spencer et al. 1990; Blessing et al. 1991; Jansen et al. 1992. [5] Nadelhaft et al. 1992; Nadelhaft and Vera 1995. [6] Marson 1997. [7] Vizzard et al. 1995. [8] Marson et al. 1993; Marson 1995; Orr and Marson 1998. [9] Marson and McKenna 1996. [10] Papka et al. 1998. [11] Vizzard et al. 2000.

Sites of labeled neurons are indicated by **X** or are specified. Location of premotor neurons is indicated by **#** on the lower margin.

Abbreviations:

Spinal cord: DCN, dorsal commissural nucleus; DH, dorsal horn; IML, intermediolateral nucleus; INNRN, interneurons; SPN, sacral preganglionic neuron; I,X, spinal laminae of the gray matter; L, lumbar; T, thoracic; S, sacral.

Dors. Med. Obl./NA: AP, area postrema; DMNX, dorsal motor nucleus of the vagus; Dors. Med. Obl., dorsal medulla oblongata; NA, nucleus ambiguus; NTS, nucleus tractus solitarii; sup.sal.n., superior salivatory nucleus.

Ventromedial medulla (VMM): GiA, GiV, nucleus gigantocellularis reticularis mecialis pars alpha and ventralis; PPN, parapyramidal nucleus; ret. n., reticular nucleus.

Ventrolateral medulla (VLM): LPGi, nucleus paragigantocellularis lateralis; RVLM, rostral ventrolateral medulla.

Raphe nuclei: M, magnus; O, obscurus; P, pallidus.

Pons: A5, A5 area (nucleus); PB, parabrachial nuclei; KF, Kölliker–Fuse nucleus; BN, Barrington nucleus (pontine micturition center); LC, locus ceruleus; SC, locus subcoeruleus; vl, ventrolateral; vm, ventromedial.

Periaqueductal gray matter (PAG): ventral tegm., ventral tegmentum; m, medial; v, ventral , vl, ventrolateral; vm, ventromedial.

Hypothalamus: DH, dorsal hypothalamus; DMH, VMH, dorso- and ventromedial hypothalamus; LH, lateral hypothalamus; perifornical, perifornical area; PVH, paraventricular hypothalamus (pc, parvocellular); retrochiasmatic, retrochiasmatic nucleus; SO. supraoptic nucleus; pc, parvocellular.

Telencephalon: BNST, bed nucleus of the striae terminalis; CeAM, central nucleus of the amygdala; MPO, medial preoptic nucleus (area).

Other: Bulbo-/Ischio-cavernosus, bulbo-ischio-cavernosus muscles; EUS, external urethral sphincter; PTPG, pterygopalatine ganglion; SM, submandibular gland.

Preganglionic neurons, premotor neurons and neurons antecedent to the premotor neurons of the parasympathetic system labeled by a neurotropic virus injected into a target tissue or target organ.

2. Parasympathetic preganglionic neurons in the sacral spinal cord are also located in the intermediate zone with some organotopic organization. Neurons innervating the urogenital tract are located laterally and those innervating the hindgut medially.

3. Parasympathetic preganglionic neurons in the brain stem are located in the external formation of the nucleus ambiguus (largely cardiomotor neurons and bronchomotor neurons), in the dorsal vagus motor nucleus (DMNX; largely gastrointestinal tract), in the salivary nuclei and in the Edinger–Westphal nucleus (eye) or related to it. Each of these nuclei projects to a distinct organ system. The preganglionic neurons in the DMNX exhibit a mediolateral columnar viscerotopic organization, those innervating the stomach being situated medially and those innervating the cecum laterally.

4. The nucleus tractus solitarii (NTS) receives peripheral synaptic input from gustatory afferents (rostral half) and from gastrointestinal, respiratory and cardiovascular afferents (caudal half of the NTS). Projections of visceral afferents from the latter three systems to the subnuclei of the NTS exhibit some topographic organization. This topography is particularly obvious for the different sections of the alimentary canal, showing a mediolateral and caudorostral organization.

5. Neurons in the NTS consist of projection neurons and interneurons. The NTS neurons project to many nuclei in the spinal cord, brain stem, hypothalamus and forebrain, and receive synaptic input from most of these brain sites. The NTS has relay and integrative functions.

6. Several groups of autonomic interneurons lie in the thoracolumbar (laminae I, II, V, VI, IX and X) and sacral spinal cord (close to the preganglionic neurons, laminae I and X, dorsal commissural nucleus), whereas propriospinal interneurons have been identified in the cervical spinal cord (lateral funiculus, lateral spinal nucleus, dorsal horn).

7. Sympathetic premotor neurons that project through the dorsolateral funiculus to the preganglionic neurons and/or the corresponding autonomic interneurons are situated in the ventrolateral medulla (mainly in the rostral ventrolateral medulla), in the ventromedial medulla, in the caudal raphe nuclei, in the A5 area of the pons, in the paraventricular nucleus of the hypothalamus and in the lateral hypothalamus.

8. Parasympathetic premotor neurons that project to the preganglionic neurons innervating the heart, pancreas, trachea or salivary glands are located in the ventral medulla in the same nuclei as sympathetic premotor neurons, but additionally in the periaqueductal gray (mostly ventrolateral). The same applies to parasympathetic premotor neurons associated with the urinary bladder and probably also those associated with the other pelvic target organs. Some of these lie in Barrington's nucleus in the pons.

9. Neurons antecedent to autonomic premotor neurons are also present in various nuclei of the pons (parabrachial nuclei, Kölliker–Fuse nucleus, Barrington's nucleus), periaqueductal gray, various hypothalamic nuclei and various nuclei of the telencephalon (preoptic nuclei, amygdaloid complex, insula, infralimbic cortex, medial preoptic cortex).

10. Attempts to relate the anatomical location of autonomic premotor neurons and those antecedent to them have so far failed to yield patterns specific for the functioning of particular target organs.

Suggested Reading

Deuchars, S. A. (2011) Spinal interneurons in the control of autonomic functions. In *Central Regulation of Autonomic Functions*, *2nd edn* (Llewellyn-Smith, I. J., and Verberne, A. J. M., eds) pp. 140–160, Oxford University Press, Oxford.

Jänig, W. (1985) Organization of the lumbar sympathetic outflow to skeletal muscle and skin of the cat hindlimb and tail. *Rev Physiol Biochem Pharmacol* **102**, 119–213.

Jänig, W. (1986) Spinal cord integration of visceral sensory systems and sympathetic nervous system reflexes. *Prog Brain Res* **67**, 255–277.

Jänig, W. and McLachlan, E. M. (1986b) Identification of distinct topographical distributions of lumbar sympathetic and sensory neurons projecting to end organs with different functions in the cat. *J Comp Neurol* **246**, 104–112.

Jänig, W. and McLachlan, E. M. (1987) Organization of lumbar spinal outflow to distal colon and pelvic organs. *Physiol Rev* **67**, 1332–1404.

Paton, J. F. (1996b) A working heart-brainstem preparation of the mouse. *J Neurosci Methods* **65**, 63–68.

Paton, J. F. and Kasparov, S. (2000) Sensory channel specific modulation in the nucleus of the solitary tract. *J Auton Nerv Syst* **80**, 117–129.

All references cited in the text are available online at www.cambridge.org/janig.

Notes

1. In rodents the central autonomic nucleus (CA) is large in the lumbar segments and mainly located dorsal to the central canal and therefore has been called the dorsal commissural nucleus (Hancock and Peveto 1979). This should not be confused with a similarly named nucleus in the sacral segments that does not contain preganglionic neurons but receives pelvic visceral and somatic afferents (Honda and Perl 1985; Roppolo et al. 1985).
2. In human probably to segment L4. In rat and mouse to segment L4. The cat has seven lumbar segments; the rat and mouse have six lumbar segments.
3. Some lumbar sympathetic preganglionic neurons project to sacral paravertebral ganglia and form synapses with postganglionic neurons that project to pelvic organs (see Costa and Furness [1973]; Jänig and McLachlan [1987]).
4. The gray matter of the spinal cord is divided into laminae by cytoarchitectonic criteria according to Rexed (1952; Molander and Grant 1995).
5. These numerical data for the rat are based on estimations described by Powley et al. (1992). In other publications by this author group, estimations of afferent and efferent (preganglionic) neurons projecting in the abdominal vagal branches of the rat, based on counting of cell bodies in the DMNX labeled by the fluorescent tracer True Blue and on counting of nerve fibers under the light and the electron microscope, resulted in the following numbers: the vagal branches contain about 22 000 nerve fibers (11 000 in each subdiaphragmatic vagal trunk); 16 000 nerve fibers are afferent and 6000 efferent. About 85% of the preganglionic neurons project through the gastric branches, 11% through the celiac branches and 4% through the hepatic branch of the subdiaphragmatic vagus nerves (Fox and Powley 1985; Prechtl and Powley 1990; Berthoud and Neuhuber

2000) (see Note 6 for the innervation territories of these branches).
6. The rostrocaudal columnar organization of the preganglionic neurons in the DMNX is based on labeling of the branches of the subdiaphragmatic vagus nerves in the rat. A one-to-one correspondence between these vagal branches and the different parts of the gastrointestinal tract does not exist. The hepatic branch also contains preganglionic axons that innervate the antrum and duodenum. The gastric branches contain preganglionic axons innervating the proximal duodenum. The celiac branches contain preganglionic axons innervating (in addition to the small intestine, cecum and proximal colon) the distal part of the duodenum (Berthoud et al. 1991). Finally, preganglionic neurons innervating the pancreas project through the gastric branches and the hepatic branch and probably not through the celiac branches (Berthoud and Powley 1990; Berthoud et al. 1990). These three points explain why preganglionic neurons to the liver and pancreas are represented more medially in the DMNX (Figure 8.10c).
7. In humans, the parasympathetic preganglionic neurons projecting to the ciliary ganglion are located dorsomedial to the Edinger–Westphal nucleus (Neuhuber and Schrödl 2011). In the rat, rabbit and cat, most oculomotor parasympathetic preganglionic neurons do not lie in the Edinger–Westphal nucleus but ventral to the oculomotor nucleus in the ventral tegmental area and in the central gray matter (see Loewy 1990b).
8. In primates, the rostral (gustatory) NTS also projects viscerotopically to the basal part of the ventromedial nucleus of the thalamus (VMb), which in turn projects to the dorsal insula (limbic sensory cortex representing interoception; see Subchapter 2.6).
9. There is some confusion about the nomenclature and the limitations of these nuclei (see Blessing [1997]; Mason [2001]). Here I will use the nomenclature of Paxinos and Watson (2014). The rostral ventrolateral medulla (RVLM) and the lateral paragigantocellular nucleus (LPGi) are subsumed under ventrolateral medulla (VLM). The ventromedial medulla (VMM) includes the medial paragigantocellular reticular nucleus, alpha and ventral (GiA, GiV) and the parapyramidal region or nucleus (PPy) (see Subchapter 7.2 and Figure 10.2).

Chapter 9

Spinal Autonomic Systems

The activity in spinal preganglionic neurons is the result of the summation of potential changes in the neuronal membrane arising from integrative processes in the spinal cord, brain stem, hypothalamus and forebrain (Note 1). As in the somatomotor system (Lloyd 1960; Baldissera et al. 1981), the spinal cord itself is a major highway of interaction between the brain and the autonomic target organs and tissues. In this chapter, I will concentrate on the thoracolumbar (sympathetic) and sacral (parasympathetic) autonomic systems. I will argue that the spinal cord contains autonomic systems, that the spinal autonomic systems are coordinated, involving function-specific interneurons, and that the spinal autonomic systems are integrated in the regulation of autonomic effector organs and tissues. Thus, I will put forward the concept that the spinal autonomic systems are integrated in the regulation of activity in preganglionic neurons by supraspinal centers.

9.1   The Spinal Autonomic Reflex Pathway as a Building Block of Central Integration

In Chapter 4, I emphasized that many components of the reflex patterns in sympathetic neurons are likely to depend on spinal circuits (see Figures 4.3, 4.4, 4.6 and 4.17). The principles of organization of the basic circuits of the parasympathetic systems in the brain stem, related to gastrointestinal function, cardiac function, function of airways, secretion of exocrine glands and to regulation of pupil diameter, are presumably organized in a similar way (see Subchapter 10.7).

9.1.1   Structure and Inputs of the Spinal Autonomic Reflex Pathway

Sympathetic preganglionic neurons receive synaptic inputs from spinal and propriospinal interneurons and sympathetic premotor neurons in the brain stem and hypothalamus (Figure 8.15). Primary afferent neurons from skin, deep somatic tissues and viscera form spinal reflex circuits with the preganglionic neurons. These reflex circuits are disynaptic or polysynaptic. The autonomic circuits in the brain stem and hypothalamus that project to the spinal cord connect via autonomic premotor neurons (see Subchapter 8.4) to the preganglionic neurons mono-, di- or polysynaptically. This spinal arrangement of preganglionic neurons, interneurons, primary afferent neurons and autonomic premotor neurons in supraspinal centers is the basic building block of spinal autonomic systems (Figure 9.1) and can be

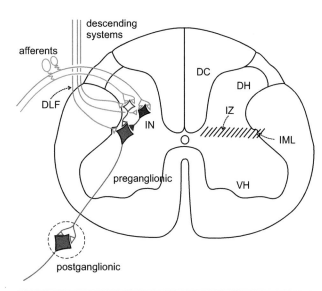

Figure 9.1 The spinal autonomic reflex pathway as the building block between supraspinal centers and final autonomic pathways. There is usually at least one (excitatory or inhibitory) interneuron (IN) between (somatic or visceral) primary afferent neurons and preganglionic neurons. Supraspinal centers in the brain stem and hypothalamus project mainly through the dorsolateral funiculus (DLF) of the spinal cord and connect synaptically to the autonomic interneurons and the preganglionic neurons. DC, dorsal column; DH, dorsal horn; IML, intermediolateral nucleus; IZ, intermediate zone; VH, ventral horn.

recognized for most if not all final spinal autonomic pathways. It probably applies to final cranial autonomic (parasympathetic) pathways as well (see Figures 10.27–10.29).

Most autonomic premotor neurons in the supraspinal centers that connect synaptically to the spinal autonomic circuits project through the dorsolateral funiculi of the spinal cord. The location of the cell bodies of these neurons has been identified by experiments in which the descending neurons have been labeled retrogradely using various types of markers, including neurotropic viruses (Subchapter 8.4; Tables 8.2 and 8.3; see Subchapter 8.4.4 for critical assessment).

The functions of most of these individual autonomic premotor pathways projecting to spinal sympathetic or parasympathetic circuits are unknown. Sympathetic premotor pathways related to the regulation of resistance vessels or heart (see Subchapters 10.2 and 10.3, Figures 10.4 and 10.7) or related to thermoregulation of cutaneous blood flow (see

Subchapter 10.5 and Figure 10.16) have been characterized. The number of different types of sympathetic premotor neurons in the brain stem and hypothalamus identified so far morphologically and histochemically (see Subchapter 8.4) is low relative to the number of postulated types of descending sympathetic premotor neurons, which appear necessary for the function of the different sympathetic systems (see Figure 4.25 for the lumbar sympathetic systems).

The situation appears to be simpler as far as the types of parasympathetic premotor neurons in the brain stem projecting to the sacral spinal cord are concerned. The sacral parasympathetic systems have basically only the major functions of defecation, micturition, penile/clitoral erection and secretion from the vagina in their regulation of elimination or storage, and erection or detumescence. Therefore, the number of types of supraspinal parasympathetic premotor neurons is smaller than that of sympathetic premotor neurons.

9.1.2 Synaptic Transmission and Transmitters

Synaptic transmission from primary afferent neurons and autonomic premotor neurons to the spinal autonomic circuits and within the spinal autonomic circuits is chemical (Note 2):

- Transmission from primary afferent neurons with myelinated and unmyelinated fibers to spinal interneurons is excitatory, the excitatory transmitters being amino acids (e.g., glutamate and possibly aspartate) and possibly neuropeptides (such as substance P and calcitonin gene-related peptide [CGRP]). The functions of these peptides in synaptic transmission in the spinal cord are not well understood, as is the case with dorsal horn interneurons related to nociception (Todd 2010).
- Transmission from descending systems to preganglionic neurons and autonomic interneurons is excitatory or inhibitory (Deuchars et al. 1997, 2001b; Llewellyn-Smith and Weaver 2001; Whyment et al. 2004; Deuchars 2011; Deuchars and Lall 2015). The main *excitatory transmitters* involved in fast synaptic transmission from many, if not most, of the autonomic premotor systems that project bilaterally through the dorsolateral funiculi are glutamate and possibly other excitatory amino acids. The *inhibitory transmitters* in fast synaptic transmission from sympathetic premotor neurons to preganglionic neurons are γ-aminobutyric acid (GABA) and

possibly glycine. Both GABA and glycine may be coexpressed in the same neurons. The functional meaning of this coexpression is unknown (Llewellyn-Smith et al. 1995, 1997; Llewellyn-Smith and Weaver 2001; Llewellyn-Smith 2011).

- 5-Hydroxytryptamine (serotonin), adrenaline, noradrenaline and dopamine and the various neuropeptides localized or colocalized in autonomic premotor neurons (see Figure 8.16) may also be transmitters. Focal electrical stimulation in spinal cord slices evokes, in addition to fast synaptic potentials elicited by release of amino acids, slow excitatory (sEPSP) and slow inhibitory postsynaptic potentials (sIPSP) in the sympathetic preganglionic neurons. The sEPSPs may be mediated by noradrenaline or adrenaline acting via α_1-adrenoceptors and the sIPSPs via α_2-adrenoceptors (Yoshimura et al. 1987a, b). Dopamine has inhibitory effects on preganglionic sympathetic neurons in vitro (Gladwell and Coote 1999). However, overall it is unclear how and whether these monoamines and neuropeptides released by sympathetic premotor neurons act as transmitters during autonomic regulation.
- Nitric oxide (NO) released by sympathetic neurons during excitation may act on nearby interneurons, causing the release of the inhibitory transmitter glycine (Yang et al. 2004).
- Synaptic transmission from interneurons to preganglionic neurons is excitatory or inhibitory, probably involving excitatory amino acids (such as glutamate) and inhibitory amino acids (such as GABA and glycine).
- Synaptic transmission from descending excitatory (glutamatergic) and inhibitory (GABAergic) pathways to preganglionic neurons or associated interneurons is modulated presynaptically by adenosine. Excitatory transmission is inhibited via A_1 adenosine receptors and inhibitory transmission enhanced via A_{2A} adenosine receptors located in the presynaptic terminals. Adenosine may be released within presynaptic terminals or as the result of extracellular breakdown of adenosine triphosphate (ATP) during local ischemia and hypoxia. This mechanism of inhibiting excitatory synaptic transmission and enhancing inhibitory synaptic transmission may protect sympathetic neurons and associated interneurons against overexcitation (Deuchars et al. 2001a; Brooke et al. 2004; Deuchars 2011).

9.1.3 Spinal Interneurons Associated With Autonomic Circuits

Up to now no autonomic interneuron has been fully and unequivocally identified by its physiological function; the best examples of reasonably well-identified autonomic interneurons exist in the sacral spinal cord (see Figures 9.8 and 9.9). However, indirect evidence for the existence of functionally different types of autonomic interneurons is overwhelming, based on several physiological and morphological investigations (see Cabot et al. 1994; Cabot 1996; Weaver and Polosa 1997; Shefchyk 2001; Deuchars 2011):

- Putative interneurons were labeled by retrograde trans-synaptic transport of compounds applied to the cut preganglionic axons or their terminals in the respective ganglia or applied to cut postganglionic axons or to their terminals in the target tissue. The compounds are actively taken up by the preganglionic fibers and conveyed by retrograde axoplasmic transport mechanisms to the preganglionic cell bodies and dendrites. Here they are released by exocytosis and actively taken up by the presynaptic terminals that innervate the preganglionic neurons. Such substances are, e.g., wheat-germ agglutinin, the B-unit of the cholera toxin or neurotropic viruses (see Subchapter 8.1). These types of studies demonstrate that interneurons associated with preganglionic neurons are located in the gray matter of the thoracolumbar spinal cord in laminae I, II, V, VII (dorsal to the intermediolateral nucleus) and X (intermediomedial nucleus, central autonomic nucleus in rats) (see Table 8.2 and Subchapter 8.2.1).
- Spinal neurons labeled by a neurotropic virus from the stellate ganglion, the adrenal medulla or the tail of rats are located in various laminae of the gray matter, in the lateral spinal nucleus and in the lateral funiculus of the cervical spinal cord (Strack et al. 1989a, b; Jansen et al. 1995a, b; Jansen and Loewy 1997; Smith et al. 1998) (see Table 8.2). These propriospinal neurons may communicate indirectly with preganglionic neurons via local interneurons, or less commonly by direct synaptic contact (Tang et al. 2003, 2004).
- In the sacral spinal cord, similar morphological investigations have been conducted using pseudorabies virus injected into the urinary bladder or urethra of rats. Interneurons were found dorsal and medial to the preganglionic neurons in the

lateral band, dorsal to the central canal (in the dorsal commissural nucleus), and in lamina I and lamina X of the dorsal horn (de Groat et al. 1996) (see Table 8.3 and references therein).

- Neurophysiological recordings demonstrate some excitatory neurons in the spinal cord close to sympathetic preganglionic neurons, which could not be activated antidromically by stimulation of preganglionic axons in the ventral root and which exhibited discharge patterns that were correlated with those in the preganglionic neurons (Barman and Gebber 1984).

- Some excitatory neurons in the intermediomedial nucleus in the cat (central autonomic nucleus in the rat) exhibit discharge patterns similar to preganglionic neurons in the intermediolateral nucleus and inhibit the preganglionic neurons (McCall et al. 1977). In vitro experiments show that these interneurons in the central autonomic area are GABAergic and form inhibitory synapses with preganglionic neurons (Deuchars et al. 2005). These inhibitory interneurons probably mediate inhibition of preganglionic neurons generated from supraspinal centers (and even the prefrontal cortex [Bacon and Smith 1993]).

- In both acutely and chronically spinalized rats (Note 3), discharges in some neurons in the dorsal horn and in the intermediate zone in the thoracic segments T10 and adjacent segments precede the efferent discharge in the renal nerve by about 60 ms. These interneurons exhibit reflex patterns similar to renal sympathetic neurons, but differ in their electrophysiological properties from preganglionic neurons (Chau and Schramm 1997; Chau et al. 2000; Krassioukov et al. 2002).

- Two weeks after transection of the spinal cord, about 30% to 50% of the synaptic inputs to sympathetic preganglionic neurons located caudal to the transection remain, about 40% of them being glutamatergic (excitatory) and 60% GABAergic (inhibitory) (Llewellyn-Smith et al. 1997; Llewellyn-Smith and Weaver 2001). In control rats, the proportions are closer to 50:50.

- Reflexes generated in preganglionic neurons to electrical stimulation of *myelinated* afferents in white rami in normal (and spinal) cats have relatively long and variable latencies, arguing that they are not elicited monosynaptically but are mediated di- or polysynaptically (see shortest latency responses in Figure 9.2b).

- Several functionally distinct groups of autonomic interneurons have to be postulated on the basis of neurophysiological investigations of reflexes elicited in functionally identified sympathetic neurons upon physiological stimulation of afferents in spinal cats (see Figures 4.3, 4.4, 4.6 and 4.17 and see Subchapter 9.2).

- Electrical stimulation of the dorsolateral funiculus, through which the axons of most autonomic premotor neurons project, or electrical stimulation of the rostral ventrolateral medulla (RVLM) in the lower brain stem, elicits monosynaptic and polysynaptic EPSPs in preganglionic neurons (in vivo experiments and in vitro experiments) (Dembowsky et al. 1985; Deuchars et al. 1997).

- Several distinct types of autonomic interneuron that are associated with preganglionic neurons innervating pelvic organs have been postulated or shown to exist on the basis of neurophysiological experimental investigations in vivo or in vitro (see Shefchyk [2001] and Figures 9.8 to 9.10).

In spite of this limited knowledge, we hypothesize that spinal cord circuits are involved in distinct discharge patterns in sympathetic and spinal parasympathetic neurons. We can therefore develop a concept about the role of spinal autonomic circuits in the regulation of activity of the final autonomic pathways by the brain.

9.2 | Spinal Reflexes Organized in Sympathetic Systems

In Chapter 4, I discussed the reflex pattern in functionally different types of sympathetic pre- and postganglionic neurons and indicated that many characteristics of these reflex patterns are dependent on spinal reflex pathways. Here I will extend this idea and show, for the lumbar sympathetic outflow, *first*, that some functionally defined sympathetic pathways are associated with several distinct spinal reflex pathways and, *second*, that there are indications for coordination of spinal autonomic reflex circuits in the spinal cord.

9.2.1 Segmental and Suprasegmental Reflexes Elicited in Sympathetic Preganglionic Neurons by Electrical Stimulation of Afferents

Sympathetic preganglionic neurons exhibit short- and long-latency reflexes to electrical stimulation of spinal afferents (e.g., in the dorsal roots or white rami). These reflexes are mediated by spinal and supraspinal pathways. The spinal reflexes are most powerful when the afferents of the same or a neighboring segment in which the preganglionic neurons are located are stimulated. Although there seems to exist some general organizing principle for reflexes in the sympathetic system at the spinal segmental and supraspinal levels, it is unclear from these investigations, *first*, which functional types of afferent are involved in these reflexes and, *second*, whether different types of sympathetic neuron exhibit functionally distinct types of segmental (spinal) and suprasegmental reflexes (Sato and Schmidt 1971, 1973; Sato 1972; Sato et al. 1997). Coote (1988) has extensively discussed the integration of spinal and supraspinal reflexes elicited in sympathetic preganglionic neurons by electrical stimulation of visceral and somatic nerves.

Spinal and supraspinal reflexes elicited by electrical stimulation of spinal afferents in functionally identified sympathetic preganglionic neurons have been examined in only one study (Bahr et al. 1986b):

- *Preganglionic visceral vasoconstrictor neurons* that project in the lumbar splanchnic nerves exhibit very powerful reflexes to electrical stimulation of lumbar somatic and visceral afferents (Figure 9.2b). The excitatory reflexes consist of several components when classified by their latencies: short-latency reflexes are probably mediated by spinal reflex circuits and long-latency reflexes by supraspinal reflex circuits. Interestingly, the reflexes with the shortest latency have the lowest threshold and are probably elicited by stimulation of fast-conducting somatic or visceral afferents. Similar powerful short- and long-latency reflexes to electrical stimulation of afferents have been reported in the cardiac and renal nerves (Coote and Downman 1966; Coote and Sato 1978; Coote 1984; for a review see Sato and Schmidt [1973]).
- *Preganglionic motility-regulating neurons* that project in the lumbar splanchnic nerves also exhibit reflexes to electrical stimulation of lumbar somatic and spinal afferents (Figure 9.2c). However, these reflexes are present in only about 60% of the functionally identified motility-regulating neurons; they are much weaker than the reflexes in visceral vasoconstrictor neurons and most of them have a short latency (i.e., are probably mediated by a spinal reflex pathway) (Bahr et al. 1986b).

Intracellular recordings from preganglionic sympathetic neurons in the spinal segment T3 of the cat (Dembowsky et al. 1985) have shown that electrical stimulation of somatic or visceral spinal afferents in the corresponding spinal nerve and white ramus, respectively, elicits early and late EPSPs in ≥80% of the neurons when the spinal cord is intact, early EPSPs in almost all neurons in spinal animals and late EPSPs in about 50% of the neurons in spinal animals. The results obtained so far on functionally identified preganglionic neurons reported by Bahr et al. (1986b) agree with these intracellular measurements. These experiments show: (1) that spinal reflexes exist for most sympathetic pathways and (2) that spinal and supraspinal reflexes are different in functionally distinct types of preganglionic neuron. Unfortunately, these results, which were obtained on functionally identified preganglionic sympathetic neurons, give only limited answers to the question of which spinal reflexes are associated with which functional type of sympathetic system because the function of the spinal afferents stimulated electrically are unknown.

9.2.2 Recovery of Spinal Reflexes After Spinal Cord Transection

When the spinal cord is acutely isolated from the brain stem, almost all reflexes in sympathetic neurons projecting to somatic tissues, including those elicited by strong noxious stimuli, disappear for days to weeks in cats and in humans, probably as a consequence of the interruption of the descending control systems. This state of the spinal cord is called "spinal shock" (Note 4) (Guttmann 1976; Jichia and Frank 2000; Mathias et al. 2013). The recovery of functionally distinct reflexes elicited by physiological stimulation of primary afferent neurons (Note 5) and of ongoing activity in those sympathetic systems that are under dominant supraspinal control takes weeks to months, depending on the functional type of sympathetic system, the type of (excitatory or inhibitory) reflex and the animal species studied (Note 6). The

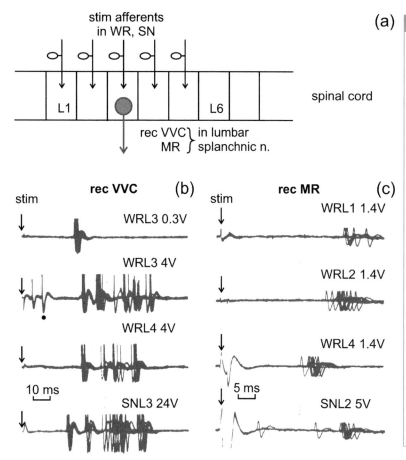

(a)

Figure 9.2 Spinal and supraspinal reflex activation of sympathetic neurons to electrical stimulation of spinal afferents in the cat. Activity was recorded from a preganglionic visceral vasoconstrictor axon (VVC in [b]) and a preganglionic axon of a motility-regulating neuron (MR in [c]), which were both isolated for extracellular recording from one of the lumbar splanchnic nerves. The functional classifications arise from the characteristic discharge patterns (see Subchapter 4.3). Spinal afferents in spinal nerves (SN, nerve containing somatic afferents) or in white rami (WR, containing visceral afferents) were stimulated electrically with single pulses (pulse duration 0.5 ms for SN and 0.2 ms for WR). Different segmental nerves were stimulated in each row (e.g., WRL3, etc.). (a) Experimental setup. rec, record; stim, stimulus. (b) VVC neuron. The neuron projected through WRL3 (axon directly excited by stimulation of WRL3, see dot). Each trace is superimposed 10 times. Note the powerful short-latency (probably segmental) and long-latency (probably suprasegmental) reflex responses. (c) MR neuron. Each trace is superimposed 11 times. Note the weak reflex activity of the reflexes in the MR neuron. (b) Modified from Bahr et al. (1981); (c) modified from Bahr et al. (1986b).

following data were obtained in cats (Horeyseck and Jänig 1974b; Jänig and Spilok 1978; Jänig and Kümmel 1981):

- Rate of spontaneous activity, proportion of neurons with spontaneous activity and excitatory reflexes to noxious stimuli of skin recover faster in postganglionic muscle vasoconstrictor neurons than in postganglionic cutaneous vasoconstrictor neurons. For spontaneous activity, the recovery is in the range of <40 (muscle) or <60 days (skin). For excitatory reflexes, the recovery is in the range of 30 to 50 days (muscle) and 60 to 90 days (skin).
- Inhibitory reflexes elicited in postganglionic neurons by cutaneous noxious stimuli (noxious stimuli; stimulation of hair follicles) take longer to recover than excitatory ones.
- Inhibitory reflexes elicited in cutaneous vasoconstrictor neurons by visceral stimuli (distension or contraction of urinary bladder or colon)

disappear, thus never recover, after transection of the spinal cord. In chronic spinal cats, these reflexes are excitatory (Figure 9.7; Jänig 1985, 1996c) (Note 7).
- Reflexes in sudomotor neurons (to stimulation of Pacinian corpuscles [vibration reflex] or of nociceptors) take >50 days to recover (see Subchapter 4.2.1 and Figure 4.11).
- Spinal excitatory reflexes and ongoing activity in some sympathetic systems that project to visceral organs and have no vasoconstrictor function (e.g., "motility-regulating" neurons in the cat [Bartel et al. 1986]; see Subchapter 4.3) change very little after acute transection of the spinal cord performed rostral to the preganglionic cell bodies of these systems. Spinal inhibitory reflexes in these neurons may be enhanced or depressed acutely after spinalization.

In conclusion, "spinal shock": (1) is present in vasoconstrictor systems and in the sudomotor system, (2) is particularly strong for inhibitory reflexes (e.g., in the cutaneous vasoconstrictor neurons) and (3) is absent or weak for excitatory reflexes in sympathetic motility-regulating neurons.

9.2.3 Spinal Reflexes Upon Physiological Stimulation of Afferents Chronically After Spinal Cord Transection

The vasoconstrictor pathways to skeletal muscle, viscera or skin, the sudomotor pathway and the sympathetic non-vasoconstrictor pathways to pelvic viscera and hindgut are connected to spinal reflex circuits that are linked to specific groups of afferent neurons. These spinal autonomic reflex circuits are

summarized in Figure 9.3 and in Table 9.1. They have been inferred on the basis of neurophysiological investigations of the reflexes in these functionally identified sympathetic neurons in chronic spinal cats (for the vasoconstrictor pathways and the sudomotor pathway) and in acutely spinal cats (for the motility-regulating pathways). It is clear from these studies that some components of the reflex patterns that were observed in these neurons in cats and rats with intact spinal cord are organized at the spinal level (see Chapter 4).

Some neurons of the five types of sympathetic final pathways that are demonstrated in Figure 9.3 and Table 9.1 have spontaneous activity in the spinal

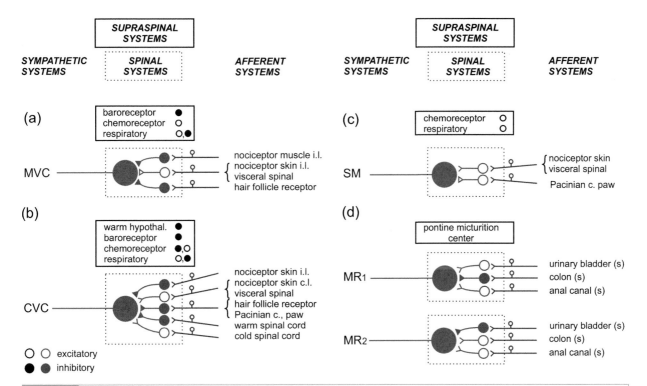

Figure 9.3 Spinal reflex pathways in lumbar sympathetic systems. These pathways were postulated on the basis of neurophysiological investigations of functionally identified pre- and postganglionic neurons projecting to skin, skeletal muscle or pelvic viscera (see Subchapters 4.1 to 4.3). They are defined by the spinal (right) and supraspinal afferent input systems and by the function (target cells, reflex patterns) of the output systems (left). The *spinal reflex systems* are shown in the dotted-line boxes. The *supraspinal systems* connecting to the spinal systems (and related to baroreceptors, chemoreceptors, respiratory generator, warm receptors or pontine micturition center) are shown in the solid-line boxes. Closed circles, inhibitory system/interneurons; open circles, excitatory system/interneurons. After chronic transection of the spinal cord, some neurons of each type of these sympathetic systems have ongoing activity. Visceral spinal, sacral afferents from pelvic organs; c.l./i.l., afferent input contralateral/ipsilateral to sympathetic outflow. (a) MVC, muscle vasoconstrictor neurons. The results in MVC neurons to noxious stimulation of skeletal muscle were obtained on anesthetized rats with intact spinal cord (Kirillova-Woytke et al. 2014). (b) CVC, cutaneous vasoconstrictor neurons. (c) SM, sudomotor neurons. (d) MR, motility-regulating neurons. Warm hypothal., warming rostral hypothalamus; Pacinian c., paw, Pacinian corpuscle in paw; s in (d), sacral afferent input. References see Table 9.1. Modified from Jänig (1996c) with permission.

state (Horeyseck and Jänig 1974b; Jänig and Spilok 1978; Bartel et al. 1986). In neurons of sympathetic pathways to the vasculature and to sweat glands, spontaneous activity is not present hours to days after interruption of the spinal cord, but may recover over weeks and months (see above). In human para- or tetraplegic patients, spontaneous activity in sympathetic postganglionic neurons innervating skin or

Table 9.1 Reflex pathways in the spinal cord associated with lumbar sympathetic systems

Sympathetic system	Afferent neuron	Reaction[a]	References
MVC	Nox. cutaneous	Excitation	3,9
	Nox. muscle	Inhibition i.l.	8
		Excitation mostly c.l.	8
	Hair follicle	Inhibition	3
	Viscera, sacral	Excitation	5,9
CVC	Nox. cutaneous	Inhibition i.l.[b]	2–7,9
		Excitation c.l.	2,4
	Low threshold mech. (Pacinian c., hair follicle)	Inhibition[c]	3,9
	Viscera, sacral	Excitation[d]	5,9
	Warm, spinal cord	Inhibition	6
	(cold, spinal cord	Excitation)	6
SM	Nox. cutaneous	Excitation[b]	7,9
	Pacinian corp. paw	Excitation	7,9
	Viscera, sacral	Excitation	5,9
MR1	Urinary bladder, sacral	Excitation	1
	Colon, sacral	Inhibition[e]	1
	Anus, sacral	Excitation[f]	1
MR2[g]	Urinary bladder	Inhibition	1
	Colon, sacral	Excitation	1
	Anus, sacral	Excitation[f]	1

All data obtained on chronic spinal (MVC, CVC, SM) or acute spinal (MR) cats. Spinal cord transected between segmental level T7 and T13 30 to 135 days before the experiments. Abbreviations: c.l., contralateral; i.l., ipsilateral; CVC, cutaneous vasoconstrictor neurons; MVC, muscle vasoconstrictor neurons; SM, sudomotor neurons; MR, motility-regulating neurons; Pacinian c., Pacinian corpuscle

[a] All reflexes that are present in the sympathetic neurons after transection of the spinal cord are also present, with two exceptions (see [c,d]), in anesthetized cats with intact spinal cord under standardized experimental conditions. Results in MVC neurons to noxious stimulation of skeletal muscle obtained on rats with intact spinal cord

[b] Inhibition and excitation outlast stimulus

[c] In cats with intact spinal cord, stimulation of hair follicle receptors elicits excitation mostly followed by depression of activity in many CVC neurons (Horeyseck and Jänig, 1974a; Grosse and Jänig, 1976)

[d] In cats with intact spinal cord, inhibition in most CVC neurons (see Häbler et al. 1992)

[e] Probably more pronounced in spinal preparation (acute) than in the intact preparation

[f] Afterdischarge sometimes present, but shorter in duration than in intact preparation (Bahr et al. 1986a); sometimes inhibition also present in acute spinal preparation to mechanical stimulation of the anal canal

[g] This pattern seems to be rare

References: 1. Bartel et al. (1986); 2. Grosse and Jänig (1976); 3. Horeyseck and Jänig (1974b); 4. Jänig (1975); 5. Jänig (1985a); 6. Jänig and Kümmel (1981); 7. Jänig and Spilok (1978); 8. Kirillova-Woytke et al. (2014); 9. Kümmel (1983) skeletal muscle of the hindlimb, recorded microneurographically, is low or absent, even many months after interruption of the spinal cord (Stjernberg and Wallin 1983; Wallin and Stjernberg 1984; Stjernberg et al. 1986) (Note 8). In many motility-regulating neurons innervating pelvic viscera or colon, spontaneous activity remains acutely after spinalization (Bartel et al. 1986).

The spontaneous activity in sympathetic neurons after spinalization is not correlated in any way with respiration or with cardiovascular parameters (e.g., with the excitation of arterial baroreceptors; see Chapter 10). The source of the spontaneous activity in these sympathetic neurons after spinal cord transection is in the spinal networks associated with the spinal pathways, possibly in activity in primary afferents (Taylor and Weaver 1993), and possibly in the preganglionic neurons themselves.

Of particular interest is the comparison of the reflex circuits of functionally related sympathetic pathways innervating skin, pelvic viscera or skeletal muscle (such as cutaneous vasoconstrictor and sudomotor neurons; muscle vasoconstrictor and cutaneous vasoconstrictor neurons; different types of motility-regulating neurons). In the chronic spinal cat, these pairs of final pathways seem to be reciprocally organized with respect to functionally distinct afferent inputs and therefore with respect to the populations of interneurons:

- Activity in postganglionic cutaneous vasoconstrictor neurons is inhibited and activity in sudomotor neurons increased during stimulation of nociceptors of the ipsilateral hindpaw in cats (Figure 9.4a1, a2). Interestingly, these reciprocal nociceptive reflexes are followed by a long-lasting decrease and increase of spontaneous activity in the neurons, respectively. The *long-lasting* depression of spontaneous activity in cutaneous vasoconstrictor neurons during noxious stimulation of ipsilateral skin is also present in animals with intact spinal cord (see Subchapter 4.1.1 and Box 4.1). Stimulation of contralateral nociceptors excites the neurons of both pathways.
- Stimulation of Pacinian corpuscles in the paw also leads to reflex excitation of sudomotor neurons and reflex inhibition of some cutaneous vasoconstrictor neurons innervating hairless skin of the same hindpaw, but there are no long-lasting changes in the spontaneous activity (Figure 9.4b1, b2).
- Reflexes in motility-regulating neurons of type 1 and type 2 are reciprocally organized with respect to the afferent inputs from the urinary bladder and from the colon. Figure 9.5 demonstrates the reciprocal reflexes in motility-regulating type 1 neurons to distension of the urinary bladder (activation) and to distension of the distal colon (inhibition). These reflexes and those elicited by mechanical stimulation of the anal canal and of the perianal skin are mediated by several distinct types of spinal sacro-lumbar reflex circuits.
- Stimulation of hair follicle afferents from skin elicits reflexes that are reciprocally organized between cutaneous and muscle vasoconstrictor neurons of the *same* distal hindlimb.
- Stimulation of warm receptors in skin of chronic paraplegic humans by high ambient temperatures (Randall et al. 1966) activates sudomotor neurons innervating the trunk skin and either inhibits cutaneous vasoconstrictor neurons or activates cutaneous vasodilator neurons innervating the trunk, which leads to increase of cutaneous blood flow. By the same token, warming the spinal cord in chronic spinal cats decreases activity in cutaneous vasoconstrictor neurons innervating the hind paws (with increase in cutaneous blood flow) and may possibly activate cutaneous vasodilator neurons (Gregor et al. 1976; Jänig and Kümmel 1981).
- Visceral stimuli (e.g. generated by contraction or distension of pelvic organs or by mechanical stimulation of the anal skin) elicit uniform excitatory reflexes in all vasoconstrictor neurons and in sudomotor neurons accompanied by a large increase in arterial blood pressure (in animals with high spinal transection) (Figure 9.6) (Note 9).

Specific spinal autonomic reflex circuits, connected to the final sympathetic pathways innervating skin, skeletal muscle or pelvic viscera, have been postulated, on the basis of neurophysiological investigations of sympathetic pre- and postganglionic neurons in spinal cats. There is strong indirect evidence (from recording of autonomic effector responses and from clinical observations) that other distinct spinal autonomic reflex circuits exist, and therefore also other groups of spinal autonomic interneurons, which are associated with the sympathetic systems innervating viscera or somatic tissues. It is

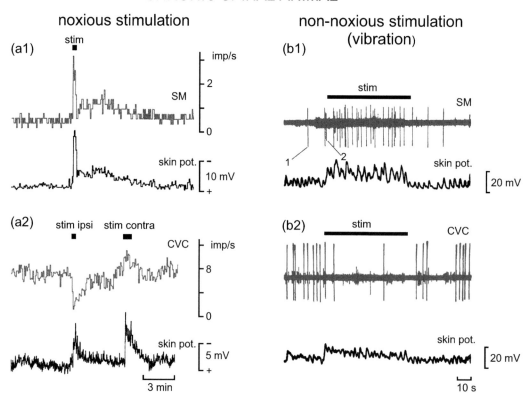

Figure 9.4 Reflexes in postganglionic cutaneous vasoconstrictor (CVC) and sudomotor (SM) neurons in chronic spinal cats. Activity was recorded from fine nerve-fiber bundles isolated from the medial plantar nerve of the cat hindpaw. Skin potential was recorded simultaneously from the hairless skin of the central pad of the hindpaw indicating sweat gland activation (for experimental setup see Figure 4.11a). (a) Reflexes to mechanical noxious stimulation of one of the toes of the ipsilateral (ipsi) hindpaw (a1) or of the ipsilateral (ipsi) or contralateral (contra.) hindpaw (a2). Single sudomotor axon in a1. CVC-multiunit activity in a2. Note: (1) SM and CVC neurons have ongoing activity, (2) long-lasting afterdischarge in SM neurons following noxious stimulation, (3) long-lasting inhibition of CVC activity following ipsilateral noxious stimulation and (4) absence of inhibition in CVC neurons following contralateral noxious stimulation. (a1) 91 days and (a2) 108 days after spinalization at the lower thoracic level. (b) Reflexes to stimulation of Pacinian corpuscles in the hindpaw by vibration. (b1), recording from a bundle with two SM axons (axons 1 and 2); (b2), recording from a bundle with one CVC axon (small signals probably also from CVC axons). Note: (1) absence of afterdischarge in SM neurons and (2) inhibition of CVC neuron, 122 days after spinalization in (b). skin pot, skin potential. (a) From Jänig and Spilok (1978); (b) from Kümmel (1983) with permission.

postulated that these spinal reflex circuits also exhibit functional specificity with respect to the primary afferent neurons and with respect to the hypothetical interneurons.

- The sympathetic innervation of the kidney influences four functions: kidney blood flow and glomerular filtration (blood vessels), renin release (juxtaglomerular cells) and sodium reabsorption by the tubules, although there is only a sparse innervation of the latter (Luff et al. 1991, 1992).

Various groups of mechano- and/or chemosensitive visceral afferents innervate the kidney. Based on physiological investigations, several types of *spinal reno-renal reflexes* have been postulated, which are involved in neural control of these renal functions (DiBona and Kopp 1997; Kopp and DiBona 2000).

- Stimulation of spinal visceral afferents from the heart (e.g., during exercise or during coronary hypoxia) leads to reflex activation of sympathetic

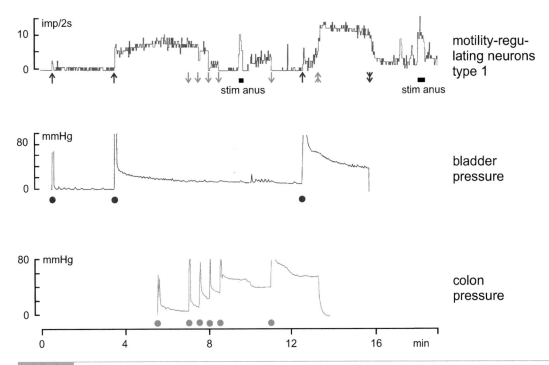

Figure 9.5 Interaction of reflex activation and inhibition of motility-regulating (MR) neurons by stimulation of sacral afferents from urinary bladder or colon in an acutely spinal cat. The spinal cord was sectioned 1 hour before the measurements at the thoracic level T8. Activity was recorded in a bundle with two preganglionic MR axons type 1 (see Subchapter 4.3) isolated from one of the lumbar splanchnic nerves. *Upper histogram*: activity in the two neurons (ordinate scale in impulses/2 s).↑, excitation produced by filling of the urinary bladder; ↓, depression of activity produced by filling of the colon; ↑, excitation following release of pressure in the colon; ↓, decrease of activity following release of intravesical pressure; stim anus, gentle mechanical shearing stimuli applied to the anal canal. *Middle record*: intravesical pressure measured through a urethral catheter in the urinary bladder. Filling of the bladder in steps with 10 ml each through the same catheter (blue dots). *Lower record*: pressure in a large flexible balloon in the distal colon connected to a catheter inserted through the anal canal. Filling of the colon balloon in steps six times with 10 ml each (green dots). From Bartel et al. (1986) with permission.

cardiomotor neurons via *spinal cardio-cardiac reflexes* (Malliani 1982; Jänig 2016).

- Stimulation of spinal visceral afferents from the gastrointestinal tract (by distension or inflammatory processes) may activate, via *spinal intestino-intestinal reflex circuits*, sympathetic motility-regulating neurons and induce immobilization of the gastrointestinal tract by inhibition of enteric circuits of the myenteric plexus. The spinal intestino-intestinal reflex circuits are connected to extra-spinal intestino-intestinal reflexes relayed through prevertebral sympathetic ganglia (see Subchapters 2.3, 4.3, 5.7 and 6.5 and Figures 2.3, 5.15, 6.10 and 6.11). In isolated preparations consisting of prevertebral ganglia attached to parts of the gastrointestinal tract inhibitory intestino-intestinal reflexes can be rather powerful (see Figure 6.10). It is debatable how much the

sympathetic preganglionic neurons contribute to these reflexes.

- Irritation of viscera (e.g., by inflammatory processes) may generate changes in blood flow, sweating and trophic changes of the skin in the corresponding dermatomes, as well as changes in blood flow and trophic changes in the corresponding myotomes and sclerotomes. These changes are thought to be generated, at least in part, by sympathetic pathways to skin and deep somatic tissues and mediated by spinal visceral afferents and spinal autonomic circuits (*viscero-cutaneous reflex circuits*; Jänig [1993]). The zones of skin in which these changes occur are identical to those to which visceral pain is referred (see Jänig and Morrison [1986]; Ness and Gebhart [1990]; Jänig and Häbler [2002]). Patients with affected viscera and visceral pain (e.g., with angina

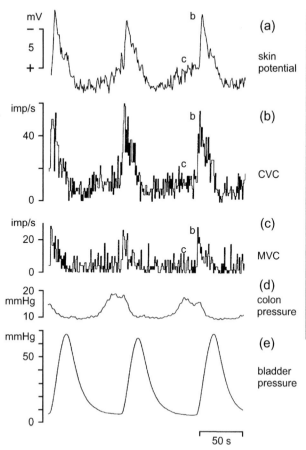

Figure 9.6 Reactions of cutaneous vasoconstrictor (CVC), sudomotor (SM, skin potential) and muscle vasoconstrictor neurons (MVC) during isovolumetric contractions of urinary bladder and colon in a chronic spinal anesthetized cat. Experiment was done 135 days after interruption of the spinal cord at T10. Activity in postganglionic neurons was recorded from multiunit bundles isolated from the superficial peroneal nerve (to hairy skin) and from a muscle branch of the deep peroneal nerve. For SM activity, the skin potential was recorded from the surface of the central pad of the ipsilateral hindpaw (see Jänig and Kümmel [1981] and Figures 4.11 and 4.12). The urinary bladder was filled with 20 ml saline and the intravesical pressure measured through a urethral catheter. The distal colon was filled with about 40 ml saline in a flexible balloon and the intracolonic pressure recorded through an anal catheter connected to the balloon in the colon. Note that CVC, SM and MVC neurons are synchronously excited during isovolumetric contraction of the urinary bladder (indicated by *b*) and colon (indicated by *c*), that the reflex activation to urinary bladder contraction starts with the beginning of the contraction, that urinary bladder and colon contract reciprocally (due to reciprocal inhibition in the spinal cord, see Figure 9.10) and that the reflex excitation of muscle vasoconstrictor neurons is not very strong in this experiment, in comparison to the reflex excitation of cutaneous vasoconstrictor and SM neurons. Jänig and Kümmel, unpublished.

pectoris, appendicitis, inflammation of pelvic viscera) may experience spontaneous pain and mechanical hyperalgesia in these cutaneous zones (Vecchiet et al. 1993; Jänig and Häbler 1995, 2002; Giamberardino 1999; Jänig 2014, 2020).

- Regulation of pelvic organs (continence of urinary bladder and hindgut, activation of internal genital organs) is dependent on special sacro-lumbar reflex circuits involving distinct groups of sacral visceral afferent neurons and distinct groups of sacro-lumbar proprio-spinal interneurons (Figure 9.10).

In *conclusion*, distinct groups of spinal autonomic interneurons have been postulated on the basis of reflexes measured in the pre- and postganglionic neurons of functionally distinct sympathetic pathways, on the basis of reflex reactions of sympathetic effector organs or on the basis of clinical observations. The question arises as to whether or not these spinal circuits are integrated with the supraspinal ones in the regulation of activity in the neurons of the final sympathetic pathways. This question will be discussed in the last part of this chapter.

9.3 | Sacral Parasympathetic Systems

Sacral parasympathetic systems are essential in the regulation of lower urinary tract, hindgut and reproductive organs. The pelvic organs receive an abundant nerve supply that arises at two levels of the spinal cord, lumbar and sacral. At both levels, the innervation has afferent (sensory) as well as efferent components; the latter are classified as sympathetic and parasympathetic, respectively. The three organ systems in this region have storage and evacuation as major functions:

1. The lower urinary tract (urinary bladder, urethra) retains and evacuates urine (continence and micturition, respectively).

2. The distal part of the large bowel (distal colon, rectum and anus) stores and evacuates feces (continence and defecation) and is involved in resorption of water and electrolytes.

3. The internal reproductive organs and erectile tissues of the external reproductive organs have basically similar functions related to the retention and transportation of semen and ova, together with, in the female, implantation of fertilized ova, storage of the developing fetus and subsequent birth of the new individual.

These specific functions are supplemented by two more general functions of the innervation of these three organ systems, namely, neural regulation of blood flow and of sensory feedback. Both of these aspects of the innervation serve to adjust the function of the pelvic organ systems to the overall behavior of the organism.

The precision of the control of the three organ systems, including their coordination and adaptation to the actual behavior of the organism, depend on the spinal afferent, spinal autonomic (sympathetic and parasympathetic) and somatomotor innervation. The central circuits are located in the spinal cord, brain stem, hypothalamus and telencephalon. The supraspinal mechanisms of the regulation of these organ systems are insufficiently understood, in particular those of the hindgut and the reproductive organs. I will describe the spinal reflex circuits in order to give an additional argument that these circuits, and the interneurons integrated in these circuits, are essential in the regulation of the three pelvic organ systems. Furthermore, the spinal circuits will be shown to be important in the coordination of spinal autonomic systems and somatomotor systems. Details and principles about the neural regulation of these pelvic systems are described in the literature (de Groat and Krier 1978; Jänig and McLachlan 1987; Loewy and Spyer 1990; de Groat and Booth 1993; de Groat et al. 1993, 1996, 1998, 2001, 2015; Blok and Holstege 1996, 1999; Jänig 1996a,b; McKenna and Marson 1997; McKenna 1999, 2000, 2001, 2002, 2013; Brookes et al. 2009; de Groat 2013; Callaghan et al. 2018).

9.3.1 Urinary Bladder: Micturition Reflexes and Spinal Circuits

Detailed neurophysiological investigations of sacral preganglionic neurons innervating the urinary tract and of other sacral neurons resulted in the postulation that at least five types of sacral interneurons, in addition to ascending neurons, are involved in the regulation of activity of these preganglionic neurons (Figure 9.7b). Two types of interneuron are inhibitory; they are activated by collaterals of sacral preganglionic axons or by perineal somatic afferents, respectively. Three types of interneuron are excitatory and activated by sacral bladder afferents and/or by perineal somatic afferents or by neurons projecting from the pontine micturition center. It is not too far-fetched to hypothesize that these groups of interneurons are synaptically connected to each other and that they receive convergent synaptic inputs from different sources. They form networks of interneurons in the sacral spinal cord that contribute to the excitation of the preganglionic neurons regulating the lower urinary tract (Figure 9.7b).

Furthermore, we have to postulate at least one type of excitatory and one type of inhibitory interneuron, each connected synaptically to the motoneurons in Onuf's nucleus innervating the external urethral sphincter (Figure 9.8b, c). The excitatory interneuron receives convergent synaptic input from primary afferents projecting through the pelvic or pudendal nerves and from supraspinal systems, e.g., from an area in the lateral pons called the pontine storage center (PSC). The inhibitory interneuron located in the dorsal commissural nucleus receives synaptic input from the pontine micturition center and possibly from sacral pelvic afferents (Figure 9.8a).

Let us undertake a brief excursion to the neural regulation of the lower urinary tract (urinary bladder [detrusor muscle], bladder neck, urethra and external urethral sphincter) as described by de Groat and coworkers (de Groat 2013; de Groat et al. 2015) and others, in order to exemplify the importance of sacral interneurons. The urinary bladder stores and periodically evacuates urine, which is continuously produced by the kidney. Long collecting phases alternate with brief emptying phases. The ability of the bladder to collect and store urine is called *continence* and the act of emptying, *micturition*. Both processes are dependent on myogenic, peripheral neural and central neural mechanisms. The essential neural control involves afferent and efferent components and a cascade of control centers in the spinal cord, brain stem, hypothalamus and forebrain. Sacral visceral afferent neurons innervating the bladder are activated during contraction or distension of the

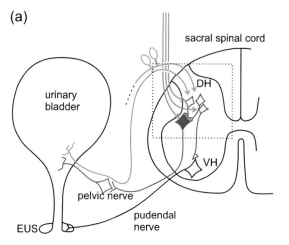

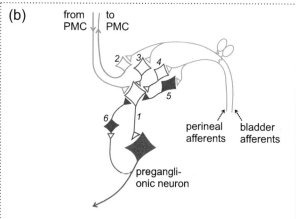

Figure 9.7 Putative role of spinal interneurons in the control of activity in the sacral parasympathetic pathway to the urinary bladder. (a) General scheme. DH, dorsal horn; VH, ventral horn; EUS, external urethral sphincter. (b) Reflex pathways connected to preganglionic neurons to the urinary bladder involving five types of local interneuron. The interneuron *1* mediating the command signals from the pontine micturition center (PMC), which are initiated from the urinary bladder via ascending neuron *2*, receives additional excitatory synaptic input from sacral interneuron *3*, activated by vesical afferents and inhibitory synaptic input from interneuron *6*, activated by collaterals of vesical preganglionic neurons. Furthermore, stimulation of perineal (pudendal) afferents may activate or inhibit the vesical preganglionic neurons via two populations of interneurons (*4, 5*). It is likely that these populations of interneurons are synaptically interconnected and that interneurons *3* to *6* also receive synaptic input from supraspinal centers. Inhibitory neurons colored violet. Data from de Groat et al. (1982) for interneuron *1*; McMahon and Morrison (1982a, b) and Coonan et al. (1999) for interneuron *2*; McMahon and Morrison (1982b) for interneuron *3*; Araki and de Groat (1996, 1997) for interneuron *4*; Araki (1994) for interneuron *5*; de Groat and Ryall (1968) and de Groat (1976) for interneuron *6*. Modified after Shefchyk (2001).

urinary bladder and encode in their activity the intravesical pressure (Figure 2.7). The detrusor muscle is innervated by a sacral parasympathetic pathway that contracts the muscle when activated, using acetylcholine as the transmitter or ATP in some species. The smooth muscles of the bladder neck and urethra are innervated by sacral parasympathetic neurons that relax both, using NO as the transmitter. The muscle of the external urethral sphincter is part of the pelvic floor musculature and thus a striated muscle. It is innervated by sacral motoneurons that project through the pudendal nerve and are situated in the lateral ventral horn in Onuf's nucleus in humans and other mammalian species (Figure 9.8a).

Bladder muscle, bladder neck and urethra are additionally innervated by noradrenergic (sympathetic) neurons that have their cell bodies in the pelvic or inferior mesenteric ganglia. These postganglionic cell bodies are innervated by preganglionic neurons in the upper lumbar segments (in the cat, segments L3 to L5 [Baron et al. 1985]; in the rat L1 to L3 [Baron and Jänig 1991]). This innervation is important for continence (inhibition of bladder muscle and contraction of bladder neck and urethra) and for contraction of the proximal urethra during emission and ejaculation of semen (Figure 9.12), but not for micturition.

In the adult under physiological conditions, the urinary bladder slowly fills and accommodates to the increasing intravesical volume. This accommodation is related to the large extensibility of the smooth musculature and is actively generated by the innervation of the urinary bladder (relaxation of the detrusor muscle and activation of the bladder base and urethral smooth musculature by the sympathetic innervation; constricted external urethral sphincter). Depending on the degree of filling of the urinary bladder and the central (cortical) command signals (acting at the spinal and supraspinal neural circuits involved in regulation of micturition and continence; see Figure 9.8), micturition is initiated. The detrusor muscle contracts and the bladder neck, urethra and external urethral sphincter relax, resulting in the evacuation of urine. These coordinated actions are initiated by activation of sacral afferents from the bladder dome and generated by: (1) reflex activation of parasympathetic neurons to the detrusor muscle, (2) reflex activation of inhibitory parasympathetic neurons to the urethra and bladder neck (leading to active relaxation of the outlet of the urinary bladder) and (3) inhibition of pudendal motoneurons. These

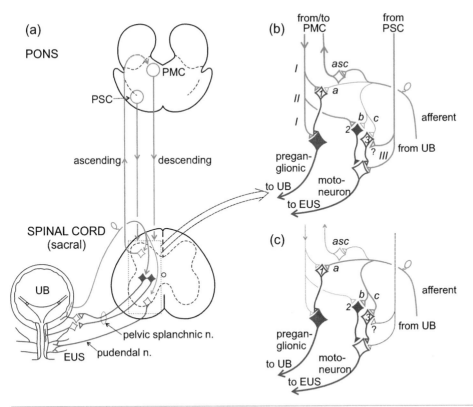

Figure 9.8 The micturition reflexes. (a) Sacral visceral afferents (blue) from the urinary bladder (UB) project to interneurons involved in micturition and to ascending tract neurons (ascending) that project (probably via the periaqueductal gray) to the pontine micturition center (PMC, Barrington's nucleus). Neurons in the PMC project to the sacral spinal cord (descending). Sacral preganglionic neurons (red) project to the bladder body, inducing, via postganglionic neurons, contraction of the urinary bladder. Other sacral preganglionic neurons project to the urethra and bladder neck, inducing, via postganglionic neurons, relaxation. Motoneurons project to the external urethral sphincter (EUS). (b) Micturition reflex pathways in intact spinal cord indicated in bold lines: neurons in the PMC project to sacral preganglionic parasympathetic neurons and interneurons (excitatory open, inhibitory filled in); they activate preganglionic neurons (directly and via interneuron *l*; pathway *I*) and inhibit motoneurons to the EUS (via interneuron 2; pathway *II*). Neurons in the pontine storage center (PSC) activate motoneurons to the EUS during continence (directly and possibly also via interneuron 3; pathway *III*). (c) Micturition reflex pathways after chronic transection of the spinal cord at the lumbar or thoracic level indicated in bold lines; dotted lines indicate degenerated pathways. Afferents from the urinary bladder form spinal reflex circuits via interneurons *1*, 2 and 3 (reflex pathways *a*, *b* and *c*).

processes are reflexly enhanced by activation of urethral afferents during urine flow through the urethra during micturition.

Figure 9.8 outlines schematically the central reflex circuits involved in micturition:

- Activity in sacral vesical afferents activates via an ascending pathway (*asc* in Figure 9.8b) neurons in the (medial) pontine micturition center (PMC; Barrington's nucleus). The output neurons of Barrington's nucleus project to the sacral spinal cord and activate the preganglionic neurons to the urinary bladder directly and via interneurons (pathway *I* to interneuron *1* and preganglionic

neurons in Figure 9.8b) and inhibit the moto-neurons projecting to the external urethral sphincter (EUS) via inhibitory interneurons (pathway *II* to interneuron 2). The pontine storage center (PSC) is inhibited during activation of the PMC.

- Chronically after interruption of the spinal cord in humans and animals, filling of the urinary bladder also leads to reflex activation of the preganglionic neurons to the urinary bladder and to micturition contractions (via pathway *a* and interneuron *1* in Figure 9.8c). However, now the pudendal motoneurons to the EUS are simultaneously activated via the spinal reflex pathway *c* and interneuron *3*, resulting in simultaneous contraction of the urinary bladder and sphincter. The bladder neck and urethra also do not relax or relax only weakly. Thus, the coordinated action between bladder body and sphincter is lost. Pathway *c* connecting via the excitatory interneuron *3* to the motoneurons seems to dominate over the inhibitory pathway *b* via the inhibitory interneuron *2*. This functional state of the lower urinary tract is called *detrusor–sphincter dyssynergia.*

- It is a matter of debate whether the spinal circuits *a*, *b* and *c* represented by the interneurons *1*, *2* and *3* are important during normal micturition when the spinal cord is intact. De Groat and his co-workers (de Groat et al. 1993; de Groat 2013; de Groat et al. 2015) believe that the spinobulbospinal reflex pathway via the PMC mediates micturition in the adult and that the spinal pathways are unimportant during normal micturition. Others propagate the concept that these spinal reflex pathways are integrated into the normal micturition reflexes (Morrison 1997; Shefchyk 2001, 2002). Thus, there is discussion as to whether the signals from the PMC are gated by the spinal interneurons activated by vesical afferents (see Subchapter 9.5 for details of the concept) (Note 10).
- During continence, motoneurons to the EUS are activated by neurons in the PSC projecting to the sacral spinal cord. This activation occurs by direct synaptic activation of the sacral motoneurons or by synaptic activation of excitatory interneurons antecedent to the motoneurons (interneuron *3* in Figure 9.8b). The neurons in the PSC are inhibited during micturition; the pathway is unknown. In animals (e.g., rats), the external urethral sphincter contracts and relaxes rhythmically during micturition resulting in rhythmic release of urine. These rhythmic contractions may be generated by alternating activation and inhibition of the motoneurons via the inhibitory interneuron *2* and the excitatory interneuron *3*.

9.3.2 Hindgut (Rectum And Anal Canal): Defecation

As already mentioned at the beginning of Subchapter 9.3, the main functions of the distal colon and rectum (here called colon-rectum) are storage (regulation of continence), defecation (elimination of waste) and, as in the more proximal parts of the colon, resorption of fluid and electrolytes. Here I will concentrate on the principles underlying the regulation of defecation, the mechanisms of which are only incompletely understood. This regulation is very precisely adapted to behavior in mammals, including humans. Macroscopically, distension of the rectum by its contents is followed by contraction of the rectum and relaxation of the internal anal sphincter (IAS). This leads to transport of the rectal content into the upper anal canal while the striated external anal sphincter (EAS) is still contracted. Filling of the rectal ampulla and the anal canal is followed by relaxion of the EAS and subsequently by elimination of the contents of the colon-rectum by contraction of the distal colon and rectum. This defecation process, which is supported by increase in intra-abdominal pressure generated by contraction of the abdominal musculature involves the coordinated activity of the following neural components (de Groat and Krier 1978, 1979; Brookes et al. 2009; Callaghan et al. 2018) (Figure 9.9):

- sacral visceral primary afferent neurons innervating the colon-rectum and the mucosa of the anal canal,
- a sacral parasympathetic pathway innervating the colon-rectum,
- the enteric nervous system (ENS) associated with the circular and longitudinal musculature of the colon-rectum and the IAS,
- sacral motoneurons in Onuf's nucleus innervating the (striated) EAS,
- reflex pathways associated with the colon-rectum in the sacral spinal cord,
- spino-bulbo-spinal reflex pathways involving the ponto-medullary defecation center, which are under cortical control, and
- a sympathetic pathway to the colon-rectum and IAS that originates from the upper lumbar spinal cord (not shown in Figure 9.9).

Figure 9.9 demonstrates graphically the different functional neural components underlying defecation:

1. Filling of the colon-rectum activates sacral visceral afferent neurons innervating the colon-rectum. This afferent activation leads to activation of a sacral pre-postganglionic pathway to the colon-rectum, to activation of the ponto-medullary defecation center (Barrington's nucleus [BN]) and to cortical activation with the urge to defecate.

(a)

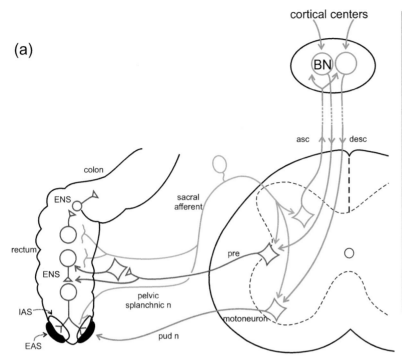

cortical centers

BN

asc   desc

colon

ENS

sacral
afferent

rectum

ENS

pre

IAS

pelvic
splanchnic n

motoneuron

EAS

pud n

Figure 9.9 Neural mechanisms underlying defecation. (a) Neural components involved in defecation: sacral visceral afferent neurons innervating the colon-rectum or mucosal skin of the anal canal (blue); a pre-postganglionic sacral (parasympathetic) pathway to the colon-rectum (red); enteric nervous system (ENS, violet); sacral motoneurons (in Onuf's nucleus, orange) to the external anal sphincter (EAS); supraspinal ponto-medullary centers (Barrington's nucleus [BN] and lateral to BN) and their cortical control centers (green). (b) Hypothetical wiring diagram of the regulation of the activity in sacral preganglionic neurons to the colon-rectum and in sacral motoneurons to the EAS involving interneurons (excitatory [interneurons 1 and 2] and inhibitory [interneuron 3]). IAS, internal anal sphincter; asc, ascending; desc, descending; pre, preganglionic; pud n, pudendal nerve. For details see text.

(b)

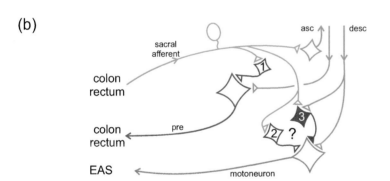

sacral
afferent

asc   desc

colon
rectum

1

colon
rectum

pre

3

2 ?

EAS

motoneuron

2. The parasympathetic preganglionic neurons are activated via interneurons (interneuron 1 in Figure 9.9b). This spinal activation is enhanced by a descending pathway from the ponto-medullary defecation center (Barrington's nucleus). The synaptic connection of the sacral preganglionic neurons innervating the colon-rectum with interneurons is sometimes called the "spinal defecation center." The structural details of this spinal defecation center are unknown.

3. Distension of the colon-rectum stimulates intrinsic primary afferent neurons of the ENS and leads to reflex activation of enteric excitatory motoneurons, generating contraction of the circular and longitudinal musculature of the colon-

rectum and of inhibitory motoneurons producing inhibition of the IAS. This inhibition is generated by nitric oxide and vasoactive inhibitory peptide released by the inhibitory motoneurons of the ENS. This enteric reflex is called the *recto-anal reflex*.

4. Sacral motoneurons located in Onuf's nucleus are inhibited during defecation, leading to relaxation of the EAS. This inhibition is produced by activation of neurons located lateral to Barrington's nucleus in the ponto-medullary area (Figure 9.9a) and most likely mediated by inhibitory sacral interneurons (interneuron 3 in Figure 9.9b). During continence of the colon-rectum, these motoneurons have ongoing activity keeping the

EAS contracted. The way spinal and supraspinal pathways, involving excitatory and inhibitory spinal interneurons, are integrated in the regulation of activity of the motoneurons innervating the EAS is poorly understood.

5. Defecation is most likely strongly enhanced by stimulation of myelinated sacral visceral afferents innervating the anal mucosa. These afferents are powerfully activated by shearing stimuli exerted by the anal contents during defecation (Bahns et al. 1987; Jänig and Koltzenburg 1991).

6. The colon-rectum and IAS are innervated by a sympathetic pathway originating in the upper lumbar segments of the spinal cord (not shown in Figure 9.9). The noradrenergic neurons of this sympathetic non-vasoconstrictor pathway innervate the ENS, presynaptically and possibly postsynaptically, and the IAS. They consist functionally of motility-regulating neurons that are entirely different from vasoconstrictor neurons (see Subchapter 4.3). Activation of them inhibits the ENS and contracts the IAS. Thus, this sympathetic non-vasoconstrictor system contributes to continence of the colon-rectum.

9.3.3 Interaction Between Regulation of Urinary Bladder and Hindgut: An Idea About the Role of Spinal Circuits

After intraluminal filling, both the urinary bladder and distal colon exhibit alternating contractions in spinal-cord-intact animals, as well as in chronic spinal animals (see Figure 9.6d,e). I hypothesize that the spinal neural circuits associated with both organ systems inhibit each other reciprocally. Activation of sacral afferents from the urinary bladder inhibits hindgut activity and activation of sacral afferents from the hindgut inhibits urinary bladder activity. This reciprocal inhibition of the two organ systems is hypothesized to be generated by the following mechanisms and involves several types of spinal interneuron:

1. As described before, many sympathetic motility-regulating (MR) neurons projecting in the lumbar splanchnic and hypogastric nerves (preganglionic and postganglionic neurons) exhibit reciprocal reflex patterns upon stimulation of sacral afferents from the urinary bladder and colon: MR1 neurons are excited from the urinary bladder and inhibited (or not affected) from the hindgut; MR2 neurons are excited from the hindgut and inhibited (or not

affected) from the urinary bladder (see Figures 4.15 and 9.5). MR1 neurons may innervate the hindgut and MR2 neurons the lower urinary tract (Bahr et al. 1986a; Bartel et al. 1986; Jänig et al. 1991).

2. Interneurons in the sacral spinal cord excited by stimulation of bladder afferents may inhibit the preganglionic neurons to the colon. By the same token interneurons in the sacral spinal cord excited by stimulation of the colonic afferents may inhibit preganglionic neurons to the lower urinary tract.

The diagrams in Figure 9.10 demonstrate the putative spinal neural mechanisms underlying the reciprocal inhibition between the two organ systems (in [a] when the sacral afferent neurons from the urinary bladder are activated, in [b] when the sacral afferent neurons from the hindgut are activated). The spinal interneurons *postulated* to be involved in this reciprocal inhibition are two types of propriospinal (sacrolumbar) excitatory neurons, two types of sacral inhibitory interneurons and two types of lumbar inhibitory interneurons.

Supraspinal control systems associated with the lower urinary tract (indicated in Figure 9.10 by the vertical dotted lines) may act at the preganglionic neurons and at the different pools of interneurons (not shown in Figure 9.10). These supraspinal autonomic premotor neurons are located in the medulla oblongata (lateral paragigantocellular nucleus, ventral part of the gigantocellular nucleus, raphe nuclei), in the pons (Barrington's nucleus, A5, subceruleus nucleus) and in the hypothalamus (paraventricular nucleus, lateral hypothalamus) (see Table 8.3). However, all or most of these areas also project to preganglionic neurons that innervate other functional types of autonomic target organs, such as the colon-rectum, reproductive organs or other organs (see Tables 8.2 and 8.3 and Subchapters 8.1 and 8.4). Neurons in Barrington's nucleus (pontine micturition center, PMC) and in the pontine storage center (PSC) lateral to Barrington's nucleus appear to be most important in the regulation of micturition and the continence of the urinary bladder.

9.3.4 Reproductive Organs and Spinal Circuits

Precise neural regulation of reproductive organs and its coordination with the regulation of somato-motor behavior is of utmost importance for the propagation of species. Most importantly, reproductive function in the male is entirely dependent on neural control. However, knowledge about the neural mechanisms

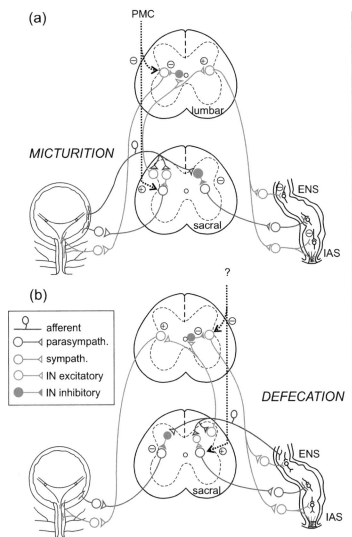

Figure 9.10 Hypothetical spinal reflex pathways involved in reciprocal contraction and inhibition of urinary bladder and distal colon (see Figure 9.6d, e). Demonstrated are neural circuits mediating inhibition of the colon during micturition contractions (a) and inhibition of the bladder during defecation contractions (b). (a) Activation of sacral bladder afferents leads to inhibition of sacral preganglionic neurons to the colon-rectum, excitation of lumbar preganglionic neurons to the colon-rectum (contraction of the internal anal sphincter [IAS] [*this is shown with a minus* −], inhibition of enteric nervous system [ENS]) and inhibition of lumbar preganglionic neurons to the urinary bladder. (b) Activation of sacral colon-rectum afferents leads to inhibition of sacral preganglionic neurons to the urinary bladder, excitation of lumbar preganglionic neurons to the urinary bladder and inhibition of lumbar preganglionic neurons to the colon. Supraspinal systems related to micturition (PMC, pontine micturition center) or defecation (?) (both indicated by dotted lines) control these spinal reflex circuits by acting at the preganglionic neurons or at the corresponding interneurons (excitation of sacral neurons; inhibition of lumbar neurons). Note that postganglionic parasympathetic neurons in the pelvic ganglion interact with the enteric nervous system to produce contraction. Inhibitory interneurons filled; +, excitation; −, inhibition; IN interneuron.

underlying the regulation of reproductive organs in the spinal cord and in supraspinal centers is still in its infancy. This applies particularly to the female, although the principles of neural regulation of reproductive organs appear to be rather similar in males and females.

In addition to the described groups of spinal interneurons associated with the regulation of the urinary tract and hindgut (Figures 9.7–9.10), we have to postulate several other types of interneuron in the sacral spinal cord and sacro-lumbar propriospinal neurons that are associated with sacral and lumbar preganglionic neurons innervating the erectile tissue and internal reproductive organs (vas deferens, prostate, seminal vesicle, proximal urethra, uterus, proximal vagina) (de Groat and Booth 1993; Jänig 1996b; McKenna and Marson 1997; McKenna 1999, 2000, 2001, 2002, 2013; de Groat 2013).

Spinal autonomic pathways involved in regulation of reproductive organs are usually divided into sacral (parasympathetic) pathways mediating erection and thoracolumbar (sympathetic) pathways mediating contraction of internal reproductive organs and secretion (emission). However, this is an oversimplification. Thoracolumbar sympathetic neurons are also involved in erection and both parasympathetic and sympathetic pathways are involved in secretion (Figure 9.12). Thus, functions assumed to be primarily associated with sacral (parasympathetic) systems are duplicated by thoracolumbar (sympathetic) pathways (Müller 1906; Semans and Langworthy 1938; Root and Bard 1947; Bors and Comarr 1960; see Jänig and McLachlan [1987]; McKenna and Marson [1997]). This shows that the division of the spinal autonomic systems into sympathetic and parasympathetic with respect to sexual functions is questionable. Theoretically it is possible that the separation of neuron groups in lumbar autonomic and sacral autonomic neurons by the expansion of the lumbar enlargement during development is incomplete (for discussion of this subject see Espinosa-Medina et al. [2016]; Jänig et al. [2017, 2018]; Neuhuber et al. [2017]).

The central mechanisms leading to the sequence of erection, emission and ejaculation are made up of several neural components. The central mechanisms that mediate erection are descriptively divided into spinal reflex mechanisms and supraspinal "psychogenic" mechanisms. This distinction is somewhat artificial, although clinically useful, since both mechanisms always work together under biological conditions (Coolen et al. 2004). Here I will focus mainly on the spinal mechanisms underlying this sequence of reproductive reflexes since they illustrate the coordination between: (1) different spinal autonomic pathways and (2) spinal autonomic systems and somatomotor systems. This coordination requires several types of interneurons.

The supraspinal control involves the paragigantocellular nucleus, the periaqueductal gray, the paraventricular nucleus of the hypothalamus, the medial amygdala and the medial preoptic area (see Table 8.3). With the exception of the latter, these supraspinal centers receive information from pelvic somatic and visceral structures by afferent neurons projecting through the pelvic splanchnic and pudendal nerves via second-order ascending tract neurons in the sacral dorsal horn. The result of the integrative activity in the supraspinal centers is channeled through the paragigantocellular nucleus, the periaqueductal gray and the paraventricular nucleus of the hypothalamus to the spinal reflex circuits, the first having inhibitory effects and the latter two excitatory effects (McKenna 2001, 2002, 2013).

Erection

The sacral preganglionic neurons involved in the generation of erection are situated in the intermediate zone of the spinal cord, probably lateral to the preganglionic neurons that are associated with the hindgut and dorsomedial to preganglionic neurons associated with the lower urinary tract (Figure 9.11, left). These preganglionic neurons have dendrites projecting medially to the interneurons in the dorsal commissural nucleus (DCN), laterally to descending systems from the brain stem and hypothalamus, and dorsally along the lateral dorsal horn. Sacral afferent neurons innervating the penis, which are important to elicit reflex erections, project to the superficial dorsal horn, medially through the dorsal horn to the dorsal commissural nucleus and also laterally to the preganglionic neurons (Figure 9.11, dotted on the left).

Mechanical stimulation of afferent receptors in the penis or in the tissue surrounding it elicits erection of the penis via a reflex pathway in the spinal cord (Figure 9.11, right). The reflex pathway in the sacral spinal cord is at least disynaptic and involves one interneuron. It functions in males with transected spinal cords as long as the interruption is rostral to the sacral segments and as long as spinal shock is over (Note 11).

Mechanical stimulation of penile afferents also activates supraspinal centers that control the spinal reflex mechanisms, resulting in sexual sensations when centers in the forebrain are activated. The supraspinal centers can also be triggered by imaginary, visual, auditory and olfactory stimuli and induce erection, apparently independently of stimulation of afferents from the penis. This "psychogenic" erection is produced not only via the sacral (parasympathetic) efferent innervation of the erectile tissue (pathway 1 in Figure 9.12) but also via the thoracolumbar sympathetic innervation (pathway 2 in Figure 9.12). Some patients with destroyed sacral spinal cord (e.g., following an accident) or in whom the spinal cord is interrupted between upper lumbar and sacral segments can still induce erection psychogenically (Kuhn 1950). This erection can only be produced by activation of thoracolumbar sympathetic neurons (pathway 2 in Figure 9.12). It is unclear to what degree excitation of the neurons of this sympathetic pathway contributes to erection in normal conditions. However, these observations on human patients are fully consistent with experiments performed on

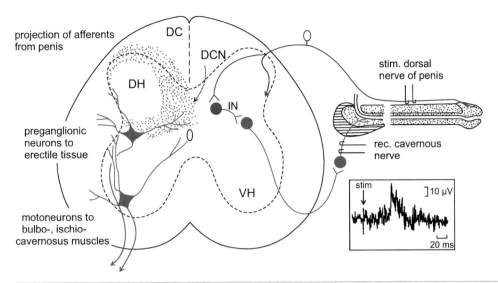

Figure 9.11 The spinal-sacral reflex pathway mediating penile erection (right) and its morphological components (left). *Left side*: anatomy of connections in sacral spinal cord. Dotted areas, sites of projection of penile afferents in the pudendal nerve determined by horseradish peroxidase tracing in the cat. These afferents project to the superficial dorsal horn (DH), medially to the dorsal commissural nucleus (DCN, which contains the interneurons) and laterally towards the preganglionic neurons. Preganglionic neurons located in the lateral part of the intermediate zone have dendrites within regions of afferent projection (medially and dorsally) and laterally into the region of termination of descending systems. Motoneurons innervating the bulbo- and ischiocavernosus muscles are situated laterally in the ventral horn (VH; Onuf's nucleus in humans) and send dendrites laterally, medially and dorsally. *Right side*: diagram of the spinal components of the erection reflex in the rat. Electrical stimulation of penile afferents with single impulses (arrow in inset) activates postganglionic neurons projecting in the cavernous nerve and innervating erectile tissues (reflex response in inset). DC, dorsal columns; IN, interneuron. From de Groat and Booth (1993) with permission.

animals (Müller 1902, 1906; Semans and Langworthy 1938; Root and Bard 1947; Dail 1993).

The pre-postganglionic pathways *1* and *2* in Figure 9.12, activation of which leads to erection, are most likely entirely separate and overlap very little (Jobling et al. 2003, 2004). Sympathetic neurons of pathway *2* must also be separate from sympathetic vasoconstrictor neurons, which can obviously override the dilation of the erectile tissue in various mental and bodily conditions (e.g., during mental stress or exercise). Whether sympathetic noradrenergic neurons projecting through the cavernous nerve are functionally different from sympathetic neurons innervating the internal reproductive organs is unknown (pathway *3* in Figure 9.12).

Emission and Ejaculation

Emission and ejaculation are the high point of the male sexual act. Emission is generated by thoracolumbar sympathetic pathways innervating smooth muscle and secretory epithelia of the internal reproductive organs (epididymis, vas deferens, seminal vesicles, ampulla, prostate, proximal urethra). The sympathetic preganglionic neurons project through the lumbar splanchnic nerves to postganglionic neurons in the caudal part of the inferior mesenteric ganglion (superior hypogastric plexus) and in the pelvic plexus (ganglion; see pathway *3* in Figure 9.12). Ejaculation is generated by pudendal motoneurons innervating bulbo- and ischiocavernosus muscles, the external urethral sphincter and other muscles of the pelvic floor.

As sacral afferents from the reproductive organs become excited during copulation, thoracolumbar sympathetic pathways to the internal reproductive organs are activated in bursts (Figure 9.13b). Contraction of the internal reproductive organs propels the semen into the urethra. Contraction of the proximal urethra prevents reflux of the secretion into the urinary bladder. The activation of sympathetic neurons to the internal reproductive organs requires powerful enhancement from supraspinal brain centers. After a delay, ejaculation starts. This is also triggered by activation of pudendal afferents

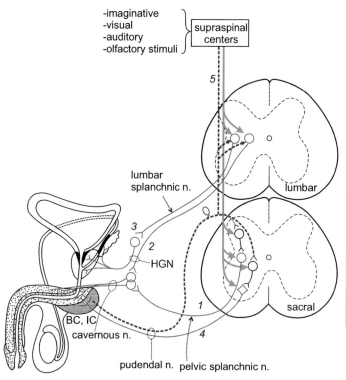

-imaginative
-visual
-auditory
-olfactory stimuli

supraspinal centers

lumbar splanchnic n.

lumbar

HGN

BC, IC
cavernous n.

sacral

pudendal n.   pelvic splanchnic n.

Figure 9.12 Peripheral neural pathways controlling erection, emission and ejaculation. *1*, efferent parasympathetic pathway to erectile tissue. *2*, efferent sympathetic pathway to erectile tissue. Preganglionic sympathetic axons in lumbar splanchnic and hypogastric (HGN) nerves and preganglionic parasympathetic axons in pelvic splanchnic nerve synapse largely with separate cholinergic (nitrergic) postganglionic neurons in the pelvic plexus/ganglion that project through the cavernous nerve to the erectile tissue. *3*, sympathetic noradrenergic pathway to internal reproductive organs (vas deferens, seminal vesicle, prostate, proximal urethra [internal vesical sphincter]). *4*, motor axons to bulbo- and ischiocavernous muscles (BC, IC). *5*, ascending spinal systems to and descending spinal system from supraspinal control centers. Sacro-lumbar interneurons and ascending tract neurons mediating the afferent activity to supraspinal centers are not shown. Vasoconstrictor neurons to blood vessels of the reproductive organs that pass through lumbar splanchnic and hypogastric nerves, as well as through the sympathetic chain and the pelvic splanchnic and pudendal nerves, are not shown.

and possibly pelvic splanchnic afferents from the urethra and consists of rhythmic contractions of the bulbo- and ischiocavernosus muscles (Figure 9.13), which enclose the proximal erectile tissue, and of the muscles of the pelvic floor. These rhythmic contractions expel the secretion from the posterior urethra through the anterior urethra.

During the ejaculation phase, the excitation of the parasympathetic and sympathetic innervation of the reproductive organs becomes maximal due to continuous afferent feedback and strong supraspinal excitation of the spinal reflex arcs. The synchronous maximal excitation of autonomic neurons and of pudendal motoneurons is rhythmic and generated by spinal interneuronal circuits. It is represented by the model of the *urethro-genital reflex* in the rat (Figure 9.13; McKenna et al. 1991; McKenna and Marsden 1997), showing that stimulation of urethral afferents leads to synchronous rhythmic activation of pudendal motoneurons to striated perineal muscles, of parasympathetic neurons innervating the erectile tissue through the cavernous nerve

and of sympathetic neurons innervating internal reproductive organs (hypogastric nerve in Figure 9.13b) and possibly the erectile tissue. Discharges in autonomic neurons always precede the discharges in pudendal motoneurons innervating the bulbo- or ischiocavernosus muscles (see insets in Figure 9.13). The rhythmic contractions are probably produced by a spinal pattern generator involving spinal interneurons. The segmental interneurons and propriospinal sacro-lumbar neurons of this hypothetical spinal pattern generator that coordinates excitation of autonomic and somatomotor neurons are unknown (Coolen et al. 2004; Chang et al. 2007).

The spinal reflex mechanisms in females leading to engorgement of the erectile tissues, rhythmic contractions of the striated perineal muscles and rhythmic contractions of vagina and uterus are probably similar to those in males. This includes strong rhythmic activation of postganglionic neurons projecting in the cavernous nerve and of preganglionic neurons projecting in the pelvic or the hypogastric nerve (McKenna et al. 1991; McKenna 2002).

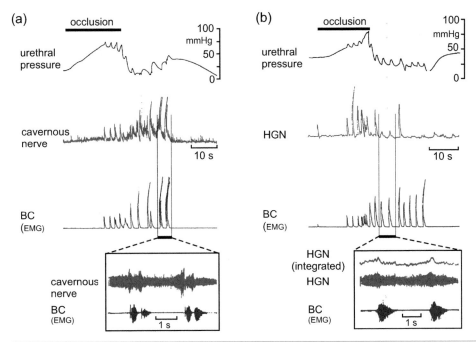

Figure 9.13 The urethro-genital reflex (coitus reflex) in the male rat elicited by stimulation of urethral afferents. Urethral afferents were stimulated by distension of the urethra (increase of intraurethral pressure) caused by infusion of saline into the urethra closed at the urethral meatus (bar above upper records) in urethane-anesthetized rats. (a) Simultaneous recording of intraurethral pressure, activity in the cavernous nerve and electromyogram (EMG) recorded from the bulbocavernosus (BC) muscle. *Inset*: original recordings from the cavernous nerve and EMG (during time period indicated by bar). (b) Simultaneous recording of intraurethral pressure, activity in the hypogastric nerve (HGN) and EMG recorded from the BC muscle. *Inset*: original recordings from HGN (plus integrated HGN activity) and of EMG during time period indicated by bar. Mechanical stimulation of the urethra leads to repetitive synchronous bursting discharges in pudendal motoneurons innervating the BC muscle (and other pelvic floor muscles [not shown]), in postganglionic neurons projecting into the cavernous nerve, which are activated by upper lumbar (HGN) and sacral preganglionic neurons. The synchronous bursting discharges in autonomic and somatomotor neurons outlast the urethral stimulation. Both signals were rectified and integrated with a time constant of 50 ms. Modified from McKenna et al. (1991) with permission.

9.4 Autonomic Dysreflexia Chronically After Spinal Cord Transection

In the chronic stage after spinal cord transection, spinal reflexes to noxious and innocuous somatic and visceral stimuli may be very strong (Horeyseck and Jänig, 1974b; Jänig and Spilok 1978; see Lee et al. [1995]; Karlsson [1999]; Mathias et al. [2013]). In animals and humans with the spinal cord interrupted at the upper thoracic or lower cervical level, which leads to high paraplegia or tetraplegia in patients, there is uniform reflex activation of various autonomic effector organs. The vasculature in the viscera, deep somatic tissues (e.g., skeletal muscle) and skin contracts following excitation of visceral afferents during bladder or hindgut contractions or distension, or excitation of deep somatic afferents, e.g., during muscle spasms, with an ensuing dramatic increase of arterial blood pressure. Furthermore, sweat glands and arrector pili muscles are reflex activated, although this may be rather irregular (Guttmann 1976; Jänig 1985, 1996a; Mathias et al. 2013). These spinal cardiovascular and other autonomic reflexes, together with reflex dysfunctions of the urinary bladder (detrusor-sphincter-dyssynergia), reproductive organs and gastrointestinal tract, are part of a condition called *autonomic dysreflexia*.

The detailed mechanisms underlying autonomic dysreflexia are only partially known (for review and literature see Weaver et al. [2002]):

- Transection of the spinal cord leads to loss of synaptic input to the preganglionic neurons and autonomic interneurons from descending excitatory and inhibitory supraspinal and propriospinal control systems. Initially, in the first days after spinal cord transection, the dendrites of preganglionic neurons shrink. Later these dendrites lengthen again.

- The density of synapses on the somata and dendrites of the preganglionic neurons decreases by about 70% and 50%, respectively, in the chronic state, arguing that interneurons do not or minimally sprout to the denervated sites of the preganglionic neurons (Figure 9.14) by two weeks after the injury. However, sprouting at longer times after injury, using electron microscopy, has not been studied.

- About 60% of the synapses on the preganglionic neurons deprived of their supraspinal synaptic inputs are GABAergic, i.e., are inhibitory, and about 40% are glutamatergic, i.e. are excitatory (Llewellyn-Smith et al. 1995; Llewellyn-Smith and Weaver 2001).

- Peptidergic small-diameter afferents may sprout in the spinal cord distal to the lesion site, possibly forming new synapses with autonomic interneurons and other neurons (Krenz et al. 1999; Weaver et al. 2001). However, only neurons containing CGRP, but not those containing substance P, sprout (Marsh and Weaver, 2004). This is surprising since CGRP is colocalized in most afferent neurons containing substance P (Lawson 2005). Since more primary afferent neurons contain CGRP than substance P (Lawson 1996; 2005) this would mean that only a subclass of primary afferent neurons containing CGRP sprout.

- The changes are probably produced by subsets of astrocytes in the injured spinal cord *and/or by entry of immune cells into the injured cord*. Whether macrophages (i.e. activated microglia) are involved is debatable. These cells are sources of nerve growth factor and other molecules, which in turn trigger sprouting of peptidergic primary afferents (Krenz et al. 1999; Krenz and Weaver 2000; Marsh et al. 2002; Brown et al. 2004). However, other processes must be involved, since substance P afferents do not sprout.

The changes occurring in the spinal cord cannot entirely explain the autonomic dysreflexia observed in

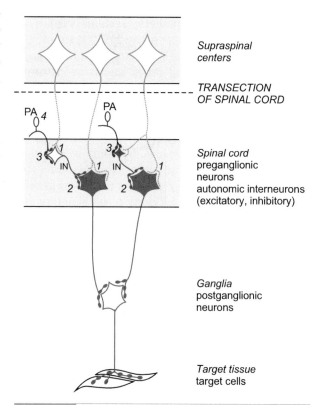

Figure 9.14 Consequences of spinal cord transection for spinal autonomic systems. *1*, denervation of preganglionic neurons and autonomic interneurons; *2*, changes in geometry of preganglionic neurons; sprouting of interneurons into the denervated territories of the preganglionic neurons seems unclear; *3*, sprouting of primary afferent neurons (PA); *4*, neurochemical changes of afferent neurons. IN, interneurons.

the patients. Responses of the rat tail artery to nerve stimulation are enhanced in chronically spinal animals. This increase in vascular responsiveness is probably related to a decrease in activity in vasoconstrictor neurons following spinal cord transection, since decentralization of the postganglionic neurons innervating the tail artery (by cutting the preganglionic axons) is also followed by increased responsiveness of the tail artery to nerve stimulation. Both pre- and postjunctional changes seem to be involved in this increased vascular responsiveness, such as increased release of noradrenaline by nerve impulse activity and increased responsiveness of the vascular smooth musculature (sensitization of the contractile mechanism to calcium entering the cells from outside), but probably not an increase in the number and affinity of adrenoceptors

(Yeoh et al. 2004a, b). These data imply that the increased reactivity of blood vessels to nerve impulses chronically after spinal cord transection could contribute to autonomic dysreflexia of the vasculature (Al Dera and Brock 2018).

Here I want to emphasize, irrespective of the plastic changes occurring in the spinal cord following spinal cord injury, that the isolated spinal cord is capable of regulating residual autonomic functions and that it is the *preservation* of these discrete spinal autonomic functions after interruption of the spinal cord that is remarkable, rather than the uniformity of the discharge of neurons of functionally different sympathetic pathways (see Figure 9.3 and Table 9.1). Thus, I want to put the main emphasis on the *differentiation* of the spinal autonomic circuits and that several reflexes elicited by physiological stimulation of somatic or visceral afferents are qualitatively similar in both normal and spinal cats. This view does not deny the importance and prominence of hyperreflexia of spinal autonomic systems after spinal cord transection, in particular, to visceral stimuli.

9.5 | The Spinal Cord as an Integrative Autonomic Organ

9.5.1 Integration of Autonomic Circuits and Supraspinal Centers

Functional characteristics of the discharge pattern in neurons of the sympathetic and sacral parasympathetic systems are dependent on spinal reflex circuits and supraspinal mechanisms (see Chapter 4). For example:

- Discharge pattern and ongoing activity ("tone") in vasoconstrictor neurons regulating resistance vessels (e.g., muscle vasoconstrictor and visceral vasoconstrictor neurons, renal vasoconstrictor neurons) largely depend on activity generated in the medulla oblongata, on reflexes associated with cardiovascular afferents (notably baroreceptor and chemoreceptor afferents; Guyenet 1990, 2006; Koshiya et al. 1993) and on the coupling between respiratory neurons and sympathetic premotor neurons in the medulla oblongata (McAllen 1987; Richter and Spyer 1990; Häbler et al. 1994; Häbler and Jänig 1995; Guyenet 2011; see Subchapters 10.3, 10.4 and 10.6).
- The discharge pattern and ongoing activity in most cutaneous vasoconstrictor neurons is dependent on

the hypothalamus (thermoregulation), on spinal circuits (nociceptive and non-nociceptive somato-sympathetic and viscero-sympathetic reflexes, thermoregulatory reflexes) and on the medulla oblongata (cardiovascular reflexes and coupling to the central respiratory generator; see Subchapters 10.3, 10.4 and 10.6).

- The discharge pattern and ongoing activity in motility-regulating neurons is dependent on sacro-lumbar reflex pathways and relatively independent of brain stem and hypothalamus.
- Discharge patterns in sympathetic neurons innervating the kidney that are involved in the regulation of blood volume and extracellular sodium concentration are dependent on: (1) the hypothalamus (paraventricular nucleus); (2) cardiovascular reflexes mediated by the medulla oblongata; (3) coupling to the central respiratory generator mediated by the rostral ventrolateral medulla (see Subchapters 10.3, 10.4 and 10.6); and (4) specific spinal reflex circuits receiving distinct afferent inputs from the kidney (Badoer 2001; Yang and Coote 2003; Yang et al. 2004).

These findings do not rule out, *first*, that spinal circuits are important for the regulation of activity in those spinal autonomic systems that are normally under predominant supraspinal control (e.g., vasoconstrictor pathways) and, *second*, that supraspinal controls are important for the regulation of activity in those spinal autonomic systems that normally depend predominantly on spinal circuits (e.g., motility-regulating pathways). Furthermore, these findings are completely compatible with experimental results showing: (1) that up to 50% (or more) of the synapses on sympathetic preganglionic neurons are formed by descending systems (Llewellyn-Smith and Weaver 2001) and (2) that some EPSPs and IPSPs elicited monosynaptically in sympathetic preganglionic neurons from descending axons are relatively large (McLachlan and Hirst 1980; Deuchars et al. 1997), this being probably more a property of the preganglionic neuron input impedance than of the synapses.

Thus, the results reported so far suggest that the autonomic circuits in the spinal cord are important for integrating information from the periphery and from supraspinal brain structures. They clearly demonstrate that the spinal cord contains neural circuits, which consist of preganglionic neurons, segmental and propriospinal interneurons, and the synaptic connections of these neurons with the afferent inflow from the periphery on one side and with supraspinal autonomic premotor neurons projecting to the spinal cord on the other side. Functionally different types of spinal final autonomic pathways may receive connections from the same spinal circuit and an individual final autonomic pathway may be associated with several spinal circuits (Figure 9.4, Table 9.1).

Here I *hypothesize* that spinal and supraspinal autonomic circuits are integrated in a function-specific way. This leads to the characteristic discharge patterns in sympathetic neurons and parasympathetic sacral neurons. The experiments described in this chapter are fully consistent with this hypothesis, but they do not prove it:

- Spinal autonomic circuits are integrative mechanisms for the control of autonomic target organs. These may be called "spinal autonomic subroutines" or "spinal autonomic motor programs." They are preprogrammed and require, for appropriate functioning, distinct afferent inputs from the periphery of the body and synaptic input from supraspinal centers.
- Higher (supraspinal) centers "use" these spinal integrative mechanisms in the control of the peripheral autonomic pathways. Signals in the supraspinal autonomic premotor neurons are finally shaped by the spinal circuits before they are channeled into the final peripheral sympathetic and parasympathetic pathways. This shaping by the spinal autonomic motor programs varies between sympathetic systems, as there are also many monosynaptic connections between supraspinal autonomic premotor neurons and preganglionic neurons (Strack et al. 1989b; Morrison et al. 1991; Zagon and Smith 1993; McAllen et al. 1994). For example, the fast baroreceptor reflexes may be mediated monosynaptically by sympathetic premotor neurons in the lower brain stem to sympathetic preganglionic vasoconstrictor and cardiomotor neurons. However, it is not excluded that baroreceptor reflexes are additionally mediated: (1) by inhibitory spinal interneurons, (2) by excitatory spinal interneurons, or (3) via inhibitory sympathetic premotor neurons projecting through the dorsolateral funiculus (McLachlan and Hirst 1980; Deuchars et al. 1997; Stornetta et al. 2004) (see Subchapter 10.3).

- Thermoreceptor reflexes, somatosympathetic reflexes, micturition reflexes, defecation reflexes, erection reflexes, etc., may be preferentially mediated by spinal autonomic interneurons that receive convergent synaptic input from supraspinal neurons and from primary afferent neurons (Figures 9.8, 9.9, 9.10). Although not readily visible in the neural regulation of several autonomic target organs (e.g., cardiovascular regulation, thermal regulation of blood flow through skin, regulation of evacuative organs, regulation of gastrointestinal functions), the spinal components are probably very important in these control mechanisms.
- Sacro-lumbar reflexes related to the sympathetic outflow involved in the regulation of pelvic organs (continence of urinary bladder and hindgut; emission of semen by the internal reproductive organs) are mediated by several types of propriospinal interneurons (Bartel et al. 1986). The supraspinal control of these spinal circuits is unknown.
- Spinal circuits may set the gain for supraspinal reflexes or supraspinal systems may regulate the sensitivity of spinal reflex circuits. For example:
  - activation (by supraspinal systems) of sympathetic cardiomotor neurons during exercise may be enhanced and maintained by the spinal afferent feedback from the heart and from the exercising skeletal muscles;
  - inhibition of cutaneous vasoconstrictor neurons during warming of the hypothalamus is enhanced non-linearly by activation of spinal thermosensitive circuits (Grewe et al. 1995), as is also predicted from thermoregulatory changes in skin blood flow during hypothalamic and spinal cord warming (Simon 1974; Simon et al. 1986);
  - nociceptive and non-nociceptive spinal reflexes in sudomotor neurons are enhanced by supraspinal systems, etc.

Preganglionic neurons, spinal autonomic interneurons, spinal afferent neurons and sympathetic premotor neurons in the brain stem and hypothalamus may be synaptically interconnected in a characteristic way according to the function of the preganglionic neurons. This is demonstrated by the two hypothetical examples in Figure 9.15. Synaptic input from autonomic premotor neurons located in the brain stem and hypothalamus can act directly on

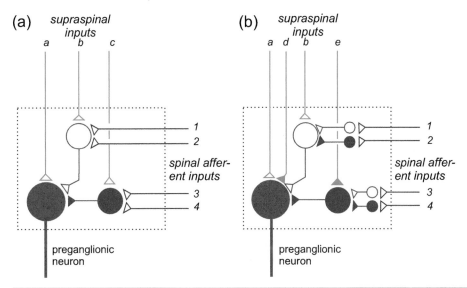

Figure 9.15 Hypothetical arrangement of autonomic interneurons and their synaptic connections with spinal afferent neurons and descending systems in the regulation of activity in preganglionic neurons. Spinal afferent inputs *1* to *4* synapse with autonomic interneurons; descending systems *a, b, c, d* and *e* synapse with interneurons or preganglionic neurons. These descending systems and the interneurons are either excitatory (open violet) or inhibitory (closed violet). This type of arrangement could represent the spinal autonomic motor programs "used" by the supraspinal autonomic centers to regulate the activity in preganglionic neurons during various autonomic activities. Modified from Jänig (1996c) with permission.

the preganglionic neurons or on autonomic interneurons. This synaptic input can be excitatory or inhibitory. Spinal afferent input from body tissues acts on spinal (excitatory or inhibitory) interneurons, which may also receive excitatory and/or inhibitory synaptic input from supraspinal centers. Thus, spinal autonomic reflex circuits may gate synaptic input from supraspinal centers or synaptic input from supraspinal centers may gate spinal reflex circuits. This shows that this principle of organization of the neural regulation of target organs by spinal autonomic systems has considerable flexibility.

We have no direct data about synaptic connections of autonomic interneurons with each other. It is conceptualized that these circuits do exist for the spinal sympathetic and parasympathetic systems, e.g., for cutaneous vasoconstrictor and sudomotor systems in the coordinated regulation of sweating and blood flow through hairless skin, for the sympathetic motility-regulating systems in the coordinated regulation of evacuative organs (lower urinary tract and hindgut) and for parasympathetic systems in the coordinated regulation of the lower urinary tract and hindgut.

Indeed, the experimental work that has so far been done on autonomic interneurons in the sacral spinal cord clearly supports this contention (Figure 9.6; Shefchyk 2001). It has not been shown so far, directly or indirectly, that different pools of autonomic interneurons are synaptically connected with each other to form networks of interneurons that are responsible for generation of the typical discharge patterns in peripheral autonomic pathways.

9.5.2 Coordination of Activity in Somatomotor Systems and Spinal Autonomic Systems

In the introduction of this book, I have described that the regulation of the autonomic nervous system is closely integrated with the regulation of activity in the somatic motor systems. Both systems (together with the neuroendocrine motor system in the hypothalamus) are hierarchically organized in the spinal cord, brain stem and hypothalamus, have common synaptic inputs from afferent systems, the cerebral cortex and the behavioral state system (see Figure 0.2), and constitute the basis for behavior

(Swanson 2000, 2003; Watts and Swanson 2002). This will be further elaborated in Chapter 11. The discussion of the spinal autonomic systems and the interneurons putatively associated with these systems has shown that spinal circuits, and therefore specific interneurons, may be important in the coordination of activity in somatic motor systems and activity in spinal autonomic systems. This is reflected in the coupling of somatomotor and sympathetic outflows from the spinal cord (Chizh et al. 1998). Putative interneurons involved in this coordination may be activated by supraspinal command signals. This coordination between somatomotor and spinal autonomic functions could be important in several functional contexts. Examples are:

- Regulation of pelvic organs (coordination between external sphincters and smooth muscle activity of urinary tract [Figures 9.7, 9.8, 9.10], hindgut and reproductive organs [Figure 9.13]).
- Regulation of sweat glands and blood flow through skin during somatosensory discrimination and manipulation (see vibration reflex in Subchapter 4.2).
- Regulation of cardiovascular system (heart rate, blood flow through skeletal muscle) during cortically induced and maintained muscle contractions (exercise; see Figures 11.3, 11.4) (Victor et al. 1995).
- Initiation of shivering, cutaneous vasoconstriction and inhibition of the sudomotor pathway during body cooling.

Future experiments, using in vitro or in vivo animal models, will have to dissect out which groups of interneurons are involved in this coordination of somatomotor and autonomic motor activity and what the underlying mechanisms are.

Conclusions

1. The spinal cord is an autonomic integrative organ in its own right, which determines several components of the discharge pattern in the spinal autonomic pathways in animals with an intact spinal cord. Preganglionic neurons, autonomic interneurons and primary afferent neurons form spinal autonomic reflex circuits, which are integrated into the regulation of preganglionic activity by supraspinal centers. Autonomic premotor neurons projecting from the brain stem and hypothalamus to the spinal cord synapse with preganglionic neurons and autonomic interneurons.

2. Analysis of the discharge patterns in the autonomic neurons under standardized experimental conditions leads to the following conclusions:

   a. The spinal cord contains distinct autonomic reflex pathways, which are integrated with supraspinal reflex pathways during normal regulation of the autonomic target organs and tissues.

   b. The discharge patterns in the different types of sympathetic neuron consist of components that are associated with integration into the spinal cord and integration into the lower brain stem, upper brain stem and hypothalamus.

   c. Reflex integration into the spinal cord is related to distinct afferent inputs from the skin, deep somatic tissues, viscera and spinal cord (thermoreceptors).

   d. Signals in supraspinal systems are integrated with spinal circuits, leading to reciprocal facilitation.

   e. Spinal circuits may be important in the coordination of somatomotor functions and spinal autonomic functions.

3. It is hypothesized that spinal interneurons and preganglionic neurons constitute spinal autonomic motor programs that are integrated into the regulation of autonomic target organs.

4. Spinal circuits, spinal afferent inflows and descending influences from the brain stem and hypothalamus often work together and determine the activity of the preganglionic sympathetic neurons. The systems may be under predominant control of the lower brain stem (e.g., the muscle and visceral vasoconstrictor pathways innervating resistance vessels), of the hypothalamus (e.g., the cutaneous vasoconstrictor pathways) or of the circuits in the spinal cord (e.g., the sympathetic motility-regulating and secretomotor pathways innervating the gastrointestinal tract or pelvic organs). However, in *all* spinal autonomic systems, the spinal component may be essential for this integration because it may set the excitability of the preganglionic neurons and/or shape the supraspinal signals according to "spinal autonomic programs."

5. This organization is particularly exemplified in the regulation of evacuation and continence of

the urinary bladder and colon-rectum, and in the regulation of the sequence of erection, emission and ejaculation of male reproductive organs. The functioning of these pelvic organs depends on multiple sacral and sacro-lumbar reflex circuits and several supraspinal integrative centers that interact with these spinal circuits.

6. In conclusion, experimental approaches that aim to clarify the central neural circuitry of the spinal autonomic systems should start at the level of the spinal cord and use functionally identified peripheral neurons of autonomic final pathways as the reference point.

Suggested Reading

Bartel, B., Blumberg, H. and Jänig, W. (1986) Discharge patterns of motility-regulating neurons projecting in the lumbar splanchnic nerves to visceral stimuli in spinal cats. *J Auton Nerv Syst* **15**, 153–163.

De Groat, W. C., Griffiths, D. and Yoshimura, N. (2015) Neural control of the lower urinary tract. *Compr Physiol* **5**, 327–396.

Deuchars, S. A. and Lall, V. K. (2015) Sympathetic preganglionic neurons: properties and inputs. *Compr Physiol* **5**, 829–869.

Häbler, H. J., Hilbers, K., Jänig, W., et al. (1992) Viscerosympathetic reflexes responses to mechanical stimulation of pelvic viscera in the cat. *J Auton Nerv Syst* **38**, 147–158.

Jänig, W., Keast, J. R., McLachlan, E. M., Neuhuber, W. L. and Southard-Smith, M. (2017) Renaming all spinal autonomic outflows as sympathetic is a mistake. *Auton Neurosci* **206**, 60–62.

Jänig, W., Schmidt, M., Schnitzler, A. and Wesselmann, U. (1991) Differentiation of sympathetic neurones projecting in the hypogastric nerves in terms of their discharge patterns in cats. *J Physiol* **437**, 157–179.

Shefchyk, S. J. (2002) Spinal cord neural organization controlling the urinary bladder and striated sphincter. *Prog Brain Res* **137**, 71–82.

All references cited in the text are available online at www.cambridge.org/janig.

Notes

1. Bypassing integrative processes, changes in excitability (conductance of membrane) of preganglionic neurons can also occur due to local low-oxygen tension and spillover of neuropeptides released in the dorsal horn, or may be intrinsic to the preganglionic neurons (as activity-dependent processes).

2. Sympathetic preganglionic neurons may be electrically coupled, as has been shown electrophysiologically in vitro on thoracolumbar spinal cord slices of rats aged 8 to 14 days (Logan et al. 1996; Nolan et al. 1999). It is unclear whether this coupling occurs between functionally related preganglionic neurons and whether it contributes to synchronized firing of sympathetic neurons in vivo.

3. Using the term spinal or spinalized rat (or any other animal), I mean an animal in which the spinal cord has been completely transected (in our experiments at the thoracic segmental level T8/T9).

4. Spinal shock describes the temporary loss or depression of reflex activity mediated by the spinal cord below the lesion of the spinal cord. The term "spinal shock" was introduced by Hall (1841) in order to differentiate hypotension following blood loss from hypotension following contusion of the spinal cord with subsequent interruption of communication between supraspinal centers and the spinal cord.

5. With "functionally distinct reflexes" I mean reflexes that are well defined according to the function (receptive properties) of the primary afferent neurons and the function (target cells) of the autonomic system.

6. Electrical stimulation of afferent axons in nerves elicits short- and long-latency reflexes in preganglionic neurons, depending on the afferent axons stimulated (A- or C-fibers) and on the central pathways (spinal or supraspinal). Spinal reflexes elicited in this way are preserved acutely after transection of the spinal cord rostral to the preganglionic neurons recorded from (e.g., those projecting into the cardiac or renal nerves) and do not appear to exhibit "spinal shock" (Coote and Downman 1966; Coote and Sato 1978; Coote 1984). It is important to emphasize that this experimental situation is entirely different from that when afferent fibers are activated physiologically (e.g., by noxious or non-noxious stimulation of the skin, by contraction or distension of a visceral organ): electrical stimulation leads to synchronous non-physiological activation of afferent neurons; physiological stimulation activates afferent neurons asynchronously.

7. This experimental finding does not argue against the existence of the spinal inhibitory pathway activated by visceral afferents. It argues that this pathway can no longer be activated after spinalization. We have studied, in the cat, the viscero-sympathetic reflexes in

cutaneous and muscle vasoconstrictor neurons to distension or contraction of the urinary bladder or distal colon 60 to 130 days after spinalization at the thoracic segmental level T8. During this time period, we did not observe inhibitory reflexes in cutaneous vasoconstrictor neurons to these visceral stimuli. We have not studied the time course of recovery of the excitatory viscero-sympathetic reflexes after spinalization (Jänig and Kümmel, unpublished).

8. This discrepancy between experimental studies on animals (mainly cats) and studies on paraplegic patients is puzzling. However, when the spinal autonomic circuits are no longer under supraspinal control after interruption of the spinal cord, postganglionic sympathetic neurons exhibit asynchronous activity. Because of the low signal-to-noise ratio in the microneurographic recordings, and since single-unit recordings from postganglionic cutaneous vasoconstrictor axons and postganglionic sudomotor axons are very difficult to obtain with this recording technique, it is probably difficult, if not impossible, to detect this asynchronous spontaneous activity in the unmyelinated postganglionic axons. Macefield and Wallin (1999a, b, 2018) succeeded in recording routinely from single muscle and cutaneous vasoconstrictor axons in humans, using high-impedance tungsten metal electrodes (see Subchapter 3.5), but this has not been done in spinally injured patients.

9. Note in Figure 9.6 that the contractions of the urinary bladder and colon are alternating. This is probably generated by activation of reciprocal inhibitory spinal reflex pathways connected to preganglionic neurons innervating the urinary bladder or the colon (see Subchapter 9.3.1 and Figure 9.10). Stimulation of bladder afferents leads to strong synchronous reflex activation of the sympathetic vasoconstrictor systems (CVC, MVC) and the sudomotor system (skin pot.) (marked *b* in Figure 9.6). Stimulation of colon afferents leads to a smaller synchronous reflex activation of the three sympathetic pathways (marked *c* in Figure 9.6).

10. The *arguments* supporting the concept of de Groat and coworkers are: (1) Lesion of the pontine micturition center (PMC) abolishes micturition. (2) Electrical or chemical stimulation of the PMC triggers micturition. (3) In cats, electrical stimulation of Aδ-afferents in the pelvic splanchnic nerve elicits long-latency reflexes in the preganglionic neurons innervating the urinary bladder mediated by the PMC. Short-latency reflexes are absent. Thus, Aδ-fibers form the afferent limb of the pontine micturition reflexes. (4) In chronic spinal cats, the afferent limb of the micturition reflexes elicited by electrical stimulation of the pelvic splanchnic nerve are C-fibers but not Aδ-fibers.

These results have considerable *implications*: (i) Sacral afferent C-fibers innervating the urinary bladder are not involved in micturition reflexes in the adult cat. This conclusion is consistent with investigations of sacral afferents innervating the urinary bladder, showing that most Aδ-fibers have low thresholds to distension of the urinary bladder and that only a few afferent C-fibers can be activated by distension of the urinary bladder at high intravesical pressures of >30 mmHg (see Figure 2.7b; Häbler et al. 1990). (ii) In chronic spinal cats, afferent C-fibers innervating the urinary bladder and their synaptic connections in the spinal cord must undergo plastic changes, serving now as an afferent limb in the micturition reflexes. Capsaicin, a neurotoxin that disrupts the function of nociceptive C-fibers that have the transient receptor potential (TRP) V1-receptor in their membrane, prevents the micturition reflex contractions when given systemically in chronic spinal cats, but not in normal cats (see de Groat et al. 1993; de Groat 2013). In rats, activation of the spinal parasympathetic pathway, which relaxes the urethra by releasing nitric oxide (NO) during distension of the urinary bladder (see Figure 9.8), appears to be dependent on a spinal reflex pathway.

11. (1) The erectile tissue of the penis (corpus cavernosum and corpus spongiosum) and the erectile tissue in females consist of trabecular tissue and sinusoids, which contain smooth muscle cells. It is vascularly supplied by branches of the internal pudendal artery via helicine arteries. The postganglionic neurons that innervate these vascular sections of the erectile tissue are cholinergic or noradrenergic. The cholinergic neurons are located in the pelvic ganglion and project through the cavernous nerve (Figure 9.12) to the erectile tissue. The noradrenergic neurons are located in the sacral sympathetic chain ganglia (and possibly the inferior mesenteric ganglion and pelvic ganglia). (2) Activation of the cholinergic postganglionic neurons dilates the helicine arteries and relaxes the sinusoids and trabecles of the erectile tissue. The pressure in and volume of the erectile tissue increase, leading to elongation of the penis. The venous outflow of the erectile tissue of the penis is reduced by passive compression of the emissary veins. The pressure in the erectile tissue reaches values that are about 10 to 20 mmHg below arterial blood pressure. It is further increased above arterial blood pressure by contraction of the bulbo- and ischiocavernosus muscles (generated by activation of pudendal motoneurons); this enhances the rigidity of the penis in humans and generates rigidity in animals. Activation of noradrenergic neurons supplying the erectile

tissue leads to subsidence of erections (detumescence). (3) Acetylcholine and the vasoactive intestinal peptide are colocalized in the postganglionic neurons generating dilation of the erectile tissue. Additionally, the neurons synthesize and release the radical NO during activation. These three substances relax the branches of the internal pudendal artery, helicine arteries and sinusoids, and work cooperatively together in the initiation, potentiation and maintenance of the active dilation, NO released by the postganglionic neurons being the principal mediator of penile erection in humans and animals. The quantitative importance of the three compounds in the generation of erection varies between species. Finally, NO released by the endothelium of the blood vessels in the erectile tissue may also be important to mediate erection (Burnett et al. 1992; Andersson 2001).

Chapter 10

Regulation of Organ Systems by the Lower Brain Stem

Sympathetic premotor neurons and cranial parasympathetic preganglionic neurons are present in the lower brain stem (medulla oblongata and pons) in addition to those located more rostrally (see Subchapter 8.4). Their cell bodies are located in the ventrolateral medulla (mainly rostral ventrolateral medulla), the ventromedial medulla, the caudal raphe nuclei and the A5 area of the ventrolateral pons (see Figures 8.15 and 8.17 and Tables 8.2 and 8.3). Premotor neurons form synapses with preganglionic neurons (and/or local interneurons associated with the preganglionic neurons) (Chapters 8 and 9). How do autonomic premotor neurons in the lower brain stem function so as to contribute to the characteristic discharge patterns of the neurons of the peripheral autonomic pathways?

On the basis of the knowledge we have about the central autonomic systems, I can partially answer this question for some systems in the lower brain stem. These answers clearly indicate that we will be able to unravel the maze of the neural organization of autonomic systems in the lower brain stem in the near future. Ways to achieve this aim are:

1. Experimental studies to record the effects of microinjection of pharmacological agents into defined regions of the lower brain stem on effector responses (e.g., arterial blood pressure, heart rate, blood flow through an organ; phrenic nerve discharge; movements or secretion in the gastrointestinal tract, etc.).

2. Experimental studies on single central neurons that combine neurophysiological, histological, neurochemical and neuropharmacological methods.

3. Correlation of these data with the firing patterns of pre- and postganglionic neurons of functional autonomic pathways in the periphery (see Chapter 4).

4. The alignment of these studies with the physiological behavior of autonomic target tissues (cardiovascular responses [e.g., heart rate, arterial blood pressure, blood flow through organs], thermoregulatory responses, gastrointestinal responses, responses of pelvic organs, etc.).

Only a cellular and neurochemical approach combined with a precise knowledge of the microanatomy and of the input–output functions of individual cell groups will advance our understanding of autonomic integration in supraspinal brain centers (Blessing 1997; Guyenet 2000). This includes various experimental techniques, some of which have been mentioned in

Chapters 3 and 8 and, to emphasize and repeat it, *the anchor of all investigations is the physiology of the regulation of autonomic effector organs and tissues (cardiovascular system, respiration, gastrointestinal tract, pelvic organs, thermoregulatory system)*. Using this approach, there have been some advances towards this aim for central autonomic neurons involved in the regulation of these systems. Here I will concentrate mainly on three topics:

1. Sympathetic premotor neurons in the rostral ventrolateral medulla and parasympathetic preganglionic neurons in the nucleus ambiguus, which have been most thoroughly studied in the context of cardiovascular regulation and its coordination with the regulation of respiration without going into detail about the mechanisms underlying respiration.
2. The role of neurons in the caudal raphe nuclei in the regulation of activity in cutaneous vasoconstrictor neurons during thermoregulation and of activity in sympathetic neurons innervating the brown adipose tissue in the rat (which I call lipomotor neurons).
3. The function of the dorsal vagus complex (nucleus tractus solitarii [NTS], dorsal motor nucleus of the vagus and area postrema) in the regulation of gastrointestinal functions.

Neurons in the ventromedial medulla and raphe nuclei are also important in the endogenous control of nociceptive impulse transmission in the spinal dorsal horn and caudal trigeminal nucleus and therefore important in protection of the body during noxious events. This function is closely associated with the regulation of peripheral sympathetic pathways and is reviewed elsewhere in the context of "Autonomic nervous system and body protection" (Jänig 2005, 2020a,b; Heinricher and Fields 2013; Jänig and Levine 2013; Heinricher and Ingram 2020).

Finally, regulation of pelvic organs involving pontine and suprapontine centers (see Chapter 9; McKenna 2013; de Groat et al. 2015), and regulation of glucose and fat metabolism involving the lower brain stem will not be covered.

10.1 | General Functions of the Lower Brain Stem

The lower brain stem contains the neuronal mechanisms for control of the cardiovascular system, the respiratory system and the gastrointestinal system (Figure 10.1). This global regulation of body systems is closely coordinated in different time domains and according to the external and internal demands on the organism. The regulation of respiration, cardiac output and peripheral blood flow resistance is adjusted in the time domain of seconds, so as to precisely adjust the gas transport into the body and to the peripheral tissues in the body. Ingestion of food and fluid and respiration are precisely regulated in the time domain of milliseconds in order to prevent nutrients and fluid getting into the lungs. Intake, digestion and absorption of nutrients are closely coordinated with regulation of blood flow through the gastrointestinal tract in the time domain of hours to guarantee the transport of nutrients to the liver and body tissues. These differentiated control systems, their coordination and their adaptation to

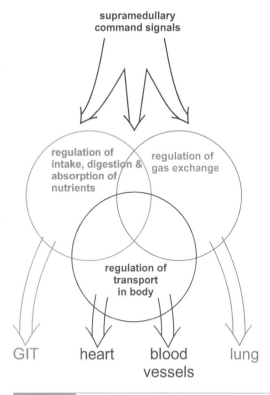

Figure 10.1 Three global homeostatic control systems and their coordination in the medulla oblongata. Regulation of the cardiovascular system, the respiratory system and the gastrointestinal tract (GIT). Each system receives specific afferent inputs from the periphery and is under the control of the upper brain stem, hypothalamus and telencephalon. The three systems are closely integrated.

the external and internal challenges of the body require:

1. functionally specialized primary afferent neurons, which continuously inform the lower brain stem centers about the internal state of these systems (see Chapter 2);
2. specialized final autonomic pathways to the effectors of the three systems (and somatic motor pathways to the respiratory muscles);
3. distinct synaptic connections between the afferent and the efferent pathways to these three systems mediated by functionally special groups of interneurons;
4. differentiated neuronal control of these reflex pathways by centers in the upper brain stem, hypothalamus and telencephalon.

It is clear that the different groups of interneuron in the lower brain stem must be synaptically interconnected in a functionally specific way, otherwise the closely coordinated control of the three systems would not be possible. We have only limited knowledge about the different types of interneuron, their transmitters, their synaptic connections and their connections with supramedullary brain centers. The specific components of these neuronal control systems become visible in the distinct reflexes elicited in peripheral autonomic neurons by physiological stimulation of different groups of afferent neurons (innervating the cardiovascular, gastrointestinal or respiratory systems). Specific reflexes obtained under standardized experimental conditions change quantitatively and qualitatively according to the state of the control systems and are therefore dependent on the command signals from suprapontine centers. Details about the specific reflexes, their integration into homeostatic regulation and their anatomical basis have been described elsewhere (Spyer 1981, 1994; Guyenet 1990, 2000; Loewy and Spyer 1990; Guyenet and Koshiya 1992; Ritter et al. 1992; Dampney 1994, 2016; Sun 1995; Guyenet et al. 1996; Blessing 1997 [see extensive literature here]; Jordan 1997; Kirchheim et al. 1998; Rekling and Feldman 1998; St.-John 1998; Chapleau and Abboud 2001; Richter and Spyer 2001; Pilowsky and Goodchild 2002; Dampney and Horiuchi 2003; Guyenet 2006; Feldman et al. 2013a,b; Romanovsky 2018; Ashhad and Feldman 2020).

Some general principles of this organization will be described here for the arterial baroreceptor reflexes, arterial chemoreceptor reflexes, reflexes in cutaneous vasoconstrictor neurons and lipomotor neurons innervating brown adipose tissue, for the respiratory modulation of activity in peripheral autonomic neurons and for gastrointestinal reflexes. This description is restricted to the short time domain of the functioning of these systems, but not the long time domain related to the adaptation of these systems during changes in the body or environmental load (e.g., thermal load, stress, exercise, fluid loss etc.).

10.2 Sympathetic Premotor Neurons in the Ventrolateral Medulla Oblongata

Neurophysiological recording from sympathetic nerves in anesthetized animals and from postganglionic axons in muscle nerves in humans using microneurography, under resting conditions, shows that many sympathetic neurons have spontaneous activity and that the discharge pattern of this activity appears to be rather similar in different nerves. The activity shows rhythmic changes that are correlated with the arterial pulse pressure wave ("cardiac rhythmicity" of the activity; see Figures 4.1, 4.7 and 4.8 in Chapter 4) and with the central respiration generator (Figure 4.2). But rhythmic changes in sympathetic activity also occur independently of cardiovascular and respiratory parameters and are hypothesized to be generated by neural oscillators in the brain stem (Gebber 1990; Malpas 1998; Barman and Gebber 2000; see Subchapter 10.6.2). Activity with cardiovascular, respiratory or similar rhythmicities occurs in sympathetic vasoconstrictor neurons innervating resistance vessels (such as in skeletal muscle, kidney and other viscera) and in sympathetic cardiomotor neurons. Vasoconstrictor neurons of this type project in many peripheral nerves and dominate the activity in them. For this reason the mass discharge patterns are rather similar in different peripheral nerves.

Spontaneous activity and its rhythmic changes in sympathetic cardiovascular neurons, being involved in blood pressure control, but not necessarily in other functional types of sympathetic neuron, are dependent on the lower brain stem. Both disappear *acutely* after transection of the spinal cord at the cervical level, paralleled by a decrease in arterial blood pressure to values of 50 to 60 mmHg (for discussion of spontaneous activity in sympathetic neurons after spinalization see Subchapter 9.2). They are little affected after transection of the brain stem at a suprapontine level. However, this is a very controversial issue and results depend very much on the experimental preparation used, whether the animal is anesthetized or awake and on the animal species. Many parasympathetic cardiomotor neurons are also spontaneously active and exhibit the same rhythmicities in their activity. What is the origin of this resting activity in sympathetic and parasympathetic cardiovascular neurons? Which mechanisms underlie these typical and universally observed phasic changes of the spontaneous activity?

10.2.1 The Discovery of the Cardiovascular Center in the Medulla Oblongata

Unethical experiments by present day standards had been performed on curarized unanesthetized animals (usually rabbits) in the late nineteenth century to explore the central origin of activity in vasomotor neurons and the central organization of blood pressure regulation (Bernard 1858; Dittmar 1873; Owsjannikov 1874). These experiments will not be discussed any further. In about the middle of the twentieth century, Alexander (1946) performed systematic experiments in anesthetized cats, lesioning and electrically stimulating different sites of the medulla oblongata. He defined the excitatory and inhibitory cardiovascular centers in the medulla oblongata. His description dominated the textbooks for many decades.

The systematic investigation of the organization of the cardiovascular center in the medulla oblongata, using various methods, started in the second half of the 1960s:

- Schläfke and Loeschcke (1967) showed that bilateral cooling of the ventrolateral medulla in the anesthetized cat dramatically reduced arterial blood pressure and respiration.
- A few years later, it was shown in the cat that application of the inhibitory amino acids γ-aminobutyric acid (GABA) or glycine to the ventrolateral surface of the medulla oblongata or bilateral lesion of this area also generated a dramatic fall in arterial blood pressure (Guertzenstein and Silver 1974; Feldberg and Guertzenstein 1976). These experiments clearly demonstrated that neurons

responsible for or mediating spontaneous activity in sympathetic vasoconstrictor neurons are present in the ventrolateral medulla.

- Amendt et al. (1979) showed in the cat that the rostral ventrolateral medulla contains neurons that project to the preganglionic neurons in the nucleus intermediolateralis of the spinal cord. They retrogradely labeled the cell bodies of these neurons by the tracer horseradish peroxidase, which was transported in the axons to the cell bodies of the sympathetic premotor neurons after its application to the nucleus intermediolateralis (see Subchapter 8.1 and Figure 8.1).
- At the beginning of the 1980s, Roger Dampney and his group demonstrated in the unanesthetized rabbit that excitation of neurons in the rostral ventrolateral medulla (RVLM) by microinjection of the excitatory amino acid glutamate increased arterial blood pressure, and that the sites of stimulation in the RVLM corresponded very closely with the location of neurons projecting to the nucleus intermediolateralis or the intermediate zone of the thoracolumbar spinal cord. This group was the first to show that bilateral lesions of the RVLM abolish the baroreceptor reflex mediated by vasoconstrictor neurons to resistance vessels. Finally, based on immunohistochemical investigations in rabbits and rats, they proposed that bulbospinal neurons that were probably involved in the generation of activity in the vasoconstrictor neurons (so-called "sympathetic vasomotor tone") and in mediating the baroreceptor reflex contain adrenaline (i.e., are C1 neurons) (Dampney et al. 1982; Goodchild et al. 1984; for early reviews see Dampney [1981], Dampney et al. [1985]).
- These experimental investigations were extended by Donald Reis and his group. They studied the changes in arterial blood pressure and heart rate: (1) to electrical or chemical stimulation of the RVLM, (2) to decreasing the activity in the RVLM neurons by topical injection of the inhibitory amino acid GABA or the sodium channel blocker tetrodotoxin or (3) to disinhibition of the RVLM neurons by topical injection of the GABA antagonist bicuculline. They compared the sites from which these responses could be elicited with the location of adrenergic (C1) neurons. Like Dampney and coworkers, they came to the conclusion that neurons in the RVLM are responsible for activity in sympathetic vasoconstrictor neurons maintaining

arterial blood pressure, are under inhibitory control and may mediate the baroreceptor reflex (Ross et al. 1984a, b; Ruggiero et al. 1989).

- The first neurophysiological recordings were made in the 1980s from bulbospinal neurons in the RVLM, which had the same discharge properties as muscle vasoconstrictor neurons and which were therefore candidates to generate the activity in these cardiovascular sympathetic neurons (Brown and Guyenet 1984, 1985; Sun and Guyenet 1985; McAllen 1987; Sun and Spyer 1991).

10.2.2 The Ventrolateral Medulla Oblongata

Sympathetic preganglionic neurons and their related interneurons obtain their supraspinal synaptic inputs from various nuclei in the brain stem and hypothalamus (Figure 8.15; Table 8.2). The sympathetic premotor neurons in the RVLM have been more thoroughly studied than the sympathetic and parasympathetic premotor neurons in other nuclei. Therefore, I will concentrate preferentially on bulbospinal neurons in the RVLM (and on parasympathetic preganglionic cardiomotor neurons [see "Heart" in Subchapter 4.8.2]). The RVLM belongs to a complex network of neurons in the ventrolateral part of the medulla oblongata (VLM), which is important in the regulation of the cardiovascular system and of respiration. The VLM contains neuronal circuits, which are part of a network generating the respiratory rhythm in respiratory and cardiovascular neurons and the spontaneous activity in sympathetic cardiovascular neurons, possibly parasympathetic cardiomotor and bronchomotor neurons. These neuronal circuits mediate various cardiovascular and respiratory reflexes, and integrate the two homeostatic control systems. Therefore the neurons that are involved in blood pressure regulation and in regulation of respiration are anatomically closely associated in the VLM (for review see Dampney [1994, 2016]; Pilowsky and Goodchild [2002]; Guyenet [2006]). Functionally, these neurons are sympathetic premotorneurons, parasympathetic preganglionic neurons, respiratory premotor neurons and various groups of excitatory and inhibitory interneurons related to these output pathways. The presympathetic neurons in the RVLM may innervate, in addition to sympathetic preganglionic neurons, several other neuronal targets in the brain stem (see Subchapter 10.2.3 and Box 10.2; Guyenet et al. 2013; Stornetta et al. 2016).

Information identifying the neurons in the VLM as components of neuronal circuits that are involved in cardiovascular regulation (or regulation of respiration) has been obtained using multiple methodical approaches:

- Effect of chemical activation (e.g., by glutamate or another excitatory amino acid) or inhibition (e.g., by GABA agonists such as muscimol) of spatially circumscribed neuron populations on arterial blood pressure (or respiration).
- Effect of local blockade of excitatory or inhibitory synaptic transmission on arterial blood pressure (or respiration).
- Recording the expression of *c-fos* mRNA or protein in neuron populations that are activated by physiological stimulation of afferents (e.g., arterial baroreceptors or chemoreceptors) (Note 1).
- The effect of selective destruction of a neurochemically specific population of neurons by a toxin that is conjugated to an enzyme or agonist. The toxin–enzyme complex or toxin–agonist–receptor complex reacts with its specific receptor in the neuron membrane and is taken up into the neuron leading to its destruction (Note 2).
- Activation by light of specific neurons that express (naturally or after genetic manipulation) a light-sensitive protein. For example, this could be an ion channel that, when opened, leads to depolarization/hyperpolarization and firing/suppression of action potentials in intact pathways in vivo, usually in mice. The light can be delivered to specific neurons or groups of neurons lying deep in the brain using optical fibers or miniaturized light-emitting diodes (Fenno et al. 2011).
- Recording of activity in single neurons in the VLM with respect to cardiovascular parameters and to activity in peripheral (post- or preganglionic) cardiovascular neurons.
- Determination of the morphology (location of cell body, orientation and projection of dendrites, projection and collateralization of axons), immunohistochemistry (putative fast transmitters, such as glutamate or GABA; monoamines, such as adrenaline, noradrenaline or 5-hydroxytryptamine [5-HT]; colocalized peptides) and pharmacology of the neurophysiologically and functionally identified neurons (Note 3).

Figures 10.2 and 10.3 illustrate, for the rat in simplified form, the functional anatomical organization of the VLM and the nucleus ambiguus (NA) between the caudal pole of the facial nucleus and the caudal pole of the lateral reticular nucleus. This is based on studies of the anatomy, the neural control of respiration and the neural control of arterial blood pressure or of perfusion of organs with blood. This anatomical organization applies with some modifications to other mammalian species too (e.g., cat, rabbit or dog, and probably also humans). The division of the VLM into subnuclei was and is still somewhat controversial since the anatomical borders, as reported by Paxinos and Watson (2014), which are based on

cytological and other anatomical criteria, do not necessarily correspond with the functional subdivision of the VLM (see Bieger and Hopkins [1987], Guyenet [1990] and Blessing [1997] for critical discussion). The nomenclature used in Figures 10.2 and 10.3 (as well as in this chapter; see also Chapter 8) is based on Paxinos and Watson (2014). Future taxonomy will be based on developmental lineage and transcriptomics. Here the VLM is defined for practical reasons as the region ventrolateral and ventral to the nucleus ambiguus (NA, compact and subcompact parts), but not including it (Note 4). Figures 10.2 and 10.3 illustrate the anatomical structures that are relevant for the topics to be discussed in this chapter. These

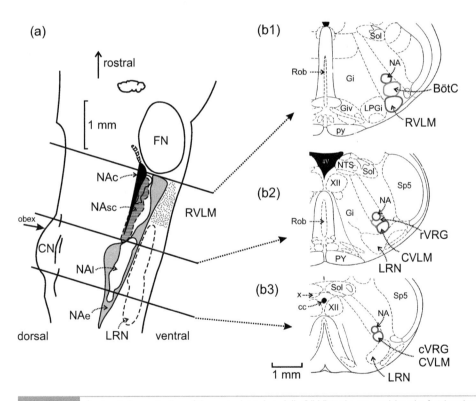

Figure 10.2 Anatomical organization of the ventrolateral medulla (VLM) in the rat caudal to the facial nucleus (FN). Location of subdivisions of the nucleus ambiguus (NA), of the rostral ventrolateral medulla (RVLM), of the caudal ventrolateral medulla (CVLM) and of cell groups involved in regulation of respiration. (a) Major subdivisions of the NA and location of the RVLM in a schematic drawing of a parasagittal section of the rat medulla oblongata. (b) Coronal (transverse) sections through the medulla oblongata (b1) just caudal to the facial nucleus (i.e. at the level 12.8 mm caudal to bregma according to the atlas of Paxinos and Watson [2014]), (b2) 300 μm rostral to the obex (13.24 mm caudal to bregma) and (b3) about 0.8 mm caudal to the obex (14.3 mm caudal to bregma). (a) Modified from Bieger and Hopkins (1987) with permission; (b1–b3) modified from Paxinos and Watson (2014). BötC, Bötzinger complex; cc, central canal; CN, cuneate nucleus; cVRG, caudal ventral respiratory group; Gi, gigantocellular nucleus; Giv, ventral part of the gigantocellular nucleus; LPGi, lateral paragigantocellular nucleus; LRN, lateral reticular nucleus; NAc/NAe/NAl/NAsc, compact/external/loose/subcompact parts of the nucleus ambiguus; NTS, nucleus tractus solitarii; PY, pyramidal tract; Rob, raphe obscurus; rVRG, rostral ventral respiratory group; Sol, solitary tract; Sp5, spinal trigeminal nucleus; 4V, fourth ventricle; X, dorsal motor nucleus of the vagus; XII, hypoglossal nucleus.

structures have been projected on a parasagittal section of the medulla oblongata (Figures 10.2a, 10.3b), on three coronal (transverse) sections (Figure 10.2 b1: just caudal to the facial nucleus; b2: just rostral to the obex; b3: about 1 mm caudal to the obex) and on a dorsal view of the VLM (Figure 10.3a) (Note 5).

The Cardiovascular Ventrolateral Cell Column

The neurons related to the regulation of the cardiovascular system involving the sympathetic nervous system are located in the cardiovascular ventrolateral cell column of the ventrolateral medulla (VLM). The sympathetic (bulbospinal) premotor neurons, which mediate and potentially generate spontaneous activity and mediate many reflexes in sympathetic cardiomotor neurons and in neurons of sympathetic pathways innervating blood vessels in skeletal muscle, kidney or other viscera, are located in the RVLM (Note 6). The VLM is situated caudal to the facial nucleus, rostral to the lateral reticular nucleus (Figure 10.4) and ventral to the rostral (compact and subcompact) part of the NA (Figure 10.3b). It extends close to the ventral medullary surface (Figure 10.2a). The RVLM overlaps dorsally with the rostral part of the external formation of the NA and of the compact and subcompact formation of the NA (Figure 10.2b1). It lies rostral to most parasympathetic cardiomotor neurons with chronotropic and dromotropic activity, which are situated in the more caudal part of the external formation of the NA, and ventral to the caudal part of the NA, which contains the motoneurons innervating the larynx (Figure 10.2a, b2).

The RVLM extends caudally into the caudal VLM (CVLM) (Figure 10.4). The CVLM is divided into a rostral part (the rCVLM) and a caudal part (cCVLM). The rCVLM is also sometimes called the intermediate VLM (IVLM, which was originally defined in the rabbit; see Dampney [1994]). The CVLM contains various groups of inhibitory and excitatory interneurons, which are important for the regulation of activity in sympathetic premotor neurons of the RVLM and which project directly or indirectly to the RVLM. Chemical stimulation of the neurons in the CVLM is followed by a decrease in arterial blood pressure. Therefore, this part of the VLM is also called the ventrolateral depressor area.

The most caudal part of the VLM is also called the caudal pressor area (CPA; Figure 10.4) since stimulation of the neurons in this area (e.g., by the excitatory amino acid glutamate) increases the blood pressure

and activity in "sympathetic" nerves (renal and splanchnic nerves), whereas inhibition of the neurons in the CPA decreases the arterial blood pressure and abolishes activity in these nerves. The CPA is situated between the caudal pole of the LRN and the medullary dorsal horn close to the transition between medulla oblongata and spinal cord (Gordon and McCann 1988; Possas et al. 1994; Campos and McAllen 1999; Natarajan and Morrison 2000; Sun and Panneton 2002, 2005; see Schreihofer and Sved 2011).

The Ventral Respiratory Column

Respiratory neurons are located in a cell column of the VLM called the ventral respiratory column (VRC). This cell column extends from the caudal border of the facial nucleus to about 1.5 mm caudal to the obex (Figures 10.2b, 10.3a). These neurons of the VRC and their excitatory and inhibitory synaptic connections are part of the respiratory network, including the dorsal respiratory group in the medulla oblongata and centers in the caudal and rostral pons (ponto-medullary respiratory network; St-John and Paton 2004; Rybak et al. 2014; Feldman and Kam 2015; Anderson et al. 2016; Del Negro et al. 2018; Ashhad and Feldman 2020). The respiratory network is responsible for the generation of the respiratory rhythm and of the different types of respiratory pattern, as present in the activity of motoneurons projecting in the phrenic nerve, glosso-pharyngeal nerve, superior laryngeal nerve, hypoglossal nerve or the pharyngeal branch of the vagus nerve (Monnier et al. 2003). During eupneic breathing in vivo, and under anesthesia, the pattern of breathing consists of three phases: inspiration, postinspiration (or stage 1 expiration) and stage 2 expiration. This is reflected in the activity of output (premotor) neurons of the respiratory network and in the discharge of inspiratory motor neurons (see discharge in phrenic nerve in Figure 10.21) (Monnier et al. 2003; Smith et al. 2013; Guyenet 2014).

The ventral respiratory column is anatomically interposed between the NA (compact and subcompact part and external formation) and the RVLM/ CVLM cell column (Figure 10.3b). It overlaps with both rostrocaudally organized cell columns and there is some intermingling between the neurons in the three columns (Pilowsky et al. 1990). The VRC has the following characteristics (Dobbins and Feldman

1994; Bianchi et al. 1995; Rekling and Feldman 1998; Monnier et al. 2003):

- The VRC is divided into four functional segments. These segments consist, in rostrocaudal order, of the Bötzinger Complex (BötC), the preBötzinger Complex (preBötC), the rostral ventral respiratory group (rVRG) and the caudal ventral respiratory group (cVRG). Each segment contains distinct groups of excitatory or inhibitory interneurons or premotor output neurons, which are synaptically connected with each other in a distinct way. Excitatory neurons are glutamatergic and inhibitory neurons glycinergic.
- Output premotor neurons of the respiratory network that project to and excite inspiratory motorneurons (e.g., phrenic motorneurons innervating the diaphragm) are located in the rVRG. Output premotor neurons that project to and excite expiratory motorneurons (e.g., innervating abdominal muscles) are located in the cVRG, which extends from the obex to the spinal segment C1.

- Neurons in the preBötC are inspiratory and generate the inspiratory rhythm. This rhythm relies on recurrent excitatory interaction between two symmetrically located clusters of special glutamatergic neurons.
- Most neurons in the Bötzinger complex are expiratory neurons. Many of these neurons are glycinergic propriobulbar neurons that inhibit respiratory premotor neurons (bulbospinal inspiratory neurons in the rVRG and/or bulbospinal expiratory neurons in the cVRG and respiratory motoneurons; Schreihofer et al. 1999; Ezure et al. 2003; Smith et al. 2013; Rybak et al. 2014).

It is important to emphasize, explicitly by referring to Figures 10.2 and 10.3, that *the anatomical substrates of the neural regulation of respiration and of the cardiovascular system are present in the same column of neurons of the VLM.* Neurons in the nuclei of the VRC are part of the ponto-medullary respiratory network that adapts respiration to the various needs of the organism (for details see Rybak et al. [2014]; Feldman and Kam [2015]; Anderson et al. [2016]; Del

---

Box 10.1 | Location of Nuclei in the Ventrolateral Medulla Oblongata (see Figures 10.2 and 10.3)

1. The motoneurons of the esophagus, pharynx and larynx are situated in the compact (NA_C), subcompact (NA_{SC}) and loose (NA_L) formations of the nucleus ambiguus (NA).
2. The external formation of the NA (NA_e) is anatomically not very well defined; it contains the parasympathetic preganglionic cardioinhibitory neurons (in particular ventrolateral at the level of the obex and extending rostrally) and the parasympathetic preganglionic bronchomotor and secretomotor neurons innervating the trachea and bronchi (located in particular at the level of the obex, but also throughout NA_C, NA_{SC} and NA_L).
3. Respiratory neurons are located between the NA_C/NA_{SC} cell column and the RVLM/CVLM cell column in the ventral respiratory column (VRC): (i) The caudal ventral respiratory group (cVRG) in the caudal third and further caudal contains expiratory premotor neurons. (ii) The rVRG in the intermediate part rostral and caudal to the obex contains inspiratory premotor neurons. (iii) The preBötC located about midway between facial nucleus (FN) and lateral reticular nucleus (LRN) contains inspiratory interneurons. (iv) The BötC located caudal to the FN contains expiratory neurons.
4. The RVLM is located caudal to the FN, rostral to the LRN and ventral to the NA. It overlaps with the BötC and preBötC (see Figure 10.3b).
5. The CVLM is situated at the level of the preBötC and further caudal.
6. The caudal pressor area (CPA) is located at the most caudal part of the VLM.

Abbreviations: BötC, Bötzinger complex; CVLM, caudal ventrolateral medulla; preBötC, preBötzinger complex; RVLM, rostral ventrolateral medulla

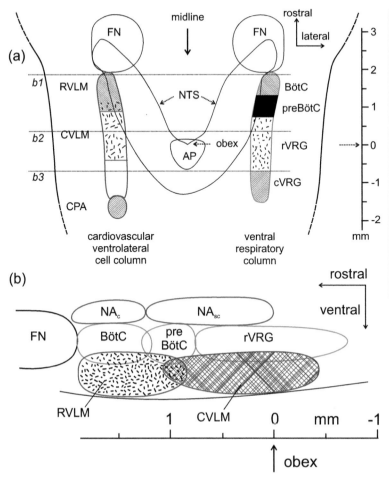

Figure 10.3 (a) Dorsal view of the medulla oblongata showing the location of neurons involved in cardiovascular regulation (left) and in regulation of respiration (right), and the outline of the nucleus tractus solitarii (NTS) and area postrema (AP). *b1, b2, b3,* location of coronal sections in Figure 10.2b. (b) Parasagittal diagram of the VLM showing in schematic outline the topographical relation between nucleus ambiguus (NA$_C$, compact NA; NA$_{SC}$, subcompact NA), groups of respiratory neurons (Bötzinger complex [BötC], preBötzinger complex [preBötC], rostral ventral respiratory group [rVRG]) and cardiovascular neurons rostralventrolateral medulla [RVLM], caudal ventrolateral medulla [CVLM]). CPA, caudal pressor area; cVRG, caudal ventral respiratory group; FN, facial nucleus. (a) After Dobbins and Feldman (1994) and Sun and Panneton (2002); (b) modified from Rekling and Feldman (1998) with permission.

Negro et al. 2018]). The "cardiovascular" neurons in the VLM appear to be organized in a *continuous column* of neurons extending from the RVLM down to the CPA (Figure 10.4). Functionally different types of cardiovascular neurons *overlap* in their location. However, as shown schematically in Figures 10.2b and 10.3a, the rostrocaudal boundaries of cardiovascular and respiration-related groups of neurons do not exactly coincide (e.g., RVLM and Bötzinger complex; CVLM and rVRG). Furthermore, it must be kept in mind that the dendrites of cardiovascular and respiratory neurons intertwine. Finally, as already mentioned, the strict anatomical borders of nuclei as described by Paxinos and Watson (2014) do not need to be identical with the exact location of the functionally determined subdivisions of neuron assemblies (Note 7) (see Figure 10.3; for details see Schreihofer and Guyenet [2002]; Wang et al. [2002]; Weston et al. [2003]; Schreihofer and Sved [2011]):

1. The RVLM overlaps with the more dorsally located Bötzinger complex and also with part of the preBötzinger complex.
2. In the rostral part of the CVLM (sometimes called the intermediate part of the VLM [IVLM]), inhibitory interneurons are located, most of which are excited by baroreceptor afferents (see Subchapter 10.3). This region contains many neurons of the preBötzinger complex and neurons of the rVRG. Both groups of respiratory neurons are located dorsally to the cardiovascular neurons and ventrally to the parasympathetic cardiomotor neurons.
3. In the caudal part of the CVLM are located mainly sympathoinhibitory interneurons and probably sympathoexcitatory interneurons, which are independent of the baroreceptor afferents. This region contains respiratory neurons of the rVRG.
4. In the most caudal part of the VLM, the CPA, are located sympathoexcitatory interneurons. This

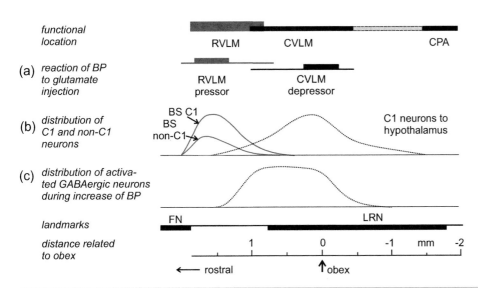

Figure 10.4 Schematic rostrocaudal distribution of the location of cardiovascular neurons in the ventrolateral medulla (VLM) with respect to the obex in the rat. The ventral landmarks are the facial nucleus (FN) and the lateral reticular nucleus (LRN). The dorsal landmark is the obex (see Note 5). Location of the rostral ventrolateral medulla (RVLM), caudal ventrolateral medulla (CVLM) and caudal pressor area (CPA) as in Figures 10.2b and 10.3a. (a) Effect of microinjection of glutamate on the arterial blood pressure (BP). (b) Distribution of adrenergic (C1) and non-adrenergic (non-C1) bulbospinal (BS) neurons. Dotted lines, distribution of C1 neurons projecting to hypothalamus and brainstem. (c) Distribution of GABAergic neurons activated during increase of BP. These neurons express c-Fos protein during activation of arterial baroreceptors generated by increase in blood pressure (see Note 1). After Schreihofer and Guyenet (2002) and Sun and Panneton (2002) for the CPA. This figure and Figure 10.3 are to the same distance scale. For references see text.

region overlaps with the caudal part of the cVRG. Cardiovascular neurons in the CPA have not been studied in detail (Sun and Panneton 2002, 2005).

10.2.3 The RVLM as a Sympathetic Cardiovascular Premotor Nucleus

The RVLM contains neurons that project to the sympathetic preganglionic neurons in the spinal cord (bulbospinal neurons; Figure 10.4). Depending on their main function, these neurons will be addressed in this subchapter either as *presympathetic neurons* or as *sympathetic premotor neurons*. Here I will describe the two functional aspects of these bulbospinal neurons:

1. The integrative function of the presympathetic neurons to protect the body in emergency situations. This is a hypothesis developed by Patrice Guyenet and his coworkers and is described in Box 10.2.
2. The role of the bulbospinal neurons as sympathetic premotor in the regulation of the cardiovascular system (neural regulation of resistance blood vessels and of the heart). These sympathetic premotor neurons are the coupling neurons

between sympathetic preganglionic neurons and the lower brainstem in the regulation of the cardiovascular system.

What is the evidence that the RVLM contains sympathetic premotor neurons (in addition to other types of projecting neurons and interneurons) that are important in the regulation of arterial blood pressure (see Dampney [1994, 2016]; Schreihofer and Guyenet [2002]; Schreihofer and Sved [2011]; Guyenet [2006])?:

- Bilateral lesions of the RVLM in the *anesthetized animal* are followed by an acute decrease in arterial blood pressure, sometimes to the same level as after transection of the spinal cord at the cervical spinal level (Dampney and Moon 1980; see Dampney [1994]; Blessing [1997]). However, using an optokinetic approach in *unanesthetized freely breathing rats* to silence the C1 neurons caused only a small reduction of blood pressure by a few mmHg (Wenker *et al.* 2017). This argues that the ongoing activity in C1 (and possibly non-C1) neurons in the RVLM contributes little to the resting activity in cardiovascular neurons

Box 10.2 | The Role of C1 Projection Neurons in the Ventrolateral Medulla to Protect the Body in Emergency Situations: A Hypothesis Formulated by Patrice Guyenet and Coworkers (Guyenet et al. 2013)

Projection neurons that are catecholaminergic and synthesize adrenaline are located in the ventrolateral medulla (VLM). They are characterized by the enzyme phenylethanolamine-N-methyltransferase (PNMT) that is necessary to convert noradrenaline into adrenaline. They also contain the other enzymes necessary to synthesize noradrenaline (tyrosine hydroxylase, dopamine-β-hydroxylase). These catecholaminergic neurons are called C1 neurons (Schreihofer and Guyenet 1997; Verberne et al. 1999). They are further characterized by various neuropeptides. However, it is unclear, but unlikely, that adrenaline and neuropeptides are released during excitation of the C1 neurons and are used as transmitters. Rather, glutamate is released during activation by C1 neurons and is used as the primary excitatory transmitter (Dampney 1994; Sun 1995; Guyenet et al. 2001; Pilowsky and Goodchild 2002; Stornetta et al., 2001, 2002). Some 33% of the C1 neurons in the rostral ventrolateral medulla (RVLM, Figure 10.4) project with their axons to the sympathetic preganglionic neurons and excite them when activated. These bulbospinal C1 neurons are barosensitive, i.e., they are inhibited during activation of the arterial baroreceptors by increased arterial blood pressure (see Figure 10.10 in Subchapter 10.3). C1 neurons within the RVLM that are located caudally to the bulbospinal C1 neurons project mostly to the hypothalamus (paraventricular nucleus, perifornical region, dorsomedial nucleus, and others), but not to the spinal cord (Figure 10.4).

Using a modified rabies virus tracing method, Stornetta et al. (2016) demonstrated in the mouse that C1 neurons innervating sympathetic preganglionic neurons in the spinal cord exhibit considerable collateral projections of their axons to various nuclei or regions of the brain stem (green in Figure 10.5) and receive monosynaptic input from neurons located mostly in these same nuclei or regions (blue in Figure 10.5). Furthermore, C1 neurons in the RVLM that do not project to the spinal cord but to other neuronal targets in the brain stem have to be postulated. C1 neurons projecting to the hypothalamus show axonal collateral projections to the brainstem nuclei and regions similar to the bulbospinal C1 neurons and receive similar monosynaptic afferent inputs (Stornetta et al. 2016). C1 neurons are most likely functionally differentiated with respect to the target neurons or neural circuits they innervate. Individual C1 neurons can project to more than one neuronal target. However, the number of functional subtypes of C1 neurons is not known.

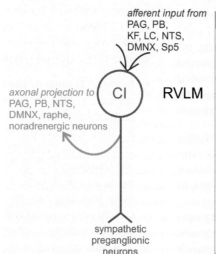

afferent input from
PAG, PB,
KF, LC, NTS,
DMNX, Sp5

axonal projection to
PAG, PB, NTS,
DMNX, raphe,
noradrenergic neurons

C1   RVLM

sympathetic
preganglionic
neurons

Figure 10.5 Axonal projection of, and first-order (monosynaptic) projection neurons to, bulbospinal C1 neurons in the rostral ventrolateral medulla (RVLM). Bulbospinal C1 neurons project collateral axonal branches to various nuclei or regions of the lower and upper brain stem (green). They receive synaptic input from neurons of nuclei or regions of the brain stem (blue), some receiving input from the collaterals of the C1 neurons (e.g., DMNX, NTS, PB, PAG). Interneurons located in or close to the RVLM and synapsing with the C1 neurons are not shown. For details see text. DMNX, dorsal motor nucleus of the vagus; KF, Kölliker–Fuse nucleus; LC, locus coeruleus; NTS, nucleus tractus solitarii; PAG, periaqueductal gray; PB, parabrachial nucleus; Sp5, spinal trigeminal tract. The figure is based on the data and argumentation of Stornetta et al. (2016).

With the exception of the bulbospinal sympathetic premotor C1 neurons that innervate sympathetic preganglionic cardiovascular neurons and possibly associated interneurons, our knowledge about the cellular mechanisms by which the C1 neurons activate their neuronal targets is poor. For example, the dorsal motor nucleus of the vagus (DMNX) contains the parasympathetic preganglionic neurons that are involved in regulation of motility, exocrine secretion, endocrine secretion and possibly immunological processes in the gastrointestinal tract (Figures 5.14, 8.10, 10.31; Subchapters 5.7 and 10.7). These preganglionic neurons must be functionally highly specific. How are they targeted and activated by the C1 neurons? The same reasoning applies to the nucleus tractus solitarii (NTS; Figure 8.14; Subchapter 8.3), which is the entrance gate to the CNS for visceral afferent

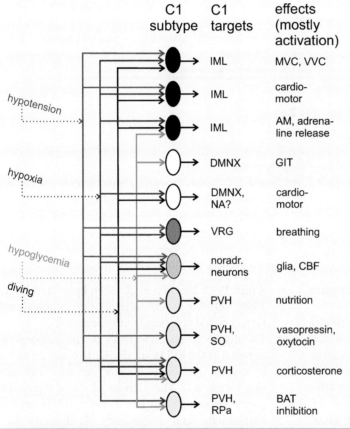

Figure 10.6 Differential recruitment of subsets of C1 neurons during emergency responses. Hypothetical scheme that illustrates how the differential recruitment of 11 subgroups of C1 neurons by hypotension, hypoxia, hypoglycemia or diving might produce a response pattern adapted to each situation of the body. The anatomical target of each type of C1 neuron and the postulated physiological effect produced by their activation are indicated. *Black:* responses mediated by C1 neurons that innervate sympathetic preganglionic neurons. *White:* responses mediated by C1 neurons that innervate parasympathetic preganglionic neurons. *Orange:* responses mediated by C1 neurons that innervate neurons of the respiratory pattern generator. *Gray:* responses mediated via activation of the CNS noradrenergic system (e.g., locus coeruleus). *Yellow:* responses mediated by C1 neurons that innervate the PVH and other hypothalamic regions. Figure and legend modified from Guyenet et al. (2013) with permission. Abbreviations: *C1 target:* DMNX, dorsal motor nucleus of the vagus; IML, nucleus intermediolateralis; NA, nucleus ambiguus; PVH, paraventricular nucleus of the hypothalamus; RPa, raphe pallidus; SO, supraoptic nucleus; VRG, ventral respiratory group. *Effects:* AM, adrenal medulla; BAT, brown adipose tissue; CBF, cerebral blood flow; GIT, gastrointestinal tract; MVC, muscle vasoconstrictor; VVC, visceral vasoconstrictor.

information from the thoracic and abdominal viscera, to the periaqueductal gray (PAG), to the parabrachial nucleus (PB) and to the other C1 neuronal targets.

What is the general function of the C1 neuron system? Guyenet, Stornetta and coworkers propagate the idea that the C1 neuron system prepares the organism to meet both internal and external threats, such as hypotension, hypoxia, hypoglycemia, hemorrhage, infection, general inflammation, noxious events and similar threatening events. These potentially dangerous bodily states produce characteristic protective patterns of responses. In initiating these protective functions, the C1 systems regulate and coordinate autonomic, neuroendocrine and immune reflexes. This is graphically expressed in Figure 10.6. The figure is an attempt to illustrate how the differential recruitment of 11 arbitrarily assumed subsets of C1 neurons might produce a response pattern that is adapted to each of the situations: hypotension, hypoxia, hypoglycemia or diving (although diving is not an emergency situation in the strict sense but a highly organized physiological response pattern observed in diving mammals [see Subchapter 11.3.1]). Each C1 neuron subtype is defined by the C1 target neuron to which the C1 neuron projects. These target neurons consist of preganglionic sympathetic or parasympathetic neurons, hypothalamic neurons, breathing neurons or central noradrenergic neurons.

Specific References for this Box

See further key references here.

Guyenet, P. G., Stornetta, R. L., Bochorishvili, G., et al. (2013) C1 neurons: the body's EMTs [emergency medical technicians]. *Am J Physiol Regul Integr Comp Physiol* **305**, R187–R204.

Stornetta, R. L., Inglis, M. A., Viar, K. E. and Guyenet, P. G. (2016) Afferent and efferent connections of C1 cells with spinal cord or hypothalamic projections in mice. *Brain Struct Funct* **221**, 4027–4044.

Stornetta, R. L. and Guyenet, P-G. (2018) C1 neurons: a nodal point for stress? *Exp Physiol* **103**, 332–336.

that are involved in regulation of blood pressure in awake rats (Note 8, Note 9).

- Bilateral inhibition of RVLM neurons by microinjection of an inhibitory amino acid or an analog of these amino acids (e.g., muscimol [a GABA agonist]) in anesthetized rats also leads to a fall in arterial blood pressure that is comparable to that after destruction of the RVLM (Ross et al. 1984b; Sun and Reis 1996; Morrison 1999; Schreihofer et al. 2000).

- Stimulation of the cell bodies in the RVLM by microinjection of glutamate generates an increase in arterial blood pressure and excites muscle, visceral and renal vasoconstrictor neurons (Ross et al. 1984b; Guyenet and Brown 1986; Schreihofer et al. 2000).

- The RVLM contains neurons that project to the intermediate zone (in particular the nucleus intermediolateralis) of the thoracolumbar spinal cord. Some of these sympathetic premotor neurons form monosynaptic connections with the preganglionic neurons (Milner et al. 1988; Zagon and Smith 1993; McAllen et al. 1994; Pyner and Coote 1998). Other connections may be di- or polysynaptic (via spinal autonomic interneurons).

- The discharge characteristics of the bulbospinal neurons in the RVLM are similar to those recorded in muscle and visceral vasoconstrictor neurons (see Figure 4.1). The activity of the sympathetic premotor neurons in the RVLM exhibits cardiac rhythmicity and respiratory rhythmicity (see Subchapter 10.6); they are inhibited by stimulation of arterial baroreceptors and excited by stimulation of arterial chemoreceptors (see Subchapter 10.5), nociceptors, and other receptors (Figure 10.7; see Guyenet [1990]; Dampney [1994]; Sun [1995]). A subgroup seems to behave like cutaneous vasoconstrictor neurons (McAllen 1992; McAllen and May 1994a).

Glutamate and GABA (in interneurons) are the fast primary (excitatory and inhibitory) transmitters to the sympathetic preganglionic neurons (Llewellyn-Smith et al. 1992, 1995, 1998). Whether a descending

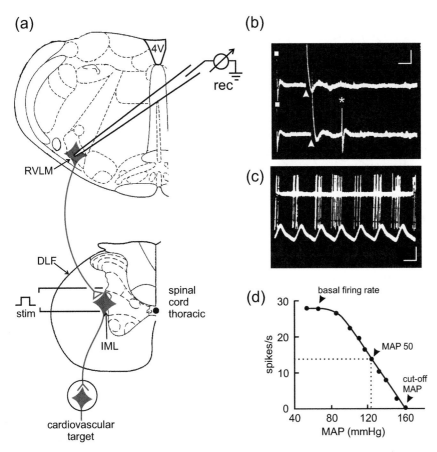

Figure 10.7 Identification and baroreceptor sensitivity of a sympathetic (bulbospinal) premotor neuron in the rostral ventrolateral medulla (RVLM) of the rat. (a) Recording (rec) the activity of a neuron in the RVLM with a microelectrode. Identification of the neuron by electrical stimulation of its axon projecting to the upper thoracic spinal cord (stim). DLF, dorsolateral funiculus; IML, intermediolateral nucleus; 4V, fourth ventricle. (b) Identification of a RVLM neuron as a bulbospinal neuron. The oscilloscope recording is triggered by spontaneous action potentials in the RVLM neuron (square). Electrical stimulation of the axon in the IML (arrow heads) with single pulses activates the neuron (marked by star) when the time interval between the orthodromic spontaneous action potential and the electrical stimulus is long (lower trace). The evoked antidromically conducting action potential collides with the orthodromically conducted spontaneous action potential when the time interval between the spontaneous action potential and the electrical stimulus is short (upper trace). Each recording five times superimposed. (c) Pulse-synchronous discharge (cardiac rhythmicity) of the RVLM neuron with the arterial pulse pressure wave (lower trace). Increased blood pressure leads to phasic inhibition of activity (six consecutive recordings superimposed). The phasic inhibition of the activity in the bulbospinal RVLM neuron starts about 50 ms after the onset of the systole. This delay in inhibition is due to the conduction time in axons of the baroreceptors, nucleus tractus solitarii neurons and neurons in the caudal ventrolateral medulla (see Figure 10.10). (d) Relation between discharge rate of an RVLM neuron (ordinate scale) and mean arterial blood pressure (MAP, abscissa scale). MAP 50, mean arterial pressure at 50% decrease in firing rate of the neuron. Time scale in (b) 5 ms and in (c) 120 ms. Vertical scale in (b) and (c) 0.5 mV. Modified from Sun and Guyenet (1985) with permission.

inhibitory pathway from the RVLM that uses GABA and/or glycine exists is very much debated but rather likely (see Miura et al. [1994]; Deuchars et al. [1997]; Whyment et al. [2004]; Stornetta et al. [2004]) (see Note 9).

Sympathetic premotor neurons in the RVLM obtain synaptic inputs from various nuclei in the brain stem and hypothalamus (CVLM, NTS, parabrachial nuclei and Kölliker–Fuse nucleus in the dorsolateral pons, periaqueductal gray [PAG], lateral hypothalamic area [LHA] and paraventricular nucleus of the hypothalamus [PVH], uvula [lobule IXb of posterior vermis of the cerebellum] [Silva-Carvalho et al.

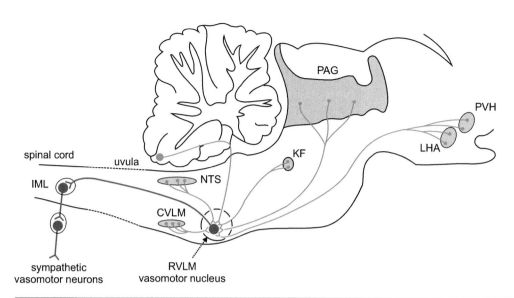

Figure 10.8 Major extrinsic synaptic inputs to sympathetic (bulbospinal) premotor neurons of the rostral ventrolateral medulla (RVLM). CVLM, caudal ventrolateral medulla; IML, intermediolateral nucleus; KF, Kölliker–Fuse nucleus; LHA, lateral hypothalamic area; NTS, nucleus tractus solitarii; PAG, periaqueductal gray of the mesencephalon; PVH, paraventricular nucleus of the hypothalamus. The sympathetic premotor neurons also receive various synaptic inputs from interneurons intrinsic to the RVLM. Modified from Dampney (1994).

1991]) and from interneurons within the RVLM (Stornetta et al. 2016). Interneurons are more frequent in the RVLM than sympathetic (bulbospinal) premotor neurons (Schreihofer et al. 1999), but seem to be rare in the corresponding subretrofacial nucleus of the cat (see Note 6; Polson et al. 1992) (Figure 10.8). Neurons in these nuclei mediate various reflexes elicited by stimulation of cardiovascular afferents (see Subchapters 10.3 and 10.5), pulmonary afferents, trigeminal afferents, nociceptive afferents and other afferents. Furthermore, they involve the RVLM in various complex homeostatic control systems and behaviors that are controlled from the upper brain stem, hypothalamus and cerebral hemispheres (e.g., defense behaviors, thermoregulation, exercise, etc.; for review see Dampney [1994, 2016]).

The synaptic inputs to RVLM neurons are excitatory or inhibitory and use glutamate, GABA and possibly other yet unknown substances as primary transmitters. Many neuropeptides, such as angiotensin II, are colocalized in neurons that form synapses with the bulbospinal RVLM neurons. The nature of the function of these peptides is now beginning to be characterized.

Sympathetic premotor neurons in the RVLM are topographically organized with respect to the functional type of vascular target innervated by the sympathetic neurons but *not* with respect to the body region. This has been demonstrated in the *cat* for the subretrofacial nucleus in the RVLM (Lovick 1987; McAllen et al. 1995, 1997). Subpopulations of sympathetic premotor neurons (and other neurons) in this nucleus were microstimulated by microinjection of small amounts of the excitatory amino acid glutamate and activity was recorded from postganglionic neurons innervating different vascular beds, or effector responses were recorded. Sympathetic renal vasoconstrictor premotor neurons or interneurons that activate the latter (RVC in Figure 10.9) are located most rostrally and sympathetic muscle premotor vasoconstrictor neurons (MVC) most caudally; sympathetic visceral premotor vasoconstrictor neurons (which regulate the mesenteric vascular bed; VVC) are located lateral to the renal neurons and sympathetic cutaneous vasoconstrictor premotor neurons (CVC) medial to the MVC neurons (Figure 10.9). Sympathetic cardiomotor premotor neurons (or interneurons that activate them) are situated in a territory rostromedial to and overlap with the sympathetic premotor neurons controlling blood flow through skeletal muscle (Lovick 1987; Campos and McAllen 1997; not shown in Figure 10.9). Furthermore, sympathetic premotor neurons controlling the adrenal medulla are located in the most rostral

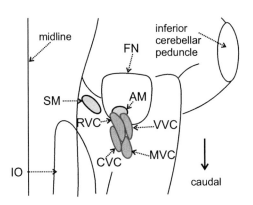

Figure 10.9 Viscerotopic organization of sympathetic premotor neurons in the subretrofacial cell column of the rostral ventrolateral medulla (RVLM) of the cat. Ventral view of the cat's left medulla oblongata showing the surface structures, inferior olive (IO) and facial nucleus (FN). The premotor neurons are organized according to the functional type of the neurons and not according to body region. The approximate locations of the premotor neurons overlap. AM, sympathetic premotor neurons associated with the adrenal medulla (release of adrenaline); CVC, cutaneous vasoconstrictor; MVC, muscle vasoconstrictor; RVC, renal vasoconstrictor; VVC, visceral vasoconstrictor (mesenteric vascular bed). Also indicated is the location of sympathetic sudomotor premotor neurons (SM). Derived from Lovick (1987), Dampney and McAllen (1988) and McAllen and May (1994a, b). Modified from McAllen et al. (1995) with permission.

part of the RVLM (Lovick 1987; see Pyner and Coote [1998]). Thus, subpopulations of sympathetic vasoconstrictor premotor neurons projecting to the respective functional types of preganglionic neurons in the spinal cord exhibit distinct though overlapping locations in the RVLM. Finally, sympathetic premotor neurons controlling sweat glands (SM) appear to be situated rostromedially to the cardiovascular premotor neurons (McAllen et al. 1995).

A similar topographic organization is also present in the RVLM of rabbits (Ootsuka and Terui 1997). Furthermore, using morphological tracing methods, it has been shown that this type of organization may also apply to the rat (Pyner and Coote 1998) although systematic functional studies in this species have not been done (Note 10).

10.2.4 Origin of Spontaneous Activity in Bulbospinal Neurons of the RVLM

An extensively discussed, controversial and unsolved issue is the origin of spontaneous (tonic) activity in the sympathetic premotor neurons of the RVLM. This spontaneous activity contributes to the ongoing activity in sympathetic cardiovascular neurons, which innervate resistance vessels (MVC, VVC, RVC neurons) or the heart. It therefore determines the height of the arterial blood pressure. Based on experimental results, alternative theories are (Dampney et al. 2000):

1. In vitro, the spontaneous activity of sympathetic premotor neurons in the RVLM is the result of intrinsic pacemaker properties of the neurons (Accorsi-Mendonca et al. 2016). Experiments on transverse sections of the lower brain stem at the level of the RVLM have shown that some RVLM neurons exhibit activity and generate action potentials after complete blockade of all synaptic inputs to the cells. This firing fulfills the criteria of intrinsic pacemaker properties (Note 11) (Sun et al. 1988a, b; see Guyenet [1990]; Sun [1995]). Using extracellular recordings from sympathetic premotor neurons in the RVLM in a working-heart-brain-stem preparation (WHBP; Paton 1996a, b) of rats three to four weeks of age, Allen could show that these neurons can generate activity (regular firing, bursting activity) without any synaptic input (Andrew Allen, personal communication). However, other intracellular measurements in sympathetic premotor RVLM neurons, performed in in vivo and in vitro experiments, could not confirm that these neurons have intrinsic pacemaker properties (Lipski et al. 1996, 1998). The ionic channels maintaining tonic activity in the neurons of the RVLM may involve low-voltage-activated calcium channels (T-type channels). Blockade of these channels (bilaterally in the RVLM) reduces spontaneous activity in the splanchnic nerve and arterial blood pressure, but does not change reflexes mediated by the RVLM (Miyawaki et al. 2003). The RVLM neurons may only show pacemaker-like activity under extreme pathophysiological conditions, e.g., when all synaptic inputs to these neurons are blocked or fail. In this case the capacity of the RVLM neurons to generate pacemaker activity may be a last "line of defense" to generate tonic activity in cardiovascular neurons to maintain arterial blood pressure (Lipski et al. 2002).

2. The spontaneous activity of the sympathetic premotor neurons in the RVLM is the result of the emergent properties of the neuronal networks and therefore depends on the inhibitory and excitatory synaptic connections between the neurons of the network, the underlying synaptic currents

and the intrinsic chemosensitivity of the neurons (related to arterial P_{CO2}, P_{O2} and pH). Thus, the generation of spontaneous activity in the sympathetic premotor neurons of the RVLM (and therefore the so-called sympathetic vasomotor and cardiomotor tone) would be generated by a neuronal network that is coupled synaptically with the RVLM neurons (Lipski et al. 2002). Evidence for the existence of such a neural network associated with the RVLM is missing. The caudal pressor area (CPA) in the caudal part of the -VLM (Figure 10.3a) may be important for the generation of activity of sympathetic premotor neurons in the RVLM. Inhibition of the activity in neurons of the CPA decreases arterial blood pressure and activity in the renal nerve to the same degree as transection of the cervical spinal cord (Possas et al. 1994; Horiuchi and Dampney 2002) and reduces the activity of the sympathetic premotor neurons in the RVLM. Whether this is generated by reduction of excitatory synaptic activity to, or by synaptic disinhibition of, the neurons in the RVLM is controversial (Natarajan and Morrison 2000; Horiuchi and Dampney 2002) (Note 12). However, what is the origin of the activity of the neurons in the CPA?

3. The RVLM neurons receive several excitatory glutamatergic synaptic inputs. Additionally, many neurons that synapse with RVLM neurons contain neuropeptides. Furthermore, substances, which are probably of non-neural cellular origin, such as nitric oxide (NO) and angiotensin II are released in the RVLM (angiotensin II also from nerve terminals). It is hypothesized that neuropeptides and local substances of unclear cellular origin modulate the excitability of the RVLM bulbospinal neurons and their synaptic inputs in a paracrine way and contribute to or are mainly responsible for the level of spontaneous activity ("tone") in sympathetic cardiovascular neurons (see Guyenet and Stornetta [1997]).

Several points in regard to the spontaneous (tonic) activity in autonomic neurons and its underlying mechanism and origin need to be emphasized:

- Practically all experimental approaches addressing the origin of spontaneous activity in autonomic neurons have concentrated so far on activity in sympathetic neurons supplying resistance vessels (in skeletal muscle, viscera including kidney) or heart.

- Many vasoconstrictor neurons innervating blood vessels in skin or skeletal muscle and sudomotor neurons develop spontaneous activity weeks and months after transection of the spinal cord at the cervical level (Horeyseck and Jänig 1974; Jänig and Spilok 1978; Jänig and Kümmel 1981; see Subchapter 9.2). Intracellular measurements in sympathetic preganglionic neurons of cats with the spinal cord acutely transected at the cervical level show subthreshold spontaneous synaptically evoked activity (mainly excitatory postsynaptic potentials) (Dembowsky et al. 1985). The ongoing synaptic activity may be related to electrical coupling between sympathetic preganglionic neurons by gap junctions. In slices, these neurons may exhibit spontaneous membrane oscillations that are transmitted to neighboring preganglionic neurons by electrical coupling. This may be a mechanism of synchronization of activity in sympathetic preganglionic neurons (Logan et al. 1996; Nolan et al. 1999). However, this coupling may only occur during development and disappear later.

- Spontaneous activity in cutaneous vasoconstrictor neurons probably depends, under normal conditions, on the activity in both premotor neurons of the RVLM and premotor neurons of the caudal raphe nuclei (McAllen, personal communication; see Subchapter 10.5 and Figure 10.17).

- Sympathetic premotor cardiovascular neurons have a target-specific viscerotopic organization in the RVLM (Figure 10.9). This organization might imply that activity in functionally different types of sympathetic neuron, which are involved in cardiovascular regulation or regulation of the adrenal medulla, can be selectively altered.

- Spontaneous activity in sympathetic non-vasoconstrictor neurons (Table 4.3; e.g., inspiration-type neurons, motility-regulating neurons, pupillomotor neurons, sudomotor neurons) probably has an entirely different central origin compared to the origin of spontaneous activity in vasoconstrictor neurons or sympathetic cardiomotor neurons. Spontaneous activity in sympathetic motility-regulating neurons may originate in the spinal cord (Bartel et al. 1986).

- The origin of spontaneous activity in parasympathetic neurons, including parasympathetic cardiomotor neurons (Table 4.6) is practically unknown.

In *conclusion*, the excitatory drive to vasoconstrictor neurons innervating resistance vessels and to sympathetic cardiomotor neurons originates partly from RVLM neurons (bulbospinal neurons and/or local interneurons synaptically connected with the bulbo-spinal neurons). This input is predominant under anesthesia, but its contribution in the absence of anesthesia is unclear. The origin of the ongoing activity of the RVLM premotor neurons remains largely unexplained and likely depends on local factors released by astrocytes or the vasculature or on inputs from multiple nuclei of the brain stem (e.g., raphe nuclei, catecholaminergic nuclei [A2, A5]), hypothalamus (e.g., paraventricular nucleus) or even the spinal cord (see Subchapter 9.2). Thus, a key problem of neural regulation of arterial blood pressure in health and disease (hypertension!), in which physiologists have been interested since Claude Bernard and Carl Ludwig in the middle of the nineteenth century, remains unsolved up to the present time.

The results show, furthermore, that discussion about the origin of spontaneous activity in sympathetic neurons should not be restricted to the RVLM. Spontaneous activity in other functional types of sympathetic and parasympathetic neurons most likely has different origins, depending on the functional type of neuron. Therefore, I find it inappropriate to use the terms sympathetic or parasympathetic "tone" in a generalized way. Spontaneous activity in autonomic systems should always be specified with respect to the functional system involved and this most likely also applies to the systems represented in the RVLM (Figure 10.8).

10.3 Baroreceptor Reflexes and Blood Pressure Control

10.3.1 Detection of Baroreceptor Reflexes

Arterial baroreceptor reflexes have fascinated cardiovascular physiologists since the second half of the nineteenth century. Cyon and Ludwig (1866) were the first to report that stimulation of the central end of the cut aortic nerve in the rabbit causes a decrease in arterial blood pressure and heart rate. They coined the term "nervus depressor" for the aortic nerve. They assumed that they stimulated afferent nerve fibers in the aortic (depressor) nerve that were linked to cardiac receptors that record intracardiac pressure. They concluded from their experiments that the decrease in arterial blood pressure following stimulation of the aortic nerve is generated by a decrease in activity (tonus) in the vascular nerves. They missed detecting that bradycardia is also generated by a reflex. These experimental results were confirmed by several experimenters in the next decades. In the 1920s Heymans and Ladon (see Heymans and Neil [1958]) performed their famous cross-perfusion experiments on dogs, finally proving that bradycardia is a reflex elicited via the vasomotor centers by activation of afferent fibers innervating the aortic arch.

The situation was more difficult for reflexes elicited by stimulation of the baroreceptors in the carotid sinus nerve. Up to the first half of the 1920s, the rise of blood pressure and heart rate after occlusion of the common carotid arteries was thought to be generated by anemia of those parts of the brain that are supplied by the carotid arteries (for a detailed description see Heymans and Neil [1958]). This situation changed dramatically when Hering performed his experiments on dogs, in which he showed that electrical stimulation of the carotid sinus nerve (which later became known as Hering's nerve) or mechanical stimulation of the carotid sinus decreases heart rate and arterial blood pressure. He formulated the concept of the baroreceptor reflex, i.e., that decreases in heart rate and blood pressure are generated by stimulation of carotid sinus afferents and mediated by reflexes via the vasomotor center (Hering 1927). It then took another 30 years to work out details about the baroreceptor reflexes, in particular the functional characteristics of the arterial baroreceptors and of their reflex effects (see Heymans and Neil [1958] for a detailed and careful description of this development). In the 1980s, various laboratories began to explore the organization of the baroreceptor reflexes in the CNS (see Guyenet [1990]; Dampney [1994]; Pilowsky and Goodchild [2002]).

10.3.2 Function of Arterial Baroreceptor Reflexes

Arterial baroreceptor afferents with *myelinated nerve fibers* encode in their activity the instantaneous level of arterial blood pressure and the rate of change of arterial blood pressure. They adapt rapidly (in less than an hour) to a change in the mean level of the arterial blood pressure, i.e., they undergo acute resetting. Thus, their main function is to encode in their activity the pressure range between diastolic and systolic blood pressures, irrespective of whether the mean pressure is low or high (Coleridge et al. 1981; Dorward et al. 1982; for review see Koushanpour [1991]). Arterial baroreceptors with *unmyelinated nerve fibers*, which have been less well studied, behave differently: they do not adapt to long-term changes in arterial blood pressure, i.e., do not exhibit resetting. Thus, these baroreceptor afferents may be responsible for signaling systemic arterial blood pressure to the nucleus tractus solitarii (NTS) in their rate of activity and therefore also for long-term changes in the level of the mean arterial blood pressure (Seagard et al. 1992). Vagal mechano-sensitive cardiovascular afferent neurons innervating the heart (notably the right atrium), which are involved in volume regulation, may be important for regulation of the level of the arterial blood pressure (Kirchheim et al. 1998).

Since the 1970s it has been believed that the function of the baroreceptor reflexes is to minimize the fluctuations of arterial blood pressure during various actions of the body (e.g., exercise, change of position of the body in the gravity of the Earth, mental activity, etc.), but not to regulate the level of blood pressure (Cowley et al. 1973; Persson et al. 1988; for review see Cowley [1992]). This belief was mainly based on continuous measurements of arterial blood pressure over three to five days in dogs with chronic denervation of the arterial (sinoaortic) baroreceptors. These dogs exhibited tremendous fluctuation of mean arterial blood pressure during their normal behavior but the average level of arterial blood pressure over 24 hours did not change or increased very little (Cowley et al. 1973). Later these experiments were reproduced using the same animal model (dogs) and also in rats (Norman et al. 1981; Persson et al. 1988). Additional denervation of the cardiopulmonary receptors leads to a long-term increase of arterial blood pressure (Persson et al. 1988). Denervation of the arterial (sinoaortic) baroreceptors in baboons leads chronically to a small increase in arterial blood pressure (Shade et al. 1990).

The dogma that arterial baroreceptors are not important in the regulation of long-term mean arterial blood pressure was seriously challenged if not refuted by Thrasher (Thrasher 2002, 2005a, b). He used dogs in which the aortic baroreceptors and the carotid sinus baroreceptors on one side were chronically denervated but leaving the carotid sinus baroreceptors on the other side intact. These dogs exhibited normal levels of mean arterial blood pressure. However, unloading of the remaining intact arterial baroreceptors by occlusion of the common carotid artery proximal to the innervated carotid sinus over seven days generated an immediate increase in arterial blood pressure and heart rate, both remaining high during the seven days of occlusion. Both returned to normal control levels after removal of the occlusion. This experiment clearly shows that arterial baroreceptors are *also* important in signaling mean long-term arterial blood pressure to the lower brain stem (see Thrasher [2005b] for a critical interpretation of his key experiments in relation to those conducted by Cowley et al. [1973]) (Note 13).

Several arterial baroreceptor reflex pathways are related to the parasympathetic and sympathetic cardiomotor neurons and to the different types of vasoconstrictor neuron innervating resistance vessels (mainly in skeletal muscle, kidney, other viscera). Phasic stimulation of the arterial baroreceptors in the carotid sinus and aortic arch with each heart beat leads to phasic activation of the parasympathetic cardiomotor neurons (McAllen and Spyer 1978) and to phasic inhibition of the sympathetic cardiomotor and vasoconstrictor neurons innervating resistance vessels. This is reflected in phasic changes in the activity of these peripheral cardiovascular neurons linked to the pulse pressure wave. This has been recorded in anesthetized and awake animals and humans (see cardiac rhythmicity of the activity in muscle vasoconstrictor neurons in Figures 4.1, 4.7 and 4.8), but not in other autonomic neurons that do not innervate resistance vessels (e.g., most cutaneous vasoconstrictor neurons innervating blood vessels in the distal skin of the extremities; sympathetic neurons innervating sweat glands or non-vascular visceral targets; see Note 14).

Some neuronal components of the baroreceptor pathways have been worked out. Figure 10.10 demonstrates a model of these baroreceptor reflex pathways that is commonly accepted. The diagram shows the essential circuitry for the baroreceptor reflex pathways, although alternative pathways may exist, as discussed below. Baroreceptor afferent neurons project to the caudal NTS (Figure 8.11). However, as already mentioned in Chapter 8, there exists no *obvious* viscerotopic organization of the second-order neurons in the caudal NTS with respect to the synaptic inputs from arterial baroreceptors, arterial chemoreceptors and gastrointestinal receptors (Paton 1999; Paton and Kasparov 2000; Andresen and Paton 2011) although there is a rough topography with respect to the projection of cardiovascular, gastrointestinal and respiratory afferent neurons to the NTS. Neurophysiological and morphological investigations of neurons in the NTS, using whole-cell patch-clamp recording in a working-heart-brain-stem preparation of the rat, clearly show that subgroups of NTS neurons are functionally almost entirely specific with respect to their afferent synaptic input from arterial baroreceptors, or arterial chemoreceptors or from receptors in the gastrointestinal tract. Only a few NTS neurons receive convergent excitatory synaptic inputs from arterial baro- and chemoreceptors, these being probably higher order neurons that received input from second-order neurons (Deuchars et al. 2000; Paton et al. 2000, 2001). Figure 10.11 demonstrates one of the first intracellular recordings from an NTS neuron that was activated by stimulation of arterial baroreceptors in the carotid sinus (Figure 10.11c, increase of carotid sinus pressure [CSP]) and identified morphologically.

10.3.3 Baroreceptor Pathway to Parasympathetic Cardiomotor Neurons

The baroreceptor pathway to the parasympathetic preganglionic cardiomotor neurons is most likely disynaptic and comparatively simple. Stimulation of arterial baroreceptors excites second-order neurons in the NTS and this in turn excites the parasympathetic preganglionic cardiomotor neurons in the external formation of the NA (see Figure 10.2a) leading to a decrease in heart rate. The transmitter from the baroreceptor afferents to the NTS neurons is glutamate and from the NTS neurons to the parasympathetic cardiomotor neurons probably also glutamate (Neff et al. 1998; Weston et al. 2003; Figure 10.10 left).

10.3.4 Baroreceptor Pathways to Sympathetic Cardiovascular Neurons

Inhibition in the RVLM

The presently most accepted baroreceptor reflex pathway to the sympathetic preganglionic cardiomotor and vasoconstrictor neurons has four synapses (Figure 10.10 right). The inhibition in this pathway occurs in the RVLM by GABAergic interneurons that are located mainly in the rostral part of the CVLM (Figures 10.2a, 10.4), i.e., at the level of the obex and rostral to it. Stimulation of arterial baroreceptors excites second-order neurons in the NTS, which project to the CVLM and excite the GABAergic interneurons synaptically. It is unclear whether these NTS neurons and those mediating the baroreceptor reflexes to the parasympathetic cardiomotor neurons are identical. What are the arguments that the inhibition in these baroreceptor pathways to the final sympathetic cardiovascular pathways occurs in the RVLM, that it is GABAergic and that it is mediated by interneurons in the rostral part of the CVLM that are monosynaptically activated by second-order neurons in the NTS? (See Guyenet [1990]; Dampney [1994]; Blessing [1997]; Pilowsky and Goodchild [2002] and Schreihofer and Guyenet [2002] for discussion and references.)

- Sympathetic premotor neurons in the RVLM are inhibited during an increase in blood pressure (which excites arterial baroreceptors). This inhibition is absent after denervation of the arterial baroreceptors and is reversibly blocked by ionophoretic application of a GABA-receptor antagonist (e.g., bicuculline) to the RVLM (Figures 10.7, 10.12).

- Activation of arterial baroreceptor afferents (by electrical stimulation of the aortic nerve [which is thought to contain only baroreceptor afferents in the rat] or by increase in arterial blood pressure) inhibits activity in "sympathetic" nerves (e.g., renal or major splanchnic nerves). An experimentally induced decrease in arterial blood pressure (which reduces the activity in arterial baroreceptors and the inhibition of RVLM neurons) generates a reflex increase in activity in "sympathetic" nerves. These reflexes are abolished after bilateral blockade of the GABA receptors in the RVLM (e.g., by ionophoretic application of bicuculline).

- Activity of barosensitive sympathetic premotor neurons in the RVLM is pulse-modulated in the same way as the activity in neurons of the sympathetic pathways innervating resistance vessels or the heart (Figures 4.1, 10.7c).

- Stimulation of neurons in the CVLM by microinjection of glutamate inhibits neurons in the

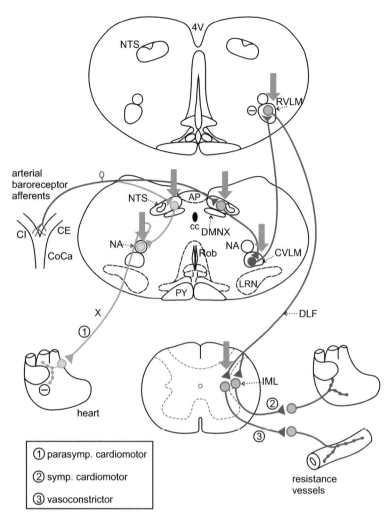

① parasymp. cardiomotor

② symp. cardiomotor

③ vasoconstrictor

Figure 10.10 Arterial baroreceptor reflex pathways. The output pathways are the parasympathetic cardiomotor (PCM) neurons (to pacemaker cells, atria and atrioventricular nodes of the heart), sympathetic cardiomotor (SCM) neurons (to pacemaker cells, atria and ventricles) and vasoconstrictor neurons (VC) innervating resistance vessels. Arterial baroreceptor afferents in the carotid bifurcation and aortic arch project to the nucleus tractus solitarii (NTS). Their activity encodes the mean arterial blood pressure and the rate of change of blood pressure. *Left*: parasympathetic baroreceptor reflex pathway to the heart. Excitatory second-order neurons of the NTS project to the preganglionic PCM neurons in the external formation of the nucleus ambiguus (NA). Activation of the baroreceptors leads to activation of the PCM neurons and subsequently to a decrease in heart rate (by inhibition of the pacemaker cells). *Right*: sympathetic baroreceptor pathways to the heart and the resistance blood vessels in skeletal muscle, kidney and other viscera (muscle, visceral and renal vasoconstrictor neurons). These baroreceptor pathways consist of a chain of at least three neurons between the baroreceptor afferents and the preganglionic neurons in the intermediolateral nucleus (IML). Sympathetic premotor neurons are located in the rostral ventrolateral medulla (RVLM), project through the dorsolateral funiculus (DLF) of the spinal cord to the preganglionic SCM and VC neurons and excite these neurons. These sympathetic premotor pathways, projecting through the DLF, are probably distinct for different final cardiovascular pathways (see Figure 10.9). Excitatory second-order neurons of the NTS project to inhibitory interneurons in the caudal ventrolateral medulla (CVLM). These inhibitory interneurons project to the sympathetic premotor neurons in the RVLM and inhibit them. Thus, activation of arterial baroreceptors leads to a decrease in activity in the SCM and VC neurons by inhibition of the neurons in the RVLM. The transmitter mediating this inhibition is GABA (γ-aminobutyric acid). The transmitter at all other central synapses of the baroreceptor pathways is glutamate. Ongoing activity in the SCM and VC neurons has its origin in the RVLM and elsewhere (see text). Signal transmission through the baroreceptor pathways can be modulated (inhibited, enhanced) from other centers in the brain stem, hypothalamus and telencephalon at all synapses (see blue arrows). AP, area postrema; cc, central canal; CE, external carotid artery; CI, internal carotid artery; CoCa, common carotid artery; DMNX, dorsal motor nucleus of the vagus nerve; LRN, lateral reticular nucleus; PY, pyramidal tract; Rob, raphe obscurus; 4V, fourth ventricle. Modified from Guyenet (1990) with permission.

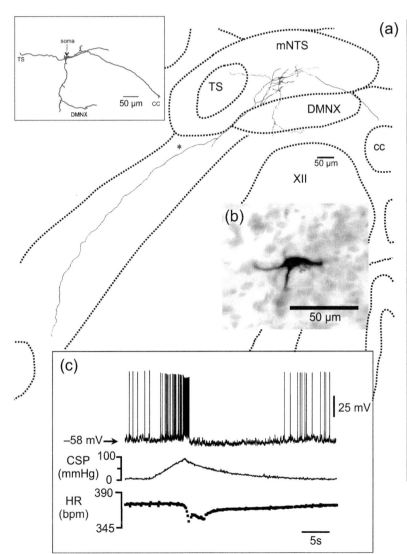

(a)

mNTS

TS

DMNX

cc

50 μm

XII

(b)

50 μm

(c)

25 mV

−58 mV→

CSP
(mmHg)

100

0

HR
(bpm)

390

345

5s

soma

TS

50 μm cc

DMNX

Figure 10.11 Functional identification and morphological characterization of a baroreceptive neuron in the nucleus tractus solitarii (NTS) in the rat. The neuron was recorded in a working-heart-brain-stem preparation (WHBP, Paton 1996a, b) using whole-cell patch-clamp recording from NTS neurons. After identification of the neuron as barosensitive it was filled with neurobiotin through the patch-clamp electrode. The neuron was reconstructed from histologically processed serial sections of 60 to 80 μm thickness. (a) The labeled soma and dendrites were located medial to the tractus solitarius (TS). Dendrites extended into the TS, into the dorsal motor nucleus of the vagus (DMNX) and across the medial NTS, where one dendrite ran close to the central canal (cc) (see upper inset left). The axon of the neuron (*) ramified in the region of the soma in the NTS and also projected toward the ventral regions of the medulla. (b) Photomicrograph illustrating the filled cell soma in a Nissl-stained section. (c) Stimulation of arterial baroreceptors by increase in carotid sinus pressure (CSP) resulted in activation of the neuron. Heart rate (HR in beats per minute [bpm]) decreased reflexly. Scale bar 50 μm. XII, hypoglossus; mNTS, medial nucleus tractus solitarii. Modified from Deuchars et al. (2000) with permission.

RVLM and sympathetic cardiovascular neurons (Figure 10.4).

- Bilateral blockade of glutamatergic transmission or functional inactivation of the neurons (e.g., by a GABA-receptor agonist) in the rostral part of the CVLM blocks the baroreceptor reflexes.
- The CVLM contains GABAergic neurons that project to the RVLM. These neurons are activated by stimulation of arterial baroreceptors and exhibit a high degree of pulse-modulated activity ("cardiac rhythmicity") (Figure 10.13b), as do bulbospinal neurons in the RVLM (see Figure 10.7) and pre- and postganglionic vasoconstrictor neurons involved in blood pressure regulation (see

Figures 4.1, 4.7, 4.8) (Jeske et al. 1993; Schreihofer and Guyenet 2002, 2003).

- Sustained increase of arterial blood pressure in awake or anesthetized rats or rabbits (e.g., produced by an α_1-adrenoceptor agonist) induces expression of *c-fos* mRNA and protein in neurons of the CVLM (see Note 1). Many of these neurons contain GABA and project to the RVLM (Li and Dampney 1994; Polson et al. 1995; Minson et al. 1997; Chan and Sawchenko 1998; Schreihofer and Guyenet 2002, 2003).
- Stimulation of arterial baroreceptors by sustained increase of arterial blood pressure activates second-order neurons in the NTS dorsomedial and medial to the tractus solitarii and in the commissural

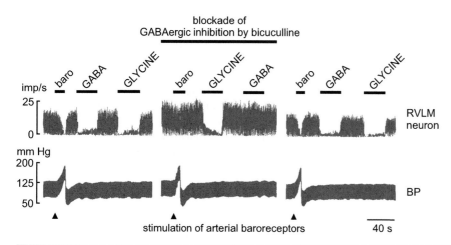

Figure 10.12 Baroreceptor reflex and γ-aminobutyric acid (GABA)-mediated inhibition of a sympathetic premotor neuron in the rostral ventrolateral medulla (RVLM). Recording from a single vasomotor neuron in the RVLM in the anesthetized rat (see Figure 10.5) with a multibarrel glass microelectrode allowing ionophoretic ejection of GABA, glycine (both inhibitory transmitters) or bicuculline (GABA-receptor antagonist) into the RVLM during recording within 40 μm of the cell body. The neuron is spontaneously active. Raising arterial blood pressure (BP, produced by constriction of the descending aorta) inhibits the activity of the neuron. Application of GABA or glycine inhibits the discharge too. During application of bicuculline, blocking the GABAergic transmission, both the inhibition during BP increase and that during GABA application are blocked but not the inhibition during application of glycine. Modified from Sun and Guyenet (1985) with permission.

nucleus (Figure 8.11). This activation is most likely monosynaptic. Some of these NTS neurons project to the CVLM; they are glutamatergic (Czachurski et al. 1988; Deuchars et al. 2000; Weston et al. 2003). The baroreceptor-sensitive NTS neurons that project to the CVLM may be those with pulse-modulated activity. But this population of neurons represents only a minority of the baroreceptor-sensitive neurons in the NTS (Deuchars et al. 2000) (Note 15).

The model of the baroreceptor pathways linked to the sympathetic and parasympathetic cardiovascular final pathways, as outlined in Figure 10.10, was synthesized on the basis of many experiments in several laboratories. It is a minimal model and there remain several open questions to be solved as far as synaptic transmission in the different "relay nuclei" (NTS, CVLM, RVLM, intermediolateral nucleus [IML]; see Figure 10.10), the specificity of these transmissions and alternative reflex pathways are concerned.

Experimental studies using *c-fos* gene expression show that there is evidence for additional baroreceptor pathways in the medulla oblongata:

(1) Barosensitive NTS neurons may project directly to the RVLM and inhibit, via local inhibitory (GABAergic) interneurons, sympathetic premotor neurons. (2) Inhibitory (GABAergic) interneurons may project to the CVLM and inhibit excitatory interneurons that project to the RVLM and activate sympathetic premotor neurons (Dampney and Horiuchi 2003). It has yet to be shown how important these alternative pathways are in relation to the pathways outlined in Figure 10.10 (Note 16).

Inhibition in the Spinal Cord

Experiments on rats and cats show that activity in sympathetic preganglionic neurons can be inhibited during stimulation of arterial baroreceptors by activation of spinal inhibitory interneurons. This possibility is not supported by most investigators (see Pilowsky and Goodchild [2002]) and has apparently been refuted in experiments conducted by Goodchild et al. (2000). However, I believe that it cannot be ignored that inhibition of activity in sympathetic neurons generated by stimulation of arterial baroreceptors may also occur at the level of the spinal cord, *first*, in view of several pieces of (mostly older) experimental data

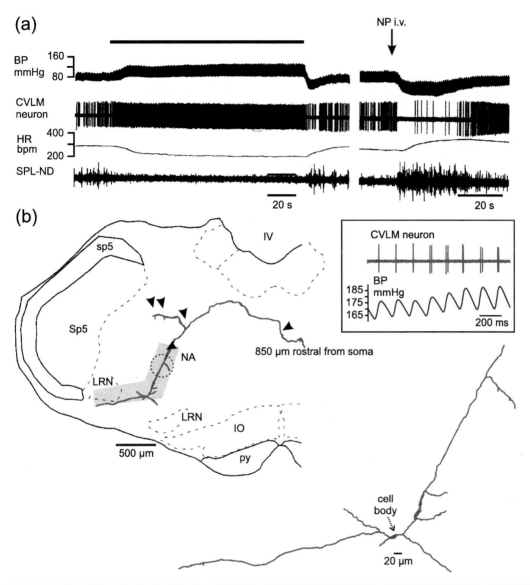

Figure 10.13 Physiology and morphology of a barosensitive neuron in the caudal ventrolateral medulla (CVLM). Experiment on a chloralose-anesthetized, artificially ventilated and immobilized rat. (a) Stimulation of arterial baroreceptors (bar; during increase of arterial blood pressure [BP] produced by constriction of the subdiaphragmatic aorta) activated the neuron. The activity in the major splanchnic nerve (splanchnic nerve discharge [SPL-ND], which occurs in visceral vasoconstrictor neurons) was inhibited and the heart rate (HR) decreased. Decrease of BP by intravenous injection of nitroprusside (NP i.v. 5 μg/kg), which dilates blood vessels (arrow), leads to unloading of arterial baroreceptors, decrease of activity in the CVLM neuron, increase of HR and increase of SPL-ND. *Inset*: pulse modulation of activity of a CVLM neuron during constriction of the descending aorta (see high BP; CVLM neuron different from that in [a]). (b) The CVLM neuron in (a) was filled through the microelectrode with biotinamide (using a juxtacellular labeling method; see Note 3). The biotinamide distributed intracellularly through the axon and dendrites of the neuron. The medulla oblongata was removed after perfusing the rat with the fixative formaldehyde and cut in 30 μm thick coronal serial sections. The labeled neuron was reconstructed from the serial sections. The axon and its collaterals (see arrow heads indicating branching points) projected dorsomedially and rostrally (in the direction of the RVLM). The lower right is a magnified view of this reconstructed neuron (see shaded part in coronal section; note the small cell body; axon reconstructed maximally 860 μm rostrally). The cell body was located 1.3 mm caudal to the facial nucleus. Most neurons in the CVLM with these physiological and morphological properties are GABAergic (i.e. inhibitory). Coronal section through the rostral part of the CVLM (intermediate VLM). IO, inferior olive nucleus; LRN, lateral reticular nucleus; NA, nucleus ambiguus; py, pyramid; Sp5, spinal trigeminal nucleus; sp5, spinal trigeminal tract; IV, fourth ventricle. Modified from Schreihofer and Guyenet (2003) with permission. For technical details see Schreihofer and Guyenet (2003).

and, *second*, in view that such an important control system may be redundant and multiple (Coote 1988):

- In the cat, activity generated in silent sympathetic preganglionic neurons by ionophoretic application of glutamate can be inhibited during stimulation of arterial baroreceptors (Coote et al. 1981).
- Activity elicited synaptically in sympathetic preganglionic neurons by electrical stimulation of descending fibers in the dorsolateral funiculus of the spinal cord can be inhibited during stimulation of arterial baroreceptors (with intact or blocked RVLM). The inhibition is mediated by GABA and possibly glycine (Lewis and Coote 1995, 1996).
- Fast hyperpolarizing postsynaptic potentials reminiscent of inhibitory postsynaptic potentials (IPSPs) were elicited in sympathetic preganglionic neurons during stimulation of arterial baroreceptors (McLachlan and Hirst 1980; Coote, personal communication). Such inhibitory potentials may also be elicited by activation of GABAergic neurons in the RVLM that project to the preganglionic neurons (Miura et al. 1994; Deuchars et al. 1997). In rabbits, some 10% of the sympathetic premotor neurons in the RVLM are excited by stimulation of arterial baroreceptors and by stimulation of neurons in the caudal ventrolateral medulla, supporting this idea (Li et al. 1991) (Note 17). Finally it has been shown that the lower brain stem contains GABAergic neurons that project to the intermediolateral nucleus of the thoracic spinal cord and form synapses with preganglionic neurons. Most of these GABAergic sympathetic premotor neurons also contain the inhibitory transmitter glycine and some 5-HT. The cell bodies of these neurons are located medial to the RVLM (in the gigantocellular reticular nucleus, ventral and alpha, and the medial reticular formation) (Stornetta et al. 2004).

The baroreceptor-induced reflex inhibition of sympathetic preganglionic neurons operating at the spinal level may duplicate the baroreceptor-induced reflex inhibition of sympathetic premotor neurons in the RVLM; the way the two baroreceptor pathways are integrated during regulation of activity in preganglionic cardiovascular neurons remains to be worked out.

10.3.5 Modulation of Baroreceptor Pathways

The baroreceptor pathways worked out so far (Figure 10.10) can only be understood within the limitations of the experimental approaches used. Under physiological ("closed-loop") conditions (Note 18), these baroreceptor reflex pathways are component parts of many complex cardiovascular regulations. They are therefore subject to many modifications during these complex regulations. This is reflected in the observation that the relays of the baroreceptor pathways are under powerful modulatory control exerted by other centers in the spinal cord, lower and upper brain stem, hypothalamus and telencephalon. This is graphically expressed in Figure 10.14 for the baroreceptor pathways to sympathetic preganglionic neurons. Depending on the functional context, these influences lead to enhancement or depression of the baroreceptor reflexes, potentially at each synaptic relay in the NTS, CVLM, RVLM and IML (Figure 10.14):

- In Subchapter 8.3 I described the NTS as anatomically reciprocally connected with various nuclei in the spinal cord, brain stem, hypothalamus and telencephalon (Figure 8.13). Electrical stimulation of the hypothalamic defense area depresses arterial baroreceptor-induced reflexes by inhibition in the NTS and probably elsewhere (Spyer 1981, 1994; Paton and Kasparov 2000). Activation of neurons in the hypothalamic perifornical defense area or in the dorsomedial hypothalamus (by disinhibition; blockade of GABAergic inhibition by bicuculline) increases the threshold of the baroreceptor control of heart rate and renal nerve activity and shifts the set point of the baroreceptor reflexes to higher pressure levels without changing their gain (Dampney, unpublished results). It is hypothesized that this shift occurs by acting in the NTS. Noxious stimulation of hindlimb, forelimb or cornea attenuates the baroreceptor reflexes. This inhibition involves GABAergic interneurons in the NTS that are activated via NK_1 receptors (Boscan and Paton 2002; Boscan et al. 2002). Only the baroreceptor pathway to parasympathetic cardiomotor neurons (but not to sympathetic cardiomotor neurons) is involved (Pickering et al. 2003). This argues that the NTS neurons are distinct for the two baroreceptor pathways.
- The inhibitory GABAergic neurons in the CVLM receive tonic excitatory (glutamatergic) synaptic input leading to tonic inhibition of the bulbospinal neurons in the RVLM, independent of the pulsatile inhibition exerted by activation of

arterial baroreceptors. The increase of arterial blood pressure following blockade of the inhibitory (GABAergic) interneurons in the CVLM is significantly higher than the blood pressure increase following denervation of the arterial baroreceptors (which removes the activation of GABAergic interneurons generated by activity in the arterial baroreceptors [Natarajan and Morrison 2000]). Furthermore, the inhibitory barosensitive neurons in the CVLM integrate activity from somatic and visceral nociceptive afferent neurons and possibly other afferent neurons. This integration is responsible for some aspects of somato- and viscerosympathetic reflexes in muscle and visceral vasoconstrictor neurons (Schreihofer and Guyenet 2003). It is likely that only a subpopulation of GABAergic interneurons in the CVLM that project to the RVLM and inhibit the sympathetic premotor neurons are activated by stimulation of arterial baroreceptors. Other subpopulations of inhibitory CVLM neurons that also project to the RVLM are not activated by stimulation of arterial baroreceptors (Cravo et al. 1991). These subpopulations of GABAergic neurons in the CVLM that project to the RVLM will be better characterized in future investigations (Wang et al. 2003).

- Sympathetic premotor neurons in the RVLM are also tonically excited by interneurons in the CVLM. The tonic activity in these excitatory interneurons is synaptically maintained by activity of neurons in the caudal pressure area (CPA) in the VLM, which is located in the most caudal part of the VLM (Figure 10.3a; Natarajan and Morrison 2000; see also Horiuchi and Dampney [2002]; Dampney et al. [2003]).
- Neurons of the respiratory network (central respiratory generator [CRG] in Figure 10.14) influence the neurons of the baroreceptor reflex pathway synaptically (i.e., the parasympathetic preganglionic cardiomotor neurons and the sympathetic premotor neurons in the RVLM). The mechanisms of this integration between respiratory and cardiovascular neurons are poorly understood. However, one type of coupling may occur between glutamatergic neurons expressing NK_1-receptors in the preBötzinger complex and GABAergic neurons in the CVLM (Wang et al. 2003; Mandel and Schreihofer 2006; see Subchapter 10.6).

- The baroreceptor reflex on heart rate is inhibited by stimulation of lung afferents (Gandevia et al. 1978).

In *conclusion*, the example of the arterial baroreceptor reflexes illustrates the complexity of the organization of the cardiovascular reflex pathways in the medulla oblongata. It shows that it is difficult to interpret the role of the baroreceptor reflexes during normal closed-loop cardiovascular regulations. Although many laboratories have concentrated and/or are concentrating on the mechanisms underlying the baroreceptor reflexes, several controversial issues

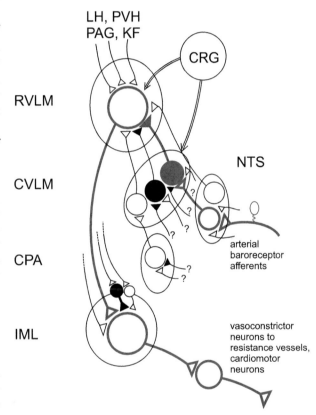

Figure 10.14 Neural influences on the nuclei of the baroreceptor reflex pathway to sympathetic cardiovascular neurons. The neurons of the baroreceptor reflex pathway are outlined in red. Excitatory neurons/synapses, open symbols. Inhibitory neurons/synapses, closed symbols. CPA, caudal pressure area; CRG, central respiratory generator; CVLM, caudal ventrolateral medulla; IML, intermediolateral cell column; LH, lateral hypothalamus; KF, Kölliker–Fuse nucleus; NTS, nucleus tractus solitarii; PAG, periaqueductal gray; PVH, paraventricular nucleus of the hypothalamus; RVLM, rostral ventrolateral medulla. Modified from Pilowsky and Goodchild (2002) with permission.

remain to be explored. These address, e.g., the function of unmyelinated baroreceptor afferents, the convergence of baroreceptor afferents on single NTS neurons, the functional types of barosensitive NTS neurons (related to parasympathetic and sympathetic cardiovascular neurons, to regulation of vasopressin release), the modulation of barosensitive NTS neurons, the projection of barosensitive NTS neurons, the neurochemistry of barosensitive NTS neurons, the differentiation of barosensitive CVLM neurons from other inhibitory CVLM neurons, alternative baroreceptor pathways, etc. (Guyenet 2006).

Similar complexities as exist for the baroreceptor pathways are present for the autonomic chemoreceptor pathways (see Subchapter 10.4) and other reflex pathways related to various types of cardiovascular, pulmonary, gastrointestinal, vestibular and somatic afferents. The organization of most of them is still unknown or incompletely understood. However, on the positive side, I want to emphasize that these complexities are the basis for the high adaptability of the homeostatic cardiovascular regulation and its distortion during disease (see Randall [1984]; Eckberg and Sleight [1992]; Rowell [1993]; Kirchheim et al. [1998]; Mathias and Bannister [2013]; Guyenet [2014]).

10.4 Arterial Chemoreceptor Reflexes in Sympathetic Cardiovascular Neurons

Reduction of oxygen tension in the blood is detected by peripheral chemoreceptors in the carotid and aortic bodies. These chemoreceptors are innervated by afferent fibers in the aortic and carotid sinus nerves that project to the commissural nucleus of the NTS. Most of these afferent fibers are unmyelinated. The primary, neurally mediated, responses to decreased arterial oxygen tension (PaO_2) are increased ventilation, arousal, aversive responses and autonomic adjustments that compensate for direct (non-neural) vasodilating effects of hypoxia on the blood vessels and redistribute blood to essential organs, including brain, heart and kidneys (Marshall 1994). Large reductions in PaO_2 are also detected directly by the brain (Reis et al. 1994, 1997) and cause sympathetic excitation. Brief stimulation of arterial chemoreceptors excites some sympathetic neurons (muscle, visceral, renal vasoconstrictor,

sudomotor, inspiratory neurons), inhibits some (many cutaneous vasoconstrictor neurons) and does not affect others (e.g., motility-regulating neurons innervating viscera) in the cat (see Chapter 4; Figures 4.1, 4.5 and 4.12). Most sympathetic premotor neurons in the RVLM are excited following stimulation of arterial chemoreceptors; some are inhibited (McAllen 1992). What are the reflex pathways for the primary excitatory responses elicited in sympathetic vasoconstrictor and cardiomotor neurons and in sympathetic premotor neurons in the RVLM?

A subgroup of neurons in the NTS can be activated by stimulation of arterial chemoreceptors. These NTS neurons do not receive convergent synaptic input from gastrointestinal tract afferents, very few can be activated or inhibited by stimulation of arterial baroreceptors and some are either activated or inhibited by pharyngoesophageal stimulation. Morphology and neurophysiological characteristics are similar to other functional types of NTS neurons (Paton et al. 2001). The chemoreceptive NTS neurons project widely to the ventral respiratory cell column and indirectly to sympathetic premotor neurons and parasympathetic cardiomotor neurons (Koshiya and Guyenet 1996; Guyenet 2014).

The following description is exemplary for chemoreceptor reflexes and based on experiments performed on rats by Guyenet's group (Koshiya et al. 1993; Guyenet et al. 1996; Guyenet 2000, 2014):

- Stimulation of arterial chemoreceptors by brief anoxia (ventilation of the rat with 100% N_2 for 4 to 12 seconds) (Note 19) activates several types of peripheral sympathetic neurons, e.g. those projecting in the major splanchnic nerve (all activated neurons probably being visceral vasoconstrictor neurons), and many sympathetic premotor neurons in the RVLM in parallel to activation of neurons of the ventral respiratory column (VRC) that is reflected in an increase in rate and amplitude of phrenic nerve activity (Figure 10.15a_1, b_1). This reflex activation of sympathetic neurons exhibits a rhythmicity correlated with the phrenic nerve discharges.
- Inhibition of the neurons in the CVLM, located caudal to the preBötzinger complex (see Figures 10.2b and 3), by topical injection of the GABA agonist muscimol, eliminates the phrenic nerve discharges (probably by inhibiting the

respiratory premotor neurons in the rVRG) but does not block the reflex activation of sympathetic premotor neurons in the RVLM (not shown) and therefore not the reflex activation of sympathetic neurons (Figure 10.15a$_2$). The respiratory rhythmicity of the activity in the sympathetic neurons is still preserved during the hypoxia-induced activation of the sympathetic neurons, probably because

the component neurons of the ponto-medullary respiratory pattern generator that are essential to generate the respiratory rhythm are situated more rostrally than the CVLM and are not inhibited (Figure 10.15a$_2$).

- After inhibition of the neurons in the rostral CVLM by local injection of muscimol, hypoxia-induced reflex activation of the sympathetic neurons, as

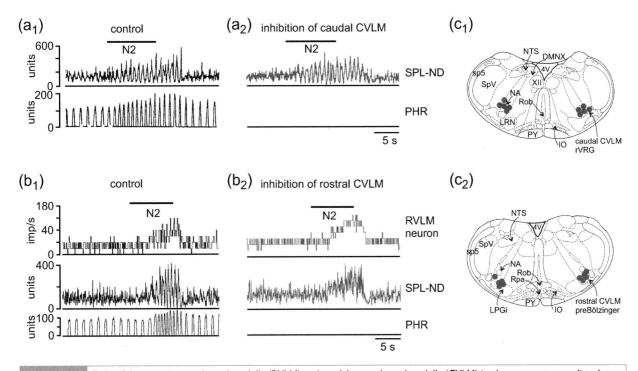

Figure 10.15 Role of the rostral ventrolateral medulla (RVLM) and caudal ventrolateral medulla (CVLM) in chemoreceptor-mediated activation of vasoconstrictor neurons projecting to the viscera. Experiments on urethane-anesthetized, vagotomized and artificially ventilated rats. Arterial carotid chemoreceptors were stimulated by ventilating the rats with 100% N_2 for 4 to 12 s. Integrated activity was recorded from the phrenic nerve (indicating activation of inspiratory neurons; phrenic nerve discharge, PHR) and from the major splanchnic nerve (mainly activity in visceral vasoconstrictor neurons; splanchnic nerve discharge, SPL-ND) in (a) and additionally from a sympathetic premotor neuron in the RVLM in (b). (a$_1$, b$_1$) Stimulation of the arterial chemoreceptors activates phrenic motoneurons, RVLM neurons and visceral vasoconstrictor neurons. During the activation of RVLM and sympathetic neurons, respiratory rhythmicity is pronounced. This activation is eliminated after denervation of the arterial chemoreceptors (not shown). (a$_2$) Inhibition of neurons in the caudal CVLM (for location see Figures 10.3, 10.4, 10.12) by bilateral injection of the GABA agonist muscimol into the CVLM eliminates the phrenic nerve activity (by inhibition of the phrenic premotor neurons in the rostral ventral respiratory group [rVRG]) but not the rhythmic reflex activation of sympathetic neurons. The arterial baroreceptor reflexes are also eliminated and the resting sympathetic activity increases (due to inhibition of the GABAergic interneurons). (b$_2$) After bilateral inhibition of the neurons in the rostral part of the CVLM (which are associated with the preBötzinger complex; see Figure 10.3a,b) by injection of muscimol, the reflex activation of the visceral vasoconstrictor neurons and of the RVLM neurons is unaffected, but the rhythmic activation and the PHR discharge are eliminated (probably because the neurons of the respiratory pattern generator are inhibited). (c$_1$, c$_2$) Typical injection sites of muscimol into the caudal CVLM for the effect shown in (a$_2$) ([c$_1$]) and into the rostral CVLM/preBötzinger complex (also called intermediate CVLM by Dampney [1994]) for the effect shown in (b$_2$) ([c$_2$]). DMNX, dorsal motor nucleus of the vagus nerve; IO, inferior olive; LPGi, lateral paragigantocellular nucleus; LRN, lateral reticular nucleus; NA, nucleus ambiguus; NTS, nucleus tractus solitarii; PY, pyramid; Rob, Rpa, raphe obscurus, pallidus; Sp5, spinal trigeminal nucleus; sp5, spinal trigeminal tract; 4V, fourth ventricle; XII, hypoglossal nucleus. (a$_1$, a$_2$) and (c$_1$) modified from Koshiya et al. (1993). (b$_1$), (b$_2$) and (c$_2$) modified from Koshiya and Guyenet (1996) with permission.

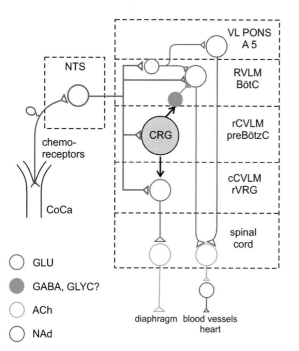

GLU

GABA, GLYC?

ACh

NAd

Figure 10.16 Hypothetical chemoreceptor reflex circuits linked to sympathetic cardiovascular neurons innervating resistance vessels or the heart. These pathways are based on experiments shown in Figure 10.15. The locations of the respiratory neurons and the sympathetic premotor neurons in the ventrolateral medulla (VLM) are shown in Figures 10.2 and 10.3. Chemoreceptor afferent neurons from the carotid and aortic bodies activate second-order neurons in the commissural subnucleus of the nucleus tractus solitarii (NTS). These second-order neurons project to phrenic premotor neurons in the rostral ventral respiratory group (rVRG) (in the caudal ventrolateral medulla [CVLM]), to neurons in the preBötzinger complex (preBötC in the rostral CVLM [rCVLM]), to sympathetic premotor neurons in the rostral ventrolateral medulla (RVLM) (monosynaptically and/or disynaptically; C1 [adrenergic] and non-C1 neurons) and (possibly disynaptically) to noradrenergic neurons in the A5 area of the ventrolateral (VL) pons. Rhythmic respiratory discharges of the sympathetic premotor neurons and peripheral sympathetic cardiovascular neurons are probably mediated via the preBötC, possibly by inhibitory interneurons. The transmitters used by the neurons are glutamate (Glu), GABA (γ-aminobutyric acid; or glycine), acetylcholine (ACh) or noradrenaline (NAd). BötC, Bötzinger complex; CoCa, common carotid artery; CRG, central respiratory generator. Modified from Guyenet (2000) with permission.

in the preBötzinger complex are inhibited) (Figure 10.15b$_2$).

These and other experiments (in particular those of Dampney's group using Fos expression of neurons in the lower brain stem during stimulation of arterial chemoreceptors [Hirooka et al. 1997; Dampney and Horiuchi 2003]) show that the primary reflex activation of sympathetic neurons generated by stimulation of arterial chemoreceptors is not only mediated via the activation of respiratory neurons (e.g., in the preBötzinger complex) but also by reflex pathways to the sympathetic premotor neurons in the RVLM that are *independent* of the respiratory neurons. Further experiments performed by Guyenet's group have shown that sympathetic premotor neurons in the A5 area of the ventrolateral pons (see Figure 8.15) may also be involved in integration of the primary chemoreceptor reflex activation of the sympathetic neurons. These A5 neurons are noradrenergic.

Figure 10.16 depicts the putative primary chemoreceptor reflex pathways to the (phrenic) inspiratory motoneurons innervating the diaphragm and to the sympathetic pathways innervating resistance vessels or the heart. The main groups of respiratory and cardiovascular neurons in the different sections of the VLM (see Figures 10.2 and 10.3) and in the ventrolateral pons are shown. The reflex pathways between the chemoreceptor afferents projecting to the NTS and the sympathetic premotor neurons are unknown, but involve at least one interneuron. These interneurons are probably glutamatergic. The synaptic connection between the neurons in the preBötzinger complex and the sympathetic premotor neurons in the RVLM, which is responsible for the increased respiratory modulation of the chemoreceptor reflex response, is possibly mediated by an inhibitory (GABAergic) interneuron.

As is the case with the baroreceptor reflex pathways (Figure 10.10), all synapses of the chemoreceptor pathways are under modulatory control of other nuclei in the lower brain stem, upper brain stem, hypothalamus and possibly telencephalon. Furthermore, the primary chemoreceptor reflexes linked to respiratory and sympathetic premotor neurons are modified by secondary cardiopulmonary reflexes connected to arterial baroreceptors, volume receptors and various types of pulmonary afferents, as well as the chemosensitivity of the neurons in the medulla oblongata (to changes in PaCO$_2$ and pH; to large changes in PaO$_2$) (Marshall 1994; Guyenet 2014).

well as of the sympathetic premotor neurons in the RVLM, is still present. However, the respiratory rhythmicity in this reflex response and the phrenic nerve discharges are eliminated (probably since neurons of the respiratory pattern generator

As described in Subchapter 4.1, most cutaneous vasoconstrictor neurons innervating hairy skin of the distal extremities (Blumberg et al. 1980) and all cutaneous vasoconstrictor neurons innervating hairless skin of the cat hindpaw (Jänig and Kümmel 1977) are inhibited following stimulation of arterial chemoreceptors generated by ventilation of the cat with a hypoxic gas mixture of 8% O_2 in N_2 or by brief stimulation of arterial chemoreceptors with a bolus of CO_2-saturated saline (Figures 4.5b, 4.12c). This inhibition is accompanied by an increase in cutaneous blood flow (Jänig and Koltzenburg 1991). The powerful inhibitory chemoreceptor reflex in the cutaneous vasoconstrictor neurons seems to be important during the diving response in diving animals (see Subchapter 11.3.1). This inhibitory chemoreceptor reflex in the cutaneous vasoconstrictor neurons is correlated with weak or absent inhibitory baroreceptor reflexes (see Chapter 4 and Figures 4.5 and 4.12). The central pathway(s) mediating the inhibitory chemoreceptor reflex in cutaneous vasoconstrictor neurons may be related to the pathway of the diving response in the medulla oblongata. However, they are most likely different from those mediating the excitatory chemoreceptor reflexes in cardiovascular sympathetic neurons that are involved in blood pressure regulation (see Figure 10.16).

Cutaneous vasoconstrictor neurons in the cat, which are normally inhibited following stimulation of arterial chemoreceptors, exhibit excitatory chemoreceptor reflexes under modified experimental conditions. This is illustrated by the following groups of experiments performed on cats:

1. Inhibition of activity in cutaneous vasoconstrictor neurons during stimulation of arterial chemoreceptors (by ventilating the animals with a gas mixture of 8% O_2 in N_2) is reversed to excitation after midcollicular (mesencephalic) decerebration, which removes reflex pathways mediated by the upper mesencephalon and hypothalamus (Gregor and Jänig 1977).
2. Weeks to months after an experimental lesion of cutaneous nerves in the cat (cutting and ligating the superficial peroneal nerve; cross-anastomizing the central stump of the superficial peroneal nerve to the distal stump of a muscle nerve or the tibial nerve) many cutaneous vasoconstrictor neurons

behave like muscle vasoconstrictor neurons: they are excited by stimulation of arterial chemoreceptors and exhibit strong inhibitory baroreceptor reflexes. These reflex changes occur both in cutaneous vasoconstrictor neurons projecting in the lesioned nerve and in cutaneous vasoconstrictor neurons projecting to intact skin nerves of the *same* extremity (Blumberg and Jänig 1983, 1985; Jänig and Koltzenburg 1991).

Both experiments demonstrate quite clearly that the central chemoreceptor circuits linked to the peripheral cutaneous vasoconstrictor pathways are complex and may change depending on the functional conditions (Note 20).

10.5 | Sympathetic Premotor Neurons in the Caudal Raphe Nuclei

Cooling the skin and/or core of the body activates cutaneous vasoconstrictor neurons, resulting in a decrease in cutaneous blood flow and heat transfer, and (in the rat) activation of lipomotor neurons (which innervate brown adipose tissue [BAT]), resulting in non-shivering thermogenesis. Both autonomic responses are part of the body's thermoregulatory cold-defense response, which is integrated into the preoptic area of the hypothalamus. The sympathetic premotor neurons mediating the responses of cutaneous vasoconstrictor neurons or lipomotor neurons to body cooling are most likely located in the caudal raphe nuclei (raphe magnus, raphe pallidus) of the medulla oblongata (Morrison 2018; Morrison and Nakamura 2019; Figure 10.2).

10.5.1 Premotor Neurons Innervating Preganglionic Cutaneous Vasoconstrictor Neurons

Several experimental investigations demonstrate indirectly that the raphe nuclei of the medulla oblongata contain sympathetic premotor neurons for the cutaneous vasoconstrictor pathway:

• Many neurons in the raphe nuclei of the medulla oblongata project to the spinal cord. Some of them project to the preganglionic neurons in the intermediolateral cell column (Morrison and Gebber 1985); they may form monosynaptic connections with the preganglionic neurons (Bacon et al. 1990).

- Transneuronal labeling of postganglionic cutaneous vasoconstrictor neurons innervating the rat tail (which is a thermoregulatory organ) with a neurotropic virus shows that many neurons are labeled in the caudal raphe nuclei (in addition to other labeled sympathetic premotor neurons, located, e.g., in the RVLM; Smith et al. 1998; see Table 8.2).
- Electrical or chemical stimulation of neurons in the caudal raphe nuclei generates vasoconstriction in skin independent of the RVLM (Blessing et al. 1999; Blessing and Nalivaiko 2000) and activates cutaneous vasoconstrictor neurons, but not vasoconstrictor neurons involved in regulation of blood pressure (such as renal vasoconstrictor neurons; Rathner and McAllen 1999).
- Many neurons in the ventral raphe nuclei of the medulla oblongata express the transcription factor c-Fos after a decrease in body temperature by whole-body cooling (Morrison et al. 1999). Expression of c-Fos indicates an increase in activity of these neurons (see Note 1).

Some neurons in the nuclei raphe magnus and pallidus that project to the intermediolateral nucleus of the spinal cord (IML; Figure 10.17a, b_1–b_2) are activated during cooling of the skin. This activation is enhanced by decreasing body core temperature (Figure 10.17b_3). Some bulbospinal neurons projecting to the IML are also inhibited by body cooling (Figure 10.17c_1), but many are not affected (Figure 10.17c_2). The bulbospinal raphe neurons that are excited during cooling exhibit a discharge pattern to other afferent inputs that is similar to that seen in cutaneous vasoconstrictor neurons innervating the rat tail or rat hindpaw (Häbler et al. 1994b, 2000; Owens et al. 2002): no or weak inhibition during stimulation of arterial baroreceptors, mostly inhibition (some excitation) to stimulation of nociceptors, respiratory rhythmicity.

These spinally projecting neurons in the nucleus raphe magnus and pallidus constitute a distinct class of cutaneous vasoconstrictor premotor neuron, being mainly involved in the regulation of cutaneous blood flow during thermoregulation. They are independent of the sympathetic premotor neurons in the RVLM. However, sympathetic preganglionic cutaneous vasoconstrictor neurons may also receive synaptic input (either directly or via interneurons) from sympathetic premotor neurons in the RVLM (Figure 10.17a; see Figure 10.9). Thus, the reflex characteristics of pre- and postganglionic cutaneous vasoconstrictor neurons depend on the discharge characteristics of two types of identified sympathetic premotor neurons in the medulla oblongata and possibly of other types of sympathetic premotor neurons that have not yet been identified [see Table 8.2 and Figures 4.6 and 8.9]. This is consistent with what has actually been measured in cutaneous vasoconstrictor neurons, in particular those innervating hairy skin of the distal extremities. Most of them exhibit no or weak cardiac rhythmicity in their activity and inhibitory reflexes to stimulation of arterial chemoreceptors and some 20% innervating (more proximal) hairy skin exhibit strong cardiac rhythmicity in their activity and excitatory chemoreceptor reflexes (Blumberg et al. 1980).

Activity in these sympathetic premotor neurons during thermoregulatory load (cooling or warming) is partly regulated via inhibitory GABAergic neurons. Blockade of this GABAergic transmission in the medullary raphe nuclei (by microinjection of the GABA$_A$-receptor antagonist bicuculline) during warming of the preoptic area of the hypothalamus prevents the inhibition of these neurons and therefore the concomitantly occurring increase in cutaneous blood flow (Tanaka et al. 2002). The reflex pathways mediating the excitatory response to cooling (and the reflexes to noxious stimulation) are so far unknown. However, they may pass through the hypothalamus as well as through a bulbospinal pathway (McAllen and McKinley 2018; Morrison and Nakamura 2019).

10.5.2 Premotor Neurons Innervating Preganglionic Lipomotor Neurons

Lipomotor neurons innervating brown adipose tissue (BAT) in the rat (see Subchapter 4.4) are also under the control of sympathetic premotor neurons located in the caudal raphe nuclei (mainly raphe pallidus) of the medulla oblongata. Excitation of postganglionic lipomotor neurons directly activates the lipocytes of the BAT, mediated by β_3-adrenoceptors. The activation of lipocytes leads to activation of an uncoupling protein in these cells and subsequently to production of heat. This mechanism of non-shivering thermogenesis is important in small mammals (like rat, mouse, guinea pig) and in hibernating animals, but less so in large-

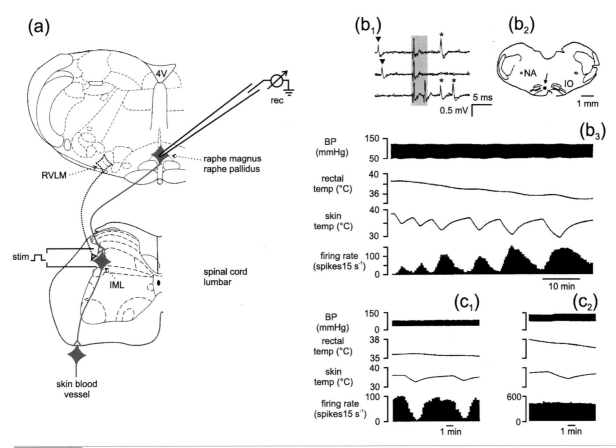

Figure 10.17 Responses of sympathetic premotor neurons in the caudal raphe nuclei of the medulla oblongata to cooling of the body surface in the rat. (a) Experimental setup for recording and identification of sympathetic premotor neurons in the caudal raphe nuclei with a microelectrode. The neuron was identified by electrical stimulation of its axon projecting to the upper lumbar spinal cord. IML, intermediolateral nucleus; 4V, fourth ventricle. Putative preganglionic cutaneous vasoconstrictor neurons may also receive supraspinal synaptic input from premotor neurons in the rostral ventrolateral medulla (RVLM) (see Figure 10.9). (b₁) Identification of a sympathetic premotor neuron in the raphe nuclei as a bulbospinal neuron: electrical stimulation of the axon of the neuron in the IML with single pulses (upper trace; stim. in [a]) or with a pair of pulses (lower trace) activates the neuron at constant latency (antidromically evoked spikes marked by stars). When the electrical stimulus occurs at ≤8 ms after a spontaneous orthodromically conducted action potential, (marked by arrowheads) the antidromic spike evoked by electrical stimulation was canceled by the orthodromic spike (second trace). This clash does not occur at a time interval of ≥9 ms between spontaneous spike and electrical stimulus (first trace). Each recording is three times superimposed. (b₂) Marked recording site for this neuron (indicated by arrow) illustrated on a transverse section of the medulla oblongata just caudal to the facial nucleus (see Figure 10.2). NA, nucleus ambiguus. (b₃) Activation of the neuron in (b₁/b₂) by lowering skin temperature on the trunk and rectal temperature. Upper trace, arterial blood pressure (BP). (c₁,c₂) Two additional raphe neurons, which are either inhibited or unaffected by skin cooling (same type of experiment as in [b₁–b₃]). Modified from Rathner et al. (2001) with permission.

sized animals and in adult humans, except in the newborn. BAT is present between the scapulae and in smaller amounts in the thoracic and abdominal cavities (e.g., around the heart, adrenal glands and kidneys; Smith and Horwitz 1969). Postganglionic axons of lipomotor neurons are present, in addition to some vasoconstrictor axons, in high concentration in nerves innervating the interscapular BAT and in low numbers in the splanchnic nerves. Therefore, sympathetic multiunit activity in the nerves to the BAT consists mainly of activity in postganglionic lipomotor axons, and activity in thoracic or lumbar splanchnic nerves is dominated by activity in visceral vasoconstrictor axons that are involved in regulation of resistance vessels and therefore in blood pressure regulation.

Figure 10.18 (Note 21) demonstrates recordings from these nerves in the anesthetized rat (in addition to recordings of arterial blood pressure and phrenic nerve activity) during various interventions in the nucleus raphe pallidus and during hypothermia) (Morrison 1999, 2001; Morrison et al. 1999):

- Activity in lipomotor neurons is low or absent, whereas vasoconstrictor activity is high, under normal thermoneutral regulatory conditions (body core temperature of 37 °C; Figure 10.18b$_1$, c$_1$).
- Hypothermia (exposure to cold with a decrease in core body temperature) activates lipomotor neurons without changing visceral vasoconstrictor activity (Figure 10.18b$_2$).
- Disinhibition of the neurons in the nucleus raphe pallidus by ionophoretic application of the GABA$_A$-receptor antagonist bicuculline activates lipomotor neurons without changing the visceral vasoconstrictor activity and arterial blood pressure (Figure 10.18b$_3$).
- Inhibition of neurons in the RVLM by the GABA agonist muscimol eliminates phrenic nerve activity (by inhibiting the neurons of the respiratory network [probably in the nearby preBötzinger complex], see Figure 10.3) and vasoconstrictor activity (by silencing the sympathetic premotor neurons in the RVLM that are involved in blood pressure regulation) with a subsequent fall in arterial blood pressure. Note there was no effect on the lipomotor neurons (Figure 10.18c$_2$).
- Disinhibition of the neurons in the nucleus raphe pallidus by microinjection of the GABA$_A$-receptor antagonist bicuculline, after inhibition of the RVLM neurons, activates the lipomotor neurons, but not the splanchnic vasoconstrictor neurons (Figure 10.18c$_3$; note some small activation in the splanchnic nerve in Figure 10.18c$_3$, which occurs synchronously with the activity in the lipomotor neurons innervating the interscapular BAT; these neurons are presumably lipomotor neurons innervating BAT in the viscera).

These elegant key experiments show that a second class of sympathetic premotor neuron in the nucleus raphe pallidus innervates preganglionic lipomotor neurons. These sympathetic premotor neurons are different from those in the same raphe nucleus that innervate preganglionic cutaneous vasoconstrictor neurons (see Figure 10.18a; Subchapter 4.4).

Figure 10.19 shows the three types of sympathetic premotor neuron that have so far been functionally identified in the medulla oblongata of the rat: (1) Premotor neurons in the raphe pallidus (Rpal) to preganglionic lipomotor neurons. (2) Premotor neurons in the RVLM to preganglionic vasoconstrictor neurons involved in regulation in peripheral vascular resistance and blood pressure control. (3) Premotor neurons in the Rpal to preganglionic cutaneous vasoconstrictor neurons involved in thermoregulation. Premotor neurons in the Rpal and in the RVLM may converge on the same preganglionic cutaneous vasoconstrictor neurons, depending on the type of target skin (distal acral skin or proximal hairy skin) (Ootsuka and McAllen 2005) (see "Vasoconstrictor Neurons in Animals" in Subchapter 4.1.1).

In the cat, premotor neurons in the RVLM are subdifferentiated with respect to different vascular beds and the heart (Figure 10.9).

In the future, other sympathetic premotor neurons will be functionally identified in the medulla oblongata (and in the pons and hypothalamus) as postulated from tracing experiments performed with neurotropic viruses (Figure 8.15 and Table 8.2) and from neurophysiological investigations of the neurons in the peripheral sympathetic pathways (Chapter 4; see Figure 4.25). For example, the nucleus raphe pallidus contains sympathetic premotor neurons that are activated during stress (via the dorsomedial hypothalamus) and generate tachycardia. These sympathetic premotor neurons are normally silent and converge with sympathetic premotor neurons in the RVLM on sympathetic preganglionic cardiomotor neurons or their associated interneurons in the thoracic spinal cord (Zaretsky et al. 2003a, b). The nucleus raphe pallidus may also contain sympathetic premotor neurons that are also under hypothalamic control and converge on preganglionic neurons to the kidney (Horiuchi et al. 2004a, b).

10.6 | Coupling Between Regulation of Autonomic Pathways and Regulation of Respiration

10.6.1 The Respiratory Network

As mentioned in Subchapter 10.2.2, respiration is the coordinated alternation of the three respiratory

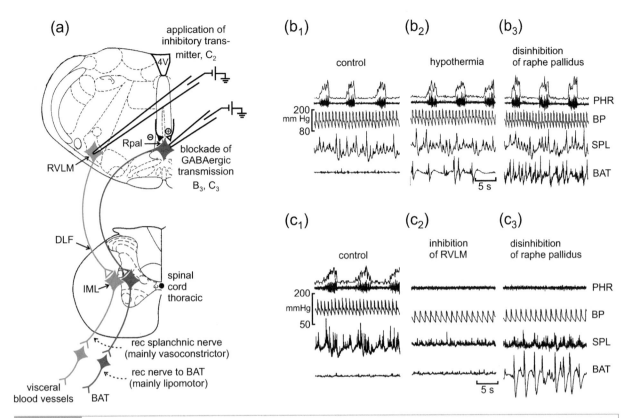

Figure 10.18 Activation of sympathetic lipomotor neurons innervating brown adipose tissue (BAT) by hypothermia and disinhibition of the nucleus raphe pallidus. (a) Arrangement of recording electrodes and electrodes for ionophoresis to inhibit activity of neurons in the rostral ventrolateral medulla (RVLM) or to block GABAergic transmission in the nucleus raphe pallidus (Rpal). Simultaneous recording of phrenic nerve activity (PHR; lower trace, original signal; upper trace, integrated signal), arterial blood pressure (BP), activity in the major splanchnic nerve (SPL), and activity in a nerve to the interscapular BAT in two anesthetized, paralyzed and artificially ventilated rats (b, c). The measurements were done sequentially. DLF, dorsolateral funiculus; IML, intermediolateral nucleus. (b_1, c_1) Control. Body core temperature 37 °C. (b_2) Hypothermia (rectal temperature 34.4 °C). (b_3) Disinhibition of neurons in the nucleus raphe pallidus by microinjection of bicuculline (antagonist to GABA) in normothermia. (c_2) Inhibition of neurons in the RVLM by microinjection of muscimol (GABA agonist). Note elimination of PHR nerve activity (probably due to inhibition of neurons of the nearby preBötzinger complex [see Figure 10.2]) and of SPL nerve activity and decrease of BP. (c_3) Subsequent disinhibition of neurons in the Rpal by microinjection of bicuculline. Note activation of BAT and small activation of SPL. Modified from Morrison (1999) with permission.

phases, inspiration, postinspiration (stage 1 expiration) and expiration (stage 2 expiration) (Richter 1982; Schwarzacher et al. 1991), which are reflected in the discharge pattern of phrenic motoneurons (see PHR in Figures 10.21 and 10.22) and other motoneurons innervating respiration-related muscles (e.g., nervus laryngeus recurrens, nervi intercostales interni). Normal respiration (eupnea) is characterized by an augmenting pattern of phrenic activity during inspiration and fully dependent in its pattern and rhythm on the ponto-medullary respiratory network of neurons (St.-John 1998; St.-John and Paton 2004).

Such coordination of the respiratory phases is important for breathing and its adaptation during muscular activity, swallowing, vocalization, thermoregulation and other motor actions. Activity in the three respiratory phases is controlled by specific classes of neuron of the ponto-medullary respiratory network. The output neurons of this network of respiratory neurons project to inspiratory or expiratory motoneurons (or to interneurons closely associated with these motoneurons) in the spinal cord (inspiratory or expiratory bulbospinal premotor neurons) or to motoneurons in the medulla

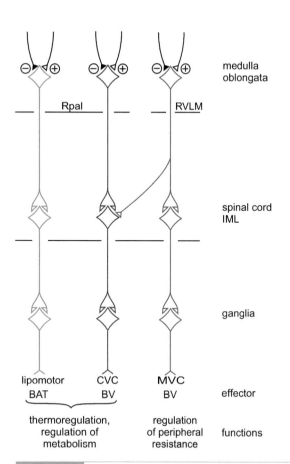

medulla oblongata

Rpal   RVLM

spinal cord
IML

ganglia

lipomotor   CVC   MVC
BAT   BV   BV   effector

thermoregulation,   regulation
regulation of   of peripheral   functions
metabolism   resistance

Figure 10.19 Three bulbospinal pathways to sympathetic preganglionic neurons. Lipomotor neurons supplying brown adipose tissue (BAT) are activated by sympathetic premotor neurons in the raphe pallidus (Rpal). Vasoconstrictor neurons (visceral and muscle vasoconstrictor, VVC, MVC) are activated by sympathetic premotor neurons in the rostral ventrolateral medulla (RVLM). Cutaneous vasoconstrictor neurons involved in thermoregulation are strongly activated by premotor neurons in the Rpal and weakly or not by premotor neurons in the RVLM. There are possibly other bulbospinal pathways in the raphe pallidus nucleus to sympathetic preganglionic cardiomotor neurons and to preganglionic neurons innervating the kidney or other viscera which have not been characterized yet. BV, blood vessel; IML, intermediolateral nucleus. Modified from Morrison (1999).

oblongata that are involved in the regulation of muscles of the upper respiratory tract (pharynx, larynx). Interneurons, proprio-brain-stem neurons and output neurons of the central respiratory network are located in the VRG (Figures 10.2b and 10.3a; Box 10.1), in the dorsal respiratory group, in the so-called pneumotaxic center in the rostral pons close to the medial parabrachial nucleus and the Kölliker–

Fuse nucleus and in scattered clusters of neurons in the pontine reticular formation between the pneumotaxic center and the rostral portion of the ventral respiratory group in the medulla oblongata (not shown in Figure 10.2; St. John 1998). Most inspiratory bulbospinal premotor neurons are located in the rVRG, the expiratory bulbospinal premotor neurons are located in the so-called Bötzinger complex and the interneurons (consisting of at least four types that are not respiratory premotor neurons) are located in the preBötzinger complex (and also in other parts of the VRG).

The functioning of the central respiratory network, the mechanism(s) of generating the respiratory rhythm and current theories on respiratory rhythm generation are discussed extensively in the literature and are still very controversial (von Euler 1986; Bianchi et al. 1995; Rekling and Feldman 1998; St.-John 1998; Smith et al. 2000; Richter and Spyer 2001; Feldman et al. 2003; St.-John and Paton 2004). Here it suffices to mention and emphasize the following:

1. Generation of rhythms and pattern of respiration (eupnea) and their adaptation to various behavioral and environmental conditions requires the ponto-medullary respiratory network. Its functioning is fully dependent on the pontine pneumotaxic center. Mechanisms responsible for rhythm generation in eupnea are controversial. They may depend on the inherent properties of the (mostly) inhibitory synaptic connections between neurons of the ponto-medullary respiratory network; they require a tonic input to the respiratory network neurons (mainly generated by the chemosensitivity [to arterial P_{CO2}] of the respiratory neurons and by neurons of the reticular formation), and they may be entirely independent of pacemaker activity of groups of neurons of the ponto-medullary respiratory network. The generation of respiratory patterns (shape and amplitude of the respiratory drive) is dependent on hypothetical pattern generators; details of the underlying mechanisms are unknown.

2. Generation of the eupneic respiratory rhythm by pacemaker neurons in the preBötzinger complex is unlikely. The pacemaker idea has been propagated based on experiments conducted on slice preparations that include the preBötzinger complex (Smith et al. 1991). However, it has been convincingly shown that pacemaker activity in

neurons of the preBötzinger complex or neighboring neurons of the ventral respiratory group of neurons appears when the medulla oblongata is isolated from the pons and/or is under severe hypoxia. Under these conditions, the activity in the phrenic nerve is steeply rising, decrementing and shows a low frequency of phrenic bursts. This pacemaker activity and the subsequent explosive activation of inspiratory neurons is the underlying mechanism of gasping. Gasping may be a respiratory mechanism of last defense during hypoxia.

3. Neurons of the ponto-medullary respiratory network are classified by their activities in reference to the activity of the phrenic nerve, i.e. in reference to the three phases of respiration. There exist at least eight types of respiration-modulated neurons (Note 22). These neurons have distinct (mostly inhibitory) synaptic connections, leading to membrane potential changes generated by distinct ionic currents for each type of neuron. This organization is the base for the coordinated activity in motoneurons supplying inspiratory or expiratory muscles or oropharyngeal muscles in various functional conditions. We do not know yet how these assemblies of functionally distinct types of neurons (including those that have the potential to generate pacemaker activity) of the ponto-medullary respiratory network function together to generate the different types of pattern and rhythm of respiration. However, taking existing data obtained on neurons of the respiratory network in vivo and in the working-heart-brainstem preparation, during normal respiration (eupnea) and during respiration when the rostral or entire pontine part of the network has been removed or deactivated, a computational model of the ponto-medullary respiratory network has been simulated (Rybak et al. 2004). This model reproduces several findings that have been observed experimentally, e.g., all changes in eupnea during increased or decreased respiratory drive, during an increase or decrease of activity in vagal lung afferents or switching of eupnea to apneusis or gasping (generated by pacemaker neurons in the preBötzinger complex) when the pontine parts of the respiratory network are inactivated. Interaction between modeling and experimental studies will finally explain the long-lasting enigma of how automatic ventilation is generated by the ponto-medullary respiratory network and how this network is controlled voluntarily (St.-John 1998; Rybak et al. 2004).

4. Only a little is known about the synaptic connections between respiratory circuits and cardiovascular circuits and therefore about the neuronal mechanisms that underlie the precise coordination of regulation of respiration and regulation of cardiovascular parameters. However, it is fair to hypothesize that this important neuronal integration does not occur by a common respiratory-cardiovascular neuronal network. It is achieved by integration of distinct reflex pathways that are defined by their afferent input, output neurons, synaptic connections, neurochemistry, etc.

10.6.2 Respiratory Generator and Activity in Autonomic Systems

The neurons in the medulla oblongata involved in regulation of blood pressure and respiration are closely organized in columns (nuclei) of the ventrolateral medulla, as demonstrated schematically in Figures 10.2b and 10.3. This tight anatomical and functional organization is reflected in the integration of the two control systems leading to a temporal adaptation under all behavioral conditions. The general framework of the integration between the two control systems is outlined in a rather simplified scheme in Figure 10.20. The ponto-medullary respiratory network and the cardiovascular neural network in the lower brain stem overlap, i.e., the two networks are connected via common interneurons. It is at present impossible to make any statement about the nature of coupling of the ponto-medullary respiratory network to neural circuits related to regulation of gastrointestinal functions, regulation of body temperature or other autonomic non-cardiovascular regulations. The cardiovascular and respiratory neural network receive multiple afferent inputs from the periphery (vagal afferents from cardiovascular organs, lung, gastrointestinal tract via the NTS; spinal afferents from the same organ systems and somatic tissues via the spinal cord). The output neurons of the ponto-medullary respiratory network project to respiratory premotor or motor neurons and to autonomic premotor neurons or preganglionic neurons. The output neurons of the cardiovascular network project to parasympathetic and

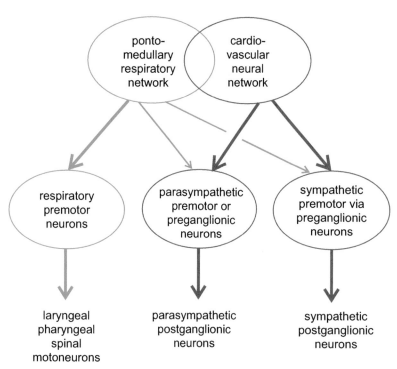

Figure 10.20 Cardiorespiratory integration in the medulla oblongata: a general conceptual framework. The ponto-medullary respiratory network (St.-John 1998; St.-John and Paton 2004) and the cardiovascular neural network overlap, i.e. the two neural networks have common interneurons. The output neurons of the ponto-medullary respiratory network activate respiratory premotor neurons and are synaptically connected with parasympathetic and sympathetic premotor and preganglionic neurons. The output neurons of the cardiovascular neural network connect synaptically to parasympathetic and sympathetic premotor and preganglionic neurons, but not to respiratory premotor neurons.

sympathetic premotor (or preganglionic) neurons, but not to respiratory motor neurons. Thus, integration between the neural regulation of respiration and of the cardiovascular system occurs mainly on more than one level. I presume that this also applies to other autonomic systems (not included in Figure 10.20).

The integration of the two control systems is reflected in respiratory oscillations of autonomic effector organ responses observed in animals and humans under standardized experimental conditions. They can be shown to exist for heart rate (respiratory sinus arrhythmia), volume of the nasal mucosa, vascular resistance in skeletal muscle, pupil diameter and tracheal air flow resistance. These neurally mediated oscillations have a central component (coupling between respiratory neurons and autonomic neurons in the medulla oblongata) and a peripheral (reflex) component. Both parasympathetic and sympathetic final pathways are potentially involved in the generation of the respiratory oscillations in effector organ regulation (for references and discussion see Häbler et al. [1994a]; for airway resistance see Paton and Dutschmann [2002]; for humans see Eckberg [2003]).

Recordings from "sympathetic" nerves in anesthetized animals (e.g., cardiac, splanchnic, renal nerves in dog, cat, rabbit, piglet), in which the vagal afferents from the lungs, heart and arterial baroreceptors have been interrupted, show that sympathetic neurons are activated during inspiration (for review and literature see Häbler et al. [1994a]). Detailed analysis of this respiratory rhythmicity in the anesthetized and artificially ventilated cat, in which vagal afferents and afferents from arterial baroreceptors have been interrupted, show that the mass activity in "sympathetic" nerves, which occurs predominantly in vasoconstrictor neurons regulating resistance vessels, exhibits a distinctive pattern, consisting of activation in inspiration, depression in postinspiration and sometimes a small depression in early inspiration (Bainton et al. 1985; Richter and Spyer 1990) (Figure 10.21; for details see below and in Figures 10.23 and 10.24) (Note 23). The respiratory pattern in sympathetic activity is due to coupling between the central respiratory network and the sympathetic system, probably occurring in the ventrolateral medulla (Richter and Spyer 1990; Richter et al. 1991; Guyenet and Koshiya 1992; see Häbler et al. [1994a]). Thus, this sympathetic pattern of discharge monitors aspects of the respiratory network during early inspiration, inspiration, postinspiration and expiration phase II.

The pattern of respiratory rhythmicity in the activity of the autonomic neurons is modulated by feedback via cardiovascular and pulmonary afferents, so that respiratory changes in the activity of these afferent neurons can lead in itself, via reflex pathways, to respiratory changes in activity in the autonomic neurons and mask the respiratory changes generated by coupling to the central respiratory rhythm generator (Figures 10.23b, 10.26). The profile of activity in sympathetic neurons during the respiratory cycle shows that this pattern is not due to a general irradiation of inspiratory activity to sympathetic premotor neurons, but the result of a specific synaptic coupling between neurons of the respiratory network and central sympathetic neurons, as will be argued in the next subchapter.

10.6.3 Early Studies of Coupling Between Regulation of Respiration and Cardiovascular System

The first evidence for the existence of a neural connection between the regulation of respiration and the regulation of autonomic systems was found by Traube (1865) and Hering (1869) in their experiments on the cardiovascular system. After stopping artificial ventilation in vagotomized and partially curarized dogs or cats, Traube was the first to observe the occurrence of large blood pressure waves. It was Hering who noticed that each blood pressure wave (later called Traube–Hering waves) was correlated with a rudimentary ineffective movement of the respiratory muscles. The waves occurred not only during asphyxia but also during artificial ventilation with a hypercapnic gas mixture. Using high-frequency artificial ventilation, centrally generated Traube–Hering waves in blood pressure could be easily distinguished from blood pressure waves produced passively by each artificial inflation. Hering pointed out that a "certain degree of venosity" of the arterial blood (generated by decrease of PaO_2 and increase of $PaCO_2$ with activation of the central respiratory generator [CRG]) was needed to evoke respiratory blood pressure waves. This, he wrote, could be accomplished by restricting the ventilation of the lungs. The heart rate mostly did not change appreciably during the blood pressure waves in vagotomized animals. Nevertheless, by isolation of the peripheral circulation from the heart, Hering excluded the heart as the cause of the observed pressure waves and showed that the vasculature alone was capable of generating respiratory blood pressure waves. From these observations he concluded that "also the vascular system performs respiratory movements." The observed blood pressure waves were thought to be caused by the rhythmic activity of the respiratory center in the medulla oblongata. In similar experiments on animals with intact vagus nerves, Traube (1865) observed an increase in heart rate during inspiration. He correctly attributed these heart rate changes to a decrease in activity in the vagal supply to the heart. With these experiments, Traube demonstrated that the sympathetic innervation of resistance vessels and the parasympathetic innervation of the heart showed a reciprocal coupling to respiration.

Respiratory sinus arrhythmia was first studied systematically by Anrep et al. (1936a, b) in animals. They proved its neural origin and showed that it is largely mediated via the vagus nerves. Anrep and coworkers postulated two contributing mechanisms: a central one being dependent on the strength of respiratory drive and a peripheral (reflex) one.

Twenty to thirty years later, the mechanisms underlying Hering–Traube blood pressure waves were studied by Koepchen and coworkers in a series of experiments on anesthetized dogs (and also on some rabbits) (Koepchen and Thurau 1959; Koepchen et al. 1968; Seller et al. 1968). They perfused a vascularly isolated gracilis muscle with intact innervation at constant flow with O_2-saturated blood at body temperature and recorded the perfusion pressure, which is a measure of the vascular resistance. Fluctuations of perfusion pressure synchronous to phrenic nerve activity (PHR) or to integer multiples of PHR were observed, mostly with the increase in vascular resistance during inspiration. The amplitude of these fluctuations paralleled the depth of breathing, being largest when inspiration was prevented by tracheal occlusion. These fluctuations of vascular resistance were still present when ventilation was stopped by muscular paralysis with curare and when the arterial baroreceptors were denervated and the vagus nerves were sectioned in order to eliminate coupling by peripheral reflexes. This observation indicates that a central mechanism was operating.

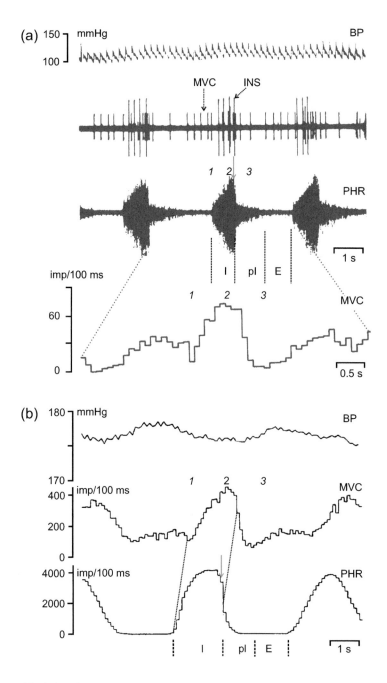

Figure 10.21 Respiratory profile in the activity of (a) preganglionic sympathetic neurons and (b) postganglionic muscle vasoconstrictor (MVC) neurons in the cat. (a) Recording from a bundle, isolated from the cervical sympathetic trunk, with a single preganglionic MVC axon and a single axon of a preganglionic inspiratory neuron (INS) in relation to phrenic nerve activity (PHR). Both vagus and aortic nerves were sectioned; in this way activity in cardiovascular and pulmonary afferents was eliminated. Upper trace, blood pressure (BP). Lower trace, histogram of the activity in the MVC neuron in 100 respiratory double cycles superimposed (bin width 100 ms) with respect to the end of inspiration on an expanded time scale (see blue arrow in PHR record). (b) Recording from a postganglionic multiunit bundle isolated from a muscle branch of the deep peroneal nerve. Vagus, aortic and carotid sinus nerves were sectioned. Activity in 100 respiratory double cycles superimposed (bin width 100 ms) with respect to the end of inspiration (blue arrow). Profile of activity in postganglionic neurons shifted to the right by 400 ms (peripheral conduction time) in the pre- and postganglionic axons with respect to PHR (dotted lines). Upper trace, blood pressure (BP). *1*, early inspiration; *2*, inspiration (I); *3*, postinspiration (pI); E, expiration. The cats were anesthetized, ventilated and immobilized. Boczek-Funcke et al. (unpublished observation).

10.6.4 Studies of Functionally Identified Sympathetic Neurons in Animals

Studies of sympathetic activity in whole nerves in animals and microneurographic recordings from bundles of postganglionic axons in human nerves may give the impression that the sympathetic neurons exhibit in their activity a more or less uniform pattern of respiratory modulation characterized by a peak in inspiration (Figure 10.21b). However, this

is not the case when one analyzes the respiratory rhythmicity of activity in *functionally identified sympathetic pre- and postganglionic neurons* in more detail in the anesthetized and artificially ventilated cat under various experimental conditions (increased/decreased respiratory drive, with/without rhythmic feedback in vagal [pulmonary] and/or arterial baroreceptor afferents). This analysis shows that the pattern of respiratory rhythmicity depends on the function of the sympathetic neuron and indicates that the coupling between the central respiratory network and the sympathetic premotor neurons in the medulla oblongata is not uniform (Boczek-Funcke et al. 1992a, b; Häbler et al. 1994a; Häbler and Jänig 1995; Jänig and Häbler 2003). Figures 10.22 and 10.23 demonstrate the main results of these studies:

- *Muscle, visceral,* a few *cutaneous vasoconstrictor neurons* and *sympathetic cardiomotor neurons* exhibit respiratory patterns in their activity that is typical for the uniform pattern seen in the "sympathetic" nerves (Figures 10.21, 10.22a, b, 10.23a). This pattern of activity has two components, one central and one peripheral (reflex): (1) The *central component* consists of an activation during inspiration (*II* in Figure 10.22b) with depression of activity during postinspiration (see *3* in Figure 10.21) and sometimes also in early inspiration (*1* in Figure 10.21). The size of activation and depression of activity increase with increasing respiratory drive (e.g., during hypercapnia). This pattern is clearly seen in vagotomized and baroreceptor-denervated animals (Figure 10.23). (2) The *peripheral reflex component* consists of a peak of activity during the declining phase of the respiratory blood pressure waves, which is associated with unloading of arterial baroreceptors (*I* in Figures 10.22b and 10.23a). In artificially ventilated cats, with intact vagus and baroreceptor nerves (and normal blood gases and pH), the activity is in many cases only related to the declining phase of the respiratory blood pressure waves, whereas the activation related to central inspiration is small or undetectable. Two factors seem to contribute to this limited evidence of coupling to central inspiration in normocapnia. *First,* the inspiratory drive to the sympathetic premotor neurons appears to be rather weak in normocapnia. *Second,* in ventilated cats with intact vagal and baroreceptor nerves the rising phase of the respiratory blood pressure wave coincides with central inspiration. Thus, the activation of sympathetic premotor neurons in the RVLM during inspiration may be attenuated by reflex inhibition via the baroreceptor reflex.
- There is no evidence from these studies that additional peripheral reflexes generated by activation of other cardiovascular or pulmonary afferent neurons directly contribute to respiration-related phasic modulation of activity in muscle and visceral vasoconstrictor activity other than by synchronizing central respiration. In *apneic hypocapnia* (decreased $PaCO_2$) generated by an increase in tidal volume, the respiration-related rhythm in the activity of muscle and visceral vasoconstrictor neurons is due to the arterial baroreceptor reflex and not, or at most only to a small extent, to the activation of cardiopulmonary vagal afferents. The neural rhythm in vasoconstrictor neurons that is related to the respiratory blood pressure waves in cats, in which only the arterial baroreceptors from the carotid sinuses are intact, is almost totally abolished by bilateral carotid occlusion when vagus nerves remain intact (Note 24).
- The respiratory modulation of activity in most *cutaneous vasoconstrictor neurons* is different from that in muscle and visceral vasoconstrictor neurons in the cat. No peripheral (reflex) component of respiratory modulation has been found that is related to rhythmic activation of arterial baroreceptor afferents or cardiopulmonary afferents. Thus, the observed patterns are due to central mechanisms. In normocapnia, most cutaneous vasoconstrictor neurons (about 80% of the postganglionic cutaneous vasoconstrictor neurons, about 40% of the preganglionic cutaneous vasoconstrictor neurons) show no respiratory modulation of their activity. The remainder exhibit some modulation in their activity, showing a weak maximum either in expiration (CVC in Figure 10.22a, c) or in inspiration (Figure 10.23). During increased respiratory drive (produced by increasing the P_{CO2} in the inspired air), some cutaneous vasoconstrictor neurons that show no respiratory modulation in their activity in normocapnia exhibit a peak of activity either in inspiration, expiration phase II or in postinspiration, whereas others maintain their unmodulated pattern. The cutaneous vasoconstrictor neurons exhibiting a peak of activity in postinspiration appear to be actively inhibited during inspiration (Figure 10.22c), which is particularly seen when the inspiratory drive is high (e.g., during hypercapnia). This respiratory activity pattern in cutaneous vasoconstrictor neurons resembles the pattern observed in parasympathetic cardiomotor neurons, which are inhibited during inspiration and excited during postinspiration (Gilbey et al. 1984). Cutaneous vasoconstrictor neurons exhibiting an inspiratory peak of activity preferentially

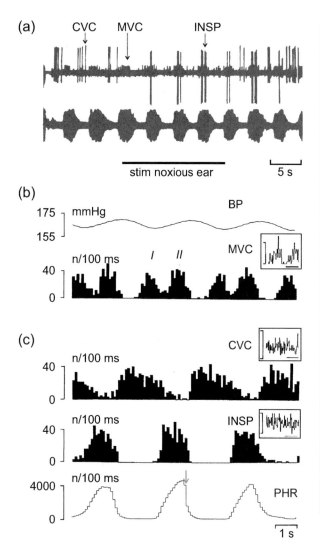

Figure 10.22 Respiratory modulation of activity in different types of functionally identified sympathetic preganglionic neurons projecting to the head or neck in the cat. (a) Original recording from three preganglionic axons isolated from the cervical sympathetic trunk. Responses (upper trace) to noxious stimulation of ear skin and correlation of activity with phrenic nerve activity (lower trace). Cutaneous vasoconstrictor (CVC) neuron (inhibited; activity in expiration). "Inspiratory" (INSP) neuron (activated: activity in inspiration). Muscle vasoconstrictor (MVC) neuron (activated; activity in inspiration and expiration). (b, c) Patterns of respiratory modulation of the activity in single preganglionic MVC, CVC and INSP neurons. Vagus and baroreceptor nerves intact. Activity in 100 respiratory double cycles superimposed (bin width 100 ms) with respect to the end of inspiration (see blue arrow in phrenic nerve activity record [PHR] in [c]). *Insets*: post-R-wave histograms of the activity ("cardiac rhythmicity"; activity in 500 cardiac double cycles superimposed, bin width 8 ms, time scale 200 ms, ordinate scales 20 imp/8 ms). Upper trace in (b), mean arterial blood pressure. (b) The activity in the MVC neuron shows two peaks, the first peak (*I*) being due to unloading of arterial baroreceptors during the falling phase of the second-order blood pressure waves (BP) and the second peak (*II*) being due to a central coupling to inspiratory neurons. Peak *I* matches the high degree of pulse rhythmicity in the activity of the MVC neuron (inset) and is increased with an increase in amplitude of the second-order blood pressure waves. Peak *II* increases during hypercapnia (increase of respiratory drive) and decreases during hyperventilation. Recorded during light hypercapnia. (c) The CVC neuron shows a pronounced expiratory peak of activity with its maximum in postinspiration. The INS neuron discharges exclusively during inspiration. Both neurons show no pulse rhythmicity in their activity (see insets). The CVC and INS neurons recorded simultaneously in normocapnia. Modified from Häbler et al. (1994b) with permission.

innervate hairless skin. The activation during inspiration in these neurons is not followed by a depression of activity in postinspiration.

- Discharges in *inspiratory neurons*, which are present only in the thoracic sympathetic outflow to the head and upper neck, are confined to central inspiration and are absent in postinspiration and expiration (INS in Figures 10.21, 10.22a, c, 10.23). These neurons are silenced during hypocapnia generated by hyperventilation and enhanced in their discharge during hypercapnia.
- Activity in *sudomotor neurons* has its maximum in postinspiration. It is enhanced during increased respiratory drive and similar to that observed in some cutaneous vasoconstrictor neurons (see Figure 10.23).
- Most *motility-regulating neurons* show no respiratory modulation in their activity. A few, however, discharge in postinspiration, similar to sudomotor and some cutaneous vasoconstrictor neurons.

In conclusion, in the cat, the respiratory profiles of activity in sympathetic neurons are not uniform, but vary according to the functional type of neuron (Figure 10.23), indicating that the central coupling between the neurons of the respiratory network and neurons associated with the sympathetic nervous system varies with the function of the sympathetic subsystem. This coupling probably depends on specific

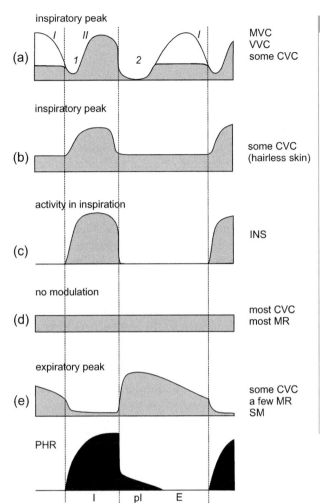

Figure 10.23 Synopsis of the various patterns of respiratory modulation exhibited by sympathetic neurons in the cat, under conditions of normal and increased respiratory drive. (a) Pattern present in almost all neurons in the cat that exhibit a high degree of cardiac rhythmicity in their activity (muscle vasoconstrictor [MVC], visceral vasoconstrictor [VVC], some cutaneous vasoconstrictor [CVC] neurons). The baroreceptor-mediated peak of activity (*I*) occurs when the ventilation pump and central respiration are entrained to each other. Inspiratory drive-dependent peak of activity (*II*) is preceded by a small and variable depression of activity (*1*) in early inspiration and followed by a pronounced depression of activity in postinspiration (*2*). These components have not been demonstrated in humans so far. (b) An inspiratory peak of activity is exhibited by a few CVC neurons (mainly supplying hairless skin). (c) Neurons discharging only in inspiration (INS) are present in the thoracic preganglionic outflow projecting into the cervical sympathetic trunk. Most of these neurons are not under baroreceptor control (see Figure 10.22a, c). (d) Respiratory modulation is absent in many CVC neurons and most motility-regulating (MR) neurons under normal respiration and neutral ambient temperature. (e) Expiratory pattern of activity with depression during inspiration and activation during postinspiration is shown by some CVC neurons, a few motility-regulating (MR) neurons and in sudomotor (SM) neurons. This pattern is also seen in parasympathetic cardiomotor neurons in the cat. E, phase II expiration; PHR, activity in the phrenic nerve: I, inspiration; pI, postinspiration. Modified from Häbler et al. (1994b) with permission. For references see Häbler et al. (1994b) and text.

synaptic connections between respiratory neurons and sympathetic premotor neurons in the medulla oblongata (e.g., in the VLM, caudal raphe nuclei, lateral paragigantocellular nuclei [McAllen 1987; Dampney and McAllen 1988; Haselton and Guyenet 1989; Guyenet 1990; Guyenet and Koshiya 1992]).

There are species differences between rodents and larger mammals, such as cats, dogs, rabbits and piglets (for discussion and literature see Häbler et al. [1994a]). The pattern of respiratory modulation that is most frequently found in the rat is depression of activity during inspiration and activation during postinspiration (Häbler et al. 1994b, 1996, 2000), whereas in larger animals the majority of sympathetic neurons shows the reverse. Similar patterns have been observed in bulbospinal barosensitive neurons of the RVLM of the rat (Haselton and

Guyenet 1989; Moraes et al. 2013) and in the activity of GABAergic barosensitive neurons in the caudal ventrolateral medulla of rats (Mandel and Schreihofer 2006). Contrary to what has been observed in cats, the patterns of respiratory modulation in rats are similar in postganglionic muscle and cutaneous vasoconstrictor neurons of the hindlimb and tail and in thoracic preganglionic neurons projecting to the head and neck (Häbler et al. 1996, 1999, 2000). Therefore, respiratory modulation cannot be used as a functional marker for sympathetic neurons in the rat projecting to skin or skeletal muscle (Häbler et al. 1993, 1994a). However, for rats it is unknown whether non-vasoconstrictor neurons (e.g., pilomotor, sudomotor, motility-regulating neurons) exhibit distinct respiratory profiles in their activity.

10.6.5 Studies of Functionally Identified Sympathetic Neurons In Humans

Respiratory changes in activity are also present in sympathetic postganglionic neurons innervating skeletal muscle or skin of humans. Figure 10.24 demonstrates one of the first microneurographic recordings from bundles of postganglionic muscle and cutaneous vasoconstrictor axons in muscle and skin nerves of an awake human subject, performed in the laboratory of Karl-Erik Hagbarth in Uppsala (Sweden). In the muscle vasoconstrictor neurons, the respiratory groupings of discharges exhibit cardiac rhythmicity (Figure 10.24b). Respiratory as well as pulsatile groupings of the multiunit activity are thought to be generated by unloading of arterial baroreceptors (decrease in baroreceptor activity) produced by the rhythmic respiratory and pulsatile decrease of arterial blood pressure. Activity in cutaneous vasoconstrictor neurons is also loosely correlated with respiration (Figure 10.24c) and during deep breathing, cutaneous vasoconstrictor neurons are strongly activated in the inspiratory phase (Figure 10.24d). This leads to rhythmic vasoconstriction of cutaneous blood vessels in the hands and feet.

Muscle Vasoconstrictor Neurons

Bursts of sympathetic activity in human muscle vasoconstrictor neurons are generated by pulsatile unloading of arterial baroreceptors and occur in groups related to the respiration (Figure 10.24a, b). They usually occur only during the falling phase of the respiratory blood pressure fluctuations (Figure 10.25a; Hagbarth and Vallbo 1968; Eckberg et al. 1985, 1988). Therefore it has been concluded that this rhythm is secondary to the blood pressure changes induced by respiration (Hagbarth and Vallbo 1968; Eckberg et al. 1985; Wallin and Fagius 1988). This rhythm appears to be analogous to the peripheral component of respiratory modulation in the activity of muscle vasoconstrictor neurons in cats when respiratory drive to the sympathetic premotor

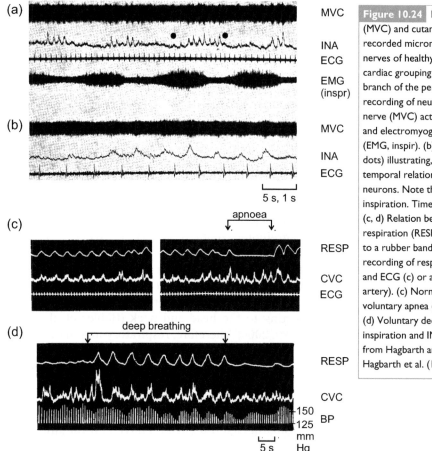

Figure 10.24 Multiunit activity in sympathetic muscle (MVC) and cutaneous vasoconstrictor (CVC) neurons recorded microneurographically in muscle or skin nerves of healthy human beings. (a, b) Respiratory and cardiac grouping of discharges in MVC neurons (deep branch of the peroneal nerve). (a) Simultaneous recording of neural activity (MVC), integrated nerve (MVC) activity (INA), electrocardiogram (ECG) and electromyogram from intercostal inspiratory muscle (EMG, inspir). (b) Part of record in (a) (between the dots) illustrating, on an expanded time scale, the temporal relation between ECG and INA in the MVC neurons. Note that some MVC activity occurs during inspiration. Time scale of 5 s for (a) and 1 s for (b). (c, d) Relation between INA in bundles of CVC fibers and respiration (RESP) (recorded by a strain gauge attached to a rubber band placed around the thorax). Simultaneous recording of respiratory movements (inspiration up), INA and ECG (c) or arterial blood pressure (BP, d; left radial artery). (c) Normal respiration (left, median nerve) or voluntary apnea (right, superficial peroneal nerve). (d) Voluntary deep inspiration. Note correlation between inspiration and INA in (c) left and (d). (a, b) Modified from Hagbarth and Vallbo (1968). (c, d) Modified from Hagbarth et al. (1972) with permission.

(a)

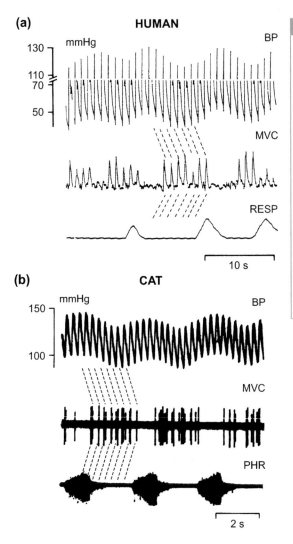

Figure 10.25 Comparison of the firing patterns of postganglionic muscle vasoconstrictor (MVC) activity in the human (a) and in the cat (b). Traces (from the top) show pulsatile arterial blood pressure (BP), neural activity (integrated MVC activity in [a] and original record of MVC activity in [b]) and central respiration (phrenic nerve activity [PHR] or pneumograph signal [RESP; inspiration upward], respectively). (a) Obtained from a conscious human being under resting conditions. (b) Obtained from an anesthetized, immobilized and artificially ventilated cat in normocapnia with intact vagus and buffer nerves and synchronized cycles of central respiration and artificial ventilation. The dashed lines indicate the close temporal relationship of the MVC action potentials and integrated MVC bursts, respectively, with the pulse pressure waves. Note that activity in the postganglionic axons is delayed by about 400 ms (cat) and 1.5 s (human) due to central and peripheral conduction time. Pulsatile muscle vasoconstrictor activity occurs mainly during the declining phase of the ventilatory oscillations of blood pressure, which coincide here with expiration. There is some, but only a little, discharge during inspiration, which is probably due to the coincidence of low inspiratory drive and the rising phase of the ventilatory blood pressure oscillations in the record on the human. (a) Modified from Eckberg et al. (1985) with permission; (b) from Häbler et al. (1994b) with permission.

neurons is relatively low (Figure 10.25b). Thus, the data obtained in conscious human subjects match those obtained in anesthetized cats.

A central respiratory component in MVC activity (i.e., activation during inspiration, equivalent to the activation of MVC neurons in cats) is absent or could not be detected in human subjects (Eckberg et al. 1985) (Note 25), probably because: (1) the respiratory drive to MVC neurons under resting conditions is relatively weak (e.g., from the sympathetic premotor neurons in the RVLM; McAllen 1987) and (2) the rising phase of the arterial blood pressure waves occurring during inspiration (activating arterial baroreceptors followed by inhibition of activity in muscle vasoconstrictor neurons) probably counteracts the inspiratory activation of these neurons (Note 26).

Cutaneous Vasoconstrictor Neurons and Sudomotor Neurons

In humans, sympathetic activity in nerves supplying distal (acral) skin, which is a mixture of vasoconstrictor and sudomotor activity, depending on the central thermoregulatory state, occurs in irregular bursts (Hagbarth et al. 1972; Wallin and Fagius 1988), which are independent of the pulsatile blood pressure oscillations. Thus, a baroreceptor-mediated reflex component of respiratory modulation is mostly not detectable in skin sympathetic activity (Hagbarth et al. 1972).

During normal quiet breathing, bursts in cutaneous sympathetic activity are loosely and variably coupled to respiration (mostly to the inspiratory phase [Figure 10.24c]; Hagbarth et al. 1972; Hallin and Torebjörk 1974). With increased vasoconstrictor activity at low ambient temperature, respiratory modulation of cutaneous sympathetic activity becomes more pronounced (Bini et al. 1980a, b). Activity of single postganglionic cutaneous vasoconstrictor or sudomotor axons innervating hairy skin of the foot in humans (superficial peroneal nerve) was investigated for respiratory rhythmicity during body cooling (skin temperature $\leq$22.8 °C; only cutaneous vasoconstrictor neurons active) or during body heating (skin temperature 31 to 33.8 °C; sudomotor neurons active [subjects were sweating] and activity in cutaneous vasoconstrictor neurons low or absent). Under these conditions, about 50% of the sudomotor neurons and two-thirds of the cutaneous vasoconstrictor neurons exhibit respiratory rhythmicity in their activity. The probability of discharge in both types of sympathetic neuron is higher in inspiration than in expiration (Macefield and Wallin 1999).

From plethysmographic measurements, it is known that deep inspiration is followed by vasoconstriction in the skin of the fingers (Bolton et al. 1936; Gilliat 1948). This is probably due to bursts of activity in skin sympathetic neurons occurring in response to deep breaths (Figure 10.24d). Activation of cutaneous vasoconstrictor neurons during deep inspiration does not correlate with the systolic blood pressure changes (Figure 10.24d). This could theoretically be due to central coupling of skin sympathetic premotor neurons to inspiratory neurons. However, since the inspiration-induced vasoconstriction was still found in patients with spinal cords transected at a high thoracic level, it was suggested that this reflex is spinal (Gilliat et al. 1948), the involved afferents being unknown. However, Hagbarth et al. (1972) also found some neural "reflex" components with long latencies following a deep breath and concluded that both spinal and supraspinal mechanisms may be involved, arguing that a central component of respiratory modulation contributes to the response of the skin sympathetic activity.

In conclusion, in humans, muscle vasoconstrictor, cutaneous vasoconstrictor and sudomotor neurons exhibit some respiratory modulation of activity. To analyze the precise temporal relationship of activity in these sympathetic neurons in relation to the different phases of central respiration in humans more closely, EMG-recordings from respiratory muscles under various experimental conditions (e.g., hypercapnia, hyperthermia, hypothermia etc.) are warranted in these studies (see Figure 10.24a).

10.6.6 Integration Between Autonomic and Respiratory Generators

The classical view on integration between autonomic and respiratory generators held by Traube (1865) and Hering (1869) was that vasomotor and respiratory centers are situated separately in the lower brain stem. In cardiorespiratory coupling, both authors gave the primacy to the respiratory system and thought that the rhythmic activity "irradiates" from the respiratory to the cardiovascular center. This concept was based on experiments performed on dogs and cats in which the coupling between the two systems was studied under extreme conditions, such as asphyxia and high CO_2 load. The term "irradiation" is now outdated, yet the concept behind it is still implicit in the term "respiratory modulation" of sympathetic activity (see Koepchen [1983]; Koepchen et al. [1987]). From the observations of respiratory blood pressure waves, a non-specific "common central rhythmicity," which is not primarily related to respiration but generates rhythmic activity in various peripheral output systems, e.g., to respiratory muscles and cardiovascular target organs, was postulated (Koepchen 1962). Later several oscillators for the respiratory, sympathetic and other output systems were proposed (Koepchen et al. 1981; Koepchen 1983). These common oscillators were thought to be entrained (Ramirez and Baertsch 2018; Baertsch et al. 2019). The neural matrix comprising the oscillators was thought to process information from cardiovascular afferents, pulmonary afferents and other types of afferent neurons and from the central chemosensitive sites that are located in the retrotrapezoid nucleus below the facial motor nucleus (not shown in Figures 10.2 and 10.3; Guyenet et al. 2019). The output of the respiratory network was believed to "irradiate" backward into the reticular formation, which then modulates the activity of the sympathetic output. Barman and Gebber (1976) suggested that the respiratory rhythm and the respiratory modulation of sympathetic activity are generated by two independent oscillators which are normally entrained to each other.

The most elaborate concept of the generation of respiratory rhythmicity in autonomic neurons in the cat has been developed by Richter, Spyer and coworkers (Richter and Spyer 1990; Richter et al. 1991). Based on their working model, it is proposed that coupling between the respiratory network and the neurons

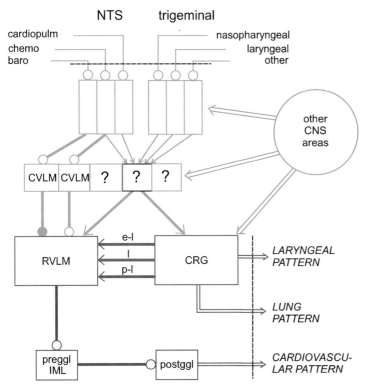

Figure 10.26 Integration of the central respiratory generator (CRG) and the rostral ventrolateral medulla (RVLM): an idea. The CRG determines the respiratory lung pattern as well as the laryngeal rhythm (which is phylogenetically equivalent to the gill rhythm in fish [see Richter et al. 1991]). The respiratory rhythm in the autonomic cardiovascular neurons is determined by the integration between the respiratory network and the cardiovascular neurons in the RVLM (constituting the so-called "common cardiorespiratory network" [Richter and Spyer 1990; Richter et al. 1991]). This system is modulated by various reflex pathways linked to cardiovascular and pulmonary afferents as well as trigeminal, laryngeal, pharyngeal and other afferents. The reflexes may influence the sympathetic premotor neurons in the RVLM either directly or via the CRG. Furthermore, the CRG may influence the RVLM indirectly via the CVLM (not shown). Other areas of brain stem, hypothalamus and telencephalon modulate RVLM, CRG and reflex pathways. CNS, central nervous system; CVLM, caudal ventrolateral medulla; IML, intermediolateral nucleus; NTS, nucleus tractus solitarii; preggl, preganglionic; postggl, postganglionic; el, early inspiration; I, inspiration; pI, postinspiration.

related to the cardiovascular autonomic systems occurs in the lower brain stem via ramp-inspiratory, early-inspiratory and postinspiratory neurons of the respiratory network. According to this model, sympathetic premotor neurons (e.g., in the RVLM) would be influenced in the following ways:

1. activation by ramp-inspiratory neurons (which activate inspiratory [bulbospinal] premotor neurons);
2. inhibition by postinspiratory neurons (which inhibit ramp-inspiratory and early-inspiratory neurons); and
3. inhibition by early-inspiratory neurons (which inhibit postinspiratory and ramp-inspiratory neurons).

This model can fully account for the respiratory activity profile in muscle, visceral, renal vasoconstrictor neurons and sympathetic cardiomotor neurons, which dominates the respiratory rhythmicity of the activity in all "sympathetic" nerves in the cat (see Figures 10.21b, 10.23a). It is supported by the finding that many sympathetic premotor neurons in the RVLM change their activity during the respiratory cycle, being activated during inspiration, although details about the depression of activity in early

inspiration and postinspiration have not yet been worked out. As emphasized by Richter and Spyer (1990), this model also accounts for the inhibition of parasympathetic cardiomotor neurons in inspiration and activation or disinhibition in postinspiration. In order to account for the various patterns of respiratory modulation seen in the activity of functionally different types of sympathetic neurons, the nature of the coupling between neurons of the central respiration generator (CRG) and the sympathetic premotor neurons must vary, depending on the function of the sympathetic neurons.

Any attempt to explain the neural mechanisms of respiratory patterns in the activity of autonomic neurons rests on the comparison between rhythmic discharges in the phrenic nerve and peripheral autonomic neurons as well as in sympathetic premotor neurons in the VLM. Thus, the explanations are based on analogy and at best on indirect arguments derived from investigations of neurons of the respiratory network with respect to the phrenic nerve. As proposed in Figures 10.20 and 10.26 the coupling between the respiratory system and the sympathetic cardiovascular pathways may occur at the level of the sympathetic premotor neurons, e.g., in the RVLM, or of neurons synaptically connected to RVLM neurons (Mandel and Schreihofer 2006; Moraes et al. 2013).

Several groups of cardiovascular, pulmonary, laryngeal, pharyngeal and other afferents can influence sympathetic premotor neurons, parasympathetic cardiomotor neurons and respiratory premotor neurons. Detailed analysis of the pathways underlying these reflexes has only been performed for a few systems (see baroreceptor reflexes and chemoreceptor reflexes in Subchapters 10.3 and 10.4). As demonstrated for the chemoreceptor reflex in sympathetic cardiovascular neurons, reflex activation and inhibition are mediated by neural pathways that are independent of the central respiratory generator (CRG) as well as via the CRG (Figure 10.26; Guyenet and Koshiya 1992; Häbler et al. 1997; Guyenet 2000; for discussion see Häbler et al. [1994a]).

The general idea of a "common cardiorespiratory network," as propagated by Richter, Spyer and co-workers, is that the neurons and their synaptic connections in the VLM (which includes the RVLM, IVLM/CVLM and VRG) represent a complex sensorimotor program that guarantees at any moment and under any physiological condition a precisely coordinated regulation of the respiratory pump, the arterial blood pressure and the perfusion of the lung. This includes the coordinated neural regulation of the right and left heart as well as of peripheral resistance. This idea requires distinct inhibitory and excitatory synaptic connections between different groups of neurons in the "common cardiorespiratory network." It requires, furthermore, that the functionally distinct types of afferent neuron involved in this coordinated regulation (see Figure 10.26) form distinct reflex circuits with the output neurons of this network. These reflex circuits may occur via the CRG or independent of it. For example, the baroreceptor pathways can normally function independently of the central respiratory rhythm generator, but clearly interact with it as well. This is still a controversial issue (Seller et al. 1968; Boczek-Funcke et al. 1991).

Overall, the distinct component parts of this neuronal network that integrates regulation of respiration and regulation of the cardiovascular system are unknown. In the rat, a main coupling may occur from the preBötzinger complex via glutamatergic interneurons (that express the NK_1-receptor) to inhibitory GABAergic and/or glycinergic interneurons in the CVLM that inhibit bulbospinal neurons in the RVLM (Wang et al. 2003). This coupling would imply that activity in vasoconstrictor neurons that are under the control of the RVLM is inhibited during inspiration. It has been shown in the rat that most barosensitive postganglionic neurons are depressed in their activity during inspiration and that this depression is enhanced during increased respiratory drive (Häbler et al. 1993, 1994a; Bartsch et al. 1999).

Command signals generated in supramedullary centers (e.g., the periaqueductal gray, hypothalamus, telencephalon) normally do not activate cardiovascular sympathetic premotor, cardiovascular parasympathetic premotor neurons or respiratory premotor neurons (nor the final autonomic and somatic motor neurons) directly. They engage instead with the "common cardiorespiratory network" (i.e., the cardiorespiratory motor program), e.g., during exercise or defense behaviors.

The idea of a "common cardiorespiratory network" should not be generalized to all sympathetic or parasympathetic systems. Most types of sympathetic and parasympathetic neurons do not have cardiovascular functions. Future experimental work is likely to show that other sensorimotor programs exist in the lower brain stem that are involved in thermoregulation (Romanovsky 2018), regulation of energy balance (see Subchapter 10.5) or regulation of gastrointestinal functions (see Subchapter 10.7). These probably include premotor pathways to motor neurons involved in body movements, sympathetic premotor neurons to cutaneous vasoconstrictor, lipomotor, sudomotor and motility-regulating pathways and parasympathetic pathways innervating the gastrointestinal tract. By the same token, it will be shown that the central autonomic systems that are not involved in cardiovascular regulation may also be coupled to the regulation of respiration. However, the underlying mechanisms of this coupling will turn out to be different from those between the neural network related to respiration and the neural network related to the cardiovascular system.

10.6.7 Synopsis and Open Questions

Neural regulation of the cardiovascular system and of respiration are closely integrated. This integration is expressed in the respiratory pattern of the activity of cardiovascular autonomic neurons involved in regulation of blood pressure, such as cardiomotor, muscle vasoconstrictor and visceral vasoconstrictor neurons. Only 10% to 20% of the sympathetic preganglionic neurons of the sympathetic outflow to the head and neck, to deep somatic tissues and to viscera are barosensitive cardiovascular neurons, as shown in detail under anesthetized conditions in the cat (Table 4.5). What is the function of the respiratory pattern in the activity of non-cardiovascular sympathetic neurons, such as cutaneous vasoconstrictor, sudomotor and inspiratory-type neurons? The patterns of activity in these sympathetic systems express a way of neural coupling to the respiratory system that is different from that of sympathetic cardiovascular systems. Is the coupling of autonomic neurons to respiration partially depressed by anesthesia and therefore mainly present in the awake state? Are autonomic functions synchronized in the awake state by the respiratory system, leading in this way to a synchronization of body functions during various types of behavior?

10.7 | Vagal Efferent Pathways and Regulation of Gastrointestinal Functions

The medulla oblongata contains the circuitry for the basic neural regulation of the cardiovascular system, the respiratory system and the gastrointestinal tract (GIT) by the brain, and their mutual integration (Figure 10.1). In the last part of this chapter, I will concentrate on some principles of regulation of the foregut by the brain, and focus particularly on the medulla oblongata. As described in Chapter 5, the GIT has an autonomic nervous system of its own called the enteric nervous system. This system is integrated into the regulation of the foregut by the brain. The dorsal vagal complex (DVC), which consists of the nucleus tractus solitarii (NTS), the dorsal motor nucleus of the vagus nerve (DMNX) and the area postrema (AP), is, in a way, the interface between the brain and the enteric nervous system in the neural regulation of the foregut. The communication from foregut to the DVC occurs via vagal afferents, hormones of the GIT and nutritive compounds; the efferent communication occurs via parasympathetic

preganglionic neurons located in the DMNX (Figure 10.27).

10.7.1 Vagal Afferents and Preganglionic Neurons

Vagal afferent neurons from the GIT, which have their cell bodies in the inferior ganglion of the vagus nerve (nodose ganglion), project topographically to the NTS. They show a distinct mediolateral as well as rostrocaudal arrangement of the projections to its subnuclei (see Figures 8.10 and 8.11). These visceral afferents monitor several parameters related to the GIT (see Subchapters 2.3 and 2.4):

1. Mechanical events related to contraction or distension of the GIT or to shearing stimuli exerted at the mucosal surface.
2. Chemical events related to decrease in pH, changes in glucose or lipid concentration or other chemical events.
3. Toxic events related to ingested food that may be harmful for the GIT and for the organism; putative afferents monitoring these toxic events may be particularly associated with the most powerful defense line in the body, the gut-associated lymphoid tissue (GALT; Mowat 2003).

The various functional types of vagal visceral afferent neurons innervating the GIT and their transduction mechanisms are only partially known and incompletely understood. The excitation of some types of vagal afferents innervating the small intestine (probably those activated by chemical stimuli such as lipids) is mediated by cholecystokinin (CCK) or 5-HT (and possibly other hormones; Richards et al. 1996; Hillsley et al. 1998; Hillsley and Grundy 1998; Kreis et al. 2002). Many afferent neurons terminate within ganglia of the myenteric plexus (Berthoud and Powley 1992; Phillips et al. 1997; Berthoud and Neuhuber 2000). These afferents are possibly mechanosensitive (Zagorodnyuk and Brookes 2000; Zagorodnyuk et al. 2001; for reviews see Brookes et al. [2013]; Spencer et al. [2016]) (for description of vagal visceral afferent neurons see Subchapter 2.3). Further afferent signals from the GIT arise via hormones of the GIT, such as cholecystokinin, glucagon-like peptide 1, pancreatic peptide, peptide YY and ghrelin and humoral substances (glucose, lipids). These substances act via the area postrema (see Subchapters 8.3 and 10.7.4) and/or via the arcuate nucleus in the

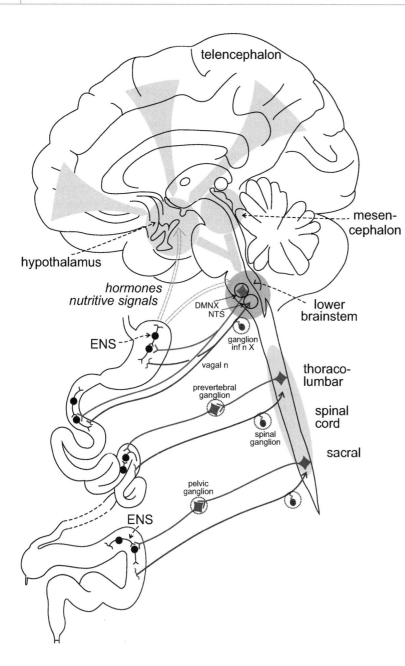

telencephalon

mesen-
cephalon

hypothalamus

*hormones
nutritive signals*

DMNX
NTS

lower
brainstem

ENS

ganglion
inf n X

vagal n

thoraco-
lumbar

prevertebral
ganglion

spinal
cord

spinal
ganglion

sacral

pelvic
ganglion

ENS

Figure 10.27 Brain and gastrointestinal tract (GIT). Reciprocal communication between the two by afferent and efferent (autonomic) systems. The centerpiece of this communication is the dorsal vagal complex in the lower brain stem, which consists of the nucleus tractus solitarii (NTS), the dorsal motor nucleus of the vagus (DMNX) and the area postrema (AP, not shown). Parasympathetic preganglionic neurons to the GIT are located in the DMNX. Signals from the GIT are transmitted by vagal afferents to the NTS as well as by hormones from the GIT and nutritive compounds (glucose, lipids) via the area postrema to the NTS or to the hypothalamus. ENS, enteric nervous system; ganglion inf n X, ganglion inferius nervi vagi (nodose ganglion).

hypothalamus in regulation of food intake, metabolism, motility and exocrine secretion of the GIT, as well as sensations (like fullness, satiety, nausea) (for hormones of the GIT acting via the area postrema).

Parasympathetic preganglionic neurons projecting to the gastrointestinal tract are situated in the dorsal motor nucleus of the vagus (DMNX). They are topographically arranged in rostrocaudally oriented cell columns according to the organ section they innervate (e.g., stomach, duodenum, small intestines and cecum; see Figure 8.10b,c). These preganglionic neurons have various functions related to:

1. regulation of motility of the GIT (several types of excitatory and inhibitory [non-cholinergic non-adrenergic] motoneurons);
2. regulation of exocrine secretion (e.g., secretomotor neurons innervating gastric parietal cells that secrete proton ions, exocrine pancreas, submucosal glands or mucosa cells);

3. regulation of hormone release (e.g., gastrin, secretin, insulin, glucagon); or possibly
4. regulation of the inner defense line of the body that is connected with the GALT (but this is rather hypothetical).

Thus, there are several functionally distinct types of vagal and spinal visceral afferent neurons and several functionally distinct types of preganglionic neuron innervating the GIT (see Figures 5.14 and 5.15). These are the peripheral substrates for the specific regulation of different functions of the GIT and their coordination by the brain (Travagli et al. 2006; Browning and Travagli 2011, 2014; Travagli and Anselmi 2016).

10.7.2 Distinct Intestino-Intestinal Reflex Circuits in the Dorsal Vagal Complex

An intimate anatomical relationship exists between nuclei in the NTS and the DMNX, implying that afferents from the GIT form disynaptic contacts with the preganglionic neurons projecting to the GIT. Therefore, as far as the GIT is concerned, the combination of NTS, AP and DMNX is called collectively the dorsal vagal complex (DVC) (see Figure 10.29). Some afferents form monosynaptic contacts with the dendrites of the preganglionic neurons in the DMNX that project dorsally into the NTS (Rinaman et al. 1989). However, these monosynaptic contacts seem to be rare compared to the disynaptic contacts via interneurons in the NTS.

Systematic neurophysiological analysis of preganglionic neurons in the DMNX that project in one of the gastric branches of the abdominal vagus nerves have shown that several functional types of preganglionic neuron can be identified by their reflex responses to physiological stimuli applied to stomach, duodenum or small intestine (e.g., distension of organ sections [esophagus, stomach, duodenum], intraluminal chemical stimulation). Figure 10.28 demonstrates two representative experiments. The preganglionic neurons exhibit various combinations of responses to the physiological stimuli. These patterns are correlated with other properties of the neurons, such as rate of spontaneous activity, morphology of dendrites and peptide content. At least four functional types of preganglionic neurons have been identified in the DMNX (see also Subchapter 4.8), indicating the functional differentiation of the parasympathetic pathways that are represented in the

DMNX and project to the GIT (Zhang et al. 1992, 1995, 1998; Fogel et al. 1996; Browning et al. 1999).

Synaptic transmission from vagal afferents to the NTS neurons is excitatory and the transmitter is glutamate. In the rostrocaudal area of the NTS where vagal afferents project to some 40% to 50% of the NTS, neurons are synaptically activated by electrical stimulation of the subdiaphragmatic vagal nerve. Inhibitory responses are practically absent. These neurons do not receive convergent synaptic input from arterial baro- or chemoreceptor afferents. Surprisingly, some 20% of the NTS neurons receiving synaptic afferent input from the GIT are activated by myelinated fibers (Paton et al. 2000) although only $\leq 1\%$ of the afferent fibers in the subdiaphragmatic vagus nerve are myelinated in the rat (Gabella 1976).

The predominant synaptic transmission between the NTS neurons and the preganglionic neurons in the DMNX projecting to the GIT is inhibitory, the transmitter being mainly GABA. Other synaptic connections between NTS neurons and DMNX neurons are excitatory, the transmitter being glutamate. Gastric relaxation induced by esophageal distension is mediated by an excitatory reflex pathway involving the central nucleus of the NTS (see "ce" in Figure 8.11a) and the DMNX. The NTS neurons involved in this reflex are noradrenergic and this receptive relaxation reflex is significantly reduced after blockade of α-adrenoceptors (α_1, α_2) in the DMNX. Seventy-five percent of neurons in the DMNX projecting to the stomach are either excited or inhibited by noradrenaline. Thus, noradrenaline is believed to be the transmitter mediating this reflex in the DMNX (Fukuda et al. 1987; Rogers et al. 2003; Martinez et al. 2004; Babic et al. 2015; McMenamin et al. 2016).

For most of the parasympathetic pathways projecting to the foregut, it is at present uncertain or a matter of speculation which target cells or functionally distinct enteric circuits they innervate (see also Chapter 5). However, it is reasonable to assume that circuits of the enteric nervous system, which are related to non-vascular smooth muscles, exocrine glands, endocrine glands or possibly even the vasculature, receive differential signals from the brain by way of the parasympathetic preganglionic neurons in the DMNX. Thus, it is also not far-fetched to assume that the number of functional types of preganglionic parasympathetic neurons in the DMNX is higher than four (see Table 1.2). Based on cyto- and chemo-

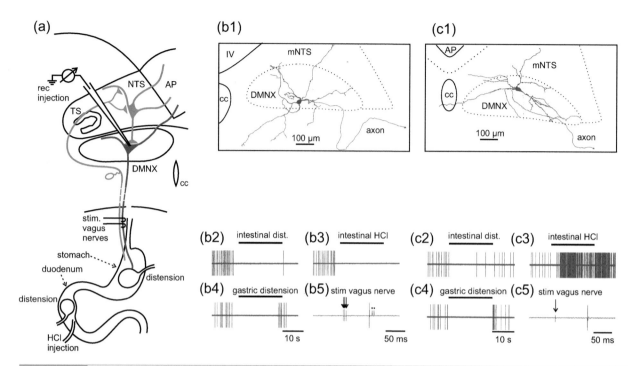

Figure 10.28 Responses of parasympathetic preganglionic neurons in the dorsal motor nucleus of the vagus (DMNX) of the rat to mechanical or chemical stimulation of the GIT and morphological identification of the neurons. (a) Experimental setup. The neurons in the DMNX were recorded extracellularly with glass microelectrodes filled with neurobiotin. After functional characterization of a neuron the micropipette was advanced until the neuron was impaled and neurobiotin was injected intracellularly. The neurons were identified by electrical stimulation of their axons in the gastric branches of the abdominal vagus nerves (see [b5] and [c5]) with pulses of 0.5 ms duration. For this purpose, both gastric branches of the abdominal vagus nerves were put on a stimulation electrode. Vagal afferents were activated by distension of the stomach or duodenum by a balloon or by intraluminal injection of HCl into the duodenum. After physiological identification of the neurons by their reflex responses, neurobiotin was injected through the recording electrode into the neurons. The rats were perfused with a fixative, the medulla oblongata was removed and its dorsomedial part containing the nucleus tractus solitarii (NTS) and DMNX was cut into serial sections, and the neuron containing neurobiotin was visualized. (b) Spontaneously active preganglionic neuron, which was inhibited by the mechanical and chemical stimuli (b_2 to b_4). (b_1) Demonstrates the morphology of the neuron in red. (b_5) Demonstrates the antidromic responses of the neuron to a train of three electrical stimuli at 150 Hz to its axon. The responses to the second and third stimulus were only electrotonically conducted (dots) since the action potentials of the axons did not actively invade the soma of the neuron. (c) Spontaneously active preganglionic neuron, which was inhibited by mechanical stimulation and excited by chemical stimulation (c_2 to c_4). (c_1) Demonstrates the morphology of the neuron in red. (c_5) Demonstrates the antidromic response of the neuron to electrical stimulation of its axon. Note that the dendrites of the neurons project into the NTS. cc, central canal; mNTS, medial nucleus of the NTS; TS, tractus solitarius; IV, fourth ventricle. Modified from Zhang et al. (1998) with permission.

architectonic criteria, the DMNX in humans contains nine types of neuron (Huang et al. 1993).

10.7.3 Integration in the Dorsal Vagal Complex: A Concept

Preganglionic neurons in the DMNX exhibit many types of functionally specific reflexes. These reflexes depend on the type of vagal afferent neuron from the GIT activated, the excitatory or inhibitory synaptic transmission from the NTS neurons to the preganglionic neurons, and on the functional type of preganglionic neuron in the DMNX. In order to account for this variety of functional reflexes, Powley and coworkers have created an interesting hypothesis on the spatial organization of the DVC (NTS, DMNX and AP) (Powley et al. 1992). This hypothesis is based on the mediolateral representation of the GIT in the DMNX (Figures 8.10c,d and 8.12) and on the rostrocaudal organization of the projections of vagal and other afferents from the tongue, pharynx and GIT to the NTS (Figure 8.12e). Powley and co-workers propose that the two layers of the DVC form a sensorimotor lattice, as illustrated in Figure 10.29. The two components of the DVC are fused. The proposed sensorimotor lattice would allow for many specific reflexes elicited in the parasympathetic preganglionic neurons by stimulation of distinct types of afferents from the GIT, pharynx and tongue and for various combinations (patterns) of reflexes (Powley et al. 1992). The functionally distinct reflex circuits formed in the DVC between the afferents from and the preganglionic neurons to the GIT are the basic building blocks for the brain to control gastrointestinal functions. The idea of the sensorimotor lattice of the DVC as proposed by Powley is a heuristic model and certainly an approximation that does not apply to all situations. For example, esophageal distension elicits proximal gastric relaxation, the basis being the "receptive relaxation reflex" arc consisting of vagal afferents from the esophagus, second-order neurons in the pars centralis of the NTS (NTS_{cen}) that receive synaptic input from these afferents and vagal preganglionic neurons projecting to the stomach. It has been shown by Rogers et al. (1999) that the neurons in the NTS_{cen} project extensively throughout the rostrocaudal DMNX.

Anatomical studies show that several nuclei in the brain stem and forebrain have reciprocal connections with the circuits of the DVC. This situation is conceptually quite similar to the role of spinal autonomic circuits in the control of spinal autonomic final pathways by supraspinal centers (see Chapter 9). Thus, these reflex pathways of the DVC are under modulatory control of neurons in supramedullary brain centers (so-called "executive" neurons, e.g., in the paraventricular nucleus of the hypothalamus [PVH], the central nucleus of the amygdala [CNA], the bed nucleus of the stria terminalis [BNST], etc.; see Figure 10.30), which also receive detailed afferent information from the GIT (via the NTS) and from other body tissues. Executive neurons and basic autonomic circuits in the DVC associated with the GIT represent the *internal state of the organism* as far as the gastrointestinal tract is concerned. This internal state is adapted to the behavior of the organism by cortex and limbic system structures, which monitor and represent the *external state of the organism*. However, the internal state also modulates the central representation of the external state, leading to changes in

sensory perception, body feelings and experience of emotions. This concept, as exemplified in Figure 10.30, shows that there is a close integration between the homeostatic regulation of GIT functions and the higher nervous system functions related to body perception, emotions and adaptation of behavior. The highly specific autonomic reflex pathways in the DVC of the brain stem (and possibly also in the spinal cord; see Figures 5.15 and 5.16) are the basis of this integration. This general concept of the control of gastrointestinal functions by the brain has been propagated and worked out by Rogers and coworkers (Rogers and Hermann 1992; Travagli and Rogers 2001). It is the biological basis for the changes in gastrointestinal function during various behaviors, including stress.

10.7.4 The Area Postrema and the Integration of Endocrine Signals

The reflex neural circuits in the DVC are also modulated by blood-borne signals, which reach the neurons of the DVC by way of the AP. These signals are hormones from the GIT, such as insulin, CCK, glucagon-like peptide 1 (GLP-1), pancreatic polypeptide (PP) or peptide YY (PYY), other hormones and nutritive substances (glucose, lipids). In the AP and neighboring parts of the DVC the blood–brain barrier is open. Thus, these parts of the DVC do not have a vascular diffusion barrier (Figure 10.31), allowing the hormonal and humoral substances to have free access to the neural circuits of the DVC. The dendrites of both NTS neurons and DMNX neurons project into the AP. Furthermore, the circuits in the DVC are influenced by neuronal circuits that use neuroendocrine hormones as transmitters or neuromodulators (such as thyrotropin-releasing hormone [TRH] or corticotropin-releasing hormone [CRH]). The following examples illustrate this integration of neuroendocrine and autonomic functions at the level of the medulla oblongata in the regulation of gastrointestinal functions:

- *Thyrotropin-releasing hormone (TRH)* induces gastric acid secretion, enhances feeding behavior, activates metabolism, enhances the neural signals to produce cutaneous vasoconstriction and induces shivering by asynchronous firing of motoneurons. This response pattern is typically induced during cold stress and is an expression of the coordination of *thermoregulation* and *control of metabolism*.

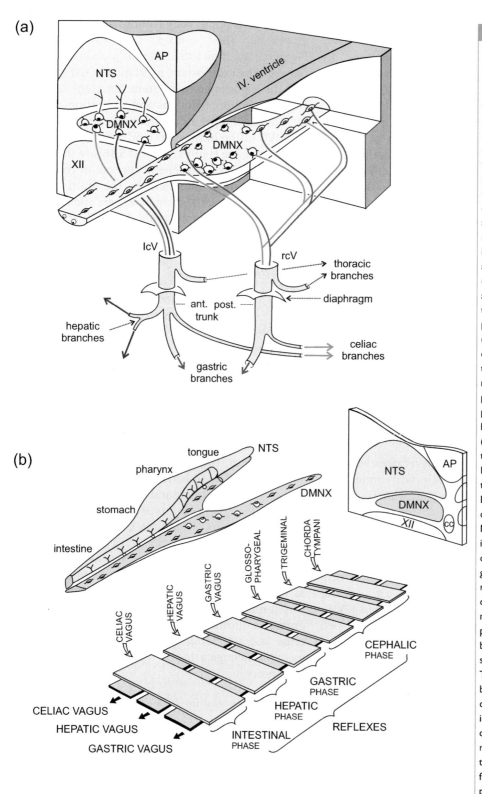

Figure 10.29 Sensorimotor spatial organization of the dorsal vagal complex (DVC): a hypothesis. (a) Schematic view of the DVC: nucleus tractus solitarii (NTS), area postrema (AP), dorsal motor nucleus of the vagus (DMNX) of the medulla oblongata seen from a caudal and lateral perspective. The DVC is shown in a transverse (frontal) section on the left and the DMNX in a longitudinal section on the right. The medial cell columns in the DMNX project in the anterior (ant.) and posterior (post.) gastric branches of the abdominal vagus nerves (red); the lateral cell columns project in the celiac branches (green); the intermediate cell column on the left projects in the hepatic branch (blue). The nucleus ambiguus, which is positioned ventrolateral and parallel to the nucleus hypoglossus (XII), is not shown. (b) The sensorimotor lattice of the DVC. Upper left, layers of NTS and DMNX. Upper right, transverse section through the DVC. Lower: mediolaterally organized cell groups in the NTS receiving distinct afferent inputs from different parts of the nasopharyngeal or gastrointestinal tract; rostrocaudally organized columns of preganglionic neurons in the DMNX that project through the different branches of the subdiaphragmatic vagus nerve. This sensorimotor lattice may be the basis for various cephalic, gastric, hepatic or intestinal reflexes. cc, central canal; lcV, left cervical vagus; rcV, right cervical vagus; TS, tractus solitarius. Modified from Powley et al. (1992) with permission.

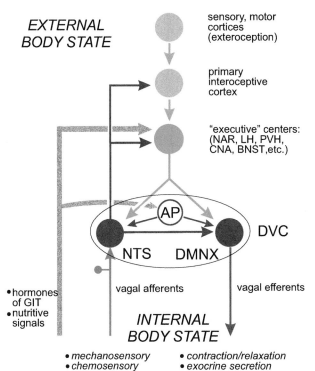

EXTERNAL
BODY STATE

sensory, motor
cortices
(exteroception)

primary
interoceptive
cortex

"executive" centers:
(NAR, LH, PVH,
CNA, BNST,etc.)

AP

NTS   DMNX   DVC

vagal afferents   vagal efferents

•hormones
of GIT
•nutritive
signals

INTERNAL
BODY STATE

• mechanosensory
• chemosensory
• sensory from
    GALT?

• contraction/relaxation
• exocrine secretion
• endocrine secretion
• defense (GALT)?

Figure 10.30 Proposed relationship between the gastrointestinal vago-vagal reflex pathways, forebrain autonomic "executive" neuronal circuits, primary interoceptive cortex and cortices involved in exteroception. Several functionally specific vago-vagal reflex pathways form the basic neuronal building blocks. They are mediated through the dorsal vagal complex (DVC). Vagal afferents record mechano-, chemo- and other sensory events, including sensing events in the gut-associated lymphoid tissue (GALT), and project to the nucleus tractus solitarii (NTS); vagal preganglionic neurons are located in the dorsal motor nucleus of the vagus (DMNX) and are involved in regulation of motility, exocrine secretion, endocrine secretion and other events (including those associated with the GALT). "Executive" centers (e.g., paraventricular nucleus of the hypothalamus, PVH; lateral hypothalamus, LH; nucleus arcuatus, NAR; central nucleus of the amygdala, CNA; bed nucleus of the stria terminalis, BNST) evaluate the state of the internal milieu (by way of inputs from vagal and other visceral afferents) as well as the current or anticipated behavioral state (via input from cortical areas being involved in exteroception). These executive centers adapt the internal state (e.g., gastrointestinal functions) to the behavioral state of the organism. AP, area postrema. Modified from Rogers and Hermann (1992).

Neurons in the raphe obscurus and in the parapyramidal nucleus of the ventromedial medulla (in which TRH and 5-HT are colocalized) project to the DVC and form synapses with neurons in the

NTS and in the DMNX (Yang et al. 2000b). These neurons are activated during cold stress. Thus, TRH, both circulatory and neuronally released, appears to be the organizing principle of the metabolic and autonomic responses to cold stress (see Rogers et al. [1995]; Travagli and Rogers [2001]).

- *Peptide YY (PYY)* released from endocrine cells in the ileum in response to fatty acids in the lumen produces, via the AP and the DVC, a decrease in acid secretion and gastric motility. Circulating PYY inhibits neurons in the DMNX that are linked to cholinergic motoneurons of the enteric nervous system innervating smooth musculature or parietal cells. The humoral effect of PYY antagonizes the activation of the preganglionic neurons by TRH/5-HT neurons in the raphe obscurus (Yang et al. 2000a and references therein).

- *Corticotropin-releasing hormone (CRH)* injected into the cisterna magna (fourth ventricle) or in to the DMNX elicits the same responses from the GIT as *stress* (decreased motility and acid secretion, decreased transit time of the small bowel, increased transit time of the large bowel). Both CRH- and stress-induced effects in the stomach and small bowel are mediated by CRH_2 receptors in the DMNX neurons and by activation of inhibitory (non-cholinergic non-adrenergic) pathways in the enteric nervous system. The neurons of the DMNX are activated during stress by neurons of the paraventricular nucleus of the hypothalamus and by neurons in Barrington's nucleus (see Chapter 8), both releasing CRH (Taché et al. 2001; Lewis et al. 2002).

- *Pancreatic polypeptide (PP)* is released by endocrine cells of the pancreas during fasting in anticipation of feeding (e.g., in the cephalic phase of the activation of stomach and duodenum) and postprandially (after a meal). Its release is primarily under reflex neural control by the DMNX. About 30% of the pancreas-projecting neurons in the DMNX respond to PP, half of them being excited and half of them inhibited (Browning et al. 2005). PP in physiological concentrations increases gastric motility, gastric acid secretion and gastric transit. These effects are produced by activation of parasympathetic secretomotor and motility-regulating neurons in the DMNX via the AP (see Rogers et al. [1995]; Browning et al. [2005]).

- *Glucagon-like peptide 1 (GLP-1)* is released by the L cells of the distal gut into the circulation. It has multiple functions, such as glucose-dependent stimulation of insulin secretion, inhibition of gastric emptying and of acid secretion, reduction of caloric intake, enhancement of satiety. Some of these functions are probably mediated by the AP. GLP-1 activates neurons in the DMNX and enhances activation of DMNX neurons generated by stimulation of the NTS (Browning et al. 2005).

- Infectious disease states involving activation of the immune system and production of cytokines may lead to autonomic disorders including gastric stasis, nausea, emesis and anorexia. These changes associated with the GIT can be mimicked by the cytokine *tumor necrosis factor α (TNFα)*, which is released from macrophages, T lymphocytes and glia cells during the disease states. TNFα inhibits gastric functions by acting on neurons in the NTS and DMNX possibly via the AP (Hermann and Rogers 1995; Emch et al. 2000, 2002; Hermann et al. 2002; see Travagli and Rogers [2001]). Alternatively, TNFα may excite vagal afferents, which then excite synaptically the neurons in NTS and DMNX (see Subchapter 2.3; Jänig 2005).

These examples clearly demonstrate the close integration of autonomic (parasympathetic) systems and neuroendocrine systems in the regulation of gastrointestinal functions.

Conclusions

Regulation of the cardiovascular system, the respiratory system and the gastrointestinal tract is represented in the lower brain stem. These control systems require precise coordination and adaptation to somatic body functions and are therefore closely integrated. This integration is reflected in the anatomy and physiology of the neural substrates of these control systems. Included in this integration are the final autonomic pathways (in addition to the enteric nervous system), described in Chapters 4 to 8, and the spinal autonomic circuits (Chapter 9). The circuits in the medulla oblongata are under the control of the upper brain stem, hypothalamus and telencephalon. They are the essential neural building blocks for complex autonomic regulation.

1. Neurons involved in regulation of arterial blood pressure (by regulation of cardiac output and

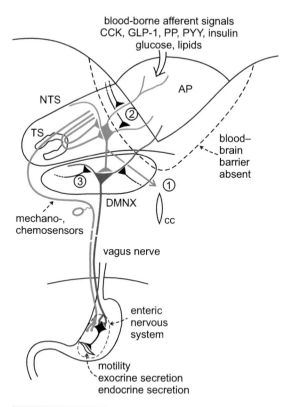

Figure 10.31 Basic vago-vagal reflex circuits involved in the regulation of the gastrointestinal tract (GIT) by the brain are modulated by gastrointestinal hormones and nutritive substances via the area postrema (AP) in which the blood–brain barrier is absent. Second-order neurons in the NTS (green) form inhibitory or excitatory synapses with preganglionic neurons in the DMNX (red) and are synaptically activated from the periphery by mechano- and/or chemosensitive vagal afferent neurons innervating the GIT (blue). The preganglionic neurons project through the vagus nerve to the enteric nervous system and have various functions. The NTS neurons project additionally to various regions of the brain stem, hypothalamus and forebrain (*1*; see Figure 8.13). Both neurons in the NTS and neurons in the DMNX are under multiple synaptic control from brain stem, hypothalamus and forebrain (*2* and *3*). cc, central canal; CCK, cholecystokinin; DMNX, dorsal motor nucleus of the vagus; GLP-1, glucagon-like peptide; NTS, nucleus tractus solitarii; PP, pancreatic polypeptide; PYY, peptide YY; TS, tractus solitarius. Designed after Rogers et al. (1995) and Travagli and Rogers (2001).

peripheral resistance) and respiration are situated in rostrocaudally organized columns of neurons in the ventrolateral medulla oblongata (VLM). These columns extend from the facial nucleus to areas caudal to the obex. The VLM includes:

- The rostral ventrolateral medulla (RVLM), containing sympathetic premotor neurons and associated interneurons.
- The caudal ventrolateral medulla (CVLM) containing excitatory and inhibitory interneurons that mediate various types of cardiovascular reflexes.
- The caudal pressor area.
- The ventral respiratory column of neurons (VRC) consisting of the caudal ventral respiratory group (VRG) (contains expiratory premotor neurons), the rostral VRG (largely inspiratory premotor neurons), the preBötzinger complex (containing the essential mechanisms underlying the central respiratory generator) and the Bötzinger complex (largely expiratory neurons).

2. The VLM is closely associated with parasympathetic cardioinhibitory and bronchomotor preganglionic neurons located in the external formation of the nucleus ambiguus. The respiratory neurons in the VLM form, together with the neurons in the dorsal respiratory group and in the pons, the ponto-medullary respiratory network.

3. The RVLM is a sympathetic cardiovascular premotor nucleus mediating reflexes to sympathetic preganglionic neurons (muscle, visceral and renal vasoconstrictor neurons, some cutaneous vasoconstrictor neurons, cardiomotor neurons). Spontaneous activity in the neurons of these cardiovascular pathways possibly originates, at least in part, in the RVLM and/or in neuronal networks associated with the RVLM.

4. Arterial baroreceptor reflexes involve parasympathetic cardiomotor neurons and sympathetic cardiovascular neurons:
- The pathway to the parasympathetic cardiomotor neurons is disynaptic between the baroreceptor input to the nucleus tractus solitarii (NTS) and the preganglionic neurons. The transmitter at both synapses is glutamate.
- The pathway to the sympathetic cardiovascular preganglionic neurons consists of four synapses between the baroreceptor input to the NTS and the preganglionic neurons in the spinal cord: second-order neurons in the NTS project to inhibitory interneurons in the rostral part of the CVLM; these project to the sympathetic premotor neurons in the RVLM. The transmitter of the inhibitory interneuron is GABA, the transmitter at the other synapses is glutamate.
- Parallel baroreceptor pathways to sympathetic preganglionic neurons may include inhibitory interneurons in the spinal cord, the transmitter being GABA (and possibly glycine), and possibly other pathways (e.g., related to a long descending inhibitory pathway).
- All components of the baroreceptor reflexes are under modulatory influence from other nuclei in the lower and upper brain stem, hypothalamus and telencephalon.

5. Excitatory arterial chemoreceptor reflexes to sympathetic preganglionic neurons are mediated both via the respiratory network and independently of the respiratory network.

6. The caudal raphe nuclei of the medulla oblongata (raphe obscurus and pallidus) contain sympathetic premotor neurons to cutaneous vasoconstrictor preganglionic neurons or to lipomotor preganglionic neurons (supplying brown adipose tissue). These premotor neurons are involved in thermoregulation and regulation of energy balance.

7. The activity of many sympathetic neurons exhibits respiratory rhythmicity. This activity profile is related to the phases of respiration and varies with the function of the sympathetic neurons. The following activity patterns are present in the cat:
- Sympathetic cardiovascular neurons are excited during inspiration and inhibited during postinspiration and sometimes early inspiration.
- Cutaneous vasoconstrictor neurons exhibit several patterns, the most common being inhibition during inspiration and excitation during postinspiration (like parasympathetic cardiomotor neurons); some cutaneous vasoconstrictor neurons are only excited during inspiration and some show no respiratory rhythmicity.
- Sudomotor neurons are excited during postinspiration. Most motility-regulating neurons do not exhibit respiratory rhythmicity.
- Inspiratory-type neurons projecting to the head (possibly to the nasal mucosa) are only excited during inspiration.

8. Respiratory modulation of activity in sympathetic neurons (muscle vasoconstrictor, cutaneous vasoconstrictor, sudomotor neurons) is also present in

humans, showing that there are differences between functionally distinct types of neurons.

9. The respiratory pattern in cardiovascular neurons is probably generated by the "common cardio-respiratory network" in the VLM. This network represents a sensorimotor program, consisting of various functionally distinct reflex pathways, that closely coordinates the regulation of arterial blood pressure and respiration under all physiological conditions. Several types of cardiovascular and pulmonary vagal afferent neurons influence the cardiovascular neurons both independent of the respiratory network and via this network. The respiratory modulation in the other types of sympathetic neuron is generated by other mechanisms in the medulla oblongata.

10. Neural control of the gastrointestinal tract (GIT) by the lower brain stem is exerted by multiple reflex circuits consisting of functionally defined vagal afferents from the GIT that project to the NTS, neurons in the NTS that project to the dorsal motor nucleus of the vagus (DMNX) and parasympathetic preganglionic neurons in the DMNX that project to the GIT. The vago-vagal reflex circuits are the basic building blocks of the central control of the GIT involving the brain stem, hypothalamus and forebrain.

11. Parasympathetic pathways to the GIT in the DMNX are under the control of hormones from the GIT via the area postrema. This hormonal modulation of the vago-vagal circuits occurs in relation to satiety, anticipation of feeding, cold and other stressors, and defense against the entry of toxic substances by way of the GIT.

Suggested Reading

Browning, K. N. and Travagli, R. A. (2014) Central nervous system control of gastrointestinal motility and secretion and modulation of gastrointestinal functions. *Compr Physiol* **4**, 1339–1368.

Dampney, R. A. (1994) Functional organization of central pathways regulating the cardiovascular system. *Physiol Rev* **74**, 323–364.

Dampney, R. A. (2016) Central neural control of the cardiovascular system: current perspectives. *Adv Physiol Educ* **40**, 283–296.

Del Negro, C. A., Funk, G. D. and Feldman, J. L. (2018) Breathing matters. *Nat Rev Neurosci* **19**, 351–367.

Feldman, J. L. and Kam, K. (2015) Facing the challenge of mammalian neural microcircuits: taking a few breaths may help. *J Physiol* **593**, 3–23.

Guyenet, P. G. (2014) Regulation of breathing and autonomic outflows by chemoreceptors. *Compr Physiol* **4**, 1511–1562.

Häbler, H. J., Jänig, W. and Michaelis, M. (1994b) Respiratory modulation of activity in sympathetic neurones. *Prog Neurobiol* **43**, 567–606.

Jänig, W. (1985a) Organization of the lumbar sympathetic outflow to skeletal muscle and skin of the cat hindlimb and tail. *Rev Physiol Biochem Pharmacol* **102**, 119–213.

Mandel, D. A. and Schreihofer, A. M. (2006) Central respiratory modulation of barosensitive neurones in rat caudal ventrolateral medulla. *J Physiol* **572**, 881–896.

McAllen, R. M. and McKinley, M. J. (2018) Efferent thermoregulatory pathways regulating cutaneous blood flow and sweating. *Handb Clin Neurol* **156**, 305–316.

Morrison, S. F. (2018) Efferent neural pathways for the control of brown adipose tissue thermogenesis and shivering. *Handb Clin Neurol* **156**, 281–303.

Morrison, S. F. and Nakamura, K. (2019) Central mechanisms for thermoregulation. *Ann Rev Physiol* **81**, 285–308.

Paton, J. F. (1996) The ventral medullary respiratory network of the mature mouse studied in a working heart-brainstem preparation. *J Physiol* **493**, 819–831.

Ramirez, J. M. and Baertsch, N. A. (2018) The dynamic basis of respiratory rhythm generation: one breath at a time. *Ann Rev Neurosci* **41**, 475–499.

Rybak, I. A., Molkov, Y. I., Jasinski, P. E., Shevtsova, N. A. and Smith, J. C. (2014) Rhythmic bursting in the pre-Bötzinger complex: mechanisms and models. *Prog Brain Res* **209**, 1–23.

Schreihofer, A.M. and Sved, A.F. (2011) The ventrolateral medulla and sympathetic regulation of arterial pressure. In *Central Regulation of Autonomic Functions*, 2nd edn. (Llewellyn-Smith, I. J. and Verberne, A. J. M., eds.) pp. 78–97, Oxford University Press, Oxford, New York.

All references cited in the text are available online at www.cambridge.org/janig.

Notes

1. Genes, such as the *c-fos* gene, that are activated rapidly within minutes, transiently, and without requiring new protein synthesis are often described as cellular immediate early genes (IEGs). Under unstimulated (resting) conditions *c-fos* mRNA and protein are nearly undetectable. Neural stimuli that activate the cAMP, Ca^{2+}, protein kinase C or other intracellular pathways produce a rapid induction of *c-fos* gene expression. Detection of c-Fos and other IEG-encoded proteins and *in situ* hybridization for the mRNA of these proteins

using immunohistochemistry have become standard tools to map neurons and neural circuits that are activated (synaptically, by drugs or otherwise) (Schulman 2013; Dampney and Horiuchi 2003).

2. Bulbospinal catecholaminergic neurons (including the C1 neurons in the RVLM) can be selectively destroyed by using the ribosomal inactivating protein (toxin) saporin conjugated to an anti-dopamine-β-hydroxylase (DBH) antibody. This immunotoxin injected in the upper thoracic segments in rats (close to the intermediolateral cell column) binds to DBH, which is expressed in the plasma membrane of the terminals of adrenergic and noradrenergic neurons. The toxin–DBH complex is internalized and retrogradely transported to the cell bodies of these catecholaminergic neurons in the lower brain stem. The neurons are selectively destroyed by blockade of protein synthesis without affecting other bulbospinal neurons (Guyenet et al. 2001). By the same token neurons with NK1-receptors can be selectively ablated by a conjugate of the toxin saporin with a selective NK1-receptor agonist (e.g. substance P). The saporin–agonist–NK1-receptor complex is internalized by the neurons and leads to their destruction (Mantyh et al. 1997).

3. Morphological identification: activity is recorded intracellularly from the neurons, to functionally characterize them, and then the neurons are filled with a marker (e.g., horseradish peroxidase, Lucifer yellow). In an alternative technique identified neurons can be labeled juxtacellularly by a dye (e.g. biotinamide) released from a microelectrode positioned extracellularly close to the cell body or a large dendrite of the neuron (Pinault 1996; Pilowsky and Makeham 2001). The labeled neurons are reconstructed from serial sections of the perfused and fixated preparation after the physiological experiment.

4. The demarcation of the VLM and its subsections may differ between different investigators. Most workers place the dorsal border of the VLM as the ventral border of the nucleus ambiguus (NA), others use the NA pars compacta (thus, including the parasympathetic cardiomotor and bronchomotor neurons). For practical reasons the medial border is taken as a line drawn from the pars compacta of the NA to the point where the pyramidal tract touches the medullary surface laterally; the lateral border is taken as a line from the pars compacta of the NA to the ventral edge of the trigeminal nucleus; the ventral border is the ventral surface of the medulla oblongata. This area includes neurons of the ventral respiratory group (Paxinos and Watson 2014).

5. Several landmarks are used to locate the groups of neurons in the medulla oblongata: (1) In the stereotaxic

atlas of Paxinos and Watson (2014) the rostrocaudal position is located with respect to the bregma. This is the point of the skull corresponding to the junction of the coronal and sagittal sutures. (2) A ventral landmark for the VLM and the column of respiratory neurons in the ventrolateral column is the caudal border of the facial nucleus. (3) Dorsal landmarks commonly used are the calamus scriptorius or the obex. The calamus scriptorius is the caudal part of the floor of the fourth ventricle towards its apex. This part presents the appearance of a pen nib; therefore it is called the calamus scriptorius. The obex is the point on the midline of the dorsal surface of the medulla oblongata that marks the caudal angle of the fourth ventricle. Anatomically it corresponds to a small transverse medullary fold and is therefore rostral to the calamus scriptorius. Most workers define the obex operationally as the rostral border of the area postrema in the midline (Figures 10.2, 10.3).

6. In the cat, the sympathetic premotor neurons involved in regulation of arterial blood pressure are located in a compact nucleus of the RVLM, sometimes called the subretrofacial nucleus (Polson et al. 1992), that is not present in the rat. For numbers of bulbospinal neurons in the RVLM in rat and cat that are related to sympathetic preganglionic neurons see Note 10.

7. The delineation of the cell columns in the transverse sections in Figure 10.2b were only done for didactic reasons and according to Paxinos and Watson (2014).

8. It is important to emphasize that decrease of activity in vasoconstrictor neurons innervating resistance vessels or in sympathetic cardiomotor neurons upon bilateral lesion of the RVLM does not prove that the ongoing activity originates *only* in the RVLM. In fact, multiple nuclei in the brain stem and hypothalamus and even the spinal cord may contribute to the generation of ongoing activity in these cardiovascular neurons (see Subchapter 10.2.4).

9. After the toxin saporin conjugated to an anti-DBH antibody is injected in the upper thoracic segments in rats (close to the intermediolateral cell column; see Note 2) about 75% to 85% of the C1 neurons in the RVLM (together with other bulbospinal adrenergic neurons and with >95% of bulbospinal noradrenergic neurons [for example in the area A5]) are lost (Schreihofer and Guyenet 2000). Rats with depleted bulbospinal C1 cells in the RVLM have normal arterial blood pressure, probably normal levels of sympathetic activity in the major splanchnic nerve and almost normal baroreceptor reflexes. However, they exhibit reduced excitatory reflexes in sympathetic neurons to stimulation of arterial chemoreceptors and to stimulation of the RVLM (Schreihofer et al. 2000; Madden and Sved 2003). Thus, the integrity of the C1 neurons is not essential

for the generation of activity in sympathetic vasoconstrictor neurons that are involved in maintenance and regulation of arterial blood pressure under resting conditions. These functions are primarily maintained by non-catecholaminergic bulbospinal neurons in the RVLM (Guyenet et al. 2001). However, the C1 neurons may well be essential for the regulation of arterial blood pressure under extreme conditions when the system is under long-term load (see Box 10.1).

10. In the rat, the RVLM contains about 600 to 800 bulbospinal sympathetic premotor neurons on both sides. From these bulbospinal neurons, about 400 to 550 neurons are adrenergic (C1) and the remaining neurons non-adrenergic (assuming that two-thirds of these bulbospinal neurons are adrenergic and one-third non-adrenergic [Sved et al. 1994; Schreihofer and Guyenet 1997]). These estimated numbers are based on counts of neurons retrogradely labeled from the spinal cord (upper thoracic segments) in serial transverse sections through the VLM (830 neurons: Schreihofer and Guyenet 2000; Guyenet et al. 2001; 800 neurons: Phillips et al. 2001; 760 neurons: Sved et al. 1994; 560 neurons: Tucker et al. 1987). Assuming that these sympathetic premotor neurons are target-specific (Figure 10.9) it follows that in the range of 100 to 150 sympathetic premotor neurons determine the activity in each sympathetic pathway to the different vascular beds (muscle, mesenteric, renal, skin), to the heart and to the adrenal medulla. Although an even distribution of sympathetic premotor neurons is unlikely, it shows that a large number of sympathetic preganglionic neurons (in the rat about 12 000 neurons on both sides, of which 20% or less may have a cardiovascular function or be related to the adrenal medullae [Strack et al. 1988; see Table 4.5 for the estimation of the proportion of preganglionic muscle or visceral vasoconstrictor neurons projecting in different "sympathetic nerves"]) is (directly or indirectly) innervated by a small number of RVLM neurons. The subretrofacial nucleus in the RVLM of the cat contains about 2000 sympathetic premotor neurons on both sides (Polson et al. 1992; McAllen, personal communication).

11. Intrinsic pacemaker properties of neurons are characterized by the following criteria (Guyenet 1990): (1) The spikes result from gradual interspike membrane depolarizations, as opposed to regularly occurring excitatory postsynaptic potentials (EPSPs). (2) After hyperpolarizing the neurons by negative current injection, pacemaker activity stops, but EPSPs are still present. (3) The pacemaker activity can be reset by a brief hyperpolarizing current or by an action potential generated by a brief depolarizing pulse or by a synaptically induced EPSP. (4) The pacemaker activity does not depend on the synaptic release of a neuromodulator.

12. The network idea to explain the generation of spontaneous activity in cardiovascular neurons appears to be least likely. It may turn out to be difficult to prove experimentally that the spontaneous activity in sympathetic cardiovascular neurons is generated by a network of neurons connected by excitatory and inhibitory synapses, independent of synaptic and other inputs from outside of the network. For example, the extracellular fluid matrix of the neurons provides continuous chemical inputs to the neurons.

13. In the experiments conducted by Thrasher (2002, 2005a) one set of carotid arterial baroreceptors was left intact. Chronic occlusion of the common carotid artery distal to the intact baroreceptor afferents abolished the rhythmic diastolic–systolic changes in the arterial blood pressure in the innervated carotid sinus, but did not lead to a significant decrease in the level of arterial blood pressure in the carotid sinus distal to the occlusion. Thus, in this experiment the rhythmic activation of the arterial baroreceptors was eliminated. In the experiments conducted by Cowley et al. (1973) all arterial baroreceptors were denervated. Chronic denervation may lead to plastic changes in the central baroreceptor pathways (e.g., in the NTS), which may explain why the mean arterial blood pressure in this preparation did not change. This clearly shows that the model of Cowley et al. (1973) is *not* a model of chronic baroreceptor unloading (Thrasher 2005a,b). It is worth mentioning that the interpretation given by Cowley and coworkers to their experiments was generally accepted by the scientific community. This is documented in textbooks of physiology for students all over the world and needs to be revised. This situation demonstrates how careful we have to be in the interpretation of experimental results as far as the normal functioning (here arterial baroreceptor reflexes) is concerned.

14. In the experiment documented in Figure 10.7c the phasic inhibition of the activity in the bulbospinal RVLM neuron starts about 50 ms after the onset of the systole. This delay in inhibition is due to the conduction time in axons of the baroreceptors, NTS neurons and neurons in the CVLM (Jeske et al. 1993; see Figure 10.10).

15. Most NTS neurons that are activated by stimulation of arterial baroreceptors have rather weak pulse rhythmicity in their activity or some even none (Spyer 1981; Mifflin et al. 1988; Rogers et al. 1993). I find this rather puzzling and an unsolved problem for the following reasons: (1) Strong pulse rhythmicity of the activity in arterial baroreceptors with myelinated axons. (2)

Strong pulse rhythmicity of the activity in all neurons of the baroreceptor reflex pathways downstream to the NTS (CVLM neurons: Figure 10.13; RVLM: Figure 10.7; pre- and postganglionic muscle and visceral vasoconstrictor neurons: Figures 4.1; 4.7, 4.8). (3) In anesthetized cats, pulsatile activation of only relatively few intact baroreceptor afferents innervating the common carotid artery (e.g., after transection of both carotid sinus nerves and both vagoaortic nerves) seems to be enough to generate cardiac rhythmicity of the activity in muscle vasoconstrictor neurons (Jänig, unpublished). The traditional explanation is that there is considerable convergence of baroreceptor afferents on NTS neurons and of NTS neurons (or interneurons synaptically connected to NTS neurons) on neurons in the CVLM. I remain skeptical whether the model outlined in Figure 10.10 can sufficiently explain the experimental observations made on sympathetic cardiovascular neurons.

16. Based on experiments performed on *cats*, Barman and Gebber propagated the idea that neurons in the so-called lateral tegmental field (LTF) of the medulla oblongata (which may correspond to the dorsal part of the medullary reticular nucleus in the rat, located medial to the spinal trigeminal nucleus [see Figure 10.2b]) mediate baroreceptor reflexes to neurons in the RVLM. These LTF neurons excite neurons in the RVLM and are inhibited upon stimulation of arterial baroreceptors. Thus, according to these authors, sympathetic premotor neurons in the RVLM are disfacilitated during stimulation of arterial baroreceptors by removal of excitatory drive from LTF neurons. Details about the putative baroreceptor reflex pathway via the LTF neurons are unknown. The depression of activity in the LTF neurons generated by stimulation of arterial baroreceptors does not occur by direct inhibition of the LTF, since selective blockade of the N-methyl-D-aspartate (NMDA)-receptors in the LTF prevents the inhibition of LTF neurons (and of the activity in sympathetic cardiovascular neurons) generated by stimulation of arterial baroreceptors (for review see Barman et al. [2001]). The view of Barman and Gebber is not accepted or is ignored by most investigators. However, this putative alternative baroreceptor pathway to sympathetic premotor neurons should also not be dismissed.

17. This idea appears to be at variance with the findings of Verberne et al. (1999): (1) Spinally projecting neurons in the RVLM in rats, that are activated by stimulation of arterial baroreceptors and would qualify as putative sympathoinhibitory GABAergic neurons were not found in the RVLM. (2) Neurons in the VLM that were activated by stimulation of arterial baroreceptors were located in the CVLM and did not project to the spinal cord. (3) Baroreceptor-activated neurons were intermixed with C1 neurons in the caudal VLM that project to the hypothalamus (or possibly to telencephalic structures) and are inhibited by baroreceptor stimulation. Furthermore, Pilowsky et al. (1994) did not find IPSPs in lumbar preganglionic neurons in cats with intact arterial baroreceptors that are correlated with blood pressure changes (increase in arterial blood pressure and activation of arterial baroreceptors). However, it must be kept in mind that preganglionic vasoconstrictor neurons to skeletal muscle and viscera in the lumbar spinal cord, which are involved in blood pressure control, (1) comprise only about 10% to 20% of all preganglionic neurons (Table 4.5) and (2) have rather slowly conducting axons (mean 3.4 ± 1.9 m/s [mean $\pm$ SD] for preganglionic muscle vasoconstrictor axons and 2.8 ± 2.5 m/s for preganglionic visceral vasoconstrictor axons [Jänig and Szulczyk 1980; Jänig 1985a; Bahr et al. 1986]). Thus, the cell bodies of these neurons are probably also very small. For these reasons it is difficult to detect these neurons in the spinal cord and to record their activity intracellularly.

18. See Note 1 in Chapter 3.

19. This is a short-lasting strong experimental anoxic adequate stimulus that does not occur under physiological conditions, but stimulates specifically arterial chemoreceptors.

20. This switch from inhibitory chemoreceptor reflexes to excitatory ones, in the anesthetized cat, in cutaneous vasoconstrictor neurons supplying the cat hindpaw, following decerebration of the animal or peripheral nerve lesion, is accompanied by a switch from inhibitory to excitatory reflexes in cutaneous vasoconstrictor neurons to noxious stimulation of the hindpaw (heating of the contralateral hindpaw with water >45 °C or noxious mechanical stimulation of the ipsilateral hindpaw [Jänig 1975; Blumberg and Jänig 1985]). These experimental results are reminiscent of observations in patients with complex regional pain syndrome (CRPS). Many patients having CRPS I (previously called reflex sympathetic dystrophy; Stanton-Hicks et al. 1995; Jänig and Stanton-Hicks 1996; Harden et al. 2001) exhibit chronic changes in thermoregulatory reflexes and respiration-related reflexes in cutaneous vasoconstrictor neurons innervating the distal extremities. The changed reflexes in cutaneous vasoconstrictor neurons are most likely due to changes in central cutaneous vasoconstrictor circuits and related to the injury that triggers the development of CRPS type I. They may reverse after successful treatment of this pain disease (Wasner et al. 1999, 2001; Jänig and Baron 2002, 2003). Patients with CRPS II, which

sometimes develops after a trauma with nerve lesion (previously called causalgia), may also exhibit dramatic changes at their distal extremities that are related to the sympathetic nervous system (cutaneous vasoconstrictor neurons, sudomotor neurons). These sympathetically maintained changes developing after nerve lesions have already been described by Mitchell (1872), who coined the term causalgia. The experimental approach to study the plastic changes of reflexes in cutaneous vasoconstrictor neurons following nerve lesions was designed on the basis of these clinical observations (Jänig 1985b, 1990; Jänig and McLachlan 1994).

21. Note that, in the experiments documented in Figure 10.18 the multiunit activity in the splanchnic nerve (SPL, most of it occurring in visceral vasoconstrictor axons) exhibits typical bursting activity (Figure 10.18b_1–b_3,c_1). The multiunit activity in the nerve to the interscapular brown adipose tissue (BAT; most of it occurring in lipomotor axons) also exhibits bursting activity during hypothermia (Figure 10.18b_2) and during disinhibition of the nucleus raphe pallidus (Figure 10.18b_3,c_3). The frequency of this bursting activity is different from that in the splanchnic nerve (Figure 10.18b_2,b_3) (Morrison 1999).

22. The nomenclature of these respiratory neurons varies somewhat between groups. The main types are: ramp-inspiratory, late inspiratory, preinspiratory, early-inspiratory, postinspiratory, augmenting expiratory, inspiratory–expiratory phase-spanning, expiratory–inspiratory phase-spanning neurons (St.-John 1998; Richter and Spyer 2001; Rybak et al. 2004).

23. In the rat the pattern of respiratory modulation of activity in sympathetic neurons is different. It mostly consists of depression of activity in inspiration and sometimes enhanced activity in postinspiration depending on the respiratory drive (Häbler et al. 1994a, b, 1996, 1999, 2000; Bartsch et al. 1996).

24. Daly and coworkers showed that activation of slowly adapting pulmonary afferents by lung inflation leads to a decrease in vascular resistance in the vascularly isolated dog hindlimb (Daly et al. 1967; Daly and Robinson 1968; Daly 1991). Thus, lung inflation is followed by a decrease in activity in muscle vasoconstrictor neurons and subsequently a decrease in vascular resistance. The most plausible explanation for this observation is that activation of lung afferents leads to a decrease in activity in inspiratory neurons (Hering–Breuer reflex) and this in turn leads to a decrease in activity in the muscle vasoconstrictor neurons (Gerber and Polosa 1978). This interpretation is contradicted by Daly et al. (1987). However, there probably is another simple reason explaining the apparent difference between the results of Boczek-Funcke et al. (1992b, c) and those of Daly and coworkers: in the experiments conducted by Boczek-Funcke et al., lung stretch afferents were stimulated phasically at low intrapulmonary pressure, whereas in the experiments by Daly et al., lung afferents were stimulated tonically at high intrapulmonary pressure. Thus, the results obtained in both types of experiment do not contradict each other.

25. The early recording of Hagbarth and coworkers in humans (Hagbarth and Vallbo 1968; see Figure 10.24a) clearly demonstrates that activity of MVC neurons occurs during inspiration (compare activity in MVC axons and EMG of inspiratory muscle in Figure 10.24a and take into account that postganglionic activity is delayed by about 2 s with respect to the EMG activity due to conduction time of the action potentials in the axons of the postganglionic muscle vasoconstrictor neurons innervating the peroneal muscles).

26. This interpretation of the changes in activity in muscle vasoconstrictor neurons with respiration in the human has been challenged by Seals et al. (1990, 1993) and Macefield and Wallin (1995). Their studies show that maximal activity in muscle vasoconstrictor neurons occurs in late expiration and early inspiration, and minimal activity in late inspiration and early expiration. This pattern is seen during normal breathing, hyperpnea and passive positive pressure ventilation, as well as in lung denervated human subjects and does not depend on unloading of baroreceptors. These data appear to be at variance with *all* published animal data showing that the central component of respiratory modulation in muscle vasoconstrictor neurons has an inspiratory peak in cats and a postinspiratory peak in rats (Häbler et al. 1994a).

Part V

The Centers of Homeostasis in the Mesencephalon and Hypothalamus and Their Telencephalic Control

This final chapter will describe how integrative neural control of most body functions is vital to allow the vertebrate/mammalian organism to survive and act in its environment. The autonomic nervous system is involved in virtually all of these functions (see Tables 11.1 and 11.2). I want to make clear:

- that the power and range of this integrative control of body functions in mammals are dependent on the mesencephalon, hypothalamus and cerebral hemispheres,
- that the mastermind of the integration of autonomic, somatomotor and endocrine systems is located in the telencephalon,
- that the functionally differentiated autonomic pathways are the slaves of this mastermind, and
- that the "wisdom of the body" is to be found within these regions of the brain.

I will strictly adhere to the autonomic systems, as described in the preceding chapters. I do not intend to describe the mechanisms underlying the integrative control systems in detail (as this would require another book or more). The chapter will not cover: (1) the functions of the hypothalamus (Table 11.2), (2) how stress and pain involve the autonomic nervous system in body protection (see Goldstein [1995, 2000]; Chrousos [1998]; McEwen [2001a]; Jänig [2020]) and (3) the neural mechanisms underlying emotional and motivational processes (Panksepp 1998; Davidson et al. 2003; Morris and Dolan 2004).

The chapter will start with some critical reflections on the concepts about the functioning of the autonomic nervous system that were propagated by Walter Bradford Cannon and Walter Rudolf Hess and are still influential in physiology and medicine. The chapter will finish with a synopsis in which I want to show that we are, again, at a new beginning in the exploration of the autonomic nervous system, with new experimental tools that have been developed in the last 10 to 20 years, and that the main focus will be on the central nervous system despite the many remaining questions about how the autonomic pathways function in the periphery.

Chapter 11

Integration of Autonomic Regulation in the Upper Brain Stem and Limbic–Hypothalamic Centers: A Summary

11.1 Functions of the Autonomic Nervous System: Cannon and Hess[1]

In the introduction of this book, I alluded to the very wide range of vital functions that are under the control of the autonomic nervous system. Here I will critically discuss the general concepts of the functions of the autonomic nervous system as they have evolved particularly from the experimental work of Walter Bradford Cannon and Walter Rudolf Hess in the first half of the last century and that still have considerable impact on our conceptual approach to this system.

The reason why I focus on Cannon and Hess is clear: both analyzed the functions of the autonomic nervous system from an integrative point of view, i.e., implicit in their descriptions and reasoning was the assumption that circuits in the central nervous system are responsible for the integrative action of the autonomic nervous system. The development of our knowledge on anatomy, physiology and pharmacology of the peripheral autonomic nervous system has been extensively described in the literature (Gaskell 1916; Sheehan 1936, 1941; Kuntz 1954; Pick 1970; see Subchapter 1.6). Aspects related to the development of knowledge on special topics and ideas have been discussed in the earlier chapters of this book.

11.1.1 Cannon and the Concept of the Sympathico-Adrenal System

In the second half of the nineteenth century, *Claude Bernard* formulated the idea that:

"It is the fixity of the 'milieu interieur' which is the condition of free and independent life" and that *"all the vital mechanisms, however varied they may be, have only one object, that of preserving constant the conditions of life in the internal environment."* No more pregnant sentence, in the opinion of J.S. Haldane, was ever framed by a physiologist (quoted from Cannon, 1939, p.38).

The American physiologist *Walter Bradford Cannon* was strongly influenced by the ideas of Claude Bernard. He called the milieu intérieur the *fluid matrix*

---

[1] This subchapter is my critical tribute to both Walter Bradford Cannon and Walter Rudolf Hess whom I admire as scientists and teachers (see my preface to this book).

of the body. Cannon described the coordinated physiological processes that maintain the steady state of the organism with the term *homeostasis* (see Subchapter 11.2). He was convinced that the automatic corrections of the physiological parameters of the body are the primary function of the autonomic nervous system, in particular the sympathetic nervous system.

Cannon's ideas about how homeostasis is achieved and the role the autonomic nervous system plays were first presented in a review "Organization for physiological homeostasis" (1929b) and culminated in his famous and influential book *The Wisdom of the Body* (1939). The title for this book was taken from the late E. H. Starling who gave a Harvey Lecture with the same title before the Royal College of Physicians in London in 1923. Starling declared that, by understanding the wisdom of the body, we shall attain the *mastery of disease and pain which enables us to relieve the burden of mankind* (quoted from the preface to Cannon's book *The Wisdom of the Body*, 1939), and that tenet also became the belief of Cannon.

Cannon was originally influenced by ideas about the role of the sympathetic nervous system in strong emotions, pain and stress. As an undergraduate he took William James' philosophy course at Harvard. James contended that the emotional state of the organism is associated with afferent feedback from the body, notably from vascular and visceral structures (James 1884). He believed that the brain triggers bodily changes by activity in the autonomic final pathways (particular the sympathetic ones) and that the activity initiated in the afferent neurons from the regulated organs leads to the emotions (see Subchapter 11.4).

Cannon was intrigued by this theory, which states that the brain generates the activity of the internal organs (including blood vessels) via the autonomic nervous system and the somatomotor system and that the various emotional states are brought about by afferent signals from these organs and transferred to the brain. The consequence of this idea is that different emotions are generated by different patterns of activity in afferent neurons from the internal organs and skeletal muscle. Interestingly, this would strictly require that the final autonomic pathways are functionally specific (as described in Chapter 4 and Chapters 8–10). If this were not the case, it would not be possible to generate the distinct basic emotions by functionally distinct patterns of afferent discharge arising from internal organs.

However, Cannon critically argued (Cannon 1914a):

If various strong emotions can thus be expressed in the diffuse activities of a single division of the autonomic nervous system . . . it would appear that the bodily conditions which have been assumed, by some psychologists, to distinguish emotions from one another must be sought for elsewhere than in the viscera. We do not "feel sorry because we cry", as James contended, but we cry because, when we are sorry or overjoyed or violently angry or full of tender affection, – when any of these diverse emotional states is present – there are nervous discharges by sympathetic channels to various viscera, including the lachrymal glands [tear formation is generated by activation of parasympathetic neurons!]. And in terror and rage and intense elation, for example, the responses in the viscera seem too uniform [and therefore the diverse discharges of sympathetic neurons to various target organs] to offer a satisfactory means of distinguishing emotional states which in man, at least, are subjectively very different. For this reason I am inclined to urge that the visceral changes merely contribute to an emotional complex more or less indefinite, but still pertinent, feelings of disturbance, in organs which we are not usually conscious of (Cannon 1914a, p.280).

Instead Cannon (1914a) proposed that the different emotional states are represented in the brain rather than being peripheral in origin, and are expressed by changes of activity in sympathetic and parasympathetic neurons.

Later, in the 1920s, this reasoning led to the famous experiments conducted by Philip Bard on diencephalic cats in Cannon's laboratory, in which he had removed the cortex and most of the structures of the limbic system. These cats exhibited behavior during stimulation of the skin which was phenomenologically very much reminiscent of a cat in rage (see Figure 4.13) as was so beautifully described by Charles Darwin (1872/1998) in the nineteenth century, in his book *The Expression of the Emotions in Man and Animals*. Bard and Cannon called the behavior of their diencephalic cats "sham rage behavior" (Bard 1928). These cats exhibited reactions with typical somatomotor components (tail arched backward, everted claws, hissing) and responses in target organs which are under control of the sympathetic nervous system (piloerection, dilation of pupils, sweating of paw pads). Had they recorded other autonomic parameters, they would have observed an increase in arterial blood pressure, heart rate, and blood flow through skeletal muscle and decreased blood flow through viscera and skin, decreased motility of the gastrointestinal tract, and increased secretion of adrenaline and noradrenaline by the adrenal medulla. These are all effects generated by activation of sympathetic pathways (see Table 1.2), but they do not involve the entire sympathetic outflow. These changes are also associated with activation of the adrenal cortex via the anterior pituitary gland and an increase of corticosterone in the blood. On the basis of their experiments, Bard and Cannon created the *thalamic theory of emotions* (Cannon 1927, 1929b; Bard 1932).

Cannon obtained the first experimental experience of the powerful influence the sympathetic nervous system can have on body functions when he studied movements of the stomach and intestines in conscious cats using X-rays. He was surprised to see that the movements of the gastrointestinal tract ceased under strong emotional stimuli, since the cats were frightened after having been fixated and forced to swallow barium solution. However, when the cats were pacified or asleep the movements of the intestine recommenced. He attributed the cessation of the movements of the gastrointestinal tract to the activation of the sympathetic nervous system (Cannon and Murphy 1906; Cannon 1911). Then, over the years, in experiments on cats, dogs and rabbits, Cannon studied the role of the sympathetic nervous system in maintaining homeostasis during various disturbances, such as hemorrhage, hypoglycemia, hypoxia, low and high body temperature, muscle exercise, emotional disturbances. On the basis of these studies, he formulated the concept of the fundamental role of the sympathetic nervous system in maintaining homeostasis: the sympathetic nervous system acts promptly and directly to prevent changes in the internal environment. It exhibits a widespread discharge through the sympathetic channels and different sympathetic outflows act simultaneously in one direction. It is organized for diffuse effects (Cannon 1939).

This generalization was extensively discussed by Cannon in his book *The Wisdom of the Body* (1939). Cannon obviously did not believe that individual sympathetic preganglionic neurons make only functional synaptic contacts with postganglionic neurons subserving the same function but, rather, that they diverge widely and form contacts with postganglionic neurons with many different functions (Note 1). Generalized activation of the sympathetic nervous system included activation of the adrenal medulla causing the secretion of adrenaline and

noradrenaline into the blood. It was assumed that the circulating adrenaline and noradrenaline reinforce the nervous effects on the target organs and mobilize glucose and free fatty acids from their stores, decrease the time for blood clotting, enhance gas exchange in the lung (by relaxation of the smooth muscles of the airways and subsequent reduction of airway resistance) and decrease fatigue of skeletal muscle (Note 2). These broad functional effects were conceptualized under the term *sympathico-adrenal system* (see Subchapter 4.5).

In contrast, the parasympathetic functions were thought to be more specific. This system serves to conserve body energies and the stability and constancy of the internal milieu of the body. It influences special viscera differentially and its discharges are directed to specific organs only. Different types of parasympathetic neurons are therefore not bound to act simultaneously but separately, depending on the organ. Individual parasympathetic preganglionic neurons influence one target organ only. The effects of the sympathetic nervous system and of the parasympathetic nervous system are generally opposite in the same organ (Cannon 1939). *This view of Cannon's, his contemporaries and followers is grossly at variance with our modern view, as outlined particularly in Chapter 4: Activation of lachrymal glands and pelvic organs is not related to conservation of body energies. Sympathetic neurons are functionally as specialized as parasympathetic ones. Functionally different types of sympathetic neurons do not act simultaneously but separately, dependent on the organ. Individual sympathetic neurons influence one group of target cells only. The effect of sympathetic neurons and parasympathetic neurons are not opposite on most target cells (see Table 1.2).* Cannon's ideas are still described in general textbooks and widely believed by many clinicians and non-specialist biological scientists.

Cannon's view of the autonomic nervous system was that of a system designed to preserve life during grave physical crises requiring extreme effort. The sympathetic division of the autonomic nervous system was considered to mobilize bodily forces during struggle, the cranial (parasympathetic) division to preserve body energies and the sacral (parasympathetic) division to function in emptying of the hollow organs and reproduction of the species (Cannon 1928, 1929a). Animals from which he had removed the entire sympathetic paravertebral chains survived, suggesting that the sympathetic nervous system might not be important at all. However, these animals lived in the protected environment of the laboratory. They would not have been able to adapt to environmental extremes, or even to maintain physiological stability in terms of body temperature, adequate arterial blood pressure for cerebral perfusion, constant fluid volume, and so forth, under more normal conditions, although this has never been experimentally tested as far as I know (Cannon et al. 1929). In this context I remind the reader that the regulation exerted by the autonomic nervous system and by the endocrine system were "designed" by nature (through natural selection during development) to cope with the extremes (e.g., living in the tropics, in Siberia, in the desert; running marathons, etc.).

Cannon was aware that the autonomic nervous system is active during small disturbances. Cannon's idea of synchronized sympathetic activity in the *fright, fight and flight responses* (Cannon 1929a, 1939) is what we would call today the *defense reaction*; however this idea was readily picked up by the scientific and clinical community, and even by lay people. The coordinated response was taken to indicate that the activity of all parts of the sympathetic nervous system was linked so as to occur in an *all-or-none* fashion without differentiation between the different effector organs. This activation of the sympathetic nervous system was thought to be generally protective and the level of arousal to be expressed in the level of sympathetic discharge or *sympathetic tone*. Some people believe the sympathetic system operates in the same way as the endocrine systems.

Cannon himself was surprised that the same unified action of the sympathetic nervous system could be useful in circumstances as diverse as hypoglycemia, hypotension, hypothermia, hypoxia, and so forth. He was aware that the unified system apparently produced responses which, although physiologically meaningful in certain states of the body, were useless in others (e.g., sweating in hypoglycemia, rise of blood sugar in asphyxia; pupillodilation in fear and love; Cannon 1939). But, he contented himself by assuming that the appearance of inappropriate features in the total complex of sympathico-adrenal function makes sense in the context of its *emergency function* (*Notfallfunktion*, Cannon 1928) if one considers *first, that it is, on the whole, a unitary system; second, that it is capable of producing effects in many different organs; and third, that among these effects are different combinations which are of the utmost utility in correspondingly different conditions of need* (Cannon, 1939, p.298).

Great emphasis was placed on the adrenal medulla in Cannon's research (Cannon 1914b). In his animals, under experimental conditions in which the body's ability to recover from major disturbances was tested, Cannon measured many effects that were responses to *catecholamines (adrenaline and noradrenaline)* released from the adrenal medulla. It is almost universally stated in textbooks that adrenaline and noradrenaline released from the adrenal medulla act on the same effector organs as the sympathetic postganglionic neurons and thereby enhance and support the effects of sympathetic neurons on target tissues. This statement is misleading as far as the function of the sympathetic nervous system is concerned, at least under normal conditions in higher vertebrates, not only because it assumes widespread and uniform actions of the sympathetic nervous system on target tissues, but also because catecholamines from the adrenal medulla often do *not* have the same effect on the target tissues as sympathetic nerve activity. About 92% to 98% of circulating noradrenaline originates from sympathetic nerve terminals (Esler et al. 1990), and all circulating adrenaline is released by the adrenal medulla. Adrenaline released from the adrenal medulla under physiological conditions is primarily a *metabolic hormone* and chiefly serves to catalyze the mobilization of glucose and lactic acid from glycogen and of free fatty acids from adipose tissue (Table 1.2, Figures 4.18, 4.19); in physiological concentrations, *it does not support* the effect of sympathetic postganglionic neurons on target tissues (see Subchapter 4.4; Celander 1954; Silverberg et al. 1978; Cryer 1980; Shah et al. 1984). In fact the physiological concentration of circulating adrenaline and noradrenaline is too low to affect the low affinity receptors on normally innervated tissues (see Subchapter 4.5) (Note 3). Furthermore, in many innervated tissues, most of the circulating catecholamines are taken up by the neuronal uptake mechanism in postganglionic nerve terminals before it can reach the target organ.

Cannon's was a puzzling way of arguing, given that the precise and distinct control of, for example, body temperature, cerebral perfusion, and so forth, by the autonomic nervous system was already known at the time. Therefore and as already mentioned in the introduction of this book, such control systems could not work if Cannon's concept about the sympathico-adrenal system were true! Cannon's argument was even more surprising given the enormous amount of detailed experimental work described by Langley between 1890 and 1920, which supported the principle that each organ and tissue is innervated by distinct sympathetic and parasympathetic pathways (Langley 1903, 1921; Chapter 1). Moreover, Langley's conclusions were strengthened by further experiments in which he studied the regeneration of preganglionic axons lesioned in the cervical sympathetic trunk to the superior cervical ganglion. He found orderly restitution of function after regeneration of the preganglionic axons (i.e., topographically correct and functionally appropriate synaptic connections between preganglionic axons and postganglionic neurons; Langley 1897).

11.1.2 Hess and the Dichotomous Organization of the Autonomic Nervous System

In the 1920s, the Swiss physiologist Walter Rudolf Hess, influenced by Karplus and Kreidle (see Akert 1981), started his famous experiments in which he studied the behavior elicited in conscious cats by local electrical stimulation of the hypothalamus. He implanted electrodes stereotactically into the hypothalamus and correlated the type of behavior (defensive behavior [Abwehrverhalten; see Subchapter 11.2], submissive, nutritive, sexual and evacuative behaviors and particular autonomic reactions, such as piloerection, sweating, pupillodilation, micturition, defecation) which he could evoke from the anatomical sites he stimulated in freely moving cats. After the experiments, he left the electrodes in position and perfused the brains of the animals in order to locate the tips of the electrodes in the diencephalon, in particular in the hypothalamus. Over several years, Hess probed the whole diencephalon and constructed maps for the different autonomic reactions, which he documented as integral components of the different elicited behaviors. Hess interpreted his results to mean that the hypothalamus integrates the activity of the autonomic nervous system so as to compose activity of body organs to somatomotor behavior (for English translations of the key publications of Hess, see Akert 1981).

Similar experiments were later conducted with chickens by von Holst and St. Paul (1960, 1962). These experimenters showed that electrical stimulation of the different areas of the hypothalamus via implanted electrodes leads to species-specific (instinctive) behavior of the birds, including

vocalization, which could not be distinguished from their natural behavior. These authors concluded that the different components of behavior, including the adaptive changes in the body that are dependent on the autonomic nervous system and the neuroendocrine system, are represented in the diencephalon.

On the basis of his experiments, Hess propagated generalizations similar to those of Cannon about the functioning of the autonomic nervous system. He believed that the cranial division of the parasympathetic nervous system promotes the conservation of energy and aids in the recovery of the body after stress (i.e., has *trophotropic* functions), while the sympathetic nervous system has *ergotropic* functions, mobilizing bodily energy and adapting the body to challenges from the environment (Hess 1948). These observations are based on the evidence that stimulation of the parasympathetic system leads to an activation of gastrointestinal tract and pelvic organs, whereas stimulation of the sympathetic branch of the autonomic nervous system generated all those reactions which are also seen during defensive behavior elicited from the caudal hypothalamus and the central gray matter of the midbrain (Hess 1954; in Akert [1981]). This generalizing belief is very similar to that of Cannon.

Hess later transferred the idea of a dichotomy of the functional organization of the autonomic nervous system to the hypothalamus (Hess 1954): he hypothesized that the rostral parts of the hypothalamus integrate somatic, autonomic and endocrine reactions and promote recovery and conservation of energy, digestion, excretion and evacuation of waste, as well as reproductive functions. He thought that these functions were associated with the excitation of the parasympathetic nervous system, and the entire process was subsumed under the umbrella term *trophotropic reaction*. He further hypothesized that activation of the caudal parts of the hypothalamus causes general excitation of the sympathetic nervous system, mobilization of body energy and enhancement of performance capacity (*ergotropic reaction*). This concept requires that the hypothalamus consists of two functionally and anatomically different systems. Thus, the unifying concept of the antagonistic function of the sympathetic and parasympathetic nervous system was extended to the hypothalamus. But the concept itself is far too general to explain the complexities of the central control of autonomic functions.

11.1.3 The Consequences of the Generalizing Concepts of Cannon and Hess

Both Cannon and Hess had enormous impact on the scientific community and in clinical medicine. Their influence was positive because it focused clinical practice, clinical research and research in systems physiology on the effects the autonomic nervous system has in regulating body functions.

The ideas of Cannon and Hess were soon accepted by physiologists and pharmacologists. Generalizations about the actions of the sympathetic nervous system also led to a change in the connotation of the terms *sympathetic* and *parasympathetic* from that originally defined by Langley. Langley's anatomical definitions were clear (see Subchapters 1.1 and 2.1; Jänig et al. 2017). However, now the terms implied particular types of function, that is, "sympathetic" function and "parasympathetic" function, in line with the generalists' ideas. This is best demonstrated by the commonly used term *sympathico-adrenal system* (Cannon 1939). However, modern research shows that the generalizations made by Cannon and Hess have functionally no justification (other than ontogenetic) and to lump all the sympathetic systems functionally together is an obsolete idea.

The concept that the sympathetic nervous system operates in a more or less unitary way was strengthened by the increase in knowledge about neurotransmitter receptors (notably adrenoceptors and muscarinic acetylcholine receptors). Drugs were developed for potential therapeutic use that interfered with or mimicked the actions of autonomic transmitter substances. This trend continues in modern molecular pharmacology:

1. A plethora of receptors in the membranes of the autonomic neurons and their target cells have been detected, cloned and their molecular structure analyzed. For example, at present, nine types of adrenoceptors and five types of muscarinic receptors have been identified on the basis of their molecular structure, their coupling to intracellular signaling pathways and their genes (Alexander et al. 2019). Subtypes of each of these receptors have been identified. The function of these different receptors in the neural regulation of autonomic target tissues is only known for some tissues and specifically for the subtypes of adrenoceptors α_1, α_2, β_1, β_2 (see Table 1.2). Unfortunately current evidence suggests that most of these receptors are not accessed by a neuronally released transmitter under physiological conditions as this often produces its effects by interacting with localized "junctional" receptors in restricted regions of the postsynaptic cell (see Chapter 7). The identification of molecularly distinct receptors will permit the development of specific antagonists for the identification of the postjunctional receptors relevant for neural control of different effector organs.

2. Many neuropeptides and other substances have been detected in autonomic neurons that are co-localized with the classical transmitters in the vesicles or the cytoplasm of the presynaptic terminals and which may have neurotransmitter functions (see Subchapter 1.4). Molecular techniques are being used to demonstrate the distribution of mRNA for a range of identified receptors/binding sites for these peptides, as well as for the pathways for synthesis and the peptides themselves (Alexander et al. 2019). Again, when specific antagonists have been developed, it may be possible to determine whether or not these peptides play a physiological role.

3. The almost exponential expansion of molecular pharmacology has not necessarily led to a better understanding of how autonomic systems work in regulating the target organs under physiological conditions. Thus, conclusions cannot be drawn from this type of research as far as the biological meaning and significance of autonomic regulations are concerned.

I do not want to dispute the scientific achievements of Cannon and Hess. Both were, over several decades, dedicated experimental scientists and observers; both were dedicated and gifted teachers (Akert 1981; Brooks et al. 1975; Benison et al. 1987). Hess was awarded the Nobel Prize for his scientific work. Cannon was somewhat unfortunate not to receive it, but this did not affect his fame. However, one wonders why both propagated their unifying and simplifying concepts on how the autonomic nervous system functions, independent of experimental tools that were rather limited. Indeed one wonders why the unifying concepts were (and still are) attractive for the medical and the public (lay) community. Reading their work carefully, in particular the book *The Wisdom of the Body* (Cannon 1939) and both of Hess' books *The Organization of the Autonomic Nervous System*

(Hess 1948) and *The Diencephalon* (Hess 1954), one is left with the impression that both were aware that the autonomic nervous system is differentiated in its organization, in particular the sympathetic nervous system. Otherwise many observations in their experiments could not have been explained. And, as mentioned above, Cannon questioned for this reason the James–Lange theory of emotions and asked himself how a system functionally as uniform in its reactions as the sympathetic nervous system can be involved in so many differentiated functions. I find the conceptual situation even more puzzling for two reasons. *First*, both of them knew Langley's work, although he is mentioned only once in Cannon's book (Cannon 1939), and not discussed in Hess' book on the autonomic nervous system (Hess 1948), despite his very important achievements. Perhaps they either did not recognize or ignored the important messages of Langley, namely that there are distinct spinal autonomic (in particular sympathetic) pathways to the effector systems. *Second*, both had extensive knowledge about the normal regulation of target systems by the sympathetic nervous system (they were teaching organ regulation over tens of years to generations of medical students!). This regulation of organs requires precise and specific autonomic nervous pathways, otherwise one could not understand how regulation is brought about.

11.2 | General Aspects of Integrated Autonomic Responses

Life of complex organisms in a continuously changing environment is only possible if the internal milieu of the body: (1) remains constant in relatively narrowly confined limits, (2) can be quickly adapted within these limits to transient brief environmental perturbations, such as the requirement for physical exertion, temperature changes, loss of blood during an accident, etc., and (3) can be semipermanently adapted to slow changes in the environment, e.g., during the changing seasons, during long-term thermal loads (i.e., in the arctic or tropics), during pregnancy, at high altitude, etc. The regulation of the internal (extracellular and intracellular) parameters for constancy in vertebrates, in particular mammals, is called *homeostasis* (Cannon 1929a, 1939). It is dependent on functioning autonomic and neuroendocrine systems. The

homeostatic control systems are represented in the brain stem and hypothalamus.

11.2.1 Homeostasis and Allostasis

The concept of homeostasis was formulated by Cannon (1929a, 1939) based on Claude Bernard's idea of the constancy of the internal milieu (Bernard 1865, 1878). This idea developed at a time that was scientifically dominated by the idea of the thermodynamic equilibrium. The formulation of the concept of homeostasis became a milestone in our understanding of how the body is controlled by the autonomic nervous and the endocrine systems. This concept was then applied to the regulation of the intracellular milieu of single cells and also to the regulation of higher brain functions.

Homeostasis is defined by the stability of physiological systems that maintain life. It applies strictly to a limited number of systems such as regulation of pH, concentration of different ions in the extracellular fluid, osmolality of extracellular fluid, glucose levels and arterial oxygen tension, etc. that are truly essential for life and are therefore maintained within a range for the current life history stage (McEwen and Wingfield 2003). This restricted definition does not allow us to understand how autonomic and endocrine controls enable the organism to adapt to severe and unpredictable environmental changes. And, in fact, physiological systems operate within a *dynamic range* of steady states which change according to the demands on the organism. Thus the concept of homeostatic control does not make clear how this adaptation during fast and slow changes in the environment occurs. The temporary deviations from the "set point" of the homeostatic control systems during adaptation to internal or external loads impinging on the organism are dependent on the forebrain. The adaptation of the homeostatic control systems to these external and internal perturbations is called *allostasis*.

The concept of allostasis, which was first formulated by Sterling and Eyer (1988) and has been elaborated on by McEwen (1998, 2000, 2001b; McEwen and Wingfield 2003), encompasses the dynamic temporary adjustments of the physiological control of body parameters. Parameters that are regulated within quite narrow limits under practically all physiological conditions, as mentioned above, are examples of homeostatic regulation in the original sense and are very similar between individuals. Parameters such as arterial blood pressure, heart rate, body core temperature, concentration of circulating hormones (e.g., glucocorticoids, adrenaline, sexual hormones), sleep–wake cycle, energy metabolism and regulation of other parameters vary more widely within and between individuals. Here allostatic adaptations minimize the duration and the magnitude of the changes of the parameters from the steady state. Thus, allostasis means achieving physiological stability through change of state. The process of altered and sustained activity during allostasis leads to changes in "set points" and boundaries of homeostatic control and is called an allostatic state. This process is fully dependent on the autonomic and endocrine regulation of body functions by the brain, in particular the forebrain (for discussion and literature see Berntson and Cacioppo [2000]; McEwen and Wingfield [2003]; Schulkin [2003a,b]; Schulkin and Sterling [2019]).

Adaptation of homeostatic regulation during changing environments is a temporary process. If the allostatic adaptations are not switched off once they are no longer needed (i.e., if they fail to habituate), if they occur too frequently or if they fail to occur at all, systemic diseases such as cardiovascular diseases, type II diabetes, obesity and metabolic syndromes, etc. may develop (Henry and Stephens 1977; Henry and Grim 1990; Björntorp 1997; Folkow et al. 1997; Henry 1997; McEwen 2001a; Robertson et al. 2012; Buijs and Swaab 2013; Mathias and Bannister 2013; Bruce et al. 2017; Guarino et al. 2017).

11.2.2 Behavioral Patterns and Autonomic Responses

Homeostatic control of the cardiovascular system, the respiratory pump and the gastrointestinal tract, as well as their moment-to-moment coordination, are represented in the lower brain stem. The integrative neural networks receive inputs from many functionally different types of visceral (spinal and vagal) afferent neurons (cardiovascular, respiratory and gastrointestinal) that trigger distinct reflexes when stimulated. The individual responses are predominantly based on anatomically and physiologically defined reflex pathways, some of which have been described in Chapter 10. It is the *coordination between these functionally distinct reflex pathways that demonstrates how these integrative networks work*. This is illustrated by the coordination of the neural regulation of the cardiovascular and respiratory systems (Subchapter 10.6), by the precise interactive control of breathing

and of the entrance to the gastrointestinal tract and by several functions discussed in this chapter in which the upper brain stem and hypothalamus are involved (Tables 11.1 and 11.2). These coordinated response patterns can be triggered or inhibited by physiological stimulation of afferents (trigeminal afferents from the nasal and oropharyngeal cavities, arterial chemoreceptors, arterial baroreceptors, unmyelinated vagal afferents from the atria and ventricles of the heart, gastrointestinal afferents, etc.).

The integrative networks in the medulla oblongata and pons are under powerful control of the mesencephalon, hypothalamus and cerebral hemispheres. They are involved in all elementary behavioral repertoires that are represented in the mesencephalon and hypothalamus (see Table 11.2). All activities of the body that are initiated from the forebrain, including those controlled by the neuronal programs in the hypothalamus and mesencephalon, co-opt the lower brain stem centers.

The mesencephalon, hypothalamus and limbic system contain the neuronal programs that generate response patterns to adjust the behavior of the organism in a continuously changing environment. These programs utilize repertoires of *somatomotor*, *autonomic* and *hormonal adjustments*, which are organized so that the motor behaviors are accompanied by changes in the viscera, metabolism etc., so as to optimize the net performance. The brain is continuously informed at all levels about the state of the environment and of the body tissues via the sensory systems and other forms of feedback from the body (e.g., hormonal, humoral and physical signals) and selects the most appropriate reaction patterns to cope with the current environmental challenges.

Figure 11.1 depicts the situation schematically. The neuronal programs representing the regulation and integration of autonomic, endocrine and somatomotor functions are at the core of the system. Their activation leads to specific responses (see Figure 11.1) and to the interoception of bodily changes correlated with the autonomic and endocrine reactions, such as during hunger, thirst, respiratory effort, satiety, muscle effort, etc. (see Subchapter 2.6). The interoceptive sensations of the body are integrated with the perception of the environmental situation. They are represented in the telencephalon (limbic system and neocortex [probably mainly insular cortex and orbitofrontal cortex]). Here I want to emphasize, by alluding to Figure 11.1:

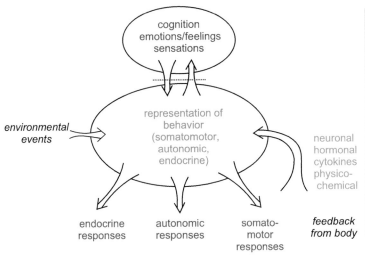

environmental
events

neuronal
hormonal
cytokines
physico-
chemical

*feedback
from body*

endocrine
responses

autonomic
responses

somato-
motor
responses

Figure 11.1 Representation of body functions in the forebrain and mesencephalon. Activation of these representations generates coordinated somatomotor, autonomic and neuroendocrine responses, body sensations and experience of emotions. The central representations continuously receive feedback information from the body (neuronal, hormonal [including cytokines], physico-chemical [e.g., glucose level in the blood, temperature of the blood]) and from the environment. The dotted line indicates the difference between "material" neural and mental processes. The central circuits representing the mental processes (cognition, body sensations, feelings, emotions) act back on the neural circuits representing motor functions of the body (somatomotor, autonomic, neuroendocrine).

- Autonomic and endocrine control systems are integrated and represented in the hypothalamus and cerebral hemispheres.

- Sensations and emotions are related to the functional state of body tissues. They are generated in close association with homeostatic autonomic and endocrine regulation and in association with the interoceptive input systems.

- The telencephalic representations, which are the basis of the mental processes, act back on the central representations of the autonomic and endocrine control systems (see upper part of Figure 11.1).

The latter topdown feedback has seldom been investigated and is a matter of intense discussion. It is important for understanding the fast adaptation of homeostatic regulations during external or internal perturbations ("stress"). The temporary adjustments that occur during challenges from the environment (or occur as a consequence of forebrain processes related to past experience and anticipation of future events) is called allostasis (see Subchapter 11.2.1). Understanding the mechanisms as to how the telencephalon initiates and modulates bodily processes involving the autonomic and neuroendocrine systems (see upper left arrow in Figure 11.1) may turn out to be the key to clarifying the mechanisms underlying psychosomatic and other behaviorally determined diseases.

The way by which the telencephalic cortex influences peripheral autonomic pathways and therefore autonomic target organs and target tissues is almost entirely unknown. This applies to all behavioral reactions organized in the upper brain stem and hypothalamus as listed in Table 11.1. However, using retrograde transneural transport of rabies virus as an experimental tool in a time-dependent manner by varying the survival time of the virus, it has been demonstrated by Strick and coworkers that there exist synaptically connected neuron chains from layer V of various cortices to sympathetic preganglionic neurons innervating the adrenal medulla (monkey; Dum et al. 2016), the kidney (rat; Levinthal and Strick 2012) and the stomach (rat; Levinthal and Strick 2020). Furthermore, there exists a pathway from the cortex to parasympathetic preganglionic neurons innervating the stomach (rat; Levinthal and Strick 2020). Most cortical output neurons are located in the motor cortices M1 and M2 and in the somatosensory cortex S1 for the sympathetic pathways to kidney and stomach, in the motor cortices and in the medial prefrontal cortex for the adrenal medulla, and in the insular cortex and medial prefrontal cortex for the parasympathetic innervation of the stomach. These elegant functional morphological experimental studies do not reveal how the cortex is directing the various target organs and tissues via autonomic final pathways. However, they open a door to work out exactly this. These future studies will lay the foundation of the neurobiological basis for the psychosocial relation between body and brain and for psychosomatic diseases.

Here, for practical reasons, I will divide the behavioral patterns into three groups: (1) Patterns that are quickly activated in minutes, seconds or less and involve somatomotor and autonomic systems

Table 11.1 Patterns of activity in neurons of sympathetic and parasympathetic pathways during different behavioral reactions organized in the upper brain stem and hypothalamus

| Organ | Autonomic Pathway | Diving Response | Exercise | Defense Reaction | | | Tonic Immobility | Vigilance | Freezing Reaction |
				Confrontation	Flight	Quiescence			
Heart	SCM	↓↓	↑↑ (tonic)	↑↑	↑↑	Ø/↓?	↓↓	?	?
	PCM	↑↑↑	↓↓ (initial)	↓↓	↓↓	↑↑	↑↑↑	↑↑	↑
Skeletal Muscle	MVC	↑↑↑	↑	↑	↑	↑	↓↓	↑↑	↑
	MVD[a]	Ø	Ø	↑↑?	↑↑	Ø	↑?/Ø	Ø	Ø
Skin	CVC (av.a.)	↓↓	↑↑	↑↑[b]	↑↑	↑?	↓↓	?	?
	CVC (nutrit.)	↑↑↑	↑↑	↑↑	↑↑	↑?	↓↑	?	?
Kidney	VVC	↑↑↑	↑↑	↑↑	↑↑	↑?	↓↓	↑↑	↑?
GIT	VVC	↑↑↑	↑↑	↑	↑↑	↑?	↓↓	↑↑	?
Art. BP		Ø	↑	↑	↑	↓↓	↓↓↓	↑↑	Ø
Card. Output		↓↓↓	↑↑	↑↑	↑↑	↓↓	↓↓	→	→
Respiration		↓↓↓	↑↑	↑/Ø	↑↑	→	↓↓↓	→	→

CVC, cutaneous vasoconstrictor neurons (to arteriovenous anastomoses [av.a.]; to nutritional vessels [nutrit.]); MVC, muscle vasoconstrictor; MVD, muscle vasodilator; PCM/SCM, parasympathetic/sympathetic cardiomotor neurons; VVC, visceral vasoconstrictor; Ø, relatively unchanged; ↑,↑↑,↑↑↑/↓,↓↓,↓↓↓, increase/decrease of activity (or of cardiovascular and respiratory parameters); ?, effect unknown; Art. BP, mean arterial blood pressure; GIT, gastrointestinal tract. Modified from Folkow (2000), Bandler et al. (2000a) and Keay and Bandler (2004, 2014).

a Probably only present in some species (see Subchapter 4.2); b Extracranial vasodilation in facial skin

(Table 11.1). (2) Patterns of somatomotor, autonomic and neuroendocrine responses that involve the hypothalamus and are mostly activated more slowly. (3) Patterns of autonomic responses occurring during experimentally generated emotions.

The main point I want to make is that the optimal activation of autonomic and endocrine responses in the behavioral patterns described in this chapter requires the telencephalon.

I will not discuss the following three groups of experimental approaches and refer the reader to the literature:

1. The Russian school beginning with Ivan Pavlov. In their experimentation on awake (non-anesthetized) animals, mostly dogs, Pavlov and his followers, notably Bykov, have clearly shown that autonomic systems are under the control of the telencephalon. Pavlov studied the neural regulation of digestive glands (salivary, gastric, pancreatic secretion). Using the paradigm of the conditioned reflexes, he clearly showed that the cranial parasympathetic pathways supplying the gastrointestinal tract are under cortical control (see Figure 10.30). Later it was shown by the Russian School (Bykov and his pupils), using the same experimental paradigm, that urinary secretion by the kidney and the cardiac output are also under cortical control, involving sympathetic systems (Bykov 1944/1959; Ádám 1967, 1998; see Dworkin [1993, 2000] for extensive discussion and literature).

2. The psychophysiologists have rendered arguments that the cortex is involved in the control of the cardiovascular system (in particular the heart) and the gastrointestinal tract via autonomic pathways. This is, e.g., expressed in the formulation of the cardiac–somatic hypothesis by Obrist (Obrist 1981). This work fully supports the points I am going to make in Subchapter 11.3 showing that regulation of autonomic target organs during body challenge in vivo is influenced by the cortex (Berntson and Cacioppo 2000, and older literature therein).

3. Brain processes underlying behavior, cognition and emotions are interdependent with bodily states that are organized by autonomic and endocrine systems. This interdependence is studied in humans by applying modern neuroimaging techniques to the brain. The overall aims of these studies are to explore the central representations of autonomic and endocrine regulation in the forebrain, to explore how cognitive and emotional processes are dependent on and interact with the autonomically determined body states, and to show that the brain processes underlying subjective experience and motivational behaviors require autonomic and endocrine control of the body, including the afferent feedback from the periphery of the body (Damasio 1994, 1999; Critchley and Dolan 2004).

11.3 Autonomic Responses Activated Quickly During Distinct Behavioral Patterns

Table 11.1 summarizes response patterns of autonomic and respiratory systems for eight behavioral reactions, including exercise, that are organized in the brain stem and hypothalamus and recruited quickly. The main emphasis is on cardiovascular parameters. The peripheral autonomic pathways involved are listed on the left. Integrated in the generation of these patterns are the various spinal and bulbar reflexes related to the cardiovascular system, the respiratory system, the gastrointestinal tract, the pelvic organs, the motor components of the eye, etc., as they have been described in the preceding chapters (Folkow 1987, 2000). The telencephalon can initiate these autonomic patterns within seconds and maintain them for some time or can shift quickly between response patterns (e.g., from an active defense reaction to a passive defense reaction or to tonic immobility). Thus, telencephalic command signals have direct access to the neural circuits of the hypothalamus and brain stem responsible for the generation of the autonomic responses characteristic for these behavioral reactions.

11.3.1 Autonomic Changes During Diving

In terms of magnitude and temporal precision, the most spectacular pattern of autonomic response is the *diving response*, which is used both for protection and for food seeking in diving species (Elsner et al. 1966; Blix and Folkow 1983; Butler and Jones 1997; Panneton 2013; Panneton and Gan 2020). Figure 11.2A illustrates the changes in blood flow and heart rate (heart beats are indicated by the pulsatile blood flow changes and the dots during diving) through the abdominal aorta and renal artery in a harbor seal during a forced dive in which the animal remained quietly restrained under water for 8 minutes (Elsner et al. 1966). This seal had experienced many dives of this type and was therefore fully habituated. The start of the dive is immediately followed by a decrease in heart rate from about 100 beats per minute to about 7 per minute. Blood flow through the abdominal aorta and renal artery almost ceased, indicating that the peripheral vascular beds (particularly of viscera, including kidney, and skeletal muscle) had virtually closed down. On surfacing, heart beat and blood flow through both arteries increased within a few seconds to their baseline levels as before diving.

Figure 11.2b shows the changes in heart rate of a harp seal during an entirely unrestrained dive (Casson and Ronald 1975). This animal had been trained to dive on command. The bradycardia (heart rate decrease from 125 to 30 beats per minute) occurred a few seconds *before* the actual dive and the heart rate increased to its predive level about 5 to 15 s

before the seal surfaced. These measurements clearly show that the dramatic changes in cardiovascular parameters during initiation, maintenance and termination of diving depend on neural signals from the telencephalon. These signals activate, probably via the lateral hypothalamus, the neural circuits in the medulla oblongata that are involved in the regulation of the heart, blood vessels and lung. The central command signals probably do not target the final autonomic and respiratory pathways directly (e.g., parasympathetic cardiomotor neurons in the nucleus ambiguus, sympathetic premotor neurons in the rostral ventrolateral medulla, bulbospinal inspiratory neurons), but rather they utilize the circuits of the neural autonomic and respiratory motor programs that are involved in the regulation of cardiovascular (and other) target organs and respiration.

The diving responses generated by the cortical signals are facilitated by stimulation of trigeminal mechano- and other receptors (of the face and nasopharyngeal mucosa), by excitation of arterial chemoreceptors (generated by decreased arterial oxygen tension) and by respiratory arrest in expiration. Excitation of trigeminal receptors by mechanical,

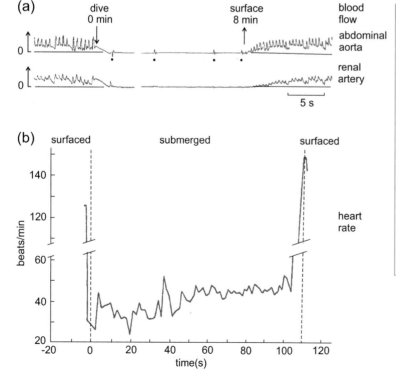

Figure 11.2 Cardiovascular changes during diving responses initiated by central signals from the telencephalon. (a) Blood flow in abdominal aorta and renal artery of a harbor seal before, during and after a forced diving of 8 min duration during which the animal remained quietly restrained under water. Note that the blood flows and heart rate decrease within 1 s after the beginning of the dive, remain low throughout the dive and increase within 2 s after termination of the dive (surface). Heart beats are indicated by the pulsatile changes in blood flow (see dots) during the dive. (b) Change in heart rate in a harp seal trained and conditioned to dive. Note the anticipatory decrease in heart rate (bradycardia) before diving and the anticipatory increase in heart rate before surfacing. (a) modified from Elsner et al. (1966) and (b) modified from Casson and Ronald (1975) with permission.

cold and other stimuli triggers reflex bradycardia too, but this bradycardia is weaker than that induced by the cortical signal in the awake animal. The autonomic pattern of the diving response can be elicited in all mammalian species and birds (even those that never dive normally) although the autonomic responses are usually much weaker than those occurring in diving animals (seals, whales, penguins). The neural mechanisms underlying the fast signaling from the telencephalon to the circuits *in the brain stem* are unknown.

The observations on diving animals show that the cardiovascular system is transformed in a few seconds into a "heart-brain circulation system." Major vascular beds (of skeletal muscle and viscera) are virtually shut off by strong activation of vasoconstrictor neurons innervating resistance vessels. The metabolism in skeletal muscle switches from an aerobic to an anaerobic mechanism. Heart rate is profoundly reduced by activation of parasympathetic cardiomotor neurons and probably withdrawal of activity in sympathetic cardiomotor neurons. In the skin, the apical non-nutritional arteriovenous anastomoses, which are under powerful neural control, are dilated during submersion by inhibition of activity in cutaneous vasoconstrictor neurons innervating these anastomoses, whereas the cutaneous vasoconstrictor neurons supplying nutritional blood vessels are activated (Note 4). This helps oxygen-containing blood in large venous "depots" to be diverted to the heart pump, without peripheral O_2 consumption, for subsequent nutritional delivery to brain and myocardium in a situation where cardiac output is reduced up to 20-fold. Furthermore, opening of arteriovenous anastomoses in skin counteracts the increase in peripheral resistance in skeletal muscle and viscera and takes away load from the heart.

11.3.2 Autonomic changes during centrally generated muscle effort

Any dynamic or tonic action involving skeletal muscle that is initiated by higher centers in the telencephalon is accompanied by fast and precise adjustments of the cardiovascular and respiratory systems to supply the exercising skeletal muscle with oxygen and nutrients. These adjustments are reflected in an increase in heart rate, arterial blood pressure and ventilation, in addition to the local metabolic changes in the skeletal muscle, and to the secondary changes involved in regulation of body temperature,

extracellular fluid volume and acid–base balance. Here I will describe that for the first seconds to minutes after the start of isometric exercise in humans the cortical signal activating the motoneurons and their associated neural circuits (see Subchapter 9.4) also access the neural circuits involved in regulation of the cardiovascular and respiratory systems.

Figure 11.3 shows an experiment on an experimentally immobilized and ventilated healthy human subject in whom arterial blood pressure and heart rate were continuously recorded. Before the experiment the subject had been systematically trained to undergo graded isometric dorsiflections of both ankles. Furthermore, he had been trained to be mentally relaxed during immobilization; therefore, he did not exhibit any sign of anxiety or stress during immobilization, as reported after recovery from paralysis. On verbal instruction by the experimenter, the subject attempted to grade his efforts to 25%, 50% and 100% of the maximum effort. Zero % effort was a sham maneuver in which the subject was encouraged by the experimenter to initiate contractions but he did not attempt to generate them. The graded attempted effort to contract the muscles, but without actual contraction due to the immobilization, was correlated with the graded increase in arterial blood pressure and heart rate. These cardiovascular responses were not correlated with the muscle mass that the subject was trying to contract but with the intensity of the central signal. Thus, the attempt to contract a large or a small muscle mass with the same effort leads to the same cardiovascular changes. The cardiovascular changes started within a few seconds after the beginning of the central command (see inset of Figure 11.3). This experiment clearly shows that the central (cortical) signal initiating muscle contraction activates neural circuits regulating the cardiovascular system within a second or less.

The central signal generated in the cortex is also important to *maintain* the cardiovascular and respiratory changes during exercise. This is shown in Figure 11.4. Tension of the biceps (b) or triceps surae (a) of the forearm was maintained at about 20% of maximum tension over three minutes. During this period, diastolic and systolic blood pressure, heart rate and ventilation increased (red curves). Stimulation of the Ia-fibers from the spindles of the biceps muscle using a vibrator applied to its tendon (a stimulus that does not generate a sensation from the muscle)

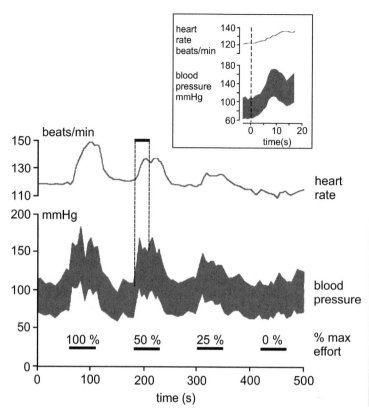

Figure 11.3 Responses of heart rate and arterial blood pressure in a paralyzed human subject during a sequence of graded attempted contractions of the dorsiflexors of the ankle. The subject was paralyzed and ventilated. Paralysis was generated by intravenous infusion of atracurium leading to neuromuscular blockade. The dose of atracurium was five times greater than required for surgical paralysis. Measurements were started about 50 min after the onset of paralysis. Attempted contractions were graded for 100%, 50% and 25% of the maximal central effort for the duration indicated by the bars. The effect of a sham maneuver was included (0% effort, verbal encouragements but no attempted contraction). *Inset:* Response of heart rate and blood pressure to an attempted contraction of 50% of maximal effort on an expanded time scale. The dashed line indicates the request to start the attempted effort. Note the rapid increase in heart rate and blood pressure after start of the effort. Arterial blood pressure and heart rate were monitored continuously with a servo-controlled device to maintain a constant volume in a finger using a cuff around the finger. The high heart rate is explained by partial blockade of the cholinergic transmission from the parasympathetic cardiomotor neurons to the pacemaker cells. Modified from Gandevia et al. (1993) with permission.

monosynaptically activates the motoneurons innervating the biceps muscle and disynaptically inhibits motoneurons of the triceps surae (the antagonist of the biceps muscle). The central signal to contract the triceps muscle is inhibited by the afferent Ia-input from the biceps muscle (Figure 11.4a) and the central signal to contract the biceps muscle is enhanced by the afferent Ia-input from the biceps muscle (Figure 11.4b). As a consequence of the activation of the Ia-fibers, either the strength of the central signal to the triceps muscle increases or to the biceps muscle decreases in order to maintain the muscle tension constant at 20% of maximum tension. These quantitative changes in the cortical signal are associated with changes in blood pressure, heart rate and ventilation. Increased central activation is followed by a larger increase in blood pressure, heart rate and ventilation (Figure 11.4a) and decreased central activation by a smaller increase in these cardiovascular and respiratory parameters than in the controls (Figure 11.4b; compare green curves with red curves).

We can conclude unambiguously from these experiments that cortical signals initiating and maintaining isometric muscle contraction access in parallel the neural circuits involved in regulation of the cardiovascular and respiratory systems. The cortical signals are important to initiate these changes quickly and to maintain them. Fast changes in heart rate are probably generated by reduced activity in parasympathetic cardiomotor neurons (i.e., these neurons are inhibited by the cortex); maintained increases in heart rate and blood pressure (during long-lasting isometric exercise) involve, particularly, activation of sympathetic cardiovascular neurons (cardiomotor neurons and vasoconstrictor neurons innervating resistance vessels). The central signals are integrated, during the static phase, with the afferent signals (1) from the exercising skeletal muscle (small-diameter myelinated [Aδ] and unmyelinated [C] afferent nerve fibers sensing muscle contraction and metabolic changes; Mitchell 1985; Rowell 1993), (2) from the lung and (3) from cardiovascular targets. The neural pathways by which the central (telencephalic) signals influence the neural regulation centers of the cardiovascular and respiratory systems have yet to be worked out.

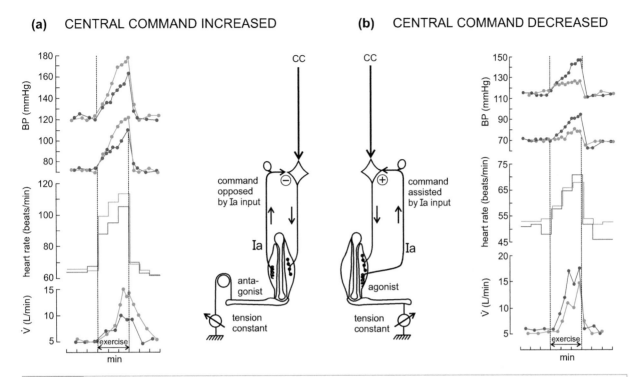

(a) CENTRAL COMMAND INCREASED

(b) CENTRAL COMMAND DECREASED

Figure 11.4 Changes in arterial blood pressure, heart rate and ventilation during changes of central command (CC) to generate isometric contractions at constant muscle tension of the biceps or triceps surae of the forearm in human subjects. Tension of the biceps (b) or triceps surae (a) generated by CC is adjusted to 20% of the maximal tension during 3 minutes. Increase in muscle tension is accompanied by an increase in systolic and diastolic blood pressure, heart rate and ventilation (closed circles and solid-line curves in red). The Ia-fibers of the muscle spindles in the biceps were stimulated by a vibrator attached to its tendon that oscillated at 100 Hz and at an amplitude of a few μm (this stimulus generates no sensation). Stimulation of Ia-fibers activates motoneurons to the biceps muscle monosynaptically and leads to a decrease in the CC necessary to maintain a biceps contraction at 20% of its maximum (right). It inhibits motoneurons to the triceps surae (antagonist) and leads to an increase in the CC to maintain a triceps contraction at 20% of its maximum (left). Changes in arterial blood pressure, heart rate and ventilation during exercise were smaller when the CC decreased (right) and larger when the CC increased (left); See closed circles and solid-line curves in green in [a] and [b]). This shows that the CC signal generated by the telencephalon has access to the cardiovascular centers in the medulla oblongata regulating the heart and peripheral resistance and to the respiratory neural network. Note the persistent and slow increase of heart rate and blood pressure after start of the effort. Modified from Goodwin et al. (1972) with permission.

11.3.3 Defense Reactions Integrated into the Mesencephalon

Responses of the autonomic nervous system to events that endanger the integrity of the body (e.g., threatening or stressful stimuli, acute blood loss, invasion of the body by microorganisms and their toxins) are well-orchestrated and their functional specificity resides in the individual responses associated with functionally discrete autonomic pathways. They enable the organism to avoid real or perceived danger and are presumably protective and adaptive under normal biological conditions. They are associated with the activation of the hypothalamo-pituitary-adrenal system, the sympatho-adrenal system, and the somatomotor system. The stereotyped patterns of these protective reactions are organized in the upper brain stem and hypothalamus and are under control of the telencephalon (limbic system, neocortex). These patterns can be recruited quickly by afferent signals from the body, by visual, acoustic or olfactory stimuli, by signals from the telencephalon (e.g., during imagined or subjectively attributed dangerous environments) or by both peripheral and central signals.

The general pattern of reaction when an individual is in pain and under stress can best be exemplified by the different types of *defense behavior.* These are integrated responses consisting of autonomic, endocrine and somatomotor components and sensory adjustments. The periaqueductal gray (PAG) in the midbrain is in a way the *final common pathway for defense behavior* as far as the somatomotor and autonomic responses are concerned. It contains the executive neural systems for brain structures located rostrally, such as the hypothalamus, amygdala, other structures of the limbic system and the prefrontal cortex (Panksepp 1998; for critical discussion and older literature see Bandler [1988] and Keay and Bandler [2014]).

Types of Defense Reaction Elicited from the PAG

Microinjection of the excitatory amino acid glutamate with a micropipette in the PAG of rats excites cell bodies of neurons in a small volume but not axons passing through. This way of stimulating neurons in the PAG elicits typical defense reactions that are characterized by their somatomotor and autonomic responses and by sensory changes. The organization of three types of defense reaction has been described by Bandler and coworkers for the rat. They called these reactions: (1) confrontational defense, (2) flight and (3) quiescence. The organization of these defense reactions has been worked out. There are good reasons to assume that the same principle of organization applies to all mammals (Bandler et al. 1991; Bandler and Shipley 1994; Bandler and Keay 1996; Bandler et al. 2000a, b; Keay and Bandler 2014). The characteristics of the three defense patterns are (Figure 11.5, Table 11.1):

1. *Confrontational defense* is characterized by hypertension, tachycardia, decreased blood flow through supporting limb muscles and viscera and increased blood flow in the face. It is activated by stimulation of the rostral part of the dorsolateral and lateral PAG and accompanied by an endogenous non-opioid analgesia.
2. *Flight* is characterized by hypertension, tachycardia, increased blood flow in the limb muscles and decreased blood flow in the face. It is initiated in the caudal part of the dorsolateral and lateral PAG. Also this defensive behavior is accompanied by an endogenous non-opioid analgesia.

3. *Quiescence* (hyporeactivity) is characterized by hypotension, bradycardia and endogenous opioid analgesia. It is activated by stimulation of the ventrolateral PAG (Note 5).

It is likely that, in addition to the cardiovascular changes, other autonomically mediated changes (e.g., related to the gastrointestinal tract or the pelvic organs) occur during the three types of defense reaction elicited from the PAG columns. Behavioral patterns elicited in this way occur independently of the hypothalamus and telencephalon. Thus, the neural circuits triggering the generation of these patterns are present in the rostrocaudally organized cell columns of the PAG.

It is important to emphasize that one component of the patterned defense reaction is the modification of sensory systems, leading, e.g., to analgesia during defense behavior in vivo. Also, functional changes in non-nociceptive somatic sensory systems, the visual system and the acoustic system occur (see Bandler [1988]). The neural circuits in the PAG are integral components of the typical defensive behaviors generated by the telencephalon via the hypothalamus. It is hypothesized that the cortically generated behavior patterns are the basis for *active behavioral coping strategies* and *passive behavioral coping strategies* in mammals (Keay and Bandler 2001, 2004).

The systemic cardiovascular changes (and probably other autonomic changes in, e.g., skin blood flow, piloerection, sweating, gastrointestinal motility, adrenal medullary secretion, pupil size, etc.) are generated by activation or inhibition of specific sympathetic and parasympathetic pathways. Some of these changes are listed in Table 11.1 for these types of defense behavior.

Systematic anatomical tracing studies of the afferent and efferent connections of the cell columns in the PAG show that these cell columns project to multiple sites in the hypothalamus, thalamus, midbrain, pons, medulla oblongata and spinal cord, and that they receive descending synaptic inputs from the cortex, amygdala and hypothalamus and ascending synaptic inputs from spinal cord, medulla oblongata and pons. With the exception of the cortex and amygdala, these connections are reciprocally organized (Carrive 1993; Bandler et al. 2000b; Carrive and Morgan 2004).

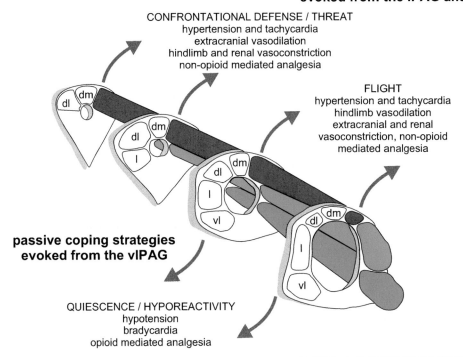

**active coping strategies
evoked from the lPAG and the dlPAG**

CONFRONTATIONAL DEFENSE / THREAT
hypertension and tachycardia
extracranial vasodilation
hindlimb and renal vasoconstriction
non-opioid mediated analgesia

FLIGHT
hypertension and tachycardia
hindlimb vasodilation
extracranial and renal
vasoconstriction, non-opioid
mediated analgesia

**passive coping strategies
evoked from the vlPAG**

QUIESCENCE / HYPOREACTIVITY
hypotension
bradycardia
opioid mediated analgesia

Figure 11.5 Representation of defense behaviors in the dorsolateral, lateral and ventrolateral periaqueductal gray. Schematic illustration of the dorsolateral (dl), lateral (l) and ventrolateral (vl) columns within the rostral, intermediate and caudal periaqueductal gray (PAG). Stimulation of neuron populations in the dlPAG, lPAG and vlPAG by microinjections of the excitatory amino acid glutamate, which only excites cell bodies of neurons, but not axons, evokes distinct defense behaviors: *Confrontational defense* is elicited from the rostral portion of the dlPAG and lPAG; *flight* is elicited from the caudal part of the dlPAG and lPAG; *quiescence* (cessation of spontaneous motor activity) is elicited from the vlPAG in the caudal portion of the PAG. These defense behaviors include typical autonomic cardiovascular reactions (changes in blood pressure, heart rate, blood flow) and sensory changes (non-opioid- or opioid-mediated analgesia). The representations of confrontational defense and flight are the basis for active coping strategies produced by the cortex. The representation of quiescence is the basis for passive coping strategies produced by the cortex. Based on experiments conducted on awake rats. dm, dorsomedial PAG. Modified from Bandler and Shipley (1994) and Bandler et al. (2000a, b).

Efferent Projections of the PAG Cell Columns to the Medulla Oblongata

As shown by anatomical tracing studies, neurons in the lateral and ventrolateral PAG columns project directly to various autonomic centers in the medulla oblongata (rostral and caudal ventrolateral medulla [RVLM, CVLM], rostral and caudal ventromedial medulla [VMM; raphe nuclei and paramedian reticular formation]). Neurons in the dorsolateral PAG column project indirectly to the same autonomic centers in the medulla oblongata: (1) via the superior lateral parabrachial nucleus and dorsomedial nucleus of the hypothalamus and (2) via the cuneiform nucleus. The way the two pathways are

integrated remains unclear, but the pathway via the hypothalamus is the more important (Figure 11.6) (van Blockstaele et al. 1991; Henderson et al. 1998; Horiushi et al. 2009; Dampney et al. 2013). These regions in the lower brain stem contain (see Chapter 10):

- the sympathetic premotor neurons and other neurons involved in regulation of the cardiovascular system, skin blood flow and other autonomic parameters;
- the parasympathetic preganglionic neurons involved in regulation of the heart and gastrointestinal tract; and

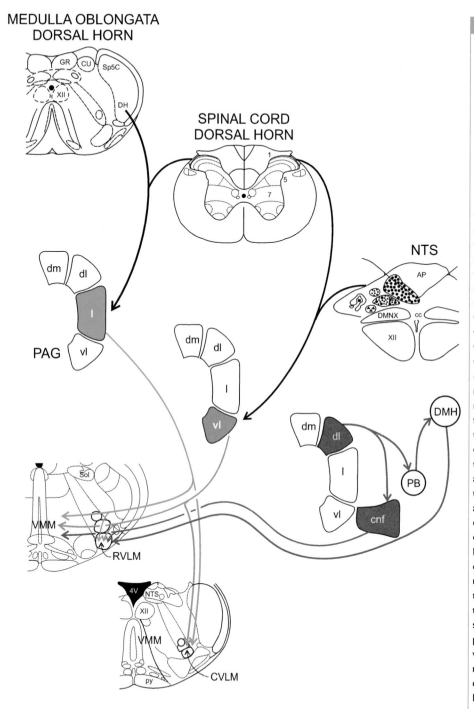

MEDULLA OBLONGATA DORSAL HORN

SPINAL CORD DORSAL HORN

NTS

PAG

Figure 11.6 Afferent inputs from the body to the cell columns in the periaqueductal gray (PAG) and efferent outputs to autonomic nuclei in the medulla oblongata from these cell columns. Second-order neurons in the spinal and medullary (trigeminal) dorsal horn (mainly lamina I and outer lamina II, but also deep laminae) project topographically to the lPAG. Second-order neurons in the spinal dorsal horn and second-order neurons in the caudal nucleus tractus solitarii (NTS) project to the vlPAG; this projection exhibits no topography. The dlPAG does not receive direct afferent input from the body. The lPAG and vlPAG project to the rostral ventrolateral medulla (RVLM), the caudal ventrolateral medulla (CVLM) and the ventromedial medulla (VMM; mainly raphe nuclei and paramedian reticular formation). The dlPAG projects to these nuclei via the cuneiform nucleus (cnf) and via the parabrachial nucleus (PB) and the dorsomedial nucleus of the hypothalamus (DMH). AP, area postrema; cc, central canal; cu, cuneate nucleus; dl, dorsolateral; dm, dorsomedial; DMNX, dorsal motor nucleus of the vagus; GR, gracile nucleus; l, lateral; NTS, nucleus tractus solitarii; py, pyramidal tract; Sol, tractus soleus SP5C, spinal trigeminal nucleus, caudal part; 4V, fourth ventricle; vl, ventrolateral; XII, hypoglossal nucleus. Modified from Bandler et al. (2000a) and Keay and Bandler (2004) with permission.

- the neurons of the respiratory network (particularly in the ventral respiratory column).

The ventromedial medulla contains the neurons controlling transmission of nociceptive impulses in the dorsal horn and caudal trigeminal nucleus (Mason 2001; Heinricher and Fields 2013; Heinricher and Ingram 2020). The lateral and ventrolateral PAG columns and the dorsomedial hypothalamus project to the *same* regions in the medulla oblongata. Thus, the anatomical and functional tracing studies, on which the concept is based, do not reveal how stimulation of the neurons in the PAG cell columns leads to the distinct autonomic reaction patterns that are characteristic for the three types of defense behavior elicited by PAG stimulation (Table 11.1).

Afferent Projections to the PAG Cell Columns From the Body (Upper Part of Figure 11.6)

Particularly second-order neurons in the superficial layer (lamina I), but possibly also in deep layers (lamina V and deeper), of the spinal and medullary dorsal horn project somatotopically to the lateral column of the PAG (see also Figures 2.11 and 2.12). These projections originate preferentially from the body surface. About 50% of the projecting neurons are located in segments C1 to C3. In the sacral spinal cord, the projecting neurons are located within the sacral parasympathetic nucleus (intermediolateral cell column) (Keay et al. 1997; Keay and Bandler 2014).

The ventrolateral column of the PAG receives direct projections from second-order neurons in the spinal cord (superficial and possibly deep dorsal horn), but not from those in the medullary dorsal horn. About 50% of these projecting neurons are located in deep laminae of spinal segments C1 to C3. The projections to the ventrolateral PAG are *not* somatotopically organized; they originate preferentially in the deep somatic and visceral body domains. Additionally, the ventrolateral PAG receives direct projections from the nucleus tractus solitarii (NTS). Other projections to the lateral and ventrolateral PAG originate in the dorsomedial, ventromedial and ventrolateral medulla. These anatomical connections are consistent with functional studies showing that deep injury (in deep somatic tissues and viscera), ischemia (during hemorrhage) or injurious stimuli exciting vagal cardiopulmonary afferents preferentially activate the neurons in the ventrolateral PAG. Injurious stimuli exciting only deep spinal afferents preferentially activate neurons in the caudal ventrolateral PAG and those exciting vagal afferents activate neurons in the rostral ventrolateral PAG (Keay et al. 1994, 1997, 2002; Clement et al. 1996, 2000).

The dorsolateral PAG does not receive direct afferent synaptic connections from the spinal cord, the NTS or other sites in the medulla oblongata.

Projections from Cortex and Hypothalamus to the PAG Cell Columns

Cortical structures and subcortical forebrain structures (e.g., the central and basal nucleus of the amygdala and the medial preoptic area) have powerful projections to the PAG and hypothalamus. These afferent projections from the forebrain also have a topical (columnar) organization, those from the neocortex being spatially more discrete than those from subcortical structures. Furthermore, many projections from subcortical structures are denser than those from the cortex (An et al. 1998; Bandler et al. 2000b).

Figure 11.7 demonstrates in the monkey the anatomical connections between the medial or orbital prefrontal cortex, the dorsolateral, lateral and ventrolateral PAG and the lateral, dorsal and ventromedial hypothalamus. There is specificity in the anatomical projections from the medial and orbital prefrontal cortex to the three cell columns of the PAG and the three hypothalamic regions. Corresponding regions in the hypothalamus and PAG communicate with each other reciprocally. This basic principle of anatomical connections between prefrontal cortex, hypothalamus and PAG has been described for the monkey and the rat (Floyd et al. 2000, 2001; Öngür and Price 2000). These (and other) anatomical studies demonstrate the powerful control of the PAG and hypothalamus by the telencephalon. However, they do not reveal the underlying mechanisms of this control (Note 6).

The attractive element of the idea of Bandler and his collaborators (notably Carrive, Keay and Shipley) and others is that the rostrocaudally organized cell columns in the PAG contain the neural networks which enable the forebrain structures to coordinate, on a moment-to-moment basis, the somatic, autonomic and antinociceptive mechanisms and other sensory mechanisms during stress and pain. These fast neuronal adjustments are critical for the survival of the organism. Primitive strategies to cope with threatening situations seem to be represented in the longitudinal cell columns of the PAG. Noxious events related to the environment and occurring at the body surface are associated with active coping strategies (e.g., confrontational defense and flight) and are represented in the dorsolateral and lateral cell columns. Noxious events in the deep body domains are associated with passive coping strategies (quiescence) and are represented in the ventrolateral cell column. The

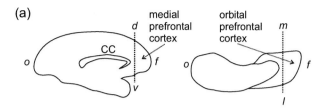

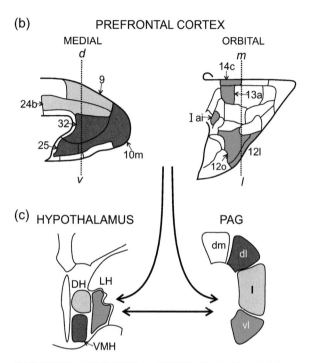

dorsolateral PAG cell column that does not receive direct afferent input from second-order neurons (in the spinal dorsal horn and in the NTS) is probably involved in active coping strategies initiated from the cortex. These fast neuronal protective mechanisms are coordinated with hypothalamic mechanisms that control homeostatic body functions, including the hypothalamo-pituitary axis and the immune system (Table 11.1). The latter may be mediated by a special sympathetic pathway (see Subchapter 4.6). The fast, neuronally directed protective adjustments of body functions require precisely functioning sympathetic and parasympathetic pathways, as described in Chapter 4.

We conclude with the words of Keay and Bandler 2014: (1) The *lateral PAG* column (and its associated neural circuits) is preferentially activated by *"escapable" physical stressors* to which an active defensive reaction is the primary response. (2) The *dorsolateral PAG column* (and its associated neural circuits) is activated preferentially by *"escapable" cortically initiated psychological stressors* to which an active defense reaction is the primary response. (3) The *ventrolateral PAG column* (and its associated neural circuits) is activated: (a) by *"inescapable" physical or psychological stressors* for which passive coping behavior is the primary response; or (b) as a delayed/secondary response, to *promote recovery and healing* following any stressor.

11.3.4 Autonomic Responses During Conditioned Emotional Responses

An important experiment, combining measurements of cardiovascular parameters with those of somatomotor parameters during conditioned emotional responses, was conducted by Orville Smith and coworkers on male baboons. In a first step, they investigated whether the cardiovascular changes occurring during an experimentally produced emotional state of the animals (using the conditioned emotional response paradigm) are integrated in the hypothalamus. They tested this by making controlled local lesions in the hypothalamus in animals that had developed emotional responses to the conditioning stimulus. They determined whether the autonomic changes could be attenuated without affecting either the "emotionality" of the animals (as indicated by their motor behavior during the conditioned emotional response) or other cardiovascular response patterns during, e.g., exercise or eating that are also organized in the hypothalamus. In a second step, they tried to work out the afferent and efferent connections of the hypothalamic area that integrates the cardiovascular changes during the conditioned emotional response (Smith et al. 1979, 1980, 2000; Smith and DeVito 1984;). Here I will only discuss the first aspect (Note 7).

During the conditioning trial, characteristic cardiovascular changes occurred in the monkeys (solid-line curves on the left side in Figure 11.8). Heart rate, arterial blood pressure and renal vascular resistance increased, whereas resistance in the terminal aorta (reflecting hindlimb resistance) decreased. The increases in heart rate and blood pressure were generated by decreased activity in parasympathetic cardiomotor neurons (particularly for the fast component) and increased activity in sympathetic cardiomotor and vasoconstrictor neurons innervating resistance vessels. The slow

increase in renal vascular resistance and decreased hindlimb resistance were assumed to be generated by adrenaline released by the adrenal medulla (via β_2-adrenoceptors in the vascular bed of skeletal muscle and α_1-adrenoceptors in the vascular bed of the kidney). This may or may not be the case, particularly in the kidney (see Subchapter 4.4) (Note 8). During the conditioned stimuli, the monkeys stopped pressing the lever (see upper red bars in Figure 11.8, left); this is the emotional motor response of the animals (they had been conditioned and expected the unconditioned electrical stimulus). The pattern of cardiovascular response was different from that during lever pressing alone (solid-line curves on right side of Figure 11.8), eating or exercise (solid-line curves in Figure 11.9).

Electrical stimulation of the perifornical region in the lateral hypothalamus produced the same pattern of cardiovascular response as that occurring during the

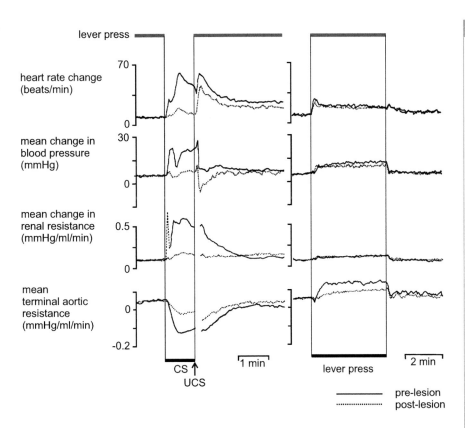

Figure 11.8 Cardiovascular reactions during a conditioned emotional response (left) and during lever pressing (right) before (solid-line curves) and after bilateral lesion of the perifornical region in the hypothalamus (dotted-line curves) in monkeys. The conditioned emotional response was elicited by a conditioned stimulus (CS, auditory signal of 2900 Hz, 80 dB interrupted 2.5 times per second) and terminated by an unconditioned stimulus (UCS, electrical shock applied to the abdominal skin; 7–12 mA, 1 s duration). Upper red bars: lever pressing; cessation of lever pressing during the CS indicates that the monkeys felt emotionally. This response is the same before and after bilateral lesion in the perifornical region in the lateral hypothalamus. Ordinate scales of cardiovascular responses indicate the changes compared to the baselines in the minute preceding the conditioned emotional response (left) or preceding the lever pressing (right). The data were averaged from five prelesion and five postlesion trials in six monkeys (baboons). Modified from Smith et al. (1980) with permission.

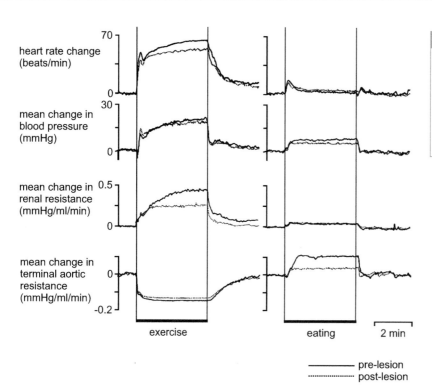

Figure 11.9 Cardiovascular response during exercise or during eating before and after bilateral lesion of the perifornical region in the hypothalamus of monkeys. For exercise the monkeys turned a wheel with their legs. For details see caption of Figure 11.8. Modified from Smith et al. (1980) with permission.

conditioned emotional response. After bilateral lesions of this region, the cardiovascular changes occurring during the conditioned stimulation were largely abolished (see dotted-line curves in Figure 11.8 left) whereas those occurring during lever pressing (dotted-line curves in Figure 11.8 right), exercise or eating did not change significantly (dotted-line curves in Figure 11.9). The monkeys with the hypothalamic lesions continued to stop lever pressing during the conditioned stimuli, indicating that they had not "forgotten" the significance of this stimulus and felt emotional. Thus, they still showed emotional behavior during the conditioning stimuli but on this occasion without the characteristic cardiovascular changes.

We can draw the following general conclusions from this experiment:

- The hypothalamus contains an area (perifornical area in the lateral hypothalamus) that controls the cardiovascular response pattern associated with emotional behavior.
- Lesioning of the perifornical area abolishes these cardiovascular responses but does not affect the cardiovascular responses during other behaviors, such as exercise or eating.

- After destruction of the perifornical region in the lateral hypothalamus the monkeys still responded in an emotional way during the presentation of the conditioned stimulus; thus the two components of the conditioned emotional response, the cardiovascular response and the emotional motor response, have been *separated* by the hypothalamic lesion.
- The cardiovascular response pattern elicited during the conditioned emotional response was mediated by sympathetic and parasympathetic pathways to the cardiovascular effector systems.
- Other changes mediated by non-vascular autonomic pathways (e.g., those to the gastrointestinal tract, to the pelvic organs, to skin) may also be generated during the conditioned emotional response.

Do the cardiovascular changes during the conditioned emotional response have underlying mechanisms comparable to those elicited by central signals during exercise? Both groups of cardiovascular changes are elicited from the telencephalon: those generated by the conditioned emotional response precede the motor responses (they occur in anticipation of the somatomotor changes in posture and locomotion), and those generated during isometric exercise start almost immediately with real or attempted motor activity (see Figures 11.3 and 11.4). This has been experimentally studied in baboons which were fully instrumented to measure cardiovascular parameters to be transmitted by telemetry and which lived entirely unrestrained in their natural habitat, in groups of four or five (Smith et al. 2000):

- The monkeys exhibited cardiovascular responses during postural or locomotor changes *without emotional content* (e.g., changes from quiet sitting to standing, walking or running) starting *within a second* of the motor activity but never longer before. The explanation must be that somatomotor and cardiovascular responses are both initiated by the same central signal (see Figure 11.3).
- Changes in motor activity during a behavior *with emotional content* (e.g., changes from quiet standing to "aggressive walking" of an alpha [dominant] male towards a subordinate beta male in the group) were *preceded* by cardiovascular changes by up to 10 seconds. These anticipatory changes in the unrestrained baboons are equivalent to those during the conditioned emotional response (Figure 11.8 left).
- After bilateral lesions of the perifornical region in the lateral hypothalamus with ibotenic acid (which destroys neuronal cell bodies but not axons), these alpha males exhibited the same aggressive behavior, but without any anticipatory cardiovascular changes.
- The cardiovascular responses occurring with postural or locomotor changes without emotional context were unchanged in the baboons with bilateral perifornical hypothalamic lesions.

These results support the idea that the central efferent signals and their pathways initiating the cardiovascular changes during the conditioned emotional response, or during postural locomotor changes in an emotional context, differ from those initiating cardiovascular changes during motor behavior without emotional context.

11.3.5 Tonic Immobility, Freezing and Vigilance

The autonomic (and somatomotor) responses during *tonic immobility* in animals are extreme (see Table 11.1). The animal drops as if dead. Its state is characterized by complete immobility (the musculature is flaccid), apnea (cessation of respiration), decreased heart rate and blood pressure, and decreased consciousness (relative lack of responsiveness to external stimuli).

Tonic immobility response is used by animals in a confrontation with a predator to increase the chances of survival (e.g., by sheep against a poaching dog). This response is therefore sometimes also called "playing-dead response" or "playing possum." This reaction is quickly activated in dangerous situations. Electrical stimulation of the anterior cingulate gyrus in the cat produces the same pattern of responses: decreased heart rate, blood pressure, respiration and skeletal muscle tone and increased blood flow in skeletal muscle. It is assumed that activity in other types of vasoconstrictor neurons (e.g., those to skin or viscera) also decreases (Löfving 1961). The response pattern elicited from the anterior cingulate gyrus is probably relayed through the central nucleus of the amygdala (Applegate et al. 1983; Cox et al. 1987; Leite-Panissi et al. 2003), the lateral hypothalamus and the depressor area of the medulla oblongata. In fact Hess had already described that electrical stimulation of some sites in the lateral anterior hypothalamus leads to adynamia, reduced reactivity, decreased arterial blood pressure and bradycardia in awake cats (Hess 1944).

In humans, tonic immobility probably corresponds to *neurally mediated syncope* that occurs without any obvious peripheral pathophysiology (Humphreys and Ruxton 2018). This syncope is characterized by quick loss of consciousness and of motor tone and decrease of peripheral arterial resistance, heart rate and arterial blood pressure. Decreased vasoconstrictor activity and increased cardiovagal activity seem to be the primary autonomic events (Hainsworth and Claydon 2013; Kenny and Grubb 2013). This neurally mediated syncope can be generated by emotional stimuli; therefore it is also called *emotional fainting/syncope*.

It is generally assumed that loss of consciousness during neurally mediated syncope is the consequence of decreased arterial blood pressure (due to centrally generated bradycardia and decreased peripheral resistance). However, it could well be that the three events, namely decreased activity in vasoconstrictor neurons innervating resistance vessels, increased activity in parasympathetic cardiomotor neurons and loss of consciousness, are generated by the *same* central mechanism. This would not be at variance with the long-held experience that syncope can be triggered by many peripheral stimuli exciting afferents (e.g., from the heart, lung, gastrointestinal tract, urogenital tract, carotid sinus) (Freeman and Rutkove 2000). Whether tonic immobility and neurally mediated syncope in humans correspond to each other and are generated by similar central mechanisms is currently controversial (Freeman and Rutkove 2000; Mosqueda-Garcia et al. 2000; van Dijk 2003).

The *freezing reaction* can also be characterized by complete immobility, yet high preparedness for sudden motor action and intense alertness (Roelofs 2017). In this respect, the freezing reaction is fundamentally different from tonic immobility ("playing-dead"). The autonomic responses are decreased heart rate (probably generated by activation of parasympathetic cardiomotor neurons and subsequent inhibition of pacemaker activity), increased muscle vasoconstrictor activity and decreased respiration. Thus, the autonomic reactions of the freezing reaction resemble those of the diving response, although they are much stronger in the latter.

The *vigilance reaction* in animals is characterized by immobility, a large decrease in heart rate (with decreased cardiac output; probably generated by activation of parasympathetic cardiomotor neurons), increased arterial blood pressure (due to increased peripheral resistance generated by activation of muscle and visceral vasoconstrictor neurons), decreased respiration and behavioral signs of increased vigilance. This response can be elicited, in rabbits, by electrical stimulation of the dorsolateral hypothalamus ("hypothalamic vigilance area") or the ventrolateral PAG ("periaqueductal vigilance area") (McCabe et al. 1994; Duan et al. 1996, 1997). As far as the autonomic pattern is concerned, the vigilance reaction is unlikely to be identical to quiescence, the freezing reaction or tonic immobility (Table 11.1).

11.4 Emotions and Autonomic Reactions

Emotional feelings and the corresponding emotional expressions generated by the somatomotor system are highly integrated components of behavior in humans and animals that are important (extero- and interoceptively) for reproduction, selection, genome protection and regulation of social behavior (Darwin 1872/1998). An influential theory of emotions that was propagated by William James (James 1884/1994; see Meyers [1986]) states that activation of emotions is closely associated with the afferent feedback from the periphery of the body (Figure 11.10a, see broad arrow B). This theory became known as the James–Lange theory of emotions (see Subchapter 11.1) (Note 9). According to this theory, the brain generates bodily changes by activity in the autonomic and somatomotor systems and the perception of these changes triggered by the afferent feedback from the viscera and somatic tissues leads to the emotional feelings. This theory of generation of emotions was not based on data obtained in experimentation but on deduction and introspection.

Its main content is strongly expressed by William James in the following statement:

" ... If we fancy some strong emotion, and then try to abstract from our consciousness of it all the feelings of its characteristic bodily symptoms, we find we have nothing left behind, no 'mind-stuff' out of which the emotion can be substituted, and that a cold and neutral state of intellectual perception is all that remains ...." (James 1884)

The James–Lange theory of emotions was vigorously contested by Cannon and Bard. They state that the emotions develop after perception and cognitive assessment of the emotional stimulus. Their theory went into the literature as the Cannon–Bard theory of emotions (Cannon 1927).

11.4.1 Basic Emotions and Autonomic Response Patterns

In its original version, the James–Lange theory is no longer tenable because it cannot be refuted experimentally. It appears to be impossible to design an experiment in which the development of emotions can be investigated without afferent feedback from the body (viscera and deep somatic structures). However, it is widely accepted that the activity in afferents from the somatic and visceral body domains shapes and amplifies the emotions. The pattern of afferent activity might be generated, via the effector tissues, by activation of the efferent autonomic systems. Finally it should be kept in mind that modern neurobiological research has shown that the autonomic pathways to the effector tissues and the neural afferent feedback from these effector tissues are functionally highly specific (see Chapters 2 and 4). These points fully support the James–Lange theory of emotions and show that this theory is not at variance with the idea that different basic emotions (or groups of related affected states) can be characterized by specific autonomic motor patterns (see below) in addition to the somatomotor patterns.

There is some, although not generally accepted, consensus that there exist six basic emotions that are the product of evolution: anger, fear, disgust, sadness, surprise, happiness (Figure 11.11). Charles Darwin formulated this idea in his famous book *The Expression of Emotions in Man and Animals* (1872/1998).

The term "basic emotion" should not be taken too literally. Each emotion is, according to Ekman and Panksepp (see Ekman and Davidson 1994), not a single discrete separable affective state, but represents a group of related affective states. These states are universal and the result of evolution. They unfold and develop in biologically specific environments. They are represented in central circuits and are not

(a) James-Lange Theory of Emotions

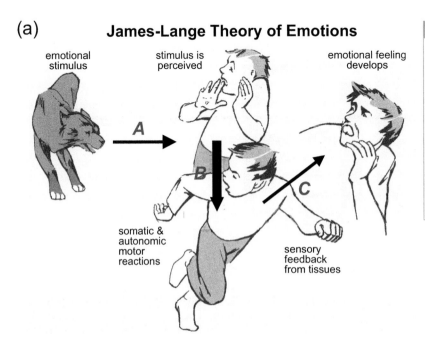

emotional stimulus

stimulus is perceived

emotional feeling develops

A

B

C

somatic & autonomic motor reactions

sensory feedback from tissues

Figure 11.10 The development of emotions after James & Lange and Cannon & Bard. (a) According to James & Lange, the emotional feelings develop by sensory feedback from the body tissues that is generated by the activation of the autonomic systems and the somatomotor systems (symbolized by the broad arrow B). (b) According to Cannon & Bard, the emotional feelings develop after perception and cognitive appraisal of the emotional stimulus. Modified after Rosenzweig and Leiman (1982).

(b) Cannon-Bard Theory of Emotions

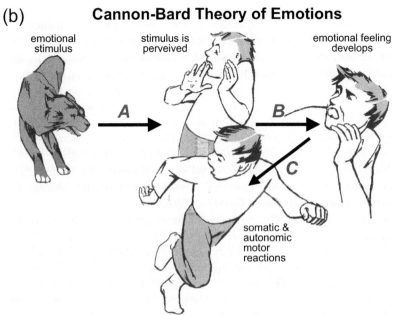

emotional stimulus

stimulus is perveived

emotional feeling develops

A

B

C

somatic & autonomic motor reactions

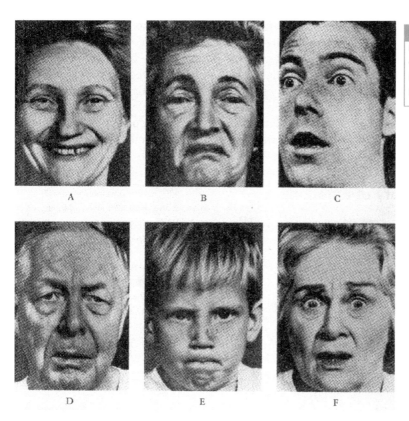

Figure 11.11 Facial expressions of the six basic emotions. A, happiness; B, disgust; C, surprise; D, sadness; E, anger; F, fear. From Darwin (1872/1998, 3rd edition edited by Paul Ekman) with permission.

the result of associative learning (for extensive discussion see Ekman and Davidson [1994]). The relatively invariant expression of these basic emotions by the somatomotor system (above all by the facial muscles in humans and primates) are represented in the neural programs of the limbic system and neocortex (notably the amygdaloid complex and the orbitofrontal cortex; see Aggleton [2000]). These central programs are also responsible for the internal experience of the emotions, i.e., the feeling of emotions (see Ekman and Davidson [1994]).

Ekman and his coworkers tested the hypothesis that each basic emotion is correlated with a distinct pattern of autonomic changes. They studied American actors, American college students, Americans in old age and indigenous people from West Sumatra, whose cultural background is entirely different from Westerners. The participants of this study had to learn to produce the facial configurations which resemble the facial expression of the different types of *basic emotions* (Figure 11.11) without knowing which basic emotion they were trained to express. For this purpose, they had to follow muscle-by-muscle

instructions of the facial musculature and undergo extensive coaching. The *autonomic parameters* recorded during the generation of the facial expression of the emotions were changes in heart rate (dependent on parasympathetic and sympathetic cardiomotor neurons), changes in acral skin temperature (dependent on cutaneous vasoconstrictor activity), and changes in acral skin conductance (dependent on sudomotor activity). Finally the subjective experiences of emotion reported by the experimental subjects during these activities were recorded (Ekman et al. 1983; Levenson et al. 1990, 1991, 1992; Levenson 1993). In the study of elderly Americans, autonomic activity was also measured while the subjects attempted to relive emotional experiences occurring during the produced facial configurations.

The patterns of autonomic reactions measured were found to be specific for each basic emotion. This specificity was independent of cultural background, age and profession, and the three parameters (expression of emotions, relived subjective emotions and autonomic reactions) correlated significantly with each other. The three outcomes, i.e., the subjective emotional feelings, the somatomotor expression of the emotions and the autonomic responses during the emotions, were therefore concluded to be parallel (not sequential) "readouts" of the same brain regions (Figure 11.12).

The authors came to the conclusion that the autonomic patterns that are specific for the different groups of emotional states are functionally distinct adaptive responses that have developed during evolution. The authors express their view by stating that "there is an innate affect program for each emotion that once activated directs for each emotion changes in the organism's biological state by providing instructions to multiple response systems, including facial muscles, skeletal muscles [of trunk and extremities] and the autonomic nervous system" (Levenson et al. 1990, 1991; Ekman 1992). Finally they came to the important conclusion that a general arousal model of the sympathetic nervous system, as originally propagated by Cannon (1927, 1939), cannot account for the differentiated autonomic responses seen during expression of the basic emotions.

11.4.2 Central Representation of Emotional States and Patterns of Autonomic Reactions

Ekman and coworkers have shown that there is a correlation between the type of basic emotions and the autonomic responses. These data are fully compatible with the findings discussed extensively in this book showing that the autonomic, and in particular the sympathetic, pathways and their central connections are functionally specific. The findings are also fully compatible with the generally accepted notion that the basic emotions (consisting of the characteristic motor expressions and the corresponding subjective emotional feelings) are distinct affective states represented in the brain, each consisting of a distinct pattern of autonomic (and possibly endocrine) responses. Future experimental investigations in humans, using modern imaging methods and more refined methods to measure autonomic responses, will have to show that emotional feeling states, autonomic response patterns and patterns of activation of forebrain areas generated during the six basic emotions correlate with each other (see Anders et al. [2004]).

Using functional imaging, it can be shown that the perception of the different basic emotions from visual stimuli (faces) or auditory stimuli are correlated

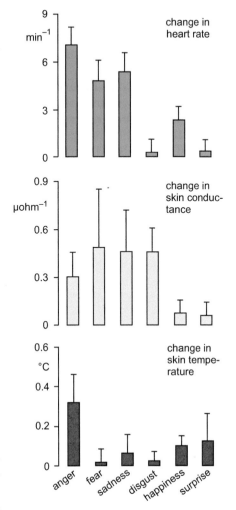

Figure 11.12 Changes in autonomic parameters during the six basic emotions (see Figure 11.11). The facial motor expression of the basic emotions was generated experimentally under visual control. The experimental subjects did not know the type of emotion they were expressing. Increase in heart rate (dependent on changes in activity of parasympathetic cardiomotor neurons), decrease in skin temperature of the finger tips (dependent on skin blood flow and therefore on activity in cutaneous vasoconstrictor neurons) and increase in skin conductance (dependent on activity of sweat glands and therefore on activity in sudomotor neurons) were measured simultaneously. The relived subjective emotions experienced by the experimental subjects were reported afterwards. The patterns of the autonomic reactions and the type of relived emotions are highly correlated with each other. Data from 12 experimental subjects. Mean + SEM. Modified from Levenson et al. (1992).

with characteristic patterns of activation of the forebrain (Damasio et al. 2003). Forebrain structures representing expression of emotions are the orbitofrontal cortex, the anterior and posterior cingulate cortex, the insular cortex, the anterior parietal cortex, parts of the anterior basal ganglia and the amygdala (see Phan et al. [2002]; Damasio et al. [2003]; Morris and Dolan [2004]).

The amygdala orchestrates mainly the expression of negative emotions, such as anger and fear, for the somatomotor, autonomic and endocrine responses, as shown in the rat by LeDoux and coworkers. Using fear conditioning in rats as an experimental model system, this group has worked out the neural circuits in the forebrain that coordinate the behavioral reactions, including those occurring in the body involving the autonomic nervous system and neuroendocrine systems, to threatening stimuli. Figure 11.13 outlines the structures in the forebrain, hypothalamus and brain stem that are activated during fear conditioning. Any environmental or intracerebral stimulus that activates these neural centers leads to somatomotor, autonomic and endocrine responses that are characteristic for the different types of defense behavior, as described in Subchapter 11.3, and also for the basic emotions fear and anger. The amygdala is a key region in the limbic system that is important to recognize dangerous environmental situations and initiate the appropriate behavioral changes. The following components of the fearful behavior in which the amygdala is involved can be distinguished (LaBar and LeDoux 2001):

- Direct subcortical connections from the thalamus (lateral and medial geniculate for the visual and auditory system, respectively) mediate a preattentive generation of fear to archetypical biologically aversive somatosensory, visual or acoustic stimuli. This activation is fast and occurs without awareness. There is no precise representation of the stimulus or environmental situation (e.g., a spider or a crocodile) (connection 1 in Figure 11.13), but only prepared response components (contours, colors, etc.) are analyzed.
- Processed and discriminated stimuli reach the amygdala from unimodal association cortices (visual, acoustic etc.). Via these synaptic connections, neutral conditioned stimuli (e.g., touch, visual, acoustic stimuli) can be paired with biologically important stimuli. The synaptic activation of neurons in the lateral amygdala by the conditioned stimuli is enhanced. Now the conditioned

stimuli can activate the neurons and trigger the fear reaction (connection 2 in Figure 11.13).
- The conditioned fear reaction (and therefore the activation of the neurons in the lateral amygdala by the conditioned stimuli) is co-activated in the context of past experience and future expectations (i.e. with regard to temporal and spatial contexts in which the stimulus occurs) with the hippocampus and medial prefrontal cortex (and probably other prefrontal areas). This leads to enhancement or extinction of the synaptic activation in the lateral and basal nuclei of the amygdala and therefore of the fear reactions (connections 3 and 4 in Figure 11.13).
- The central nucleus of the amygdala is the output nucleus to neural circuits in the hypothalamus and brain stem that are involved in somatomotor, autonomic and neuroendocrine responses, resulting in the typical defensive and arousal responses. Furthermore, the nucleus basalis (Meynert) is activated via the central nucleus of the amygdala which activates the neocortex resulting in cortical arousal and attention.
- Monkeys with bilateral lesion of the amygdala (or of the prefrontal cortex) are no longer able to learn to recognize harmful situations in their environment. They are not able to acquire the "meaning" of exteroceptive (visual, auditory, somatosensory or olfactory) stimuli in the social context of the behavior of the other members of the social group and cannot associate these stimuli with their own affective states. Humans with bilateral lesions of the amygdala are not able to recognize faces that signal anger or fear, yet they have no or little difficulty in recognizing the emotional content of faces signaling happiness or surprise. These patients exhibit changed patterns of cortical activation when shown faces signaling anger or fear (Damasio et al. 2003). This shows that the amygdala is not only important for somatomotor, autonomic and neuroendocrine expression, and for recognition of the emotional states of anger and fear, but also for the generation of the corresponding emotional feelings.

How do these experimental findings connect to the results of Ekman and coworkers, as described above, in terms of the regulation of autonomic pathways? Is the central nucleus of the amygdala, that orchestrates the autonomic and neuroendocrine responses

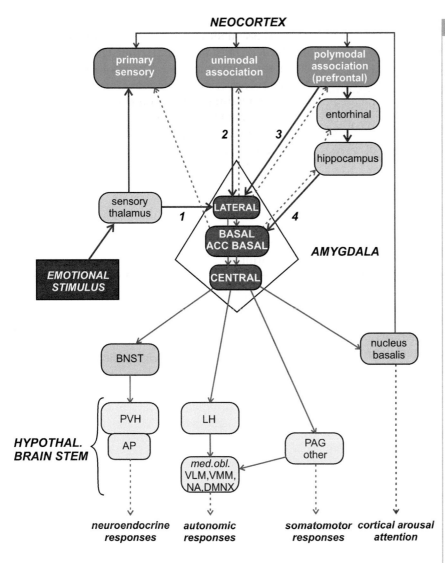

Figure 11.13 Amygdala, fear conditioning and autonomic systems. Emotional somatosensory, visual, acoustic or olfactory stimuli in the environment signaling danger elicit fear behavior consisting of defensive motor behavior, central emotional feeling state, autonomic responses and endocrine responses. The lateral nucleus of the amygdala receives afferent information about the environmental stimuli via synaptic input directly from the thalamus (pathway *1*) and from unimodal and polymodal association cortices (pathways *2* and *3*), as well as from the hippocampus (pathway *4* to the basolateral amygdala). These synaptic inputs are processed in parallel during fear conditioning. Simple cues that do not require discrimination are relayed via pathway *1*. The emotional event is discriminated from other events and evaluated in the context of past and future expectations and relayed by pathways *2* to *4* to the amygdala. The amygdala projects virtually to every cortical region and to the hippocampus (red interrupted arrows).

The somatomotor, endocrine and autonomic responses elicited during fear conditioning are mediated by the central (output) nucleus of the amygdala. Cortical arousal and attention are generated by the central nucleus via the nucleus basalis (Meynert). ACC basal, accessory basal nucleus; AP, area postrema; BNST, bed nucleus of the stria terminalis; DMNX, dorsal motor nucleus of the vagus; LH, lateral hypothalamus; NA, nucleus ambiguus; PAG, periaqueductal gray; PVH, paraventricular nucleus of the hypothalamus; VLM, ventrolateral medulla; VMM, ventromedial medulla. Modified from LaBar and LeDoux (2001) with permission.

during fear conditioned behavior in rats, also responsible for generating the autonomic response patterns during anger and fear in humans? The finding that humans with bilateral lesions of the amygdala recognize the emotional content of faces expressing happiness or surprise but no longer those showing anger or fear argues that the amygdala is not involved in the former recognition process. It would be interesting to know whether the autonomic response patterns during the basic emotions of happiness, surprise, disgust or sadness are normal in these patients with lesioned amygdalas, whereas those occurring during anger and fear are absent. These studies have yet to be done.

11.5 Integrative Responses Organized in the Hypothalamus

The volume of the hypothalamus is about 1% of the brain (Swanson 1995). An individual in whom the periventricular and medial parts of the hypothalamus are destroyed (the latter extending about 800 μm lateral to the midline in rats), but with intact spinal cord, brain stem and cerebral hemispheres, is not able to survive because the basic control of the body temperature, reproduction, fluid matrix, food intake and metabolism, temporal organization of body functions and body protection fail (Table 11.2). The hypothalamus is directly or indirectly connected to every part of the brain (including the brain stem and spinal cord). Anatomically at least 2000 projections of the hypothalamic nuclei have been recognized due to the enormous development of neuroanatomical methodology. Experimental anatomical work, using modern tracing techniques (conducted particularly by Larry Swanson and coworkers [Note 10]), tells us that the hypothalamus consists of about 50 to 100 differentiable groups of neurons (nuclei), each being characterized by the projection of their axons, their synaptic inputs and their histochemistry (Rishold et al. 1997; Swanson 2000; Petrovich et al. 2001; Thompson and Swanson 2003; Watts and Swanson 2002). Thus, we have detailed knowledge about the microstructure of the hypothalamus (at least of the periventricular and medial parts) and about the multiple physiological functions of the hypothalamus; however, it remains difficult to connect the microstructure and the physiology.

11.5.1 Anatomy and Functions of the Hypothalamus

Figure 11.14 illustrates the location of the hypothalamus as the ventral part of the diencephalon (interbrain; the dorsal part being the thalamus) that is situated between the brain stem and the cerebral hemispheres. The preoptic nuclei are considered to belong to the forebrain ganglia. Based on cytoarchitectonic and topographical criteria, the hypothalamus is conventionally divided into three longitudinal zones (periventricular zone, medial zone and lateral zone). Rostrocaudally, the hypothalamus is divided, for practical reasons, into the preoptic, anterior, tuberal and mammillary parts (Saper 2004).

Based on the patterns of connections between neuron assemblies and on the functional systems involved (Swanson 2000; Thompson and Swanson 2003), the hypothalamus is functionally divided into the neuroendocrine motor zone, the periventricular region generating visceromotor patterns, the suprachiasmatic nucleus generating behavioral states, the behavior control column in the medial hypothalamus, and the lateral hypothalamus. Thus, the longitudinal zones are roughly identified with integrative functions, the classical medial zone being further divided into three parts.

- The *neuroendocrine motor zone* contains mainly the endocrine motor neurons projecting to the posterior pituitary gland or to the median eminence (Figure 11.15a). The magnocellular neurons secreting either vasopressin or oxytocin are located in the magnocellular division of the paraventricular nucleus, in the supraoptic nucleus and in some accessory supraoptic cell groups in between. They project to the posterior pituitary gland. In the median eminence, the axons of the secretomotor neurons release excitatory or inhibitory releasing hormones (RH, IRH) to the anterior pituitary gland. The parvicellular neurons projecting to the median eminence and releasing corticotropin RH (CRH), growth-hormone RH (GHRH), dopamine (DA), somatostatin (SS) or thyrotropin RH (TRH) are located in a continuous zone around the third ventricle, including the anterior periventricular, the parvicellular (neuroendocrine) paraventricular and the arcuate nuclei. The parvicellular neurons secreting gonadotropin RH (GnRH) are located more rostrally due to their unusual embryologic origin (Markakis and Swanson 1997; Thompson and Swanson 2003).

- The *periventricular region* is interposed between the neuroendocrine motor zone and the medial nuclei in the behavior control column. In this region, the rostral part of the medial zone of the hypothalamus contains several small nuclei that constitute, together with the dorsomedial nucleus (DMN), the *hypothalamic visceral pattern generator (HVPG; Figure 11.15c)*. The rostral nuclei involved are the median preoptic nucleus (MePO), the parastrial nucleus (PS), the anterior dorsal preoptic nucleus (ADP), the anteroventral preoptic nucleus (AVP), and the anteroventral periventricular nucleus (AVPV). The medial part of the medial preoptic nucleus (MPNm) and the

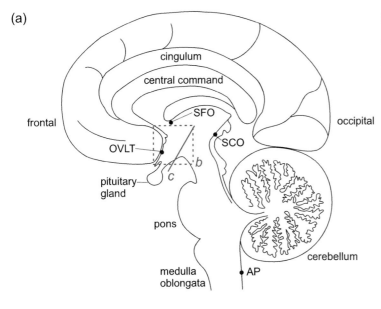

(a)

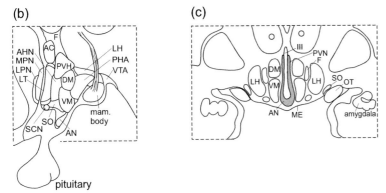

(b)   (c)

Figure 11.14 Location and components of the hypothalamus. (a) Sagittal section through the brain. The circumventricular organs are indicated (AP, area postrema; OVLT, organum vasculosum laminae terminalis; SCO, subcommissural organ; SFO, subfornical organ). (b,c) Magnified parts as indicated in (a) showing the nuclei of the hypothalamus. AC, anterior commissure; AHN, anterior hypothalamic nucleus; AN, arcuate nucleus; CC, corpus callosum; DM, dorsomedial nucleus; F, fornix; LH, lateral hypothalamic area; LPN, lateral preoptic nucleus; LT, lamina terminalis; mam. body, mammillary body; ME, median eminence; MPN, medial preoptic nucleus; OT, optic tract; PHA, posterior hypothalamic area; PVH, paraventricular nucleus; SCN, suprachiasmatic nucleus; SO, supraoptic nucleus; VM, ventromedial nucleus; VTA, ventral tegmental area; III, third ventricle. Modified from Iversen et al. (2000).

presubchiasmatic preoptic nucleus (PSCN) probably also belong to this neural network (Figure 11.15c, which has three general characteristics):

- Each component of the HVPG innervates differentially the pools of neuroendocrine motor neurons, autonomic premotor neurons located in the dorsal, ventral and lateral parts of the paraventricular nucleus of the hypothalamus (PVH), possibly other autonomic premotor neurons in the hypothalamus and possibly, e.g., via the PVH and the lateral hypothalamus or directly, autonomic circuits in the periaqueductal gray, pons and medulla oblongata.
- The synaptic inputs to the nuclei of the HVPG consist of four components: (1) Sensory inputs from the nucleus tractus solitarii via the ventrolateral medulla and parabrachial nuclei, from the spinal and medullary dorsal horn, most of them also via the parabrachial nuclei, and from the subfornical organ (osmolality, angiotensin II). (2) Synaptic input from the suprachiasmatic nucleus (SCN) which determines the behavioral state during the circadian rhythm of the organism. (3) Synaptic input from the behavior control column, each nucleus having a distinct pattern of projection. (4) Synaptic input from the cerebral hemispheres related to cognitive and affective (emotional) processes (infralimbic area [area 25 in Figure11.7b] of the medial prefrontal cortex; ventral subiculum, medial and posterior amygdala nucleus, ventral lateral septal nucleus, bed nucleus of the stria terminalis).

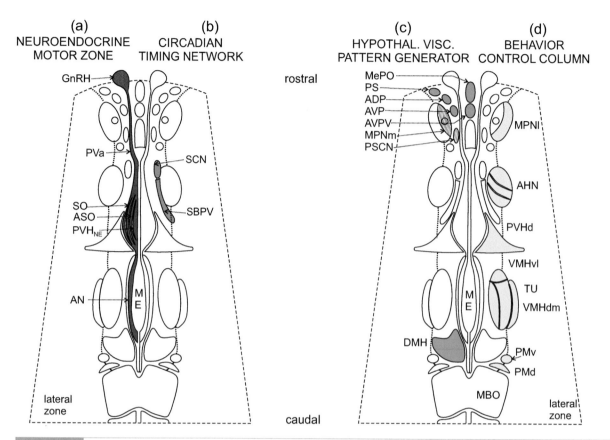

Figure 11.15 Organization of the hypothalamus into functionally different types of networks or zones. This division is based on systematic morphological studies using tracing techniques conducted on rats. The results of these studies were interpreted in the context of hypothalamic functions. The nuclei belonging to the respective network or zone are indicated in color. (a) The neuroendocrine motor zone. This zone is centered in the periventricular area of the hypothalamus and contains the endocrine motor neurons related to the posterior pituitary or the anterior pituitary gland. (b) The circadian timing network consists of the suprachiasmatic nucleus (SCN) and the subparaventricular zone (SBPV) which organizes the temporal structure of hypothalamic functions. (c) The hypothalamic visceral motor pattern generator (HVPG) network coordinates neuroendocrine and autonomic response patterns. (d) The behavior control column represents regulation of defensive behavior, ingestive behavior (nutrition, fluid balance), reproductive behavior and thermoregulatory behavior. *Abbreviations*: (a) AN, arcuate nucleus; ASO, accessory supraoptic cell groups; GnRH, nucleus synthesizing gonadotropin-releasing hormone; PVa, periventricular nucleus anterior; PVHne, neuroendocrine part of the paraventricular nucleus. (b) SBPV, subparaventricular zone; SCN, suprachiasmatic nucleus. (c) ADP, anterodorsal preoptic nucleus; AVP, anteroventral preoptic nucleus; AVPV, anteroventral periventricular nucleus; DMH, dorsomedial nucleus; MePO, median preoptic nucleus; MPNm, medial part of medial preoptic nucleus; PS, parastrial nucleus; PSCN, presuprachiasmatic preoptic nucleus. (d) AHN, anterior hypothalamic nucleus; MPNl, lateral part of the medial preoptic nucleus; PMd, dorsal premammillary nucleus; PMv, ventral premammillary nucleus; PVHd, dorsal part of the paraventricular nucleus; TU, tuberal nucleus; VMHdm, dorsomedial part of the ventromedial nucleus; VMHvl, ventrolateral part of the ventromedial nucleus. MBO, mamillary body; ME, median eminence. Modified from Thompson and Swanson (2003).

- The location of the HVPG between the various input systems, related to reflexes, behavioral state, behavioral context and cerebral (cognitive and emotional) activity, and the output system to the neuroendocrine and autonomic circuits allows a selection of variable patterns of autonomic and endocrine responses.

- The *suprachiasmatic nucleus (SCN)* in the medial zone is the dominant *mammalian circadian pacemaker*. Its endogenous rhythm is entrained by the retina via the retino-hypothalamic tract to the light–dark cycle of the environment and determines the temporal organization of virtually all body functions. Most of its projections are confined to intrahypothalamic nuclei, some of them via the subparaventricular zone (SBPV); some projections are to the basal forebrain and the thalamus. The SCN nuclear complex is the *circadian timing network* of the body and involved in the organization of the *behavioral states of the organism* (sleep and wakefulness, arousal) (Figure 11.15b) (Weaver and Emery 2013).

- The *medial zone* contains several anatomically defined nuclei of neurons that constitute according to Swanson and coworkers the *behavior control column* (Figure 11.15d). These nuclei project to the somatomotor centers and autonomic centers in brain stem and spinal cord, to the lateral hypothalamus and to the thalamus. This column includes the medial preoptic nucleus (MPN), the anterior hypothalamic nucleus (AHN), large parts of the paraventricular nucleus (dorsal, lateral and ventral parvicellular parts of the PVH), the ventromedial nucleus (VMN or VM), the supraoptic nucleus (SO), the posterior hypothalamic area and some other small premammillary nuclei. The neuron assemblies in the behavior control column determine, *first*, the somatomotor programs in the brain stem and spinal cord that underlie elementary behaviors related to defense, reproduction, ingestive behavior (nutritive substances, fluid) and thermoregulatory behavior, *second*, the autonomic motor programs adapting the body organs during these behaviors (cardiovascular and respiratory systems, gastrointestinal tract, pelvic organs, immune system), and, *third*, the neuroendocrine output systems (Figure 11.15a). Single nuclei or subnuclei cannot be identified to have any of these integrative functions. However, groups of nuclei constituting networks can be roughly identified with particular functions (Table 11.2):
  - *Defensive (agonistic) behavior* is organized in the anterior hypothalamic nucleus (AHN), the dorsomedial part of the ventromedial nucleus (VMHdm), the ventrolateral part of the ventromedial nucleus (VMHvl) and the dorsal part of the premammillary nuclei (PMd).
  - *Reproductive behavior* is organized in the medial preoptic nucleus (MPNm), the ventrolateral part of the ventromedial nucleus (VMHvl) and the ventral part of the of the premammillary nuclei (PMv). Both the defensive and the reproductive behavior are the basis for the social behavior.
  - *Ingestive behavior* is organized by those parts of the paraventricular nucleus that do not belong to the periventricular neuroendocrine motor zone (dorsal part, PVHd; lateral part, PVHl).
  - *Thermoregulatory behavior* is organized in the preoptic region, the anterior hypothalamus and posterior parts of the hypothalamus (Kanosue et al. 1998; Nagashima et al. 2000; McAllen and McKinley 2018; Morrison 2018; Romanovsky 2018).

- The lateral zone of the hypothalamus does not contain well-defined nuclei of neurons, but appears to be a *liaison structure* or crossroad connecting forebrain structures, medial and periventricular zones of the hypothalamus, brain stem and spinal cord. The lateral hypothalamus has been little explored.

The hypothalamic nuclei receive multiple afferent inputs: (1) Neural afferent inputs involving the spinal and medullary dorsal horn, the nucleus tractus solitarii (NTS), the parabrachial nuclei. (2) Non-neural inputs from the body via the circumventricular organs (Figure 11.14a; plasma osmolality, angiotensin II, cytokines). (3) Afferent inputs via neurons that are thermosensitive or sensitive to hormones of peripheral endocrine organs (adrenal cortex, thyroid gland, sexual glands, gastrointestinal endocrine glands [insulin, glucagon, ghrelin, pancreatic peptide YY, glucagon-like -1 peptide, cholecystokinin], adipose tissue [leptin]). (4) Multiple synaptic inputs from the forebrain related to cognitive and emotional activity. These include projections from the nuclei in the amygdala, septal nuclei, bed nuclei of the stria terminalis, subiculum, medial and orbital prefrontal cortex and infralimbic cortex.

11.5.2 Functional Model of the Hypothalamus

The anatomical characterization of the hypothalamus in longitudinal (rostro-caudal) zones arranged mediolaterally, by the different types of nuclei (in the medial hypothalamus) and by their afferent and efferent neural connections, does not reveal the mechanisms by which such a small part of the brain is able to regulate the multiple integrative body functions (Table 11.2). Swanson and coworkers have proposed a model to explain the general mechanisms underlying the

Table 11.2 Integrative functions of the hypothalamus

Function	Behavior	Nuclei in hypothalamus	Afferent systems hormones, cytokines	Autonomic systems	Endocrine systems, hormones
Thermoregulation	Thermoregulatory behavior	Preopt. region, AH, posterior H, OVLT (pyrogenic zone, fever)	Peripheral thermoreceptors, central thermosens. (preopt.), cytokines (fever)	SyNS (skin [CVC, SM]), (BAT [rodents])	TRH/Thyr (anterior pituitary)
Reproduction	Sexual behavior and sexual orientation	MPNl (male; human dimorphic), VMvl (female), TU, PMv	Afferents from sexual organs, afferents from sensory systems	SyNS (thor.-lumb.), PaNS (sacral) (sexual organs)	GnRH, FSH/LH (anterior pituitary)
Volume and osmoregulation (fluid homeostasis)	Drinking behavior, thirst	PVHmc, SOmc, AVPV, MePO, OVLT, SFO	Osmorecept. in OVLT & liver, volume rec. ri. atrium (vagal) angiotensin II via SFO	NTS, SyNS (kidney)	Vasopressin (posterior pituitary)
Regulation of nutrition and metabolism	Nutritive behavior, hunger/satiety	AN, PVHd,v,l, VMH (insulin secretion)	Vagal afferents and hormones from GIT (CCK, ghrelin, glucagon, GLP-l, insulin), leptin from WAT, glucose	Enteric nervous system, PaNS (DMV), SyNS, WAT	Orexin
Temporal organization of body functions	Sleep–waking behavior, circadian/ endogenous rhythm of body functions	SCH, SBPV	Afferents from retina (Tr. retino-hypothalamicus)	SyNS, PaNS, SyNS to gl. pinealis	Melatonin (gl. pinealis)
Body protection (acute, e.g., during pain and stress)	Defense behavior (fight, flight, quiescence)	AHN, VMHdm, PMd, PAGdll,vl	Nociceptive afferents	SyNS, PaNS (cardiovascular system [CMN, MVC, VVC etc.])	CRH/ACTH (anterior pituitary gland), adrenaline (SA system)
Immune defense	Defense from toxic substances and situations (sickness behavior)	PVH, ?	Cytokines	SyNS (to immune tissue)	CRH/ACTH (anterior pituitary gland), adrenaline (SA system)

Listed are the behavior, the nuclei in the hypothalamus, the afferent systems, the autonomic (parasympathetic and sympathetic) pathways (shaded) and the endocrine systems (including the hormones) that are involved in these hypothalamic functions. The function "body protections" includes fast defense behaviors (see Table 11.1), as well as immune defense.

Abbreviations: AH, anterior hypothalamus; AHN, anterior hypothalamic nucleus; AN, arcuate nucleus; AVPV, anteroventral periventricular nucleus; BAT, brown adipose tissue; CCK, cholecystokinin; CRH/ACTH, cortocotropin-RH/adrenocorticotropic hormone; CMN, cardiomotor neurons (symp., parasymp.); d, dl, dm, dorsal, dorsolateral, dorsomedial; CVC, cutaneous vasoconstrictor neurons; DMNX, dorsal motor nucleus of the vagus; FSH/LH, follicle-stimulating hormone/luteinizing hormone; GIT, gastrointestinal tract; GLP-1, glucagon-like peptide 1; GnRH, gonadotropin RH; H, hypothalamus; l, lateral; mc, magnocellular; MePO, median preoptic nucleus; MPNl, lateral part of the medial preoptic nucleus; MVC, muscle vasoconstrictor neurons; NTS, nucleus tractus solitarii; OVLT, organum vasculosum laminae teminalis (osmosensors); PAG, periaqueductal gray; PaNS, parasympathetic nervous system; PM, premammillary nucleus; PVH, paraventricular nucleus of the hypothalamus; PYY, pancreatic peptide YY; RH, releasing hormone; SA system, sympatho-adrenal system (adrenal medulla); SBPV, subparaventricular zone; SCN, suprachiasmatic nucleus; SFO, subfornical organ (angiotensin sensibility); SM, sudomotor neurons; SOmc, magnocellular part of supraoptic nucleus; SyNS, sympathetic nervous system; thor.-lumb., thoracolumbar; TRH/Thyr, thyrotropin-RH/thyroxine; TU, tuberal n; v, vl, ventral, ventrolateral; VMH, ventromedial nucleus; WAT, white adipose tissue; VVC, visceral vasoconstrictor neurons.

References: Gore and Roberts (2003); Moore (2003); Stricker and Verbalis (2003); Woods and Stricker (2003); McKinley et al. (2004)

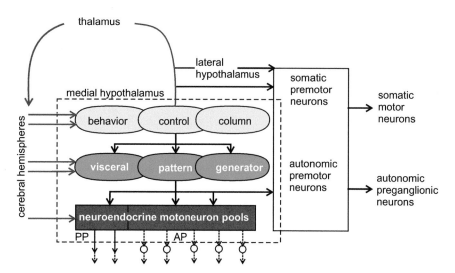

Figure 11.16 A model of the functional organization of the hypothalamus. 1. Neurons of the behavior control column project (see Figure 11.15d), *first*, to regions in brain stem and even spinal cord, that are associated with somatic and autonomic motor systems (descending projections), *second*, to thalamocortical loops (ascending projections), *third*, to the adjacent hypothalamic area (being involved with modulation of the behavior state), and *fourth*, to nuclei of the hypothalamic visceral pattern generator (HVPG) network. 2. Neurons of each nucleus of the HVPG project to characteristic combinations of neuroendocrine motor neuron pools and pools of autonomic premotor neurons in the paraventricular nucleus. Neurons in the behavior control column, in the HVPG and in the neuroendocrine motor zone are under multiple influences of the cerebral hemispheres. AP, anterior pituitary gland; PP, posterior pituitary gland. Modified from Swanson (2000) and Thompson and Swanson (2003).

basic integrative functions of the hypothalamus (Figure 11.16). This explanatory model is an approximation and helps us to understand how somatomotor, autonomic and neuroendocrine responses are integrated to control body temperature, fluid matrix, nutritional state, reproduction and defense and to adapt these complex regulations to the needs of the organism. These needs change during challenges from the environment that are related to the search for nutritive substances and water, to environmental temperature changes, to an aggressor, to toxic substances or to reproductive cues (mating and raising the next generation).

The model as outlined in Figure 11.16 includes the four functional components of the hypothalamus discussed before: (1) the neuroendocrine motor zone; (2) the periventricular zone representing the hypothalamic visceral pattern generator (HVPG); (3) the behavior control column (medial nuclei) representing the basic functional states (regulation of defense, nutrition, body fluid, body temperature, reproduction and temporal organization); and (4) the lateral hypothalamus as an intersection of communication between cerebral hemispheres and circuits

regulating body functions (somatomotor, autonomic, neuroendocrine):

- The behavior control column has descending projections to somatomotor and autonomic circuits, ascending projections to thalamocortical circuits and projections to the lateral hypothalamus.
- The behavior control column projects topographically and in a functionally specific way (i.e., related to the basic hypothalamic functions represented in the nuclei of this control column [see Table 11.2]) to the HVPG. This guarantees a coordinated activation of neuroendocrine and autonomic circuits (in the paraventricular nucleus and probably in other nuclei).
- The behavioral state (circadian, diurnal, ultradian, mensual, seasonal rhythms) is modulated in the nuclei of the behavior control column and of the HVPG by the suprachiasmatic nucleus without changing the functions of these nuclei (not shown in Figure 11.16).
- The nuclei of the HVPG network are reciprocally connected with each other. This visceral

pattern-generating network determines the patterns of activation of neuroendocrine channels (pools of neuroendocrine motor neurons) and of final autonomic pathways (Table 11.2). The mechanisms underlying the generation of the function-specific patterns by this network are poorly understood.

- The hypothalamic complex consisting of behavior control column, hypothalamic visceral pattern generator, periventricular neuroendocrine motor zone and autonomic premotor circuits (in the lateral hypothalamus and paraventricular nucleus) is under multiple control by the cerebral hemispheres. This powerful hemispheric input coordinates the hypothalamic functions with the cognitive and emotional state of the organism.

This general model, based on anatomical tracing studies and functional considerations, is speculative. However, it helps us to understand the complex control of integrative functions of the hypothalamus. It will serve as a platform for future functional studies, using in vivo and in vitro animal models. This model of the functioning of the hypothalamus connects to the explanatory model outline in Figure 0.2 in the introduction of this book which is also based on Swanson's argumentation.

11.6 Synopsis: The Wisdom of the Body Revisited

11.6.1 Autonomic Nervous System and Behavior

As already mentioned in the introduction of this book, the behavior of vertebrates (including humans) consists of the somatic, autonomic and neuroendocrine motor responses generated by the target tissues of the motor neurons of these three systems. The pattern of activity in the three categories of output channels is dependent on: (1) The behavior control programs in the spinal cord, brain stem and hypothalamus that orchestrate the somatomotor, autonomic and endocrine output channels. (2) The afferent feedback from the body (hard-wired neural and hormonal, as well as humoral) to all levels of central integration. (3) The input from the cerebral hemispheres related to cognitive and emotional processes. (4) Intrinsic processes in the central nervous system that determine the behavioral state of the organism

(sleep stages, arousal) and the activity in output channels that are not dependent on afferent activity or activity in the cerebral hemispheres (e.g., the resting activity of neurons of peripheral autonomic pathways occurring either randomly or in relation to intrinsic oscillators, such as the respiratory pattern generator in the medulla oblongata, the circadian pattern generator in the suprachiasmatic nucleus, etc.). This basic conceptual plan underlying the behavior of the individual is graphically depicted in Figure 0.2 in the introduction of this book. It has been developed by Swanson (Swanson 2000, 2013) and serves as a framework to understand the integrative action of the autonomic and neuroendocrine systems generated by the brain. As has been detailed in Chapter 4 and repeatedly emphasized and exemplified in Chapter 5 (enteric nervous system), Chapter 9 (spinal cord) and Chapter 10 (medulla oblongata), reflexes, generated in functionally distinct autonomic neurons, are components of the readouts of the central "sensorimotor" programs.

11.6.2 Integrative Autonomic Responses and Forebrain

In this book I have described the organization of the peripheral and central autonomic nervous system. I focused on the functional specificity of the final autonomic pathways with respect to the target organs or tissues and used as a basis neurophysiological investigations. Wherever we looked in the periphery of the body, in the spinal cord, in the lower brain stem or, more generally, in the upper brain stem and hypothalamus, we concluded that the regulation of the target organs and tissues by the autonomic nervous system can only be understood if the generation of the electrical signals in the peripheral autonomic pathways by the central nervous system is function-specific. In view of the many specific peripheral autonomic pathways and the precise transmission of signals in them generated by the central nervous system, as described in Chapters 3 to 8, the question arises: *How is the central nervous system able to distinguish between these many autonomic channels and to activate them differentially?*

The discharge patterns generated in the neurons of the peripheral autonomic pathways clearly demonstrate that the central nervous system is capable of differential activation. What are the principles of organization in the spinal cord, brain stem and hypothalamus that enable the autonomic systems to function precisely during the behavioral repertoire that is available to the forebrain? How does the forebrain master these many autonomic systems? Looking at the microstructure of the central systems related to autonomic regulations, we are astounded by the neurobiological differentiation, yet we are barely able to bring these complex anatomical central structures together with the functions they are involved in.

There are four sets of independent data from different disciplines that teach us that the secret of the precise autonomic control systems in relation to the somatomotor behavior of the organism has to be found in the brain:

1. Precise regulation of the inner milieu and organ systems. This regulation is traditionally described by the concept of homeostasis (see Table 11.2).
2. The specificity of the neurophysiological response patterns of the peripheral autonomic neurons and of the central neurons associated with the peripheral autonomic pathways (e.g., sympathetic or parasympathetic premotor neurons in the brain stem; autonomic interneurons in the spinal cord and lower brainstem).
3. The detailed microstructure (location, projection of axons and dendrites, synaptic inputs, histochemistry) of neuron assemblies in the spinal cord, brain stem and hypothalamus that are involved in regulating the activity in the peripheral autonomic pathways.
4. The temporary adaptation of the regulation of the inner milieu during extreme challenges of the body from outside, as well as inside the body (e.g., during extreme climatic and other environmental changes; during bacterial or viral infection), a process called allostasis (see Subchapter 11.2). Adaptation of the autonomic control systems during external load occurs in anticipation of somatomotor actions. This anticipatory adaptation of autonomic control is dependent on the cerebral hemispheres and reflected in the dense reciprocal communication between the autonomic centers in the brain stem and hypothalamus on one side and the cortical and subcortical structures of the cerebral hemispheres on the other side.

The principles of autonomic integrative action already apply to the sympathetic and parasympathetic systems at the level of the spinal cord (Chapter 9). It contains many autonomic sensorimotor programs that underlie the coordinated activation of spinal autonomic pathways to physiological stimulation of spinal afferents. These sensorimotor programs are represented in pools of interneurons that are synaptically connected to preganglionic neurons and to each other. Spinal afferent systems form distinct synapses with these pools of interneurons. Autonomic premotor neurons in the brain stem and hypothalamus access these spinal autonomic programs by forming synapses with the interneurons and/or preganglionic neurons (see Subchapter 9.4). A further characteristic already seen at the level of the spinal cord is that some of these autonomic systems generate intrinsic activity independent of the afferent and supraspinal inputs. Finally, activity in the autonomic systems and the somatomotor systems is coordinated in the spinal cord (see sacral spinal systems; Subchapter 9.3). Thus, three of the four components of neural regulation of behavior by the brain as defined by Swanson (Swanson 2012; Card and Swanson 2013) are already present in the spinal cord (Figure 0.2): autonomic sensorimotor programs coordinated with somatic sensorimotor programs; multiple sensory feedbacks; intrinsic generators of activity.

The same applies to the lower brain stem. The reader is reminded of the discussion on the origin of spontaneous activity and its pattern in peripheral autonomic neurons and the coordination between autonomic and somatic sensorimotor programs during the regulation of respiration and gastrointestinal function in Chapter 10. However, this coordination is incomplete and does not instigate behavior. Full coordination of autonomic, somatomotor and sensory changes can be generated from the periaqueductal gray and from Barrington's nucleus in defense behavior and in the evacuation of pelvic organs (urinary bladder and hindgut), respectively. Furthermore, the basic neural machineries coordinating autonomic and somatomotor responses are probably present in the mesencephalon and pons for the diving response, tonic immobility, freezing reaction, the vigilance reaction and other types of response pattern. But these fast-initiated coordinated response patterns too either cannot be elicited on their own or only in a rudimentary way by physiological afferent stimuli when the hypothalamus and forebrain have been removed or inactivated. In order to be fully effective these mechanisms that lead to coordinated somatic and autonomic motor responses need differential activation from the hypothalamus. Chronic hypothalamic cats exhibit apparently normal homeostatic behaviors consisting of coordinated neuroendocrine, autonomic and somatomotor responses (see Table 11.2) (Note 11).

Both Cannon and Hess, and others like Bard, Brooks, Fulton (Fulton 1949) (Note 12) and Ranson (Ranson and Magoun 1939; Ranson and Clark 1959) were fascinated by the integrative behavior of the autonomic nervous system throughout their scientific lives. The brain's role in the integrative action of the autonomic nervous system remained a mystery to them. However, they knew intuitively and believed that the secret of autonomic regulation is buried in the integration: (1) of signals generated in the cerebral hemispheres that are related to the environment (which includes memory and anticipation in the context of cognition and emotions), (2) of the behavioral state of the organism, (3) of the afferent feedback from the body and (4) of the efferent autonomic and neuroendocrine pathways to the body organs and tissues. From this viewpoint, it is clear why the afferent feedback systems from deep somatic and visceral tissues cannot be considered to be part of the autonomic systems, although they are indispensable for their function (see Subchapter 2.1). Furthermore, it is now clear that a dichotomous concept of the autonomic nervous system as sympathetic and parasympathetic systems, being antagonistically organized, could never explain how the brain directs the control of the body's organs.

Conclusions

In Chapters 8–10 I have described that the spinal cord and medulla oblongata contain neural circuits linked to the final autonomic pathways. The circuits are integral components of regulation of the cardiovascular system, the gastrointestinal tract, the respiratory tract, the pelvic organs, the eye and some other targets. In this chapter, the role of the mesencephalon and the hypothalamic–limbic system in the regulation of body functions by the autonomic nervous system has been summarized.

1. The hypothalamus and cerebral hemispheres contain the representations of elementary motivational behaviors. These representations receive multiple afferent feedback and are responsible for the integration of regulation of autonomic, neuroendocrine and somatomotor systems. In parallel, they generate affective body states and emotional feelings closely associated with the autonomic control systems that are represented in the telencephalon. The telencephalic structures representing emotions are connected with the central representations involved in autonomic and neuroendocrine control.

2. The dorsolateral, lateral and ventrolateral cell columns in the periaqueductal gray of the mesencephalon contain the neural circuits representing the autonomic and somatomotor components of the defense behaviors, confrontation, flight and quiescence. These circuits are reciprocally connected with the autonomic centers in the medulla oblongata (rostral and caudal ventrolateral medulla, ventromedial medulla), with the hypothalamus and with the medial and orbital prefrontal cortices. They are quickly activated by the cortex during dangerous situations in the environment or in the body and represent the basic neural machinery for active and passive coping.

3. Coordinated autonomic responses are quickly generated by signals from the telencephalon during diving, freezing, tonic immobility, exercise, vigilance or other behaviors. These autonomic responses occur in anticipation of the somatomotor responses, demonstrating that the cortical signals have direct access to the autonomic centers, independent of the afferent feedback, but in conjunction with it. The underlying mechanisms of these cortical effects may involve the hypothalamus and midbrain.

4. Conditioned emotional responses are accompanied by distinct cardiovascular changes mediated by autonomic pathways. Lesions in the perifornical region of the lateral hypothalamus in monkeys abolish cardiovascular changes during the conditioned emotional responses without affecting emotional responses.

5. The basic emotions in humans are accompanied by automatically mediated response patterns characteristic for each emotion. Emotional states, somatomotor patterns (facial expression) and autonomic patterns are connected. The adaptive autonomic patterns during anger and fear are generated and mediated by the amygdala. The central structures involved in the generation of the autonomic patterns of the other basic

emotions (happiness, surprise, sadness, disgust) are less well understood.

6. The hypothalamus contains the neural structures that integrate and coordinate autonomic, neuro-endocrine and somatomotor responses to basic (elementary) behaviors such as defensive, repro-ductive, nutritive, drinking, thermoregulatory and sleep–waking behavior. The organization of these behaviors depends on the neuroendocrine motor zone, the periventricular zone constituting the hypothalamic visceral pattern generator, the behav-ior control column in the medial hypothalamus (representing hypothalamic functional states), the suprachiasmatic nucleus representing the behavior states and the lateral hypothalamus as the intersec-tion of communication to and from the brain stem, spinal cord and cerebral hemispheres.

7. The hypothalamic centers that are responsible for the homeostatic control mechanisms are under complex control of the telencephalon. This is the basis for the adaptation of these homeostatic con-trol systems to external and internal challenges that is described by the concept of allostasis.

8. The homeostatic regulation of body functions by the autonomic nervous system and its adaptation during short- and long-term changes in the environ-ment or in the body require functionally differenti-ated peripheral autonomic pathways and specific central circuits connected to them. The underlying central mechanisms of these homeostatic and allo-static regulations are still a puzzle and a challenge for future research in neurobiology.

Suggested Reading

Cannon, W. B. (1939) *The Wisdom of the Body, 2nd revised and enlarged edn.*, Norton, New York

Card, J. P. and Swanson, L. W. (2013) The hypothalamus: an overview of regulatory systems. In *Fundamental Neuroscience, 4th edn* (Squire, L. R., Berg, D., Bloom, F. E., et al., eds.) pp. 717–727, Elsevier and Academic Press, Amsterdam.

Casson, D. M. and Ronald, K. (1975) The harp seal, *Pagophilus groenlandicus* (Erxleben, 1777). XIV. Cardiac arrhythmias. *Comp Biochem Physiol A* **50**, 307–314.

Darwin, C. (1872) *The Expression of the Emotions in Man and Animals. Introduction, Afterword and Commentaries by Paul Ekman, 3rd edn.*, 1998, Harper Collins, London.

Gandevia, S. C., Killian, K., McKenzie, D. K., et al. (1993) Respiratory sensations, cardiovascular control, kinaes-thesia and transcranial stimulation during paralysis in humans. *J Physiol* **470**, 85–107.

Goodwin, G. M., McCloskey, D. I. and Mitchell, J. H. (1972) Cardiovascular and respiratory responses to changes in central command during isometric exercise at constant muscle tension. *J Physiol* **226**, 173–190.

James, W. (1884) What is an emotion? *Mind* **9**, 188–205.

Keay, K. A. and Bandler, R. (2014) Periaqueductal gray. In *The Rat Nervous System, 4th edn* (Paxinos, G., ed) pp. 207–221, Elsevier Science and Technology, Amsterdam.

Levenson, R. W., Ekman, P. and Friesen, M. V. (1990) Voluntary facial action generates emotion-specific autonomic nervous system activity. *Psychophysiology* **27**, 363–384.

Schulkin, J. and Sterling, P. (2019) Allostasis: a brain-centered predictive mode of physiological regulation. *Trends Neurosci* **47**, 740–752.

Sheehan, D. (1936) Discovery of the autonomic nervous system. *Arch Neurol Psychiat* **35**, 1081–1115.

Swanson, L. W. (2013) Basic plan of the nervous system. In *Fundamental Neuroscience, 4th edn* (Squire, L. R., Berg, D., Bloom, F. E., et al., eds) pp. 15–38, Elsevier and Academic Press, Amsterdam.

All references cited in the text are available online at www.cambridge.org/janig.

Notes

1. We still do not know whether or not this is true for some or all weak synaptic inputs by preganglionic axons to sympathetic postganglionic neurons. As described in Subchapter 6.2 and Box 6.2, these synaptic inputs may be incorrect connections that are function-ally not important under *in vivo* conditions.

2. As described in Subchapter 4.5, these functions are poorly or not at all mediated by nerves, but are the functions of the adrenal medulla. They do not reinforce the effects of sympathetic nerves at all; they may com-plement them.

3. Part of Cannon's problem may have been the condition of the animals on which they worked. The anesthetics of the time often may have depleted the adrenal medulla of catecholamines and removed or attenuated reflex control of autonomic outflow. This meant that the only responses that could be detected were the enor-mous ones produced by extreme stimuli (like asphyxi-ation). This corresponds to the experience in my laboratory showing that extensive surgery, deep anes-thesia, inexperienced handling of the animals before

the experiments and massive afferent stimulation during the experiments tend to suppress or eliminate the differentiated reflexes in sympathetic neurons.

4. In this context I remind the reader that many cutaneous vasoconstrictor neurons are inhibited by stimulation of arterial chemoreceptors or trigeminal receptors in the anesthetized cat (see Figures 4.2, 4.5 and 4.12 and Subchapter 4.1) and a few are excited by these stimuli, these possibly innervating nutritional blood vessels. Muscle and visceral vasoconstrictor neurons are always excited (Figures 4.1, 4.2).

5. The stereotype of confrontational defense is the defense behavior of the cat described by Darwin in his book *The Expression of the Emotions in Man and Animals* (1872/1998) (see Figure 4.13), the sham-rage behavior occurring spontaneously or evoked by cutaneous stimuli in hypothalamic cats (Bard 1928), and the defense behavior ("Abwehr-Reaktion") elicited by electrical microstimulation of the caudal perifornical area of the hypothalamus in cats (Hess and Brügger 1943; Hess 1948; Akert 1981). Hess has described sites in the hypothalamus from which he could evoke flight ("Fluchttrieb") or a sequence of confrontational defense followed by flight during electrical stimulation (Hess 1948). Later Hunsperger (1956), in his careful study of the "affective" defense reaction in awake freely moving cats (which he considered to be an intermediary reaction between attack and flight), showed that electrical stimulation of the midbrain central gray at sites that correspond approximately to the dorsolateral and lateral cell columns elicits attack or flight (depending on the stimulus strength). He concluded that the periaqueductal gray represents a relay for the affective reaction evoked from the perifornical region of the hypothalamus. He extended this study using systematic lesions in the periaqueductal gray, hypothalamus or amygdala in cats and came to the conclusion that these three subcortical structures are important in the shaping of the defense behavior elicited from the cortex (Fernandez de Molina and Hunsperger 1962).

6. The morphological studies on monkeys demonstrate that the viscerosensory and visceromotor prefrontal cortices connected to the autonomic regulation of body organs are much more differentiated than generally believed (for discussion see Öngür et al. [1998] and Öngür and Price [2000]).

7. In the *conditioned emotional response* paradigm, a neutral stimulus (here a tone as the conditioned stimulus) is paired with an aversive stimulus (here electrical shocks applied to the abdominal skin as the unconditioned stimulus). The animals learn that the conditioned stimulus is followed by the aversive stimulus and as consequence the originally neutral conditioned stimulus generates a *state of fear* in the animal. This emotional state of fear is indicated by the suppression of an appetitive behavior performed by the animal (here suppression of lever pressing to obtain apple juice as a reward).

The monkeys were first trained with operand techniques to perform mild dynamic exercise (turning a wheel with their legs) and to press a small lever; in doing so they were rewarded with juice. Then the conditioned emotional response was elicited in the monkeys by the classical conditioning paradigm. The procedure began by presenting the signal for lever pressing. After stable lever pressing was reached, an auditory signal was applied for 1 min as a conditioned stimulus. This stimulus was terminated by an unconditioned stimulus consisting of electrical shocks of 7 to 15 mA, applied for 1 to 2 seconds to the abdominal skin. The command signal for lever pressing remained constant throughout the conditioned stimulus and afterwards. Only *one* classical conditioning trial was applied during a one-day training period at intervals of 2 to 4 days. After the training procedures, the animals were instrumented in order to measure heart rate, arterial blood pressure, renal blood flow (resistance) and terminal aortic blood flow (resistance), the latter mainly as a measure of blood flow through the skeletal musculature of the hind limbs. Furthermore, electrodes were stereotactically placed bilaterally in the perifornical regions of the lateral hypothalamus for electrical stimulation or lesioning (for details see Smith et al. 1979).

8. The argument that the decrease in renal blood flow is generated by adrenaline released by the adrenal medulla is based on two measurements: a chronically denervated kidney showed the same slow response (1) during the conditioned emotional response and (2) when 5 µg adrenaline was injected intravenously (Smith et al. 1979). The problem is that the vascular bed of a denervated kidney develops denervation hyper-reactivity and that 5 µg adrenaline is a very high concentration compared to the physiologically occurring plasma concentrations of adrenaline (see Subchapter 4.5).

9. Based on the examination of peripheral physiological changes that occur during emotions, the Dane Carl S. Lange came to the conclusion that vascular changes (dilation of blood vessels and increase of blood volume in the organs) are the primary effects that trigger emotions (Lange 1887).

10. The reasoning in the subchapter is largely based on the experimental work of and the concepts developed by

Larry Swanson and his group (Swanson 1987, 2000, 2013; Watts and Swanson 2002; Thomson and Swanson 2003; Card and Swanson 2013).

11. Philip Bard, together with his student Rioch, conducted systematic studies on four chronically diencephalic cats (cerebral cortex and most subcortical structures of the cerebral hemispheres were removed). These animals could be kept alive for 1, 1.5, 13 or 28 months. The authors showed that these animals exhibit, in addition to the so-called sham-rage behavior, various types of behavior that are typical for the integrative hypothalamic functions (Table 11.2; thermoregulatory behavior, urination, defecation, reproduction, sleep) (Bard and Rioch 1937). Later Bard and his student Macht also studied chronic pontine (bulbospinal), low mesencephalic or high mesencephalic cats (1 to 5 months after transection of the brain stem). These animals require utmost care because of the absence of the hypothalamically organized control systems (Bard and Macht 1957).

12. Ten percent of Fulton's textbook *Physiology of the Nervous System* was devoted to the autonomic nervous system and the hypothalamus.

The Autonomic Nervous System in Future Research: Some Personal Views

Wilfrid Jänig, Elspeth M. McLachlan

In the field of the autonomic nervous system, the most exciting future research developments are likely to be, on the one hand, in the subcellular world and, on the other hand, in the world of the brain's control of the body's multicellular machines by way of individual neural programs into a unity of somatomotor, autonomic and neuroendocrine behavior. Today we would rephrase the title of Cannon's book *The Wisdom of the Body* to *The Wisdom of the Brain in Regulating the Body*. It is now clear that a dichotomous concept of the autonomic nervous system divided into sympathetic and parasympathetic and being antagonistically organized could never explain how the brain controls the body's organs and tissues.

We feel that the field "neurobiology of the autonomic nervous system" is again at a turning point and we hope for a new beginning. Over the last half century, there has been a great contrast, to compare all the advances from investigations into the control of human movement and posture, with the state of knowledge about the control of all the other organs of the body, most of which are embedded in our daily activities and are the sites of disorders of lifestyle and ageing. Together with the difficulties of measuring organ functions deep inside the body, what is not seen seems to be largely ignored. In view of the importance of understanding the functions of our body in health and disease, and of the advances in technology that are occurring, this field seems due to explode.

The future most interesting and promising scientific activity in autonomic system research[1] is to work out how all of the functionally distinct autonomic pathways are directed by the brain to influence the target tissues. This will involve revealing the complex cellular and subcellular mechanisms by which each functional type of autonomic postganglionic neuron influences its target cells and tissues in the periphery. These mechanisms include not only how the classical transmitters, acetylcholine and noradrenaline, excite or inhibit the effector cells, most of which are unknown, but also the putative roles of the various other substances such as peptides colocalized in, and released from, autonomic neurons. The interactions of local and circulating hormones and cytokines with the neuroeffector processes will also need to be unraveled.

These studies will pursue fundamental questions related to the organization of the peripheral nervous pathways to the target organs and tissues in the tradition of the research conducted in the last 20–40 years (see Chapters 3 to 7), i.e., by deconstructing the elements of the pathways and

---

[1] This is our personal and somewhat subjective view

investigating their resting behavior and responses to natural reflexes. Such studies have included, and will inevitably continue to include, utilizing biochemical and genetic techniques to define the components of these pathways at a molecular level, as well as more traditional neurophysiological techniques of electrophysiological recording, pharmacological and optokinetic interventions to interrupt normal physiological functions, and immunohistochemical identification of peptide and protein components of individual cells. Further understanding will probably come from neural network analysis of the effects of firing patterns once one knows how the target tissues are regulated by the activity of the functionally specific postganglionic neurons. Such investigations will give us clues to understanding why autonomic control runs so smoothly under healthy conditions, or, to put it the other way round, why the failure of autonomic control in disease can have catastrophic consequences.

A few examples of autonomic function that we barely understand are:

- The mechanisms by which the sympathetic innervation of the kidney regulates resistance, renin release and sodium reabsorption differentially.
- The mechanisms by which the different functions of the gastrointestinal tract related to motility, absorption of fluid and nutrients, endocrine and exocrine secretion and defense are regulated via parasympathetic and sympathetic pathways and how they involve the enteric nervous system.
- The organization of parasympathetic pathways supplying the airway smooth musculature (excitatory and inhibitory bronchomotor pathways) or airway glandular tissue (bronchial secretomotor pathway) (Subchapter 4.8.2).
- The mechanisms by which activity in parasympathetic sacral pathways and sympathetic lumbar pathways is integrated in the control of each of the pelvic organ systems with distinct functions (Subchapter 9.3).
- The mechanisms of autonomic control of exocrine gland secretion (salivary glands, pancreas, etc.).
- The mechanisms by which cutaneous vasodilation in the proximal extremities or trunk during body warming, or in skin of the face during emotional stimuli, is generated by the sympathetic innervation. This vasodilation is not produced by withdrawal of activity in vasoconstrictor neurons.

- Related to the last point, nerves innervating the proximal skin of the extremities and most likely of the trunk contain five functionally different types of postganglionic axons:
  - cutaneous vasoconstrictor (CVC) axons that are normally silent and differ from CVC axons innervating acral skin;
  - sudomotor (SM) axons that differ from SM axons innervating acral skin;
  - cutaneous vasodilator axons;
  - pilomotor axons;
  - lipomotor axons innervating white adipose tissues (see Subchapters 4.1.2 and 4.2.1).

  How does the central nervous system differentiate between these five types of sympathetic pathways?

- The concept of a cardiac nervous system consisting of local afferent neurons, local cardiac interneurons and cardiac (postganglionic) motor neurons (Subchapter 6.5.4). Is there a neuronal plexus within the heart that is equivalent to the enteric nervous system in the gut? Connected to this point is the unknown function of parasympathetic preganglionic cardiomotor neurons with unmyelinated fibers located in the most lateral part of the dorsal vagal motor nucleus (Subchapter 4.8.2).

- The convergent inputs to postganglionic vasoconstrictor neurons (muscle or cutaneous) in anesthetized animals from many silent sympathetic preganglionic neurons, as well as active preganglionic neurons that do not trigger action potentials. The function of these various inputs is unknown.

- About half (40–70%) of the sympathetic preganglionic neurons in the lumbar outflow to somatic tissues, in the lumbar outflow to viscera and in the thoracic outflow to the head and neck of anesthetized cats lack both ongoing and reflex activity (Table 4.5). The silence of so many preganglionic neurons is hard to ascribe to the anesthesia. This has to be seen in the context that only 10–20% of active sympathetic preganglionic neurons in these preparations exhibit classical cardiovascular functional properties.

- The function of non-nicotinic (muscarinic and/or peptidergic) transmission to postganglionic vasoconstrictor neurons innervating skin or skeletal muscle and whether it has a physiological function at all in mammals (Subchapter 6.6).

- The role of adrenaline released by the adrenal medulla in yet unappreciated functions such as nociceptor sensitization and regulation of synovial plasma extravasation (Subchapter 4.5).

Some specific areas that merit focused attention are:

1. A special and up to now entirely unsolved problem is the interaction between the autonomic and the immune systems (see Subchapters 4.6 and 5.6). Unraveling this communication is important so that we learn how the brain controls and orchestrates protective body reactions involved in the regulation of inflammation and hyperalgesia (see Subchapters 4.5 and 4.6). It is unlikely that this problem can be elucidated by measuring venous plasma levels of adrenaline and noradrenaline, as is often done in humans. We hypothesize that special sympathetic pathways probably exist by which the brain sends its signals to the immune system and related cells. Connected to this problem is the question of the nature of the afferent messages from the immune tissue to the brain. Vagal afferents may be important in this function, in addition to cytokines (Subchapter 2.3.1).

2. An interesting problem only marginally or not addressed in this book (Subchapter 4.9, and references therein) is the development and maintenance of the functional specificity of the peripheral autonomic pathways. The origin of the autonomic neurons from the neural crest, that has been extensively studied using various methods, is established (le Douarin and Kalcheim, 1999). Details of the migration routes and differentiation of precursor cells and the signaling molecules involved have partially been worked out (Anderson 1993; Ernsberger et al. 2005; Cane and Anderson 2009). Considerable progress has been made in the search for the molecular signals that are important in the differentiation of autonomic neurons by the characterization of BMP (bone morphogenetic protein) growth factors and Phox2 (paired-like homeobox-containing) transcription factors (Ernsberger 2000; Goridis and Rohrer 2002). Questions about the development of the functional diversity of autonomic neurons are beginning to be studied (Rohrer 2011; Furlan et al. 2016; Ernsberger and Rohrer 2018), resulting in the description of transcriptomes of postganglionic and preganglionic neurons with distinct biological functions. Which conditions enable the different functional classes of autonomic neurons to "know" what they are and to which target cells they should be connected? What are the long-term trophic interactions between target cells and postganglionic neurons that maintain their functional specificity?

3. What are the factors that regulate the plasticity of autonomic innervation throughout life as the body grows or shrinks? What determines the ability of autonomic pathways to survive and recover after damage or disease? What are the signals that determine regeneration after lesions and lead to recovery from, or maintenance of, disordered function?

4. As is obvious from the descriptions in Chapters 8 to 11, we have, despite considerable progress in the last 40 years, only just begun to unravel the central circuits in the spinal cord, brain stem and hypothalamus that control the peripheral autonomic pathways. Functional anatomical studies, using tracing, histochemical, genetic, optokinetic and other methods, have resulted in an enormous wealth of data about the layout and connections, mainly in the brainstem and hypothalamus. However, in most cases, these data do not tell us how the circuits work in the control of the autonomic pathways.

The results so far clearly show that any attempt to conduct this research on the basis of a unifying concept of the functioning of sympathetic and parasympathetic nervous systems is going to fail. Some examples from Chapters 9 and 10 illustrate this:

- It is hypothesized in Chapter 9 that spinal integration is important in order to understand the central regulation of autonomic systems. This has to be shown for the various spinal autonomic systems, including their interneurons, with different functions.
- The nucleus tractus solitarii, the afferent input gate for all information from the viscera via the vagus nerves, consists of a collection of integrative and integrated nuclei. How this integration and its modulation by other centers in the brainstem and forebrain work is barely understood (Subchapter 8.3).
- How the regulation of respiration and the regulation of autonomic (in particular cardiovascular) systems are integrated is still an enigma.

- The origin of resting activity in sympathetic neurons involved in cardiovascular regulation has been discussed for almost 150 years and is still entirely unclear. Further, the origin of resting activity in nonvascular sympathetic pathways and in parasympathetic systems has barely been considered.
- The baroreceptor reflex pathways are the best explored central autonomic pathways although the way these reflex pathways work in phasic and tonic control of arterial blood pressure is still not entirely clear. Furthermore, it is not clear whether alternative pathways exist (Subchapter 10.3). Reflex pathways related to other cardiovascular afferents, including chemoreceptor afferents, have been little explored.
- Research on the central regulation of gastrointestinal function via the dorsal vagal motor complex and its (parasympathetic) output pathways, and via sympathetic non-vasoconstrictor pathways, is still in its infancy (Subchapters 5.7 and 10.7). Unraveling the functioning of this organ system is necessary to understand how the forebrain (including the hypothalamus) controls gastrointestinal functions.

5. As described in Chapter 11, the mesencephalon and hypothalamus are relatively unexplored neural territories as far as the cellular mechanisms underlying their functions are concerned. However, detailed behavioral studies, studies of systems physiology and functional anatomical studies have paved the way for studies at the single neuron level, combined with studies addressing whole systems, that will clarify the neural mechanisms underlying integrative functions as listed in Tables 11.1 and 11.2. These functions are related to:
   - fast behavioral reactions such as the diving response, exercise, defense reactions, tonic immobility, vigilance or freezing reaction, and
   - complex hypothalamic functions, such as thermoregulation, volume and osmoregulation, regulation of reproduction, regulation of nutrition and metabolism, regulation of body protection including immune defense, and regulation of temporal organization of all body functions.

6. An enormous challenge will be to work out, first, which parts of the forebrain represent the autonomic functions; second, the neural connections between these cortical representations and the subcortical circuits in spinal cord, brain stem and hypothalamus; and, third, how this network functions during regulation of distinct autonomic functions. Daily and clinical experience suggest that maintaining health and recovery from disease are very much dependent on mental processes, i.e., on activity in the forebrain related to cognition and emotions. However, we have no neurobiological concept as to how this is brought about. It is not far-fetched to predict that systematic research on the forebrain structures in relation to the peripheral autonomic pathways and the corresponding circuits in the spinal cord, brain stem and hypothalamus will solve this problem. This will result in the formulation of the neurobiological basis of psychosomatic relations and diseases and will provide answers about how the brain influences the body in health and disease. The autonomic and endocrine systems will be at the center of this concept.

7. Connected to the last point, systematic research on the peripheral autonomic nervous system and related central circuits will lead to a new understanding of the relation between mind, brain and body. It will show, as expected, that mental activity does not exist independently of the multiple autonomic and endocrine regulators of body tissues in the brain. We are still in the situation that René Descartes described in *L'Homme* (1664). We describe the material neural processes and the mental processes using different languages. Descartes expressed this point as follows in the introductory sentences of *L'Homme*: "*Ces hommes seront composez, comme nous, d'une Ame & d'un Corps. Et il faut que je vous décrive, premierement, le corps à part, puis apres, l'ame aussi à part; & enfin, que je vous monstre comment ce deux natures doivent estre iointes & unies, pour composer des hommes qui nous ressemblent.* [Humans consist (as do we) of a soul/psyche and a body. I have to describe first, separately, the body and after that, also separately, the soul; then I will demonstrate to you how the two things must be interconnected and united together to make up the humans who resemble us].

8. A final important and interesting point that needs to be raised is the generation of emotions. As

beautifully described by Damasio (2003), the expression of emotions plays out in the theater of the body and the feelings of emotions in the theater of the mind. The expression of emotions always precedes the corresponding emotional feelings. We hypothesize that both expression and feeling are very much dependent on the differential activation of the peripheral autonomic pathways. This differential activation leads to distinct activation patterns of autonomic target tissues and organs in the different (cutaneous, deep somatic and visceral) body domains (see Subchapter 11.4). As in James–Lange theory, the body responses lead to differential activation of afferent feedback from the body tissues and subsequently to the generation or enhancement of emotional feelings. This is schematically expressed in Figure 11.10a. Thus, the generation of expression and feeling of emotions is absolutely dependent on the functional specificity of the peripheral autonomic pathways, as described in Chapter 4, and on the functional specificity of the interoceptive afferent feedback from the different body domains, as described in Chapter 2. Autonomic output pathways with their central representations and the interoceptive afferent feedback to the central representations of the body domains form multiple body loops. What is the nature of the coupling between the autonomic outflow to the different body tissues and the interoceptive afferent feedback from these body tissues to their subcortical and cortical central representations? This hypothesis does not explain how emotional feelings are mechanistically generated. But it emphasizes that the differential activation of autonomic systems appears to be essential in the generation of emotional feelings.

Conclusions

Future research to unravel the various mechanisms related to the functioning of the autonomic nervous system will make clear how the "wisdom of the brain" directs the regulation of body fluids and organs. This research will focus on, e.g.:

- The subcellular and cellular mechanisms by which the peripheral autonomic pathways distribute the brain's signals and regulate the cells and tissues of the body.
- The neural circuits in the spinal cord, brain stem and hypothalamus that are the basis of autonomic regulation of organ systems.
- The representation of autonomic regulation in the forebrain and its connection with the circuits in the spinal cord, brain stem and hypothalamus. This will result in the formulation of the neurobiological basis of the enormous bodily and mental activities we are able to go through in both health and disease.
- Regulation of the immune system by the sympathetic nervous system, this being the basis to understand the mechanisms by which the brain is involved, together with the nociceptive system, in the protection of the body from invasion and injury.
- The way the autonomic nervous system is involved in generating the expression of emotions, on the one hand, and via afferent feedback from the target tissues and organs to the brain in generating emotional feelings, on the other.

The autonomic nervous system is the essential participant in all our physiological and psychological responses to the world around us.

References

Anderson, D. J. (1993) Molecular control of cell fate in the neural crest: the sympathoadrenal lineage. *Ann Rev Neurosci* 16, 129–158.

Cane, K. N. and Anderson, C. R. (2009) Generating diversity: mechanisms regulating the differentiation of autonomic neuron phenotypes. *Auton Neurosci* 151, 17–29.

Damasio, A. (2003) *Looking for Spinoza: Joy, Sorrow, and the Feeling Brain*, Harcourt, Orlando, Florida.

Ernsberger, U. (2000) Evidence for an evolutionary conserved role of bone morphogenetic protein growth factors and phox2 transcription factors during noradrenergic differentiation of sympathetic neurons. Induction of a putative synexpression group of neurotransmitter-synthesizing enzymes. *Eur J Biochem* 267, 6976–6981.

Ernsberger, U., Esposito, L., Partimo, S., et al. (2005) Expression of neuronal markers suggests heterogeneity of chick sympathoadrenal cells prior to invasion of the adrenal anlagen. *Cell Tissue Res* 319, 1–13.

Ernsberger, U. and Rohrer, H. (2018) Sympathetic tales: subdivisons of the autonomic nervous system and the impact of developmental studies. *Neural Dev* 13, 20.

Furlan, A., La Manno, G., Lubke, M., et al. (2016) Visceral motor neuron diversity delineates a cellular basis for nipple- and pilo-erection muscle control. *Nat Neurosci* 19, 1331–1340.

Goridis, C. and Rohrer, H. (2002) Specification of catecholaminergic and serotonergic neurons. *Nat Rev Neurosci* 3, 531–541.

Le Douarin, N. M. and Kalcheim, C. (1999) *The Neural Crest, 2nd edn.*, Cambridge University Press, Cambridge.

Rohrer, H. (2011) Transcriptional control of differentiation and neurogenesis in autonomic ganglia. *Eur J Neurosci* 34, 1563–1573.

All references cited in the text are available online at www.cambridge.org/janig.

Index